Behavioral Aspects of Epilepsy

Principles and Practice

Behavioral Aspects of Epilepsy

Principles and Practice

EDITED BY

STEVEN C. SCHACHTER, MD
Director of Research
Department of Neurology
Beth Israel Deaconess Medical Center
Professor of Neurology
Harvard Medical School
Boston, Massachusetts

GREGORY L. HOLMES, MD
Chairman
Department of Neurology
Dartmouth Medical School
Hanover, New Hampshire

DOROTHÉE G.A. KASTELEIJN-NOLST TRENITÉ, MD, MPH
Professor
Department of Neuroscience
University "La Sapienza"
Rome, Italy
Department of Medical Genetics
University of Utrecht
The Netherlands

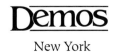

New York

Acquisitions Editor: R. Craig Percy
Cover Designer: Aimee Davis
Compositor and Indexing: Publication Services, Inc.
Printer: Sheridan Press

Cover: "Field Study" (2000; oil; 12×12 inches) by Klaas Verboom (1948–2006), an artist who lived with epilepsy.

Visit our website at www.demosmedpub.com

Library of Congress Cataloging-in-Publication Data

Behavioral aspects of epilepsy : principles and practice / edited by Steven C. Schachter, Gregory L. Holmes, Dorothée Kasteleijn-Nolst Trenité.
   p. ; cm.
  Includes bibliographical references and index.
  ISBN-13: 978-1-933864-04-4 (hardcover : alk. paper)
  ISBN-10: 1-933864-04-4 (hardcover : alk. paper)
  1. Epilepsy—Pathophysiology. 2. Epilepsy—Complications. I. Schachter, Steven C. II. Holmes, Gregory L. III. Kasteleijn-Nolst Trenité, Dorothée.
  [DNLM: 1. Epilepsy—physiopathology. 2. Neurobehavioral Manifestations. 3. Neuropsychology—methods. WL 385 B416 2008]
  RC372.5.B44 2008
  616.8'53—dc22

2007032316

Medicine is an ever-changing science undergoing continual development. Research and clinical experience are continually expanding our knowledge, in particular our knowledge of proper treatment and drug therapy. The authors, editors, and publisher have made every effort to ensure that all information in this book is in accordance with the state of knowledge at the time of production of the book.

Nevertheless, this does not imply or express any guarantee or responsibility on the part of the authors, editors, or publisher with respect to any dosage instructions and forms of application stated in the book. Every reader should examine carefully the package inserts accompanying each drug and check with a physician or specialist whether the dosage schedules mentioned therein or the contraindications stated by the manufacturer differ from the statements made in this book. Such examination is particularly important with drugs that are either rarely used or have been newly released on the market. Every dosage schedule or every form of application used is entirely at the reader's own risk and responsibility. The editors and publisher welcome any reader to report to the publisher any discrepancies or inaccuracies noticed.

Special discounts on bulk quantities of Demos Medical Publishing books are available to corporations, professional associations, pharmaceutical companies, health care organizations, and other qualifying groups. For details, please contact:

Special Sales Department
Demos Medical Publishing, LLC
386 Park Avenue South, Suite 301
New York, NY 10016
Phone: 800–532–8663 or 212–683–0072
Fax: 212–683–0118
Email: orderdept@demosmedpub.com

Made in the United States of America
07 08 09 10 5 4 3 2 1

Dedication

We dedicate this book to Norman Geschwind, MD (1926–1984) in recognition of his seminal contributions to the understanding of epilepsy and behavior.

Contents

CLINICAL SCIENCE

III   SEIZURES AND BEHAVIOR

IV   NEUROPSYCHOLOGIC FUNCTION

IX OTHER DISORDERS ASSOCIATED WITH EPILEPSY THAT IMPACT BEHAVIOR, MOOD, AND COGNITION

X CONCLUSION

Preface

The field of epilepsy is broadening as the goal of therapy expands from seizure control to minimizing the full range of epilepsy's negative medical and psychosocial consequences. Accordingly, in addition to determining seizure type and epilepsy syndrome and selecting appropriate antiseizure therapies, clinicians are increasingly taking the behavioral aspects of epilepsy into consideration in their evaluation and treatment of patients.

In recent years, psychiatric disorders have perhaps received the most attention among epilepsy-related behavioral conditions. *Behavioral Aspects of Epilepsy: Principles and Practice* builds on this widely recognized and studied group of comorbidities to encompass the complementary findings and insights of behavioral scientists from allied fields such as neuropsychiatry, neuropsychology, psychology, social science, and cognitive neuroscience.

This volume begins with the work of animal experimentalists and neurophysiologists. Their topics include the assessment of behavior in animal models of epilepsy, effects of environmental and social factors on the expression of seizures, animal models of mood disorders, cognitive and affec-

tive associations of seizures in young and mature animals, and neurophysiologic mechanisms underlying epilepsy and related behaviors.

Subsequent chapters highlight clinical topics across the age spectrum, including seizure-related behaviors, neuropsychologic function, interictal behavioral disorders, and effects of seizure therapies and epilepsy surgery on mood and cognition. The final section explores other disorders associated with epilepsy that have behavioral features, such as nonepileptic events, autism, and attention deficit disorder.

The editors and contributors have organized the topics in *Behavioral Aspects of Epilepsy: Principles and Practice* to emphasize the importance and interrelatedness of multiple perspectives from the laboratory to the clinic in understanding the behavioral aspects of epilepsy and translating research findings into clinical practice. We hope this integrative approach will bring us closer to the day that health care professionals can help their patients successfully overcome all of the debilitating consequences of epilepsy, thereby enabling them to achieve their full potential.

Steven C. Schachter
Gregory L. Holmes
Dorothée G.A. Kasteleijn-Nolst Trenité

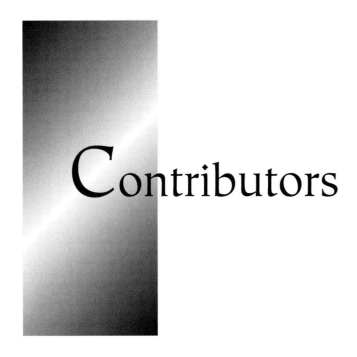

Contributors

Frederick Andermann, MD, FRCP(C)
Professor of Neurology and Pediatrics
McGill University
Director, Epilepsy Service
Montreal Neurological Hospital and Institute
Montreal, Quebec, Canada
Chapter 59: Migraine in Adults

Paul B. Augustijn, MD
Child Neurologist
Dutch Epilepsy Clinics Foundation (S.E.I.N)
Heemstede, The Netherlands
Chapter 57: Attention Deficit Hyperactivity Disorder

Joan K. Austin, DNS, RN
Distinguished Professor and Sally Reahard Chair
Indiana University School of Nursing
Indianapolis, Indiana
Chapter 43: Psychiatric Aspects of Epilepsy in Children
Chapter 50: Academic Achievement

Giuliano Avanzini, MD
Research Director
Department of Neurophysiology
Foldazione Istituto Neurologice "C. Besta"
Milan, Italy
*Chapter 63: Historical Perspectives and Future
Opportunities*

Gus A. Baker, PhD, FBPs'S
Professor of Clinical Neuropsychology
Consultant Clinical Neuropsychologist
Head of Division of Neurosciences
University of Liverpool
Fazakerley, Liverpool, United Kingdom
Chapter 11: Neuropsychologic Effects of Seizures

Sallie Ann Baxendale, Bsc (Hons), MSc, PhD
Consultant Clinical Neuropsychologist
Department of Clinical and Experimental
  Epilepsy
Institute of Neurology, Queen Square
London, United Kingdom
*Chapter 38: Neuropsychologic Outcomes after
  Epilepsy Surgery in Adults*

Carl W. Bazil, MD, PhD
Associate Professor of Clinical Neurology
Department of Neurology
Columbia University
New York, New York
Chapter 62: Sleep

Ann M. Bergin, MB, ScM, MRCP (UK)
Assistant Professor
Department of Neurology
Children's Hospital
Boston, Massachusetts
*Chapter 48: Effects of Antiepileptic Drugs on
  Psychiatric and Behavioral Comorbidities in
  Children and Adolescents*

Andrea Bernasconi, MD
Director
Neuroimaging of Epilepsy Lab
Montreal Neurological Institute
McConnell Brain Imaging Centre
Montreal, Quebec, Canada
Chapter 59: Migraine in Adults

Frank M.C. Besag, MB, ChB, FRCP, FRCPsych, FRCPCH
Professor
Child and Adolescent Mental
    Health Service
Bedfordshire and Lutton Partnership NHS Trust and
    Institute of Psychiatry
Bedford, Bedfordshire, United Kingdom
*Chapter 42: Behavioral Aspects of Pediatric Epilepsy
    Syndromes*

Helge Bjørnæs, PhD
Chief Psychologist
The National Center for Epilepsy and Department of
    Neuropsychiatry and Psychosomatic Medicine
Division of Clinical Neuroscience
Rikshospitalet University Hospital
Sandvika, Norway
*Chapter 22: Neuropsychologic Aspects of Frontal Lobe
    Epilepsy*

Peter F. Bladin, MD, BS, BSc, FRACP, FRCPEd
Professorial Fellow
Comprehensive Epilepsy Program
Epilepsy Research Centre
Austin Hospital
Victoria, Melbourne, Australia
*Chapter 40: Indicators of Psychosocial Adjustment and
    Outcome after Epilepsy Surgery*

Hillary J. Blakeley, BA
Graduate Student
Department of Psychology and Neuroscience
Baylor University
Waco, Texas
*Chapter 8: Regulation of Neuronal Excitability in the
    Amygdala and Disturbances in Emotional Behavior*

Dietrich Peter Blumer, MD
Professor and Head of Neuropsychiatry
University of Tennessee Health Science Center
Memphis, Tennessee
Chapter 26: Interictal Dysphoric Disorder

Oliviero Bruni, MD
Assistant Professor
Department of Child and Adolescent Neuropsychiatry
University of Rome, "La Sapienza"
Rome, Italy
*Chapter 58: Migraine in Children and Relation with
    Psychiatric and Sleep Disorders*

Gaetano Cantalupo, MD
Neurology Resident
Department of Neurosciences
University of Bologna
Bologna, Italy
*Chapter 28: Biting Behavior as a Model of Aggression
    Associated with Seizures*

Rochelle Caplan, MD
Professor
Department of Psychiatry and Biobehavioral
    Sciences
Semel Institute for Neuroscience and Human Behavior
Los Angeles, California
Chapter 49: Social Competence

Andrea Eugenio Cavanna, MD
Neuropsychiatrist
Department of Neuropsychiatry
Institute of Neurology
London, United Kingdom
Chapter 12: Seizures and Consciousness

Jose E. Cavazos, MD, PhD
Assistant Professor of Neurology, Pharmacology, and
    Physiology
Director of Research and Education
South Texas Comprehensive Epilepsy Center
University of Texas Health Science Center
San Antonio, Texas
*Chapter 7: The Role of Sprouting and Plasticity in
    Epileptogenesis and Behavior*

Bernard S. Chang, MD, MMSc
Assistant Professor
Department of Neurology
Harvard Medical School
Beth Israel Deaconess Medical Center
Boston, Massachusetts
Chapter 54: Cortical Malformations

Devin J. Cross, MS
Research Assistant
South Texas Comprehensive Epilepsy Center
Departments of Medicine (Neurology) and Pharmacology
University of Texas Health Science Center
San Antonio, Texas
*Chapter 7: The Role of Sprouting and Plasticity in
    Epileptogenesis and Behavior*

J. Helen Cross, MB, ChB, PhD, FRCPCH, FRCP
Professor and Clinical Lead (Epilepsy)
UCL-Institute of Child Health
Great Ormond Street Hospital for Children
    NHS Trust
London, United Kingdom
*Chapter 37: Neuropsychologic Outcomes after
    Epilepsy Surgery in Children*

JoAnne C. Dahl, PhD
Associate Professor in Clinical Psychology
Department of Psychology
Uppsala University
Uppsala, Sweden
*Chapter 30: Conditioning Mechanisms,
    Behavior Technology, and Contextual
    Behavior Therapy*

Susanna Danielsson, MD
Child Neurologist
Department of Child Neuropsychiatry Center
Sanhigrenska University Hospital
Göteborg, Sweden
Chapter 56: Autism

Antonio V. Delgado-Escueta, MD
Professor
Epilepsy Genetics/Genomics Laboratories
Comprehensive Epilepsy Program
David Geffen School of Medicine at UCLA
VA GLAHS-West Los Angeles
Los Angeles, California
*Chapter 28: Biting Behavior as a Model of Aggression
    Associated with Seizures*

John C. DeToledo, MD
Professor of Neurology
Chief, Comprehensive Epilepsy Program
Wake Forest University School of Medicine
Winston Salem, North Carolina
*Chapter 17: Behaviors Mimicking Seizures in
    Institutionalized Persons with Epilepsy*

Orrin Devinsky, MD
Professor
Departments of Neurology, Neurosurgery, and Psychiatry
Director
Comprehensive Epilepsy Center
New York University School of Medicine
New York, New York
*Chapter 41: The Myth of Silent Cortex and the
    Morbidity of Epileptogenic Tissue: Implications for
    Temporal Lobectomy*

David W. Dunn, MD
Professor of Psychiatry and Neurology
Indiana University School of Medicine
Indianapolis, Indiana
*Chapter 43: Psychiatric Aspects of Epilepsy in Children
Chapter 50: Academic Achievement*

Christian E. Elger, MD, PhD, FRCP
Director
Hospital of Epileptology
University of Bonn
Bonn, Germany
*Chapter 52: Psychogenic Nonepileptic Seizures:
    An Overview*

Maurizio Elia, MD
Director
Unit of Neurology and Clinical Neurophysiopathology
Oasi Institute for Research on Mental
    Retardation and Brain Aging
Troina, Italy
Chapter 55: Chromosomal Abnormalities

Kai Juhani Eriksson, MD, PhD
Head, Pediatric Neurology Unit
Department of Pediatrics
Tampere University Hospital and Pediatric
    Research Centre
University of Tampere
Tampere, Finland
*Chapter 46: Learning and Behavior:
    Neurocognitive Functions in Children*

Kevin Farrell, MB, ChB, FRCPC
Professor
Department of Pediatrics
University of British Columbia
British Columbia Children's Hospital
Vancouver, British Columbia, Canada
*Chapter 45: Family Factors and Psychopathology in
    Children with Epilepsy*

Karen Fernandez
Student
Department of Physiology and Pharmacology
SUNY Downstate Medical Center
Brooklyn, New York
*Chapter 9: Computer Simulation of Epilepsy:
    Implications for Seizure Spread and Behavioral
    Dysfunction*

Frederica Galli, PhD
Clinical Psychologist
Department of Child and Adolescent
    Neuropsychiatry
University of Rome, "La Sapienza"
Rome, Italy
*Chapter 58: Migraine in Children and Relation with
    Psychiatric and Sleep Disorders*

Norberto Garcia-Cairasco, BSc, MSc, PhD
Assistant Professor of Physiology
    (Neurophysiology)
Director of the Neurophysiology and Experimental
    Neuroethlogy Laboratory (LNNE)
Department of Physiology
Rebeirão Preto School of Medicine
University of São Paulo
Rebeirão Preto, São Paulo, Brazil
*Chapter 10: Neuroethology and Semiology
    of Seizures*

Alexandra J. Golby, MD
Assistant Professor
Harvard Medical School
Department of Neurosurgery
Brigham and Women's Hospital
Boston, Massachusetts
*Chapter 20: Atypical Language Organization in
    Epilepsy*

Rachel Goldmann Gross, MD
Resident
Department of Neurology
Hospital of the University of Pennsylvania
Philadelphia, Pennsylvania
*Chapter 20: Atypical Language Organization in
Epilepsy*

Arthur C. Grant, MD, PhD
Assistant Professor of Neurology
Comprehensive Epilepsy Center
New York University School of Medicine
New York, New York
Chapter 21: Interictal Perceptual Function

Marilisa M. Guerreiro, MD, PhD
Professor of Child Neurology
Department of Neurology
State University of Campinas (Unicamp)
Campinas, São Paulo, Brazil
Chapter 60: Brain Tumors in Children

Vincenzo Guidetti, MD
Professor of Child and Adolescent Neuropsychiatry
Department of Child and Adolescent Neuropsychiatry
University of Rome, "La Sapienza"
Rome, Italy
*Chapter 58: Migraine in Children and Relation with
Psychiatric and Sleep Disorders*

Stavros Hadjiloizou, MD
Instructor in Neurology
Harvard Medical School
Division of Epilepsy and Clinical Neurophysiology
Children's Hospital
Boston, Massachusetts
*Chapter 47: The Landau-Kleffner Syndrome and
Epilepsy with Continuous Spike-Waves During Sleep*

Jonathan J. Halford, MD
Assistant Professor
Department of Neuroscience
Medical University of South Carolina
Charleston, South Carolina
*Chapter 33: Neurophysiologic Correlates of Psychiatric
Disorders and Potential Applications in Epilepsy*

Stephen C. Heinrichs, PhD
Research Associate
Department of Neuropharmacology
VA Medical Center
Boston, Massachusetts
*Chapter 1: Behavior-Seizure Correlates in Animal
Models of Epilepsy*
*Chapter 2: Influence of Environment and Social
Factors in Animal Models of Epilepsy*

David H. Herman, BS
Graduate Student
Department of Psychology and Neuroscience
Baylor University
Waco, Texas
*Chapter 8: Regulation of Neuronal Excitability in the
Amygdala and Disturbances in Emotional Behavior*

Bruce P. Hermann, MA, PhD
Professor and Director
Matthews Neuropsychology Lab
Department of Neurology
University of Wisconsin School of Medicine and
Public Health
Madison, Wisconsin
*Chapter 18: Memory Impairment and Its Cognitive
Context in Epilepsy*

Audrey Ho, PhD
Clinical Psychologist
Department of Psychology
British Columbia Children's Hospital
Vancouver, British Columbia, Canada
*Chapter 45: Family Factors and Psychopathology in
Children with Epilepsy*

Gregory L. Holmes, MD
Chairman
Department of Neurology
Dartmouth Medical School
Hanover, New Hampshire
*Chapter 5: Cognitive and Behavioral Effects of
Seizures: Adult Animals*

Cathryn Rene Hughes, BS
Medical Student
Baylor College of Medicine
Houston, Texas
*Chapter 8: Regulation of Neuronal Excitability in the
Amygdala and Disturbances in Emotional Behavior*

Satish Jain, MD, DM, FRCP
Director
Indian Epilepsy Centre
New Delhi, India
*Chapter 36: Presurgical Evaluation for Epilepsy
Surgery*

Barbara C. Jobst, MD
Associate Professor of Medicine (Neurology)
Director, Neurophysiology and EEG
Dartmouth-Hitchcock Medical Center
Lebanon, New Hampshire
Chapter 32: Frontal Lobe Behavioral Disorders

Andres M. Kanner, MD
Professor of Neurological Sciences and Psychiatry
Rush Medical College
Director, Laboratory of EEG and Video-EEG-Telemetry
Associate Director of Epilepsy and
    Rush Epilepsy Center
Department of Neurological Sciences
Rush University Medical Center
Chicago, Illinois
Chapter 13: Postictal Phenomena in Epilepsy
Chapter 25: Mood Disorders in Epilepsy:
    Two Different Disorders with Common
    Pathogenic Mechanisms?

Peter W. Kaplan, MB, FRCP
Professor
Department of Neurology
Johns Hopkins Bayview Medical Center
Baltimore, Maryland
Chapter 14: Behavioral Aspects of Nonconvulsive
    Status Epilepticus

N. Bradley Keele, BS, PhD
Associate Professor
Department of Psychology and Neuroscience
Institute of Biomedical Studies
Baylor University
Waco, Texas
Chapter 8: Regulation of Neuronal Excitability in the
    Amygdala and Disturbances in Emotional Behavior

Michael Kerr, MRCGP, MRCPSYCH
Professor
Chair in Learning Disabilities and Honorary
    Consultant in Neuropsychiatry
Department of Psychological Medicine
Cardiff University
Cardiff, Wales, United Kingdom
Chapter 44: Behavioral and Psychiatric Effects in
    Patients with Multiple Disabilities

Ennapadam S. Krishnamoorthy, MD, PhD, FRCP
Director and TS Srinivasan Chair
Consultant in Neurology, Neuropsychiatry, and
    Rehabilitation
The Institute of Neurological Sciences
Voluntary Health Services
Taramani, Chennai, India
Chapter 24: Classification of Neuropsychiatric
    Disorders in Epilepsy

W. Curt LaFrance, Jr, MD, MPH
Director of Neuropsychiatry
Rhode Island Hospital
Assistant Professor of Psychiatry and
    Neurology
Brown Medical School
Providence, Rhode Island
Chapter 53: Conducting Treatment Trials for
    Psychologic Nonepileptic Seizures

Pål Gunnar Larsson, MD
Head of Department
The National Center for Epilepsy
Department of Neurodiagnostics
Division of Neuroscience
Rikshospitalet University Hospital
Sandvika, Norway
Chapter 22: Neuropsychologic Aspects of
    Frontal Lobe Epilepsy

Tobias L. Lundgren, MA
Doctoral Student
Department of Psychology
Uppsala University
Uppsala, Sweden
Chapter 30: Conditioning Mechanisms, Behavior
    Technology, and Contextual Behavior Therapy

William W. Lytton, MD
Associate Professor
Department of Physiology and Pharmacology
SUNY Downstate Medical Center
Brooklyn, New York
Chapter 9: Computer Simulation of Epilepsy:
    Implications for Seizure Spread and Behavioral
    Dysfunction

Kristina Malmgren, MD, PhD
Professor of Neurology
Institute of Neuroscience and Physiology
Sahlgrenska Academy at Götenburg University
Göteborg, Sweden
Chapter 39: Psychiatric Outcomes after Epilepsy
    Surgery in Adults

Pavel Mareš, MD, DSc
Professor of Pathophysiology
Department of Developmental Epileptology
Institute of Physiology
Academy of Sciences of the Czech Republic
Prague, Czech Republic
Chapter 4: Cognitive and Affective Effects of Seizures:
    Immature Developing Animals

Michelangelo Stanzani Maserati, MD
Neurology Resident
Department of Neurosciences
University of Bologna
Bologna, Italy
Chapter 28: Biting Behavior as a Model of Aggression
    Associated with Seizures

Hiroo Matsuoka, MD, PhD
Professor
Department of Psychiatry
Tohoku University
Graduate School of Medicine
Sendai, Japan
Chapter 16: Behavioral Precipitants of Seizures

Brenna C. McDonald, PsyD, MBA
Assistant Professor of Radiology and Neurology
Center for Neuroimaging
Indiana University School of Medicine
Indianapolis, Indiana
Chapter 32: Frontal Lobe Behavioral Disorders

Kimford J. Meador, MD
The Melvin Greer Professor
Department of Neurology
University of Florida
Gainesville, Florida
Chapter 34: Cognition

Stefano Meletti, MD
Neurologist
Department of Neurosciences
University of Bologna
Bologna, Italy
Chapter 28: Biting Behavior as a Model of Aggression Associated with Seizures

Seth A. Mensah, MSc, DPM, MRCPsych
Neuropsychiatrist
Academic Department of Neuropsychiatry
Welsh Neuropsychiatry Service
Whitchurch Hospital
Cardiff, Wales, United Kindgom
Chapter 44: Behavioral and Psychiatric Effects in Patients with Multiple Disabilities

Maria Augusta Montenegro, MD, PhD
Assistant Professor of Child Neurology
Department of Neurology
State University of Campinas (Unicamp)
Campinas
São Paulo, Brazil
Chapter 60: Brain Tumors in Children

Gholam K. Motamedi, MD
Associate Professor
Department of Neurology
Georgetown University Hospital
Washington, DC
Chapter 34: Cognition

Marco Mula, MD
Neuropsychiatrist
Department of Neurology
Amedeo Avogadro University
Novara, Italy
Departments of Psychiatry, Neurobiology, Pharmacology and Biotechnologies
University of Pisa
Pisa, Italy
Chapter 35: Mood

Thien Nguyen, MD, PhD
Assistant Professor
Department of Neurology
Johns Hopkins Hospital
Baltimore, Maryland
Chapter 14: Behavioral Aspects of Nonconvulsive Status Epilepticus

Pirkko Nieminen, PhD
Lecturer
Department of Psychology
University of Tempere
Tampere, Finland
Chapter 46: Learning and Behavior: Neurocognitive Functions in Children

Rena Orman, PhD
Research Associate
Department of Physiology and Pharmacology
SUNY Downstate Medical Center
Brooklyn, New York
Chapter 9: Computer Simulation of Epilepsy: Implications for Seizure Spread and Behavioral Dysfunction

Federica Pinardi, MD
Neurology Resident
Department of Neurosciences
University of Bologna
Bologna, Italy
Chapter 28: Biting Behavior as a Model of Aggression Associated with Seizures

Robert M. Post, MD
Professor of Psychiatry
Penn State College of Medicine
Hershey, Pennsylvania
Chapter 3: Animal Models of Mood Disorders: Kindling as a Model of Affective Illness Progression

Rema Reghu, MBBS, MSc (Lond)
Research Fellow and Junior Consultant
The Institute of Neurological Sciences
VHS Hospital
Chennai, India
Chapter 24: Classification of Neuropsychiatric Disorders in Epilepsy

Markus Reuber, MD, PhD
Senior Clinical Lecturer and Honorary Consultant
Academic Neurology Unit
University of Sheffield
Royal Hallamshire Hospital
Sheffield, United Kingdom
Chapter 27: Epilepsy and Anxiety
Chapter 52: Psychogenic Nonepileptic Seizures: An Overview

Hazel J. Reynders, D Clin Psychol, MSc, BA (Hons)
Consultant Clinical Neuropsychologist
Neuropsychology Unit
Royal Hallamshire Hospital
Sheffield, United Kingdom
*Chapter 23: Social and Emotion Information
    Processing*

James J. Riviello, Jr., MD
Chief of Neurophysiology
Director of Epilepsy and Neurophysiology Program
Texas Children's Hospital
Houston, Texas
Professor of Pediatrics
Section of Neurology and Developmental Neuroscience
Baylor College of Medicine
Houston, Texas
*Chapter 47: The Landau-Kleffner Syndrome and
    Epilepsy with Continuous Spike-Waves During Sleep*

Guido Rubboli, MD
Neurologist
Department of Neurosciences
University of Bologna
Bologna, Italy
*Chapter 28: Biting Behavior as a Model of Aggression
    Associated with Seizures*

Michael M. Saling, BA (Hons), MA, PhD
Associate Professor
Department of Psychology
School of Behavioral Sciences
University of Melbourne
Comprehensive Epilepsy Program
Epilepsy Research Centre
Austin Hospital
Melbourne, Victoria, Australia
*Chapter 40: Indicators of Psychosocial Adjustment and
    Outcome after Epilepsy Surgery*

Josemir W. Sander, MD, PhD, FRCP
Department of Clinical and Experimental Epilepsy
Institute of Neurology
University College London
London, United Kingdom
Chapter 35: Mood

Bettina Schmitz, MD, PhD
Professor
Department of Neurology
Charité, Campus Virchow-Klinikum
Berlin, Germany
Chapter 29: Psychosis and Forced Normalization

Dr. Martin Schöndienst
Neurologist and Psychotherapist
Head, Department of Psychosomatic Epileptology
Bethel Epilepsy Center
Bielefeld, Germany
Chapter 27: Epilepsy and Anxiety

Michael Seidenberg, PhD
Professor
Department of Psychology
Rosalind Franklin University
North Chicago, Illinois
*Chapter 18: Memory Impairment and Its Cognitive
    Context in Epilepsy*

Megan Selvitelli, MD
Epilepsy Fellow
Department of Neurology
Beth Israel Deaconess Medical Center
Boston, Massachusetts
Chapter 54: Cortical Malformations

Harlan E. Shannon, PhD
Research Advisor
In Vivo Pharmacology
Lilly Research Laboratories
Indianapolis, Indiana
Chapter 6: Cognitive Effects of Antiepileptic Drugs

Gigi Smith, MSN, APRN, CPNP
Pediatric Nurse Practitioner
Assistant Professor, College of Nursing
Medical University of South Carolina
Charleston, South Carolina
*Chapter 51: Psychosocial Intervention in
    Pediatric and Adolescent Epilepsy*

Carl E. Stafstrom, MD, PhD
Professor
Departments of Neurology and Pediatrics
Section of Pediatric Neurology
University of Wisconsin
Madison, Wisconsin
*Chapter 5: Cognitive and Behavioral Effects of
    Seizures: Adult Animals*

Lesley C. Stahl, PsyD
Staff Research Associate at UCLA
Department of Psychiatry
Child and Adolescent Division
Neuropsychiatric Institute
Los Angeles, California
Chapter 49: Social Competence

Hermann Stefan, MD, PhD
Director of the Epilepsy Center
Neurological Clinic
University of Erlangen
Erlangen, Germany
Chapter 61: Brain Tumors in Adults

Mark Stewart, MD, PhD
Associate Professor
Department of Physiology and Pharmacology
SUNY Downstate Medical Center
Brooklyn, New York
*Chapter 9: Computer Simulation of Epilepsy: Implications
    for Seizure Spread and Behavioral Dysfunction*

Carlo Alberto Tassinari, MD
Professor
Department of Neurosciences
University of Bologna
Bologna, Italy
*Chapter 28: Biting Behavior as a Model of
    Aggression Associated with Seizures*

Joanne Taylor, BSc
Postgraduate Student
Division of Neuroscience
University of Liverpool
Fazakerley, Liverpool, United Kingdom
Chapter 11: Neuropsychologic Effects of Seizures

Dorothée G.A. Kasteleijn-Nolst Trenité, MD, MPH
Professor
Department of Neuroscience
University "La Sapienza"
Rome, Italy
Department of Medical Genetics
University of Utrecht
The Netherlands
Chapter 15: Reflex Epilepsies

Michael Trimble, MD, FRCP, FRCPsych
Professor Emeritus
Institute of Neurology
London, United Kingdom
Chapter 29: Psychosis and Forced Normalization
Chapter 31: Personality Disorders and Epilepsy

Manjari Tripathi, DM
Associate Professor
Department of Neurology
All India Institute of Medical Services
New Delhi, India
*Chapter 36: Presurgical Evaluation for
    Epilepsy Surgery*

Guy Vingerhoets, PhD
Professor of Neuropsychology
Department of Internal Medicine
Laboratory for Neuropsychology
Gent University
Gent, Belgium
Chapter 19: Cognition

Charles Kyriakos Vorkas, BA
Weill Cornell Medical College
New York, New York
*Chapter 41: The Myth of Silent Cortex and the
    Morbidity of Epileptogenic Tissue: Implications for
    Temporal Lobectomy*

Janelle L. Wagner, MS, PhD
Assistant Professor
Department of Pediatrics
Medical University of South Carolina
Charleston, South Carolina
*Chapter 51: Psychosocial Intervention in Pediatric and
    Adolescent Epilepsy*

Sarah J. Wilson, BSc (Hons), PhD, MAPS, CCN
Senior Lecturer
Department of Psychology
School of Behavioral Science
University of Melbourne
Senior Clinical Neuropsychologist
Comprehensive Epilepsy Program
Epilepsy Research Centre
Austin Hospital
Melbourne, Victoria, Australia
*Chapter 40: Indicators of Psychosocial Adjustment and
    Outcome after Epilepsy Surgery*

Joanne Wrench, BA (Hons), MPsych
Clinical Neuropsychologist
Department of Psychology
University of Melbourne
Austin Health, Royal Talbot Rehabilitation Centre
Melbourne, Victoria, Australia
*Chapter 40: Indicators of Psychosocial Adjustment and
    Outcome after Epilepsy Surgery*

Alexei E. Yankovsky, MD
Assistant Professor
Department of Internal Medicine
Neurology Section
Health Sciences Centre
University of Manitoba
Winnipeg, Manitoba, Canada
Chapter 59: Migraine in Adults

I

ANIMAL MODELS

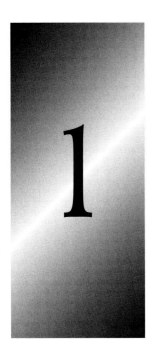

1 Behavior-Seizure Correlates in Animal Models of Epilepsy

Stephen C. Heinrichs

In-depth characterization and refinement of animal behavioral models of seizure susceptibility and reactivity have been identified as a pressing requirement for current and future research on epilepsy (1). These initiatives are paying dividends, judging by the recent publication of a behavioral assessment scale for seizure-prone rodents in a leading manual of core techniques for the neuroscientist (2). Perhaps the greatest utility for research related to assessment of seizure-related behaviors in animals is the potential yield of noninvasive tools for detecting subtle anomalies that precede and predict ictogenesis and epileptogenesis. For instance, the neurobiological basis for seizures cannot yet be studied ethically in human patients, and the examination of postictal behaviors in epileptic patients is complicated by preexisting secondary neuropathologies that arise as a result of prior seizure activity. In one possible solution to this quandry, Stafstrom identifies behavioral modeling in animals as a workable means of making the critical distinction between factors involved in the etiology of seizures as opposed to those arising as a consequence of prior seizures (3). A concrete goal would be to advance a particular behavioral test, or battery of such tests, capable of discriminating among various types of seizure disorders in the absence of electroencephalographic measures. For example, specific utility of such a behavioral test battery has been achieved using spatial, learning, locomotor, and social interaction tests to assess the long-term behavioral and cognitive effects of seizures on the developing brain (3).

A wealth of animal models is available for the study of epilepsy. These models have proven utility in advancing the understanding of basic mechanisms underlying epileptogenesis and have been instrumental in the screening of novel antiepileptic drugs (4). A review by Sarkisian (4) addresses criteria that should be met in a valid animal model of human epilepsy and provides an overview of current animal model characteristics that are relevant to human epilepsy symptoms. While most human disorders are without any animal model, those models that are clinically relevant have strengths and weaknesses. One weakness of animal models is that behavioral manifestations of different animal models can differ and may not at all resemble the behavior of an individual with epilepsy (4). The goal of the present chapter is thus to present, in abbreviated fashion, the latest advances in assessment of behavior-seizure correlates in animal models of epilepsy while integrating preclinical and clinical perspectives.

BEHAVIORAL ASSAYS RELEVANT FOR RODENT SEIZURE MODELS

Reflexive and Motor Functions

In epilepsy research a principal aim is to ensure that motor, sensory, or reflexive alterations do not explain performance differences during behavioral or cognitive testing (3). Assessment of early developmental sensorimotor norms as well as juvenile/adult motor capabilities relevant for seizure susceptibility is therefore critically important. When the unborn organism is exposed to potential pathogens during gestation, monitoring of these same developmental endpoints in offspring can be termed "behavioral teratology." One advantage for the epilepsy investigator of applying developmental measures in a predisposition (genetic or otherwise) model of epilepsy is that the postnatal period of time over which data are collected represents the earliest phase of postpartum ontogeny in seizure-prone animals.

Measurement of Developmental Norms.   Developmental test batteries have been used to examine morphological and behavioral ontogeny in inbred and mutant mice or following prenatal exposure to traumatic stimuli. For example, reflexive surface righting, forelimb-grasping reflex, and negative geotaxis assessments can be employed as very nonspecific markers of neurologic dysfunction impacting proprioception, visual acuity/muscle strength, and goal-directed locomotion, respectively (5). For example, seizure-susceptible EL mice exhibit delayed surface righting (transitioning from supine to prone positions) on postnatal days 3–7 and delayed negative geotaxis (crawling against the force of gravity) on postnatal days 5–9 relative to non-seizure-susceptible control mice (5). It is also important to note that testing procedures implemented during this early postpartum period that disturb maternal/pup interactions can have a lifelong and even transgenerational impact on adult phenotype (6) and should be instituted cautiously.

Locomotor and Circadian Rhythm Measures.   Locomotor activity is used to assess the neural bases of arousal and circadian rhythm as a dependent measure with considerable clinical validity. The study of locomotor activity in rodents does not involve learning or conditioning required for other behavioral tasks and is often used as an initial screen when describing a behavioral phenotype (7). Photobeam grid, observation checklist, and radiotelemetry-dependent measures of activity can determine spatial position very precisely, monitoring the animal as it rests, runs, walk, rears, or performs stereotyped behaviors. More than any other single behavioral dependent measure described in the present chapter, locomotor activity represents a single, seminal output system in the rodent that is likely influenced by a host of separate afferent and motivational systems. An important implication of this statement is that long-term, circadian locomotor measures are perhaps more sensitive than any other single behavioral endpoint to neurologic changes accompanying the various forms of epilepsy. Moreover, animal models of neurologic disorders and mental illness are increasingly reliant on such simple and fundamental "endophenotypic" measures in making substantive progress on questions of etiology and pharmacotherapeutic efficacy.

Basic activity monitoring has high utility for distinguishing seizure-prone from control strains of mice. For example, locomotor hyperactivity has been reported in adult, seizure-susceptible EL mice. Moreover, evidence suggests that epileptic seizures are modulated by the circadian timing system as revealed by locomotor output. For example, daily rhythms of spontaneous locomotor activity in rats were studied before and after an episode of pilocarpine-induced convulsive status epilepticus. Although both chronic epileptic and control groups displayed near-24-hour activity patterns under light-dark conditions, significant delays in phase transition were observed after spontaneous seizures had developed. The phase delay was positively correlated with seizure history and was likely the result of postictal hyperactivity associated with seizures during the normal rest period. In the absence of damage to brain areas directly involved with the regulation of behavioral rhythms, chronic seizure activity presumably alters the timing of activity patterns through an endogenous, non-light-sensitive mechanism. One additional experiment used a kindled animal model of epilepsy to investigate whether seizures could be a cause of the hyperactivity sometimes associated with brain hyperexcitability. Twenty-four hours after a seizure, kindled rats indeed displayed a greater level of exploratory behavior than did the controls. These preclinical results are consistent with the suggestion that the hyperactivity seen in some children with epilepsy may also result from recent seizure activity.

Lasting Impact of Past Experience

Human epilepsy and seizure management using antiepileptic drugs are often accompanied by some degree of cognitive decline, typically expressed as learning or memory deficits. Cognitive deficits have developmental significance in diagnosing seizure susceptibility, are relevant for seizure prognosis, and likely reveal much about hippocampal brain mechanisms that underlie seizure susceptibility (3). Similarly, certain anticonvulsant drugs are distinguished by their ability to suppress seizure incidence or severity without exerting learning- and memory-related side effects.

Assessment of Learning/Memory Capacity. Rats bred selectively for differences in amygdala excitability, manifested by "fast" or "slow" kindling epileptogenesis, display several comorbid features related to learning and memory performance. Regardless of whether the location of the platform was fixed or varied over days, the fast-kindling rats displayed inferior performance in the Morris water maze test, suggesting both working and reference memory impairments. This finding is consistent with the report that rats with status epilepticus perform significantly worse in the water maze than control rats at all time points. Furthermore, when the position of the platform was altered after the response was acquired, fast-kindling rats were more persistent in emitting the previously acquired response. The poor performance of fast-kindling rats was also evident in both cued and uncued tasks, indicating that their disturbed learning was not simply a reflection of a spatial deficit. Moreover, fast-kindling rats could be easily distracted by irrelevant cues, suggesting that these animals suffered from an attentional disturbance. These results suggest that the performance disturbance in fast-kindling rats may reflect difficulties in forming a conceptual framework under conditions involving some degree of ambiguity, as well as greater distractibility by irrelevant cues. Nonassociative memory deficits are also characteristic of the seizure-susceptible EL mouse (5). Clinical evidence for comorbidity of seizure and learning disorders is consistent with findings in animal models of epilepsy, since children with epilepsy, as a group, have a greater risk for developing learning problems as comorbid disorders.

Tests of Affiliative Behavior. Alterations in sexual receptivity, both hypo- and hypersexuality, and aggression have been reported in animal models of epilepsy. For example, investigation of mating behavior on the first night of proestrus, corresponding to the height of female sexual receptivity in rodents, revealed fewer mounts, intromissions, or ejaculations from the untreated males that were caged with previously epileptic females (8). Similarly, one notable characteristic of seizure-prone rodents is the potential for enhanced intra- and interspecies aggression. One set of experiments reported abnormal behavior in rats with a chronic epileptiform syndrome induced by the injection of tetanus toxin bilaterally into the hippocampus. The abnormal behavior included hyperreactivity to a novel environment, intermittent aggression on handling, and abnormally passive response to a strange rat introduced into the home cage. The intermittent aggressive behaviors can be so extreme as to require one group of investigators to employ chain-mail "raptor gloves" for protection against biting injuries when handling rats treated previously with an excitotoxin (2). Consistent with these findings from the animal literature, behavioral alterations associated with epilepsy in some patients include changes in sexual behavior and aggressivity.

One critical form of social contact among mammals with epilepsy is the interaction between mother and offspring. In particular, familial distributions of epilepsy reflect a higher risk for offspring of affected women, compared to the risk for offspring of affected male parents. There are also examples in the clinical literature of significant associations between family stress and seizure intensity in predicting behavior problems. One possible mechanism for generational transmission of an adult seizure phenotype is the quality of parenting provided to developing offspring. In particular, the quality of maternal behavior has been implicated as an environmental determinant in rodent neurochemical and behavioral development. For example, evaluation of parental investment in seizure-susceptible EL mice using a novel apparatus for passive observation of undisturbed mice revealed that EL dams were slower than controls to initiate pup retrieval and spent less time nursing/crouching over pups (5). The results also suggested that EL mothers exhibit an overabundance of motor activities that compete with crouching/nursing and retrieval behaviors required for viability of the litter (Figure 1-1). Maternal care appears to be relevant for cognitive deficits and neuropathology accompanying recurrent seizures in rodents, as these indices of impairment are worsened by a prior history of maternal deprivation.

Reactivity to Reinforcing and Aversive Stimuli

Interesting parallels arise between irregularities in eating behavior, such as food aversion, and seizure-related neurologic disorders, including autism and Rett syndrome. There is an increased but variable risk of epilepsy in autism, reflected by common factors including genetic susceptibility, epileptiform electroencephalograms, and behavioral symptoms such as cognitive impairment and developmental delay. In support of the association between clinical autism and food consumption, one study of eating behaviors in children with and without autism, using a questionnaire pertaining to food refusal and acceptance patterns, indicated that children with autism have significantly more feeding problems and eat a significantly narrower range of foods than children without autism. Similarly, a comprehensive study of nutrition and eating behavior revealed that patients with Rett syndrome exhibit lower body weights, more gastrointestinal symptoms interfering with eating, less self-feeding, and lower texture tolerance for chewy and crunchy foods compared with a developmental disability comparison group. While autism and Rett syndrome do not reflect major diagnostic categories among the spectrum of epilepsy disorders, detection of comorbid anomalies in such a basic and ubiquitous vegetative function as food intake regulation provides an impetus for monitoring ingestive behaviors in future epilepsy research.

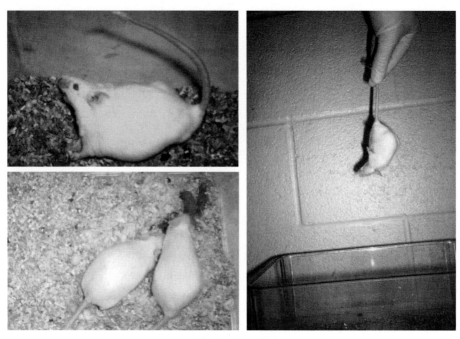

FIGURE 1-1

This panel of photos exhibits (top left) characteristics of the ictal phase of seizures in EL mice including Straub Tail, (right) the handling-induced seizure susceptibility procedure used as a seizure trigger in EL mice, and (bottom left) an example of post-partum biparental care in a home cage litter of EL pups.

Quantification of Appetite and Food Intake. Adult rodents in the laboratory consume discrete meals regularly over the course of the circadian cycle, and the meal size is proportional to meal frequency. Food intake measures may be a particularly attractive means of studying bioenergetic substrates such as plasma glucose as potential covariates for seizure-susceptibility. This is especially true since basic aspects of feeding behavior, including carbohydrate intake, are relevant for anticonvulsant efficacy of the ketogenic diet. For example, seizure management techniques, such as ketogenic diet exposure, that fundamentally alter brain energy homeostasis (9) would likely alter glucose or saccharine taste thresholds or preference if these psychometric measures of palatability were measured. Taken together, these considerations suggest that there is some functional overlap in brain systems regulating feeding behaviors, bioenergetics, and seizure susceptibility.

A more practical means of obtaining a better understanding of potential causal relationships between energy balance regulation on the one hand and seizure-related disorders on the other would be to predict efficacy of anticonvulsant drugs using measures of body weight or food intake. For example, there is evidence that the antiepileptic drug topiramate, designed originally as an oral hypoglycemic and approved subsequently as an anticonvulsant, is effective in producing weight loss sufficient to treat binge eating disorder, bulimia nervosa, and obesity. Topiramate is also reported to be effective in seizure reduction among patients with refractory focal epilepsy. Similarly, Rett syndrome patients show improvement in seizure control on topiramate. Moreover, patients receiving topiramate pharmacotherapy for a variety of neurologic disorders experience anorexia, body weight loss, and a reduction in body mass index (a coarse measure of adiposity). These intake and weight control characteristics of topiramate efficacy may promote long-term adherence to treatment among psychiatric patients. A compelling possibility is that negative energy balance manifesting a beneficial change in brain energy metabolism is one of the direct mechanism by which drugs such as topiramate exert seizure control.

Measures of Arousal and Emotionality. The finding of increased anxiogenic-like behavior in animal models of epilepsy appears to be highly reproducible. One representative study investigated the effects of amygdala kindling in Wistar rats on behavior in the elevated plus maze test of anxiety (10). It was found that kindling to stage five seizures increased anxiogenic-like responses in the plus maze for at least a week following the last seizure. Long-term amygdala kindling in rats resulted in large and reliable increases in affective behavior that model the interictal emotionality often observed in patients with temporal lobe epilepsy. The results suggest that neural changes underlying the genesis of interictal emotionality may be related closely to those mediating epileptogenesis itself. Another study evaluated the exploratory activity of an inbred rat strain derived from progenitors that have been selected for audiogenic seizure susceptibility. The exploratory activity of audiogenic seizure-susceptible and -resistant rats was measured using the open field and the elevated plus maze models of anxiety. Susceptible animals displayed a reduced exploration in both the open field (reduced total distance moved) and the elevated plus maze (reduced number of enclosed-arm entries). Therefore, available results indicate that seizure predisposition or history confers caution and behavioral restraint when faced with a novel environment. Not surprisingly, hyperemotionality is thought to underlie the majority of behavioral problems in some individuals with temporal lobe epilepsy and animal models of temporal lobe epilepsy.

CONCLUSIONS

Several animal models of seizure disorders have contributed greatly to the understanding of physiology, neuronal mechanisms, and behavioral changes associated with human epilepsy (4). However, most human conditions do not have well-characterized animal models, although select characteristics of animal models are analogous to diagnostic criteria for human epilepsy (1). One animal model characteristic that is analogous to clinical symptoms of epilepsy is the appearance of observable behavioral signs, which are often quite distinctive and exhibit face validity. For example, automatisms are de novo behaviors involving involuntary, repetitive, and meaningless movements of the face, limbs, and trunk that appear in seizure-prone organisms and can be quantified by a trained clinical observer or in animals using stereotypy rating scales. Similarly, the frequent and robust appearance of frank emotionality and disturbance of social interactions in both rodent models of seizure disorders and human epilepsy suggests that there are common, cross-species functional consequences of the neurologic hyperexcitability characteristic of epilepsy. Thus, the thesis presented earlier in this chapter that behavioral endpoints represent a kind of "meta-variable" with utility for achieving a more general understanding of seizure mechanisms, as opposed to an understanding based upon idiosyncratic features of specific seizure induction models, is supported by the available data.

Very few studies have quantified functional changes just prior to seizure onset in the case of ictogenesis or prior to the first lifetime seizure in the case of epileptogenesis, and this unexplored niche represents an opportunity for future research in the area of behavioral phenotyping. For example, auras that precede focal seizures in a clinical population have been given particular emphasis in order to localize the point of seizure origin in the brain, but subjective aura reports have no animal model counterpart. Long-term, automated behavioral dependent measures could be devised to detect some deviation in animal models of epilepsy that occurs at a preseizure latency synchronized with the occurrence of auras in a clinical population. For example, one study documented a decrease in expression of glial and neuronal glutamate transporters observed prior to the onset of epileptic seizures in cortex and thalamus of GAERS rats—an animal model of absence epilepsy. The findings suggest an impairment in maturation of the glutamatergic thalamocortical network, which may contribute to the establishment of epileptic circuitry. This hypothesis could perhaps be tested noninvasively by probing the ability of GAERS rats to perform behavioral functions, such as motor learning or attentional tasks, for which thalamocortical glutamate pathways are known to be critical. Finally, prodromes are long-lasting changes of disposition in humans in the form of anxiety, irritability, withdrawal, and other emotional aberrations that indicate a forthcoming seizure. In dogs, the most common prodromal sign described is motor restlessness. Perhaps the results from a battery of behavioral tests could be subjected to multiple regression analysis in order to devise a prodromal fingerprint for impending seizure occurrence in rodent models of epilepsy.

Available evidence suggests that anxiogenic-like reactions observed using classical tests of anxiety may be controlled by different neurobiological substrates than control those that govern defensive/social behaviors. Thus, implementation of a single animal model of anxiety as a means of assessing emotionality has a higher risk of producing misleading results than a phenotyping/characterization strategy, such as one possible algorithm (Figure 1-2) that employs multifactorial and convergent exploratory and social endpoints. The epilepsy researcher is therefore encouraged to employ as many convergent dependent measures of a particular construct of interest as available time and resources allow; adoption of a multifactorial approach is an excellent way to avoid "pitfalls" alluded to at the beginning of this chapter.

Even a concerted behavioral phenotyping effort incorporating the present methodical approach may reflect inherent limitations in sensitivity or precision of available tools. For example, one clinically relevant distinction between simple (without loss of consciousness) and complex (including loss of consciousness) partial seizures may be entirely beyond the reach of the animal model endpoints. In animals, signs of confusion or difficulties in recognizing familiar objects may be misinterpreted as signs of impaired consciousness. Rather than attempting to identify animal characteristics that are analogous to human target behaviors, the most fruitful

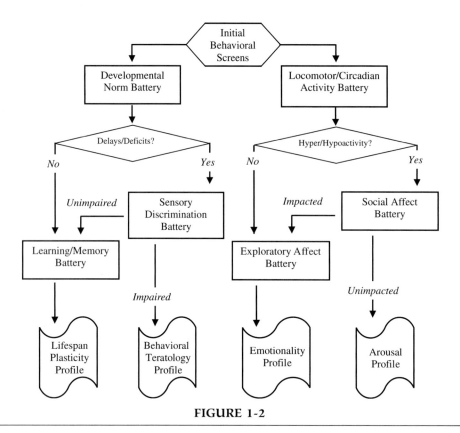

FIGURE 1-2

Behavioral phenotyping/characterization algorithm. Four branches of one possible strategy for characterizing the learning/memory, reflexive/sensory impairment, emotionality, and arousal characteristics of rodents. A learning/memory test battery is implemented once animals are found to develop normal reflexes or sensory capabilities. Reflexive/sensory impairment is present in the event that early postnatal developmental delays persist in the mature animal. A determination of emotionality can be made in the absence of overt alterations in home cage locomotor activity or in the event of altered locomotor activity following positive results in an activity-independent social affect test. An arousal profile can be deduced from alterations in motor activity in the absence of efficacy in a social affect test.

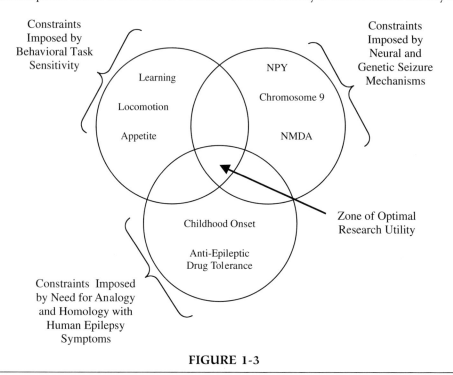

FIGURE 1-3

Venn diagram depicting the potential and desirable confluence in a "sweet spot" of behavioral task sensitivity, biological seizure mechanism specificity, and human epilepsy characteristics. Labels appearing within each circle reflect examples of phenomena that illustrate each of the three respective behavioral, neurobiological, and clinical realms, but their selection and position within the circle is arbitrary. NPY, neuropeptide Y; NMDA, N-methyl-D-aspartate receptor.

application of behavioral characterization efforts in seizure-prone animal models may well be provided by a rational approach that is sensitive simultaneously to the array of convergent behavioral dependent measures, the neural/genetic mechanisms for seizure induction/ maintenance, and the similarities between animal and human epilepsies (Figure 1-3). Such an approach can be described as flexible, causality–based, and mindful of the opportunities for translational research provided by the modern tools of behavioral neuroscience.

*R*eferences

1. Stables JP, Bertram EH, White HS, Coulter DA, et al. Models for epilepsy and epileptogenesis: report from the NIH workshop, Bethesda, Maryland. *Epilepsia* 2002; 43(11):1410–1420.
2. Hellier JL, Dudek FE. Chemoconvulsant model of chronic spontaneous seizures. In: Crawley J, Gerfen CR, Rogawski MA, Sibley DR, et al, eds. *Current Protocols in Neuroscience*. John Wiley & Sons, 2005:9.19.1–9.19.2.
3. Stafstrom CE. Assessing the behavioral and cognitive effects of seizures on the developing brain. *Prog Brain Res* 2002; 135:377–390.
4. Sarkisian MR. Overview of the current animal models for human seizure and epileptic disorders. *Epilepsy Behav* 2001; 2(3):201–216.
5. Heinrichs SC, Seyfried TN. Behavioral seizure correlates in animal models of epilepsy: a road map for assay selection, data interpretation, and the search for causal mechanisms. *Epilepsy Behav* 2006; 8(1):5–38.
6. Francis D, Diorio J, Liu D, Meaney MJ. Nongenomic transmission across generations of maternal behavior and stress responses in the rat. *Science* 1999; 286: 1155–1158.
7. Crawley JN. What's wrong with my mouse? Behavioral phenotyping of transgenic and knockout mice. New York: Wiley-Liss, 2000.
8. Mellanby J, Dwyer J, Hawkins CA, Hitchen C. Effect of experimental limbic epilepsy on the estrus cycle and reproductive success in rats. *Epilepsia* 1993; 34(2):220–227.
9. Mantis JG, Centeno NA, Todorova MT, McGowan R, et al. Management of multifactorial idiopathic epilepsy in EL mice with caloric restriction and the ketogenic diet: role of glucose and ketone bodies. *Nutr Metab (Lond)* 2004 Oct 19; 1(1):11.
10. Adamec RE. Amygdala kindling and anxiety in the rat. *Neuroreport* 1990; 1(3–4): 255–258.

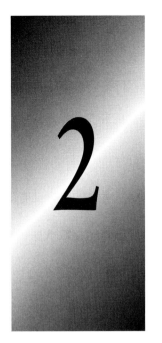

2

Influence of Environment and Social Factors in Animal Models of Epilepsy

Stephen C. Heinrichs

Whereas deterministic arguments such as the rather disturbing statement in the foregoing quotation link inherited genes with neurologic disorders, mouse and rat models of epilepsy serve as an excellent platform for testing the complementary hypothesis that the ontogeny of seizure-related disorders is subject to revision according to environmental forces to which genetically susceptible mice are exposed. Idiopathic epilepsy is most often expressed as a multifactorial disorder in which more than one gene acts in concert with environmental factors to mold the disease phenotype. The hypothesis of plasticity in animal models of epilepsy exposed to environmental and social manipulations will thus be evaluated critically in the present chapter while at the same time preclinical and clinical perspectives are integrated.

THE ROLE OF THE ENVIRONMENT IN SEIZURE ONSET

The term *environment* can be defined as a complex of surrounding circumstances, conditions, or influences in which an organism lives, modifying and determining its life or character. In animal models of epilepsy, environment is typically manipulated by altering the complexity of the home cage, by adjusting nutrition, or by adding or removing cagemates; an entire section of this chapter on socialization is devoted to this final instance of environmental change. For example, one series of studies has established the efficacy of adjusting the diversity and complexity of the home cage environment for altering subsequent seizure susceptibility (2). Seizure-prone rats were first housed from weaning in housing environments either without a companion in a standard shoebox cage (nonenriched) or in a group of 8–10 rats in a complex enclosure (enriched). The enriched environment led to worsening of seizure activity, assessed in terms of the proportion of rats exhibiting spontaneous spike-wave discharges as well as the duration of discharge (2). Moreover, exposure to the enriched environment later in life, at 3 months of age, also enhanced seizure activity, suggesting that the

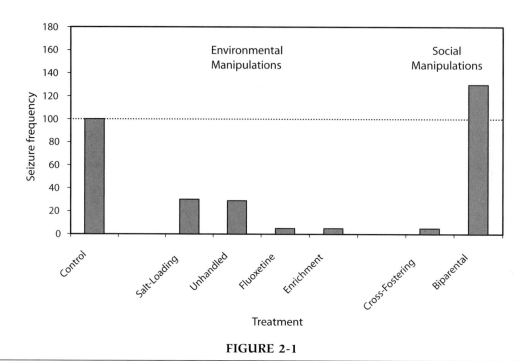

FIGURE 2-1

Seizure frequency in handled EL mice (control) as compared to EL mice exposed to a variety of environmental or social manipulations. The environmental manipulations that all decreased seizure frequency were (1) providing hyperosmotic saline as the only drinking fluid, (2) eliminating developmental contact with humans, (3) adulteration of the chow diet with fluoxetine, and (4) enriching the postweaning home cage environment. The social manipulations that modulated seizure frequency biphasically were (1) maternal cross-fostering and (2) supplemental paternal care. Values reflect percent of respective untreated control groups; the latter are exhibited at 100% seizure frequency in order to compare results drawn from six separate studies from our laboratory.

window of opportunity for environmental modulation of seizure activity is quite broad. While it is not possible to disentangle the social from the nonsocial components of enrichment in these studies, the results nonetheless provide evidence of the efficacy of daily living arrangements in altering seizure-related pathology in a genetically seizure-susceptible rat model (Figure 2-1).

Conditioned Effects of Seizure Occurrence

Mild periodic electrical stimulation to any one of several brain sites leads to the development and progressive intensification of elicited motor seizures. This phenomenon, known as kindling, has been studied widely, both as a model of epileptogenesis and as a form of neuroplasticity, and there has been increasing interest in kindling as a model of the interictal (i.e., between-seizures) changes in emotionality that accompany certain forms of epilepsy. Despite the extensive use of the kindling model, little consideration has been given to the role played by the environmental cues regularly associated with the delivery of the kindling stimulations. However, it has been demonstrated that cues associated with the standard kindling protocol

(e.g., the stimulation environment) produce conditioned effects on both the motor seizures and interictal behaviors, such as food avoidance, that are defensive in nature. The phenomenon of kindling-induced conditioning highlights how arbitrary contextual cues can produce a self-perpetuating set of seizure-related behaviors in the absence of ongoing seizure activity. One alarming possibility consistent with this finding is that increased seizure susceptibility could be induced as a conditioned response to the approach of a white-coated investigator, as first demonstrated by Pavlov using a salivation response in dogs, if some subsequent action of the investigator leads reliably to seizure onset.

Another conditioned effect of seizures is the increased likelihood of recurrent seizures arising as a facilitative consequence of seizure history (3). The conditioned nature of this plasticity is evident in that every episode is to some extent an effect of preceding ones and a cause of subsequent ones. Proposed mechanisms for such seizure facilitation include loss in inhibitory neurotransmission via hippocampal pathology. Thus, the aims of any laboratory study examining the efficacy of causal environmental factors in seizure induction are perhaps best served by minimizing the number of prior seizures in experimental animals or, alternatively, employing a time-to-first-seizure-dependent measure to remove this potential confound (4).

Adverse Consequences of Human-Animal Interaction

In performing behavioral characterization work, the testing apparatus, the experimental room, and the experimenters themselves are significant environmental variables that can impact the functional dependent measures. For instance, one complication of functional dependent measures relates to the idiosyncratic behavioral phenotype characteristic of a particular laboratory (5). In an eye-opening set of studies, mouse exploratory behaviors were found to differ significantly according to the laboratory in which the test was performed in spite of rigorous standardization of apparatus, test protocol, and environmental variables (5). Validation and application of a phenotyping battery for rodents can guard against errors in interpretation produced by uncontrolled sources of variance by providing multiple convergent measures of behavior. Similarly, innovative automated-home-cage approaches have been proposed for advancing mouse phenomics into the information age.

Stimulation-Induced Seizures. Perhaps the most convincing demonstration that noninvasive laboratory interventions are capable of modifying seizure phenotype is provided by the phenomenon of audiogenic seizure induction in nonsusceptible rodents (6). Rodents are typically exposed to loud (120 dB), high-frequency (12 kHz) pure tones in a closed environment for the purpose of inducing convulsions. Audiogenic seizures are induced in animal strains that are susceptible to epilepsy, although seizure-resistant strains of both rat and mouse can also be induced to seize with sufficiently intense or prolonged auditory stimulation. For instance, mice not susceptible to audiogenic seizures on initial exposure to an acoustic stimulus (priming) exhibit audiogenic seizures upon subsequent exposure to the acoustic stimulus as a function of age at priming and the prime-to-test interval in days. The ability of sensory overstimulation to induce seizures appears to be a general comparative phenomenon, since *bangsenseless* and *slam-dance* epileptic mutant flies respond with earlier and more pronounced postictal paralysis following mechanical shock relative to wild-type flies, and this behavioral feature can be attenuated by administration of antiepileptic drugs.

Impact of Animal Handling by Human Investigators. The term *handling* can be defined for the purposes of the present chapter as any noninvasive manipulation that is part of routine husbandry, including lifting an animal by the tail, cage cleaning, or moving an animal's cage. One comprehensive meta-analysis documented that handling procedures induce multifaceted physiologic and endocrine stress responses regardless of the skill with which they are performed (7). The consequences of handling are judged to be noxious and substantial, based upon the fact that the activation state induced in the rodent can persist for hours. While functional measures of emotionality are well suited to detecting affective responses to routine handling procedures, such measures are only infrequently collected. Thus, adverse consequences of human/animal contact on dependent-measure variability or animal welfare are a necessary evil of laboratory animal science, unless rodents can be conditioned as juveniles to accept the touch of a human hand (7) or contact can be minimized or eliminated.

The role of human/animal interactions in seizure induction can be illustrated effectively in the case of seizure-prone EL mice. Todorova and colleagues monitored a group of EL mice for seven days using 24-hour video surveillance and observed no evidence of spontaneous seizures or other behavioral abnormalities (3). In contrast, at the conclusion of the surveillance period, each mouse seized when picked up by the tail and moved from the observation cage to a cage with fresh bedding. These findings suggest that spontaneous seizures do not occur in EL mice and instead that environmental stimulation is necessary for seizure induction. Similarly, in GAD65 knockout mice, which lack the ability to synthesize gamma-aminobutyric acid (GABA) and exhibit deficiencies of this inhibitory neurotransmitter in cortex, cerebellum, and hippocampus, seizures can be induced by exposure to mild stressors such as brief confinement in a transparent acrylic plastic restraint tube or removal of the home cage lid for routine handling. Accordingly, a modified shoebox cage apparatus and a no-handling husbandry procedure have obvious utility both for examining the significance of human contact during rodent development and for behavioral phenotyping of undisturbed seizure-prone mice (8). A simple modified-cage husbandry and testing procedure allows mice to be born, be reared, and mature without the known short-term and permanent changes in behavior and neurobiology resulting from human contact and/or maternal separation.

The prediction that seizure-prone EL mice would be hypersensitive to human handling is supported by physiologic dependent measures. In particular, heart rate is elevated significantly in young EL mice by a tail suspension procedure involving exposure to an ordinarily innocuous and routine stimulus that did not impact heart rate in control mice 15 minutes following stressor onset. These results suggest that genetic and environmental risk factors establish a mechanism for overreaction to a tail suspension stressor that is capable ultimately of inducing seizure activity in mature EL mice (3). Indeed, the neural substrates for preictal tachycardia are currently being investigated as potential trigger zones for seizure onset. Together with the elevated core body temperature and increased overall activity exhibited throughout testing in EL mice relative to controls, it is clear that EL mice are faced with significant allostatic demands in which both physiologic and behavioral setpoints have been adjusted away from the normal homeostatic range. In this context, the tail suspension handling stressor can be thought of as a releasing stimulus rather than an inducing stimulus for seizure onset in EL mice (Figure 2-2).

The significant impact of human/animal contact on the phenotype of the seizure-prone mouse just described allows some clear recommendations regarding colony maintenance and experimental procedures. Firstly, it is important to know which personnel are handling experimental animals and what manipulations are being employed. If husbandry is performed by animal vivarium staff using flat-bottom caging, then the procedure used to transfer animals from cage to cage and the frequency of this manipulation should be reported. Moreover, the investigators may wish to specify for vivarium staff the

mechanism of cage transfer because the commonly used tail suspension procedure, for example, could well produce a sensitized response to this form of tactile stimulation over time, as is the case with the seizure-prone EL mouse (3). Finally, the distress of a systemic injection procedure itself induces anxiogenic-like behavioral effects in both kindled and control rats. Thus, it may be judicious to limit unnecessary experimental procedures such as handling for drug administration when other routes of hands-free administration are available (e.g., per os via adulteration of food or water). The most alarming form of investigator-induced variance in experimental outcome is one in which a latent change in results is induced unbeknownst to the investigator by implementation of within-subjects procedures. For example, the performance of wild-type mice on rotarod and emotionality tests can be altered unintentionally when mice are used previously for other experimental purposes. One way to address this concern constructively is to perform a desired sequence of tests using both within-subjects (same mice tested sequentially) and between-subjects (different mice tested at each time point) designs in an initial validation

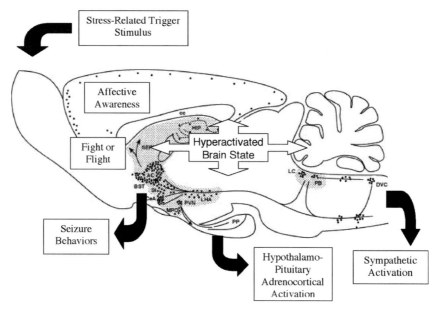

FIGURE 2-2

Schematic diagram of rat brain activity during ictogenesis in which the rat detects a seizure trigger stimulus that drives brain activation to a high level that is suprathreshold for seizure induction. Efferent responses to threat could include seizures and seizure-related behaviors, hypophysiotropic release of adrenocorticotropin (ACTH), amygdalo-medullary increases in heart rate, septo-hippocampal avoidance learning, and septo-amygdalar emotionality. Black dots reflect the distribution of corticotropin-releasing factor (CRF) neurons; the thesis that stress neuropeptide systems in the brain are agents for developmental epileptogenesis is developed in more detail elsewhere (9). The present stress diathesis hypothesis is described more thoroughly in a previously published review (8).

experiment in order to shed light on potential latent carryover effects.

THE ROLE OF SOCIAL INTERACTION IN SEIZURE ONSET

The interactive influences of biology and environment on seizure susceptibility in rodents as described in the preceding section can certainly be exerted in an isolated organism. However, a more naturalistic and necessarily more complex view of risk, etiology, and maintenance of seizures should consider the impact of conspecific interactions of individual seizure-susceptible organisms with other organisms in a social context. Indeed, the first such interaction between mother and offspring in the ontogeny of altricial rodent species represents a "critical period" for the patterning of adult characteristics, including reactivity to stressors, brain neurobiology, and the quality of parental care provided to the next generation. Similarly, affiliative events such as mating, pair bonding, and dominance hierarchy formation can be viewed as critical adaptive skills for rodent species living in a social context.

Preclinical evidence suggests an inverse relationship between social interaction and seizure susceptibility. For example, seizure-susceptible EL dams exhibit social withdrawal and neglect in caring for offspring, and an increase in the quality of dam-pup social interaction by cross-fostering attenuates seizure susceptibility (8). Similarly, juvenile recognition, an innate form of short-term social working memory, is also reported to be deficient in seizure-susceptible EL mice of both genders. Consistent with these findings from the animal literature, changes in sexuality and aggressivity associated with human epilepsy provide evidence of strained interpersonal relations. A second rationale for suspecting that an inverse relationship exists between social status and seizure outcome is the ability of stressor exposure to modulate these states in opposing directions. In organisms with a predisposition for epilepsy, early-life stress and traumatic events are associated with an increase in occurrence of seizures. Both the development of the disorder and the repeated occurrence of seizures are facilitated by environmental stressors (9). The co-occurrence of social deficits, seizure susceptibility, and altered stress reactivity implicates the proconvulsive neuromodulator corticotropin-releasing factor (CRF), which acts as an anxiogenic agent in brain to suppress social interaction (Figure 2-2). In addition, CRF receptor antagonists exert complementary prosocial and seizure-protective actions. Thus, available evidence suggests that normal social interaction is impaired in seizure-prone organisms and that centrally mediated stress-coping responses

may modulate the severity of these psychosocial and neurologic deficits.

Nongenomic Maternal Transmission

One critical form of social contact among mammals with epilepsy is the interaction between mother and offspring. In particular, population studies of epilepsy demonstrate a higher risk of epilepsy in offspring of affected women, as compared to the risk for offspring of affected men. One possible mechanism for the so-called nongenomic transmission (i.e., heritability not determined by genes alone) of an adult seizure-prone/hyperactive phenotype is the quality of parenting provided to developing offspring. In particular, the quality of maternal behavior has been implicated as an environmental determinant in rodent neurochemical and behavioral development. For example, offspring of mothers that exhibit relatively less vigorous maternal behavior mature with a high-emotionality, stress-hyperreactive phenotype, whereas the opposite result is produced in offspring reared by more vigilant mothers. Cross-fostering of offspring results in mature adults with maternal and anxiety-related behavioral characteristics of the foster mother, essentially trumping the relevant characteristics of the biological mother.

Considering the significance of mother-infant interactions in molding the behavioral phenotype of offspring, one testable hypothesis is that seizure-susceptible EL mice would suffer adult hyperexcitability as a result of differential maternal behavior provided by EL mothers. In support of this hypothesis, EL dams exhibit deficits in maternal behavior, including longer latencies to retrieve pups and decreased time spent crouching/nursing, when compared to control dams. It is hypothesized that the deficits may result from the locomotor hyperactivity of the EL dam, because locomotor activity competes with motivated maternal behaviors such as crouching or nursing and pup retrieval. Studies also reveal a striking dissociation in EL dams between two components of maternal behavior: nursing on the one hand and pro-nurturant behaviors on the other. EL dams spend less time nursing and crouching over pups than control mothers, yet they dedicate sufficient effort to build nests of quality equal to those of control dams. Maternal behavior of EL females is apparently not a coherent constellation of component behaviors that all rise or fall together, as could be predicted from some studies. Note that the relative decline in nursing by EL dams predicts high infant mortality, which is confirmed by the fact that only about 25% of EL dams in a breeding colony raise their litters successfully to the age of weaning.

A link between seizures/epilepsy and maternal behavior has been established in research using species other than the mouse. For instance, one study performed using rats induced seizures, together with postseizure multifocal neurotoxicity, by administration of lithium/pilocarpine 2 months prior to assessment of reproductive and maternal capacity. Exposure to these convulsants completely abolished maternal behavior, judged using crouching, retrieval, and nest quality measures, without altering reproductive capacity or litter size. Clinical studies have also examined the extent to which maternal behaviors could impact children with epilepsy. Investigators interested in the psychosocial support systems of families affected by childhood epilepsy studied intellectual competence of children with epilepsy aged 7–13 years in a problem-solving task using an observational technique that measured the degree of maternal involvement. The results indicated that maternal support for a child's success in a task and the degree of self-reliance produced in the child both significantly improved problem-solving performance. Taken together, these studies are consistent with the notion that the quality of maternal behavior is positively correlated with offspring adjustment and viability in seizure-prone organisms.

Conspecific Interactions

Behavioral and seizure phenotypes of seizure-susceptible mice should also be altered following exposure to meaningful and enduring changes in the nonparental social environment. In one experiment, the normal group housing condition that exists in the litter prior to the age of weaning was perpetuated in mice housed in groups of three per cage but was interrupted at the time of weaning in the case of single housing, a manipulation that could also be termed "isolation" housing. The consequence of an approximately 10-day period of post-weaning individual housing was detected using a locomotor activity measure in which group-housed, but not single-housed, seizure-susceptible EL mice exhibited significant decreases in activity during the final portion of the nocturnal phase of the circadian cycle relative to controls (8). Thus, alteration in postweaning social grouping condition alters behavioral phenotype in seizure-prone EL mice. Social enrichment can also be considered a risk factor for seizure susceptibility, to the extent that such enrichment is accompanied by persistent increases in motor activity. Indeed, social enrichment has been reported to augment seizure severity in a genetically susceptible rat model of absence epilepsy (2).

The degree to which rodents express an innate affinity to interact with members of their own species has been studied using the social interaction test as an animal model of emotionality. The degree of socialization is characteristic of a particular animal strain/species and can be modulated up and down by exposure to anxiolytic and anxiogenic drugs, respectively. A recent study tested the hypothesis that seizure-prone EL adults would exhibit diminished social investigation of juvenile and adult conspecifics relative to controls investigating conspecifics of their own strain. The hypothesis was supported when control mice spent significantly more time in social investigation than mice of the EL strain. Although it is not yet clear whether this decline in investigation among EL mice results from blunted affiliative motivation on the one hand or to incompatible locomotor hyperactivity effects on the other, this result is consistent with the maternal dam/pup finding that EL mice spend less time interacting with conspecifics than do non-seizure-susceptible controls. In additional to serving as a marker for seizure susceptibility in genetic models of epilepsy, diminished sociability could lead to deficits in social working memory and poor parental investment.

CONCLUSIONS

Findings reviewed in the foregoing sections support a diathesis-stress hypothesis (3) in which genetically seizure-susceptible rodents exhibit a multifaceted hyperreactivity to environmental and social stimuli. According to this conceptual model, seizures arise in organisms subject to both innate vulnerability and exposure to a noxious environmental event(s). In the EL mouse model of epilepsy, a variety of stress-protective and augmenting treatments are indeed reported to modulate seizure susceptibility (Figure 2-1). Consistent with this notion, stress is often noted by patients as a precipitating factor in seizure induction. One retrospective study investigated the influence of a forced evacuation on the seizure frequency of patients with epilepsy, compared with patients of the same age and type of epilepsy living outside the evacuation area at the time of a threatening flood. Of 30 evacuees, eight exhibited an increase and one a decrease in seizure frequency during or shortly after the evacuation period, compared with one and zero control patients, respectively. Consistent with these findings, 62% of 400 patients of a tertiary-care epilepsy center cited at least one seizure precipitant. In order of frequency, stress (30%), sleep deprivation (18%), sleep (14%), fever or illness (14%), and fatigue (13%) were noted by at least 10% of patients. These data support the hypothesis that there is a reliably reported relation between a stressful life event and seizure frequency. Implicit in this argument is the suggestion that stressful stimuli are potent stimulants for affective regulatory activation in the brain, a conclusion that is certainly supported by the present results (Figure 2-2). The affective character of seizure triggers is noted metaphorically by Bowman, who states that "like old volcanoes, the simmering emotions lay partially dormant until painful life context and immediate precipitants jolt them to life" (10).

The present results guide the rational design of animal colony husbandry procedures for investigators working with epilepsy models. First, prohibition of human tail suspension handling for the purpose of providing weekly cage change husbandry effectively extends for up to 60 days the time to first seizure in dam-reared EL mice (Figure 2-1). This is consistent with the known sensitivity of EL mice to tail suspension handling, which acts to increase seizure frequency and shorten seizure latency over the lifetime (3). Second, biparental rearing resulted in expression of the handling-induced seizure phenotype in EL mice that was latent in mice raised by a single dam (Figure 2-1). Phrased in a different way, biparental rearing reduced time to first seizure in genetically susceptible EL mice, consummating the process by which a normal brain is converted into a hyperexcitable brain (4). Thus, investigators working with environmental seizure triggers in animal models of genetic seizure susceptibility such as the EL or GAD65 mouse strains could potentially maximize baseline seizure incidence through biparental rearing combined with regular husbandry and minimize baseline seizure incidence through single-dam rearing combined with infrequent or alternative methods of husbandry.

References

1. Myerson A. Eugenical sterilization: a reorientation of the problem. New York: Macmillan; 1936.
2. Schridde U, van Luijtelaar G. The role of the environment on the development of spike-wave discharges in two strains of rats. *Physiol Behav* 2005; 84(3):379–386.
3. Todorova MT, Burwell TJ, Seyfried TN. Environmental risk factors for multifactorial epilepsy in EL mice. *Epilepsia* 1999; 40(12):1697–1707.
4. Dichter MA. Models of epileptogenesis in adult animals available for antiepileptogenesis drug screening. *Epilepsy Res* 2006; 68(1):31–35.
5. Crabbe JC, Wahlsten DW, Dudek BC. Genetics of mouse behavior: interactions with laboratory environment. *Science* 1999; 284:1670–1672.
6. Ross KC, Coleman JR. Developmental and genetic audiogenic seizure models: behavior and biological substrates. *Neurosci Biobehav Rev* 2000; 24:639–653.
7. Balcombe JP, Barnard ND, Sandusky C. Laboratory routines cause animal stress. *Contemp Top Lab Anim Sci* 2004; 43(6):42–51.
8. Heinrichs SC, Seyfried TN. Behavioral seizure correlates in animal models of epilepsy: a road map for assay selection, data interpretation, and the search for causal mechanisms. *Epilepsy Behav* 2006; 8(1):5–38.
9. Baram TZ, Hatalski CG. Neuropeptide-mediated excitability: a key triggering mechanism for seizure generation in the developing brain. *Trends Neurosci* 1998; 21(11): 471–476.
10. Bowman ES. Relationship of remote and recent life events to the onset and course of non-epileptic seizures. In: Gates JR, Rowan AJ, eds. *Non-epileptic Seizures*. Boston: Butterworth-Heinemann, 2000:269–283.

3 Animal Models of Mood Disorders: Kindling as a Model of Affective Illness Progression

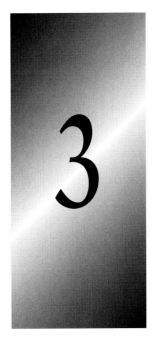

Robert M. Post

The classic animal models of depression or mania typically involve an environmental precipitant followed by a subacute period of abnormal behavior. For example, learned helplessness or depressive-like behavior in animals can be induced by a series of avoidable, mild, foot-shock stressors in which the resulting behavioral abnormalities last for a brief period of time and then return to normal. Similarly, in the defeat stress model of depression, a naïve rodent is subject to attack by a resident rodent that viciously protects its territory, resulting in short periods of depressive-like behavior in the naive animal (1).

Conversely, in animal models of mania using psychomotor stimulants, an injection of cocaine or amphetamine results in brief periods of increased activity in animals and hypomanic-like activity in humans. Interestingly, a repetition of some stressors will induce increased reactivity (stress sensitization) and cross-sensitization to psychomotor stimulants, resulting in increased degrees of motor activation compared with naïve animals that have been injected (2).

In this chapter, we focus on different aspects of the affective disorders, specifically their tendency to recur and progress. Some forms of seizure disorders, particularly complex partial seizures involving the medial temporal lobe structures, can also show this tendency for faster recurrence and progression to pharmacoresistance and intractability. In this regard, amygdala-kindled

seizures have been widely considered as a useful model for some aspects of complex partial seizure induction and progression. We take advantage of these characteristics of the animal model of amygdala-kindled seizures to examine some of the potential mechanisms underlying affective illness progression that may be useful in considering the differential pathophysiologies of both the recurrent affective disorders and complex partial seizures, as well as the potential development of loss of efficacy (tolerance) to previously effective pharmacological interventions (3).

It therefore becomes crucial to emphasize that amygdala-kindled seizures are a nonhomologous model of mood disorder recurrence, because many of the important criteria of a traditionally valid animal model of mood disorders are not met (4). Amygdala-kindled seizures do not model mood disorders in their behavioral characteristics or inducing factors, nor do they precisely parallel the pharmacotherapeutic measures that suppress or prevent them. Given this lack of direct homology, one must infer that the neurobiological substrates underlying amygdala-kindled seizures and the recurrent affective disorders are also dissimilar (5).

With such major disjunctions from a valid or typical homologous animal model of mood disorder, one might immediately question the potential relevance of such an animal model of seizure progression to that of affective illness progression. The models are useful in the following areas: (1) the progressive development to full-blown episodes; (2) regular recurrence; (3) the emergence of spontaneity; and

(4) the tendency to develop tolerance to previously effective medications. In these aspects of episode progression, some indirect predictive validity, particularly concerning the principles involved in such a progression, may be useful in conceptualizing clinically therapeutic maneuvers. The predictive validity of the amygdala-kindling model is only indirect, because there is not a direct extrapolation of the effects of the specific medications themselves that are therapeutically effective in both amygdala-kindled seizures and affective episodes (even though they may both involve anticonvulsant drugs).

AMYGDALA-KINDLED SEIZURE PROGRESSION AND PARALLELS WITH AFFECTIVE ILLNESS RECURRENCE AND PROGRESSION

Amygdala-Kindled Seizures

In animals, repeated once-daily stimulation of the amygdala with intensities below the amygdala afterdischarge (AD) threshold will eventually lower that threshold and result in the presence of amygdala ADs. With repeated stimulations, these ADs progressively become longer, more complex, and more widely distributed throughout a variety of brain structures, first unilaterally and then bilaterally in limbic structures and cortex. In association with this AD progression is the development of increasing behavioral seizure stages in rodents, beginning with behavioral arrest (stage 1), then chewing and head-nodding (stage 2), followed by unilateral forepaw clonus (stage 3), and finally bilateral seizures with rearing and falling (stages 4 and 5) (6, 7).

Following a sufficient number of these stimulation-induced seizures, full-blown seizures begin to appear spontaneously; that is, in the absence of exogenous stimulation through the amygdala electrode. Thus, three major phases or stages of amygdala-kindled seizure progression are evident. Phase I is amygdala-kindled seizure development and progression from no effect to full-blown seizures. Phase II is the mid phase, or repeated expression of completed amygdala-kindled seizures after each amygdala-kindled stimulation. Phase III, the late stage of spontaneity, involves seizures in the absence of stimulation.

What is most intriguing about these three separate phases of amygdala-kindled evolution is that they each have a different pharmacoresponsivity. As illustrated in Figure 3-1, some medications, such as the high-potency benzodiazepines, valproate, and levetiracetam, all appear to be effective in the prevention of both the phase I development and phase II completed phases of kindling. In contrast, carbamazepine, phenytoin, and lamotrigine are examples of drugs that are ineffective in preventing the development of amygdala-kindled seizures but are highly effective in preventing the full-blown or completed phase

of amygdala-kindled seizures. Conversely, other drugs are effective in preventing the development of amygdala-kindled seizures but do not suppress those that are fully developed, such as the glutamate N-methyl-D-aspartate (NMDA) receptor antagonists.

Pinel (8) and others have demonstrated that the late (phase III) spontaneous seizures also have a differential pharmacoresponsivity compared with the earlier phases. In this regard, phenytoin is not effective in preventing amygdala-kindled seizure development and is of ambiguous potency and utility in the mid phase but is highly effective in preventing spontaneous seizures. Conversely, diazepam prevents the first two phases but is without effect on spontaneous seizures. Thus, the behaviorally similar seizures of phases II and III show a marked double dissociation in responsivity and further suggest that the underlying neurobiological substrates are also quite different.

Affective Episode Recurrence and Progression

Kraepelin (9) made some of the initial observations that have now been widely replicated using a variety of modern methodologies. He observed that successive affective episodes tend to recur on average after a shorter interval between recurrences, and they progress from being triggered by psychosocial stressors to occurring more autonomously (in the absence of obvious environmental precipitants). The tendency for episodes to recur with increased frequency and shorter well intervals, as mirrored in the amygdala-kindling process, we have termed episode sensitization.

Stress sensitization involves two components. The first component is similar to the initial (phase I) developmental stage of kindling, in which psychosocial stressors may be inadequate to produce clinical manifestations of affective illness but, with increasing stressor recurrence, may be sufficient to induce brief and then full-blown episodes. A second component of stress sensitization is related to the late (phase III) stage of kindling: autonomy, in which precipitated episodes can then begin to occur more spontaneously. In contrast to some interpretations in the literature, stress sensitization therefore involves increased reactivity to a stressor over time, resulting in more full-blown episodes. However, the animal or human may continue to be highly reactive to some environmental stressors during the spontaneous phase, even though stressors are no longer necessary for the induction of affective episodes. Thus, the prediction is not that late-phase episodes are nonreactive to stressors but just the opposite—that is, stressors are not required (10).

Pharmacoresponsivity as a Function of Phase of Illness Evolution

Thus, both animals subject to amygdala-kindled seizures and many patients with recurrent affective disorders progress through the three general phases of seizure or episode progression. Based on the pharmacological

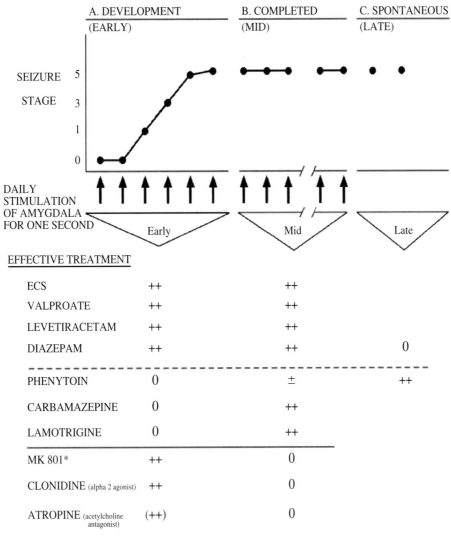

EFFECTIVE TREATMENT	A. DEVELOPMENT (EARLY)	B. COMPLETED (MID)	C. SPONTANEOUS (LATE)
ECS	++	++	
VALPROATE	++	++	
LEVETIRACETAM	++	++	
DIAZEPAM	++	++	0
PHENYTOIN	0	±	++
CARBAMAZEPINE	0	++	
LAMOTRIGINE	0	++	
MK 801*	++	0	
CLONIDINE (alpha 2 agonist)	++	0	
ATROPINE (acetylcholine antagonist)	(++)	0	

* glutamate NMDA$_R$ antagonist

FIGURE 3-1

Pharmacologic responsivity as a function of stage of kindling. Top: Schematic illustration of the evolution of kindled seizures. Initial stimulations (development) are associated with progressively increasing afterdischarge (AD) duration (not shown) and behavioral seizure stage. Subsequent stimulations (completed) produce reliable generalized motor seizures. Spontaneous seizures emerge after sufficient numbers of triggered seizures have been generated (usually >100). Bottom: Amygdala–kindled seizures show differences in pharmacological responsivity as a function of kindled stage (++, very effective; ±, partially effective; 0, not effective). The double dissociation in response to diazepam and phenytoin in the early versus the late phases of amygdala kindling, as described by Pinel, is particularly striking. ECS, electroconvulsive seizures; NMDAR, N-methyl-D-aspartate receptor.

disjunctions outlined in Figure 3-1 for kindled seizure evolution, one may ask whether such dissociations in therapeutic effectiveness also occur in different phases of affective disorder evolution. Currently, only a modicum of data directly support such differences in efficacy as a function of stage of illness progression, but the consideration of these differences may be important for clinical pharmacotherapeutics.

To date, all of the clinically effective interventions for affective illness were developed for acute treatment of affective episodes (mania or depression) and then were continued for prophylaxis (prevention of recurrence). As one begins to consider the possibility of primary prevention (i.e., intervention in the illness prior to its full-blown emergence in those at high risk), one needs to be aware that the same drugs that are effective against full-blown episodes and capable of preventing them in that phase may not successfully prevent the initial or developmental phases of the illness, as was found for lamotrigine and carbamazepine in the kindling model.

Similarly, there is considerable indirect support for the observation that many of the drugs that are effective earlier in the illness are no longer effective in the late or more spontaneous phases. Although it is difficult to directly extrapolate to the late or spontaneous phases of the illness in the recurrent affective disorders, those patients with a high number of episode recurrences or a pattern of rapid cycling (four or more episodes per year) tend to be more resistant to most psychopharmacological interventions. These medications include nonanticonvulsant drugs such as lithium and some of the typical and atypical antipsychotics, and perhaps the unimodal antidepressants. Also included on the list of medications that appear to be less effective in those with a greater number of episodes or more rapid cycling include carbamazepine, lamotrigine, and perhaps valproate (3).

It is important to make the point again that in comparison with a nonhomologous model, we are not making the assumption that the same drugs that are effective in different stages of amygdala-kindled seizures will be the same drugs that show parallel responsivity in the different stages of affective illness evolution. We are only using the clearly revealed general principle of differential pharmacoresponsivity as a stage of illness evolution (Figure 3-1) to examine whether this proposition is maintained or not for individual agents used in the treatment of the affective disorders. This distinction is most clearly seen with lithium carbonate and the traditional unimodal antidepressants, which are largely not effective against amygdala-kindled seizures but, in bipolar disorder, show a change from relative effectiveness early in the illness to relative ineffectiveness in the late or rapid-cycling phases. Also demonstrating this point are the data that a potent anticonvulsant drug such as levetiracetam, which is effective in phases I and II of amygdala-kindling evolution, has not yet been demonstrated in a controlled study to have efficacy in any stage of bipolar illness (11).

Contingent Tolerance and Cyclic Phenomena

Carbamazepine, lamotrigine, the benzodiazepines, and, to a slightly lesser extent, valproate are all associated with a progressive loss of anticonvulsant efficacy when administered immediately prior to an amygdala-kindled stimulation (12, 13). Some animals treated with the same dose of drug rapidly progress to full-blown nonresponsivity, whereas other animals show intermittent and recurrent periods of responsivity and nonresponsivity, often in a cyclic fashion that eventually proceeds to complete tolerance.

This progression represents a unique form of pharmacodynamic tolerance that we have called "contingent tolerance" because it is based on the drug's administration prior to each amygdala-kindled stimulation (12). Interestingly, if the drug is administered immediately after each amygdala-kindled seizure has occurred, and animals thus receive the same amount of drug on a daily basis, they do not become tolerant. The tolerance is therefore contingent on the drug's presence at sufficient levels at the time of the intended seizure. It is not the mere repeated presence of the drug in the body that is being adapted to and is associated with tolerance development, but its presence during the kindling stimulation.

Tolerance Reversal.   Accordingly, if an animal has completely lost responsivity to a given anticonvulsant via contingent tolerance, a period of daily amygdala-kindled stimulations in the drug-free condition, or even the experience of full-blown seizures occurring with the drug administered immediately after the seizures have occurred, will result in tolerance reversal and a transient regaining of effectiveness.

We believe this medication-free and seizure-induced tolerance reversal is related to the reinduction of endogenous anticonvulsant substances that were not induced when seizures had occurred in the tolerant state. These endogenous adaptations were likely prevented from occurring by the presence of the drug, even when a full-blown seizure in the tolerant condition was elicited.

Pathological versus Adaptive Changes in Gene Expression.   Each amygdala-kindled seizure elicits a wide variety of changes in gene expression, which can be assessed by alterations in mRNA or by subsequent changes in protein levels. Many of these adaptations can be divided into two categories (Figure 3-2). One category includes those adaptations that are putatively part of the primary pathophysiology of kindling and are related to increased excitability and seizure susceptibility, represented by increases in corticotropin releasing hormone (CRH), glutamate receptor upregulation, or gamma-aminobutyric acid (GABA) receptor inhibition. Conversely, other changes appear to represent endogenous anticonvulsant adaptations such as those represented by increases in the peptide thyrotropin-releasing hormone (TRH), or upregulation of GABA receptors or their subunits.

This model has obvious important clinical implications in distinguishing between neurochemical alterations associated with seizures and affective disorders that are part of the primary pathophysiological process from those that are secondary and endogenous mechanisms that have potential antiepisode effects. This distinction is vital because one would presumably want to enhance the abnormalities associated with the positive adaptations

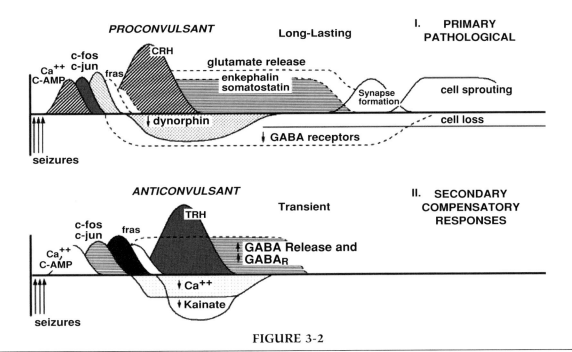

FIGURE 3-2

Competing pathological and adaptive endogenous responses to kindled seizures. This figure is a schematic illustration of potential transcription factor, neurotransmitter, and peptidergic alterations that follow repeated kindled seizures. Putative mechanisms related to the lasting primary pathological drive (i.e., kindled seizure evolution) are illustrated (top), as are those thought to be related to the more transient secondary compensatory responses (i.e., anticonvulsant effects) (bottom). The horizontal line represents time. Sequential transient increases (above the line) or decreases (below the line) in second messengers, immediate early genes, and neurotrophic factors are followed by longer-lasting alterations in peptides, neurotransmitters, and receptors or their mRNAs. Given the unfolding of these competing mechanisms in the evolution of seizures and their remission, the question arises as to whether parallel opposing processes also occur in the course of secondary and primary affective disorders or other psychiatric disorders. Such endogenous adaptive changes may be exploited in the design of new treatment strategies. CRH, corticotropin-releasing hormone; GABA, gamma-aminobutyric acid; Ca, calcium; cAMP, cyclic adenosine monophosphate; fras, fos-related antigens; TRH, thyrotropin-releasing hormone.

and suppress the abnormalities that are part of the primary pathophysiological processes in both the affective and the seizure disorders (14).

This conceptual view suggests the availability of an entirely new potential range of therapeutic tools in attempting to enhance some of the abnormalities already present in these illnesses, while suppressing others. These tools include not only ones in the pharmacological realm, but perhaps also in the physiologic realm, in which increases or decreases in brain activity in a certain region may represent either pathological or adaptive mechanisms. For example, in an abnormal area of hyperactivity in the brain that represents a positive or secondary adaptation, one might want to enhance this change further with targeted treatments such as high-frequency stimulation with repetitive transcranial magnetic stimulation (rTMS). Conversely, suppressing this hyperactive area (with low-frequency rTMS) would theoretically be appropriate if such a change were part of the primary pathophysiology of the illness process.

Tolerance Associated with Failure of Some Episode-induced Endogenous Adaptations. We discovered that selected anticonvulsant adaptations failed to occur in tolerant compared with nontolerant animals, which could help explain a loss of anticonvulsant responsivity (Table 3-1). For example, during contingent tolerance to the anticonvulsant effects of carbamazepine, we found that the normal seizure-induced increases in TRH mRNA or in the alpha-4 subunit of the $GABA_A$ receptor selectively failed to occur. This endogenous anticonvulsant hypothesis has been partially validated by studies in which TRH was administered bilaterally into the hippocampus in tolerant animals, who then showed better responsivity to the anticonvulsant effects of carbamazepine (15). Similarly, in tolerant animals, the failure of the alpha-4 subunit of the $GABA_A$ receptor to be upregulated by seizures may make the rat more susceptible to seizures and less drug responsive.

When seizures are then induced in the absence of carbamazepine, these positive adaptations are again generated and are likely to be associated with renewed anticonvulsant efficacy. We believe this phenomenon of transient

TABLE 3-1

Selective Failure of Some Kindled Seizure-induced Neurochemical Changes in Carbamazepine Contingent Tolerance

SEIZURE-INDUCED ADAPTATIONS (IN NONTOLERANT[a] ANIMALS)	IN CBZ–TOLERANT ANIMALS, SEIZURE-INDUCED ADAPTATIONS ARE	
	PRESENT	ABSENT
↑ c-fos mRNA		↑ c-fos
↑ Diazepam receptors	↑ Diazepam-R	
↑ GABA$_A$ receptors [3H] musimol		↑ GABA$_A$-R
↑ alpha-4 subunit		↑ alpha-4 subunit
↑ beta-1 and-3 subunits	↑ beta 1 and 3 subunits	
↑ TBPS binding		↑ TBPS
↑ Glucocorticoid R mRNA		↑ Glucocorticoid R
↑ Mineralocorticoid R mRNA	↑ Mineralocorticoid R	
↑ BDNF mRNA	↑ NT3 mRNA	↑ BDNF
↑ TRH mRNA		↑ TRH
↑ CRF mRNA		↑ CRF
↑ CRF-BP mRNA		↑ CRF-BP
↑ NPY-mRNA		(↑ NPY)
↑ enkephalin mRNA		(↑ enkephalin)
↓ dynorphin mRNA	↓ dynorphin	

[a]Treated with CBZ after each daily amygdala kindling stimulation; nontolerant animals were matched for amount of drug and number of seizures seen in tolerant animals. CBZ, carbamazepine; DZp, diazepam; GABA, gamma-aminobutyric acid; TBPS, [(35)S]*tert*-butylbicyclophosphorothionate; BDNF, brain-derived neurotrophic factor; NT3, neurotrophin-3; TRH, thyrotropin-releasing hormone; CRH, corticotropin-releasing hormone; CRH-BP, CRH binding protein; NPY, neuropeptide Y; ( ), partial loss; R, receptor.

tolerance reversal by seizures that are elicited in the absence of medication may be related to observations by Engel and Rocha (16) and others: that treatment-refractory patients who discontinue their medications prior to considering epilepsy surgery, experience a number of seizures in the unmedicated condition, and are subsequently found not to be good surgical candidates may show reresponsivity to their previously ineffective anticonvulsants. This prediction would be made only if a tolerance phenomenon had been involved in the eventual development of drug refractoriness, and it would not be pertinent to those patients who never had a period of good response to that drug.

These observations of both tolerance and cyclic phenomena in between seizure occurrence and suppression during drug treatment in the kindling model may be pertinent to similar periodic episode emergence that can occur during the long-term prophylaxis of the recurrent affective disorders (17).

Tolerance Development in the Course of Treatment of the Recurrent Affective Disorders. In recurrent unipolar depression, tolerance can occur in the long-term

preventive effects of the tricyclic antidepressants, the monoamine oxidase inhibitors, or the newer second-generation antidepressants. In these cases, patients show an initial excellent preventive response for a period of years and then begin to show progressively more frequent or severe episode breakthroughs (18).

The same tolerance phenomenon can occur with most of the mood stabilizing drugs for the prevention of manic and depressive episodes. These drugs include carbamazepine, valproate, lamotrigine, and the nonanticonvulsant lithium. We postulate that parallel phenomena occur, similar to that observed in the contingent tolerance model of anticonvulsants used in the prevention of amygdala-kindled seizures, and that there is a dissipation of the full range of episode-induced positive endogenous adaptations during tolerance. At the same time, there continues to be a progression of the primary pathophysiological alterations driving episode recurrence, and the convergence of these two processes could lead to gradual loss of drug effectiveness (Figure 3-3).

In this regard, there is considerable evidence that TRH possesses endogenous antidepressant and antianxiety effects

Postulate: pathological vs. adaptive changes drive episode cycling

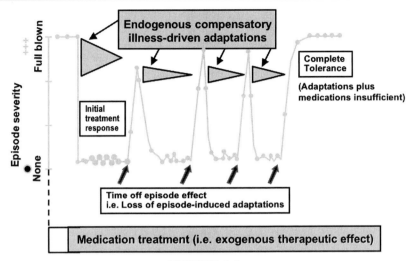

FIGURE 3-3

Hypothetical schema of the role of endogenous regulatory factors in the generation and progression of illness cyclicity. After an illness episode (A), adaptive compensatory mechanisms are induced (large triangle) that, together with drug treatment (B, bottom shaded line), suppress the illness (initial treatment response; box). The endogenous compensatory adaptations dissipate with time (i.e., the time-off seizure effect), and episodes of illness reemerge. Although this reelicits illness-related compensatory mechanisms, the concurrent drug treatment prevents some of the illness-induced adaptive responses from occurring (smaller triangles). As tolerance proceeds (associated with the loss of adaptive mechanisms), illness reemergence occurs more rapidly. Thus, the drug is becoming less effective in the face of less robust compensatory adaptive mechanisms. The primary pathology is also progressively reemerging, driven by additional stimulations and episodes (i.e., the kindled memory trace of the primary pathological mechanisms). Since this cyclic process is presumably driven by the ratio of primary pathological to secondary compensatory responses at the level of changes in gene expression, we postulate that such fluctuations arising out of illness- and treatment-related variables could account for the wide variations in individual patterns of illness cyclicity.

in patients with affective disorders as well as in normalizing both hyper- and hypoactivity in animal models. There is also evidence that TRH is hypersecreted during some affective episodes, as revealed by increases of TRH in cerebrospinal fluid (CSF) or by the downregulation of the thyroid-stimulating hormone (TSH) response to TRH during endocrine testing (19).

Thus, we postulate that TRH is an example of a positive endogenous psychotropic compound and that its failure to be induced by affective disorder episodes could be typical of a range of positive adaptations that fail to occur during tolerance development. Similarly, if a patient became tolerant to carbamazepine, and it was removed from the treatment paradigm, episodes of affective illness may again be capable of inducing TRH, which could be associated with a transient renewal of psychotropic prophylaxis. This effect has not been systematically studied in patients, although several case vignettes have been reported that are consistent with these observations.

The observations from the amygdala-kindled seizure model of cyclicity (14) and tolerance (3) have direct clinical implications for therapeutics in both the seizure and affective disorders. The model suggests the potential utility of switching to medications with different mechanisms of action that do not show cross-tolerance in the model, a potentially useful approach to the loss of clinical anticonvulsant responsivity in the epilepsies. However, the mechanisms underlying tolerance development in the seizure disorders may not be the same ones pertinent to tolerance in the affective disorders, and a specific assessment of drugs that do and do not show cross-tolerance in both the clinical epilepsies and the affective disorders needs to be directly assessed and verified.

Cross-Tolerance Phenomena. Cross-tolerance, or lack thereof, demonstrated in the contingent tolerance paradigm of amygdala-kindled seizures may be a good starting place for considering the same phenomena in the clinical seizure disorders (20) (Table 3-2). Similarly, manipulations that are associated with slowing the development of tolerance in the amygdala-kindled seizure model may be worth considering in the clinical affective disorders. We have found a variety of manipulations that appear to slow tolerance development in the kindling model,

TABLE 3-2
Cross-Tolerance Patterns in Contingent Anticonvulsant Effects on Amygdala Kindled Seizures

DRUG; TOLERANCE FROM	CROSS-TOLERANCE TO	NO CROSS-TOLERANCE TO
Carbamazepine (CBZ)	• PK11195 • CBZ-10,11-epoxide • Valproate (?via ↓ alpha-4 subunit of GABA$_A$ R)	Clonazepam Diazepam Phenytoin Levetiracetam*
Lamotrigine (LTG)	• Carbamazepine	Valproate MK801[a] Gabapentin[a]
Levetiracetam (LEV)	• Carbamazepine*	

*Unidirectional cross-tolerance from LEV to CBZ; not CBZ to LEV.
[a]These drugs slow the development of tolerance to LTG.

including using consistently higher drug doses or two previously marginally effective drugs in combination (Table 3-3). Each of these propositions requires specific testing in the clinical arena, however, to demonstrate its potential applicability and utility.

Contingent Inefficacy. One variation of the contingent tolerance phenomenon is that if a drug is administered before (but not after) each amygdala-kindled stimulation during the early phase of kindling development (when it is ineffective), the drug may no longer be effective in the fully developed stage of kindled seizures when it would

TABLE 3-3
Ways of Preventing or Slowing Tolerance to Anticonvulsant Effects on Once Daily Amygdala Kindled Seizures in Rodents

Higher doses (VPA)	More effective drugs
Steady, nonescalating doses	(VPA > CBZ, LTG)
Drug combinations (CBZ + VPA)	Alternating high and low dose (LTG)
Early rather than late initiation of treatment	For LTG, adding MK801 or Gabapentin
Decreasing stimulation intensity	

Potential Ways of Reversing Tolerance

Add drugs with different mechanisms of action (i.e., without cross-tolerance).

Discontinue now-ineffective drug; seizures occur in medication-free state and med-free episodes; responsiveness is re-achieved.

otherwise be highly effective. We have observed this phenomenon with both lamotrigine and carbamazepine pretreatment during kindling development (12, 21). The ineffective pretreatment with these drugs subsequently precludes their efficacy once the full-blown phase of completed seizures has occurred.

It is important to note that it is not the presence of the drug in the animal during kindling development that accounts for the drug's inefficacy, because the administration of these drugs after each amygdala-kindled seizure during development still results in normal anticonvulsant efficacy in completed kindled seizures. It is the treatment immediately prior to the kindling stimulation that is crucial. These observations raise a number of clinical concerns for the epilepsies and affective disorders. For example, it is theoretically possible based on the model that pretreatment with phenytoin—which has been most widely studied in the potential prevention of posttraumatic epilepsy and was found to be ineffective—would also interfere with its effectiveness in suppressing completely developed posttraumatic seizures.

Such attempts at primary prophylaxis have not yet been systematically attempted in the affective disorders, but the contingent inefficacy observations raise the caution that administering a drug that is ineffective in this early developmental prevention could also interfere with its overall efficacy when it is known to work in suppressing and preventing full-blown affective episodes. This theoretical possibility makes it even more important to discern which drugs are effective in the early developmental stages and which ones may not be, so that they can be appropriately used in these early phases of illness evolution.

Similarly, in posttraumatic seizures, it may be worth reexamining drugs that are effective during amygdala-kindling development for their potential efficacy in clinical seizure prevention following head trauma, rather than using drugs such as carbamazepine, phenytoin, and lamotrigine that are ineffective in the early developmental phases (at least in the amygdala-kindling model). Thus, assessing the usefulness of valproate and levetiracetam in the prevention of posttraumatic epilepsy would appear worthy of further consideration.

CONCLUSIONS

There are obviously a number of caveats in the application of a nonhomologous model, such as amygdala-kindled seizures, to the recurrent mood disorders. There are marked limitations in the ability to extrapolate from one to another in most realms. However, we hope we have illustrated that a variety of the principles involved in seizure progression that are revealed in the kindling model may also be pertinent for clinical consideration in the affective disorders and their therapeutics, even if the specific manipulations differ in the two illnesses.

The potential division of illness-related abnormalities into those that are pathological and those that are adaptive may be of considerable clinical importance in conceptualizing new approaches to therapeutics, as well as in the prevention or reversal of tolerance phenomena. Loss of responsiveness to many of the long-term prophylactic treatments in the affective disorders is more common than previously recognized, and the contingent tolerance model may be helpful in conceptualizing some of the processes involved and ways of circumventing them. This is of particular importance because a variety of recent observations have indicated that minor breakthrough affective episodes appear to predict more major-episode recurrence, and appropriately targeting these early phenomena with therapeutics may help prevent more serious subsequent untoward events. This course of action would not only address a generally accepted long-term goal of the treatment of the current affective disorders (i.e., achieving and maintaining long-term remission), but also aid in the conceptualization of some novel principles that may help ensure this desired long-term outcome.

Thus, while the inferences from a nonhomologous model (such as amygdala-kindled seizures) to recurrence in the affective disorders have many inherent limitations, the model may still have applicability and indirect predictive validity in the specific area of illness recurrence and progression. It is increasingly common and recognized as scientifically useful to describe illness "endophenotypes," which then can be examined in their own right, even if they are not illness-specific. In a similar fashion, we would suggest that principles of illness recurrence and progression may have similar utility in conceptualizing therapeutic approaches to both the recurrent seizures and affective disorders. Whereas amygdala-kindled seizures are not a good or homologous model for affective episodes in relationship to most characteristics—their inducing factors, the behaviors manifest, the comparative temporal relationships (seconds to minutes for seizures versus weeks to months for affective episodes), or in most cases, the pharmacological interventions—the seizures may nonetheless have considerable heuristic utility in considering variables associated with the course and prevention of these highly recurrent illnesses.

References

1. McKinney WT. Animal models of depression: an overview. *Psychiatr Dev* 1984; 2:77–96.
2. Post RM, Weiss SR, Pert A. Cocaine-induced behavioral sensitization and kindling: implications for the emergence of psychopathology and seizures. *Ann N Y Acad Sci* 1988; 537:292–308.
3. Post RM, Weiss SRB. Convergences in course of illness and treatments of the epilepsies and recurrent affective disorders. *Clin Electroencephalogr* 2004; 35:14–24.
4. Weiss SR, Post RM. Caveats in the use of the kindling model of affective disorders. *Toxicol Ind Health* 1994; 10:421–447.
5. Post RM. Neurobiology of seizures and behavioral abnormalities. *Epilepsia* 2004; 45 Suppl 2:5–14.
6. Goddard GV, McIntyre DC, Leech CK. A permanent change in brain function resulting from daily electrical stimulation. *Exp Neurol* 1969; 25:295–330.
7. Racine RJ. Modification of seizure activity by electrical stimulation. I. After-discharge threshold. *Electroencephalogr Clin Neurophysiol* 1972; 32:269–279.
8. Pinel JPJ. Effects of diazepam and diphenylhydantoin on elicited and spontaneous seizures in kindled rats: a double dissociation. *Pharmacol Biochem Behav* 1983; 18:61–63.
9. Kraepelin E. Manic-depressive insanity and paranoia. Edinburgh: ES Livingstone, 1921.
10. Post RM. The status of the sensitization/kindling hypothesis of bipolar disorder. *Current Psychosis and Therapeutics Reports* 2004; 2:135–141.
11. Muralidharan A, Bhagwagar Z. Potential of levetiracetam in mood disorders: a preliminary review. *CNS Drugs* 2006; 20:969–979.
12. Weiss SR, Clark M, Rosen JB, Smith MA, et al. Contingent tolerance to the anticonvulsant effects of carbamazepine: relationship to loss of endogenous adaptive mechanisms. *Brain Res Brain Res Rev* 1995; 20:305–325.
13. Mana MJ, Kim CK, Pinel JP, Jones CH. Contingent tolerance to the anticonvulsant effects of carbamazepine, diazepam, and sodium valproate in kindled rats. *Pharmacol Biochem Behav* 1992; 41:121–126.
14. Post RM, Weiss SRB. A speculative model of affective illness cyclicity based on patterns of drug tolerance observed in amygdala-kindled seizures. *Mol Neurobiol* 1996; 13:33–60.
15. Wan RQ, Noguera EC, Weiss SR. Anticonvulsant effects of intra-hippocampal injection of TRH in amygdala kindled rats. *Neuroreport* 1998; 9:677–682.
16. Engel J, Jr., Rocha LL. Interictal behavioral disturbances: a search for molecular substrates. *Epilepsy Res* 1992; 9:341–349.
17. Post RM. Do the epilepsies, pain syndromes, and affective disorders share common kindling-like mechanisms? *Epilepsy Res* 2002; 50:203–219.
18. Post RM, Ketter TA, Speer AM, Leverich GS, et al. Predictive validity of the sensitization and kindling hypotheses. In: Soares JC, Gershon S, eds. *Bipolar Disorders: Basic Mechanisms and Therapeutic Implications*. New York: Marcel Dekker, 2000:387–432.
19. Winokur A. The thyroid axis and depressive disorders. In: Mann JJ, Kupfer DJ, eds. *The Biology of Depressive Disorders*. New York: Plenum Press, 1993:155–170.
20. Post RM, Zhang ZJ, Weiss SRB, Xing G, et al. Contingent tolerance and cross tolerance to anticonvulsant effects in amygdala-kindled seizures: mechanistic and clinical implications. In: Corcoran ME, Moshe SL, eds. *Kindling VI*. New York: Springer, 2005:305–314.
21. Postma T, Krupp E, Li XL, Post RM, et al. Lamotrigine treatment during amygdala-kindled seizure development fails to inhibit seizures and diminishes subsequent anticonvulsant efficacy. *Epilepsia* 2000; 41:1514–1521.

4 Cognitive and Affective Effects of Seizures: Immature Developing Animals

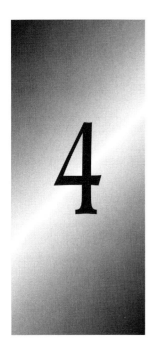

Pavel Mareš

There is general agreement about the fact that the immature brain is more prone to generation of epileptic seizures than the adult brain. In contrast, there has been a long-lasting discussion on the possible consequences of seizures in immature brain. Attention has focused primarily on morphological damage. The initial observation that the immature brain was resistant to seizure-induced morphological damage has been progressively overruled by data demonstrating age- and model-specific brain damage even if seizures are elicited at early stages of development (1–8). Less attention has been given to functional consequences of early-life seizures; there are only a few laboratories working in this field. Experimental studies were begun by Wasterlain (9, 10), and then this topic was systematically studied in Holmes' laboratory (11). At present not only Holmes' but three other laboratories are regularly publishing data in this field (Stafstrom, Kubová, Huang), and there are isolated papers from other laboratories. All these studies have been performed in rats; two strains are mainly used: Wistar and Sprague-Dawley. It is rather difficult to compare published results because different models are used, seizures are elicited at different postnatal ages (from the day of birth—postnatal day 0, or PD0—to PD45); severe status epilepticus (SE) or single or recurrent seizures are induced; and the age when the animals are tested also differs (from PD15 to PD180; mostly in adulthood). The only point common to many papers is the Morris water maze (MWM), but in various modifications as to the number of exposures, as a method to detect possible deficits in learning; other methods (open field, eight arm maze, elevated plus maze, handling test) are used far less commonly.

MOTOR PERFORMANCE

The necessary prerequisite for behavioral testing in the aforementioned tests is sufficient motor performance. Delayed development of reflexes was described by Wasterlain (9, 10) after long-lasting flurothyl-induced seizures at PD4 as well as after repeated electroshocks during the first 10 postnatal days. Phasic changes of motor abilities differed according to the age when SE was elicited, as demonstrated by Kubová et al. (12). Rotorod performance of adult rats was found to be impaired in some studies—after recurrent bicuculline seizures at PD5–7 (13), after lithium-pilocarpine (LiPILO) SE at P12 (12), but not after recurrent pentylenetetrazol (PTZ)-induced seizures at PD10-14 (14) or after LiPILO SE at P14 (15). Locomotor activity was increased in adult rats exposed to repeated PILO SE at PD7–9 (16, 17), to LiPILO SE at the age of 25 days (12), after kainic acid (KA) at PD22–26 (11), at PD30 (18) and at PD35 (19, 20), but not after KA at PD1, 7, 14 or 24 (21) and after 55 seizures induced repeatedly by flurothyl at P0–12 (22). Transient changes were demonstrated in studies checking motor activity repeatedly: LiPILO SE at PD12 (12), repeated PTZ at PD16–20 (23). Swimming speed in the MWM was not found to be a factor in the spatial impairment observed (24).

COGNITIVE CHANGES

Consequences of Status Epilepticus

Continuous Hippocampal Stimulation.   This model, originally elaborated by Lothman, was used only in one study (25). Long-lasting continuous hippocampal stimulation was performed at PD20, 30, or 60. The rats were tested in the MWM at PD 80. There were no changes in animals stimulated at the age of 20 or 30 days; impairment was found only in the PD60 group.

Kainic Acid.   The data for the KA model are at variance. Whereas Holmes et al. (11) described slower learning and worse results in the probe test in the MWM (in which, after the rat masters the MWM, the platform is removed and time spent in the quadrant where the platform was originally localized is compared to time spent in other quadrants) in adult rats exposed to KA at PD22–26, Stafstrom et al. (18) did not find any difference in the MWM test in adult rats exposed to KA at PD5 or PD10; the only difference in animals given KA at PD20 or PD30 was poorer results in the probe test. Rats exposed to KA at the age of 60 days were slow in learning and failed in the probe test. Similar results were described by Koh et al. (26) for animals exposed to KA at PD15. In contrast, Sayin et al. (21) found differences in latencies to find a platform in the MWM in adult rats exposed to KA at PD7 or PD24 and failure in probe test also in animals injected with KA at PD1. These authors also demonstrated poor performance of adult rats given KA at PD1, PD7, PD14, or PD24 in the radial arm maze and shorter time spent in the open arms of the elevated plus maze. The eight-arm radial maze was used also by Lynch et al. (27): Adult rats injected with KA at PD1, PD7, or PD14 were able to learn, though much more slowly than controls, but animals with KA-induced SE at PD24 or PD75 rarely reached criterion. As far as other tests are concerned, de Feo et al. (28) demonstrated that rats exposed to KA at PD10 or PD25 were significantly worse than controls in an active avoidance test at PD45. Adult rats after KA SE at PD22–26 exhibited worse performance in the T-maze (11). Administration of a subconvulsive dose of KA at PD12 resulted in an impaired nonassociative learning: PD25 rats exposed to open field for the second time did not exhibit (in contrast to controls) signs of habituation (29).

Discrepancies are also found in results obtained with repeated administration of KA. Tandon et al. (30) did not find any difference between controls and rats given KA repeatedly at PD12, 16, 20, and 24, and Sarkisian et al. (31) described no difference between MWM performance before and after KA injected repeatedly at PD22, 24, and 26. Koh et al. (26) described worse performance in the MWM in rats given KA repeatedly at PD15 and 45 than in animals exposed at PD45 only, suggesting that repeated seizures early in life "prime" the brain for injury with a second insult—the so-called "second hit hypothesis."

A study of Liu and Holmes (19) demonstrated that intracerebroventricular infusion of basic fibroblast growth factor during KA-induced seizures in 35-day-old rats prevented behavioral effects in the MWM, open field, and handling tests observed after these seizures in control adult rats. Animals with KA SE at PD35 treated with gabapentin up to PD75 and tested in the MWM at PD80–PD87 did not differ from nontreated KA SE rats (32).

Pilocarpine.   There are two modifications of this type of status: SE induced by a high dose of pilocarpine (PILO), and by 5–10 times lower dose in rats pretreated with lithium chloride (LiPILO). There are no marked differences in the pattern of SE induced in these two ways.

Liu et al. (33) found that adult rats exposed to PILO at PD20 performed worse in the MWM than controls but better than animals with SE at PD45. Data from the LiPILO model demonstrated no (34) or only minor (35) worsening of performance of adult rats with SE at PD12. If SE was elicited at the more advanced developmental stage—PD14 (15), PD16 or PD20 (34), or PD25 (35, 36)—performance of adult rats in the MWM was worse than that of control animals. Serious impairment of MWM performance was demonstrated also in rats undergoing LiPILO SE at PD20 and tested at PD22, PD25, or PD50 (37). Adult rats with a history of LiPILO SE between PD18 and 21 exhibited impairment of reference memory in the eight-arm radial maze (38).

Auditory testing of adult rats demonstrated a difference between animals with SE at PD20 and at PD45. The former group exhibited only moderate impairment in location discrimination, whereas rats exposed to PILO at PD45 had marked deficit in location as well as sound-silence discrimination (39).

Repeated elicitation of PILO SE at PD7, 8, and 9 resulted in marked deficits in adult rats; they were impaired in the Skinner box and exhibited longer latencies in the step-down test (16, 17).

There are also studies of possible ways to influence the consequences of severe epileptic activity in developing rats. Paraldehyde was used to interrupt seizures in studies by Kubová et al. (12, 35). If two different doses were used in PD12, animals with the lower dose tended to perform worse in the MWM; this difference was significant in rats with SE induced at PD25.

Malnutrition in the very first postnatal days neither worsened nor improved MWM performancce of adult rats with a history of LiPILO SE at PD21 (40). Akman et al. (41) reported similar results, causing food deprivation by isolating pups from dams for 12 hours daily from PD2 to PD19 and LiPILO SE at P20. At variance with Akman's data were the results of Lai et al. (42), in which shorter isolation (daily from PD2 to PD9) and LiPILO SE at PD10 led to worse learning in the MWM at adulthood. The administration of metyrapone (an inhibitor of corticosterone synthesis) immediately after SE reversed this detrimental effect.

If the LiPILO SE was elicited at PD20 and these rats were exposed to an enriched environment for 4 hours daily since PD21, they performed in the MWM better than SE controls in spite of a similar extent of neuronal damage (37, 43).

Performance in the MWM was positively influenced by choline supplementation administered with a normal diet to pregnant female rats. Their offspring were trained in the MWM at PD29–32, then PILO SE was elicited at PD34 and the rats were retrained in the MWM at PD41–44. Rat pups of choline-supplemented dams exhibited at PD41 the same latency as at PD32, whereas control SE rats had to learn from the beginning (44).

Aminophylline pretreatment just before elicitation of LiPILO SE at PD12 (45) or at PD14 (46) resulted in much worse performance of adult rats in the MWM.

The combination of LiPILO SE at PD11 with subsequent flurothyl seizures (25 seizures at PD12–16) resulted in worsening of learning in the MWM at the age of 30 days (47). This combination was modified in another study from Holmes' laboratory: LiPILO SE was induced at PD20, MWM training started at PD25, and when asymptotic performance was reached, single flurothyl seizures were elicited. Animals were exposed to the MWM at different intervals (from 15 to 360 minutes) after seizures; SE rats needed longer time for recovery than controls exposed to flurothyl seizures only (48).

Corticotropin-releasing hormone is able to induce seizures when administered to infant rats (49). These animals exhibit progressive worsening of performance in the MWM if tested at the age of 3, 6, and 10 months, as well as an impairment of short-term memory in the object recognition test (50).

Consequences of Single Seizures

Hypoxia-Induced Seizures. Nearly all 10-day-old rats exposed to hypoxia exhibited epileptiform EEG activity, but 60 days later they did not differ from control siblings in the MWM, open field, and handling tests (51).

Focal Ischemia-induced Seizures. Focal ischemia elicited by local application of endothelin-1 in the dorsal hippocampus induced acute seizures in both PD12 and PD25 rats. When tested as adults in the MWM, only the younger group exhibited significantly longer latencies than controls (52).

Tetanotoxin-induced Seizures. Rats with tetanotoxin applied into hippocampus at PD10 exhibited changes in the MWM at PD57–PD61: They learned the maze, but latencies to reach the platform were always longer than those of controls (53).

N-methyl-D-aspartate (NMDA). Stafstrom and Sasaki-Adams (54) elicited seizures by systemic administration of NMDA in 100 PD12 to PD20 rats; after 30 minutes, seizures were arrested with ketamine. Slower learning in the MWM was observed in all these animals during adulthood, but there was no difference in the probe trial.

Consequences of Repeated Seizures

Flurothyl. Rats were exposed at PD6 to flurothyl for 30 min; during this period all animals exhibited repeated seizures. A control group was exposed to flurothyl only for a short time sufficient to elicit a single seizure. Adult rats from the group with repeated seizures exhibited impaired learning in the the MWM (55). Repeated short flurothyl-induced seizures were first studied by Holmes et al. (24); 25 seizures during neonatal period resulted in impaired learning in the MWM. Three studies with 45 to 55 short flurothyl seizures during the first 9 or 12 postnatal days (22, 56, 57) found impaired learning in the MWM studied at different ages (from PD20 to PD82). Even 15 short flurothyl seizures elicited at PD15–19 were sufficient to worsen performance of adult rats in the MWM and impair auditory location discrimination, but not auditory quality discrimination (58).

Chronic administration of topiramate after repeated flurothyl seizures at PD10–14 (59) improved performance of PD48–52 rats in the MWM. The combination of repeated flurothyl seizures at PD0–4 with LiPILO SE at PD20 led to poor learning of adult rats in the MWM; chronic topiramate administration starting at PD5 improved this learning, especially at the first day of training (60).

PTZ. Daily administration of PTZ (fractionated doses up to elicitation of SE) at PD10–14 led to impairment of learning in the MWM. At the age of 35 days worse learning was observed at all four training days, whereas if MWM was trained at the age of 60 days, there was a difference only during the first day (14). If these animals were fed with fish oil (but not with corn oil) from PD3 to PD21, they performed better (61).

Bicuculline. Bicuculline administered daily at PD5–7 resulted in moderate impairment of performance in the MWM in adulthood; impairment was more severe in rats injected with kainic acid at PD53 and worse in a group with combined bicuculline and KA administration (42).

AGGRESSIVITY

All published data demonstrated increased aggression in rats undergoing SE in the fourth postnatal week and later.

Increased aggression toward the experimenter was observed in adult rats exposed to KA-induced SE at PD30 or PD60 (18) as well as in animals exposed to PILO SE at PD35 (19) or PD45 (33). Rats with LiPILO SE at PD25 treated with the oxygen radical scavenger PBN exhibited extreme aggressivity not only toward the experimenter but also to other rats in the cage, such that they were kept in isolation. Such high levels of aggressivity were not observed in rats with LiPILO SE and PBN at PD12 (Kubová et al., in preparation).

ANXIETY

Results are contradictory. Three studies demonstrated decreased anxiety, but the fourth one speaks in favor of increased anxiety.

Behavior of rats in the elevated plus maze was examined in three studies. A decrease in entries into arms was found in both laboratories, but dos Santos et al. (16) described a longer time spent in open arms in rats exposed repeatedly to PILO SE at PD7–9, whereas Kubová et al. (35) observed longer time spent in closed arms and an increase of risk assessment in rats with LiPILO SE at PD25. Transfer latency from the open to the closed arm was increased 60 minutes, 24, 48 as well as 72 hours after nonconvulsive seizures induced by KA at PD18 (62), which is in agreement with the finding that daily PTZ administration at PD16-20 (again fractionated doses up to SE) led to shorter latency to enter the open arm in an elevated T-maze (23).

GENERAL CONCLUSIONS

The basic question whether seizures are harmful to the immature brain (63, 64) can be answered without any hesitation: Yes, they impair the developing brain. Recent review articles make the same conclusion (4, 5, 65–69). The present review shows that behavioral consequences were demonstrated in adult rats exposed to severe epileptic activity at early stages of brain development. Severity of impairment is different; the age at which epileptic seizures are elicited plays an important role. It is necessary to take into account that even the morphological damage depends on this factor and that it is not the same as in adult animals. The unifying point, the MWM used to test cognitive functions, has both advantages—that it provides some possibility to compare data from different studies—and drawbacks—that it is a test only of spatial memory (66) and other aspects of cognition are studied only exceptionally. Another aspect still missing is possible phasic development of impairment. Longitudinal studies analyzing dynamics of changes are necessary not only to confirm or exclude phasic development of changes, to establish levels of maturation necessary for appearance of individual effects, but also to distinguish simple developmental delay from real damage as well as to find the optimal method and timing of therapy.

References

1. Babb TL, Leite JP, Mathern GW, Pretorius JK. Kainic acid induced hippocampal seizures in rats: comparisons of acute and chronic seizures using intrahippocampal versus systemic injections. *Ital J Neurol Sci* 1995; 16:39–44.
2. Sankar R, Shin DH, Liu H, Mazarati A, et al. Patterns of status epilepticus-induced neuronal injury during development and long-term consequences. *J Neurosci* 1998; 18:8382–8393.
3. Sankar R, Shin DH, Mazarati A, Liu H, et al. Epileptogenesis after status epilepticus reflects age- and model-dependent plasticity. *Ann Neurol* 2000; 48:580–589.
4. Holmes GL, Ben-Ari Y. Seizures in the developing brain: perhaps not so benign after all. *Neuron* 1998; 21:1231–1234.
5. Holmes GL, Ben-Ari Y. The neurobiology and consequences of epilepsy in the developing brain. *Pediatr Res* 2001; 49:320–325.
6. Kubová H, Druga R, Lukasiuk K, Suchomelová L, et al. Status epilepticus causes necrotic damage in the mediodorsal nucleus of the thalamus in immature rats. *J Neurosci* 2001; 21:3593–3599.
7. Lado FA, Laureta EC, Moshé SL: Seizure-induced hippocampal damage in the mature and immature brain. *Epileptic Disord* 2002; 4:83–97.
8. Druga R, Kubová H, Mareš P. Degenerative neuronal changes in the rat thalamus induced by status epilepticus at different developmental stages. *Epilepsy Res* 2005; 63:43–65.
9. Wasterlain CG. Effects of neonatal status epilepticus on rat brain development. *Neurology* 1976; 26:975–986.
10. Wasterlain CG. Effects of neonatal seizures on ontogeny of reflexes and behavior: an experimental study in the rat. *Eur Neurol* 1977; 15:9–19.
11. Holmes GL, Thompson JL, Marchi T, Feldman DS. Behavioral effects of kainic acid administration on the immature brain. *Epilepsia* 1988; 29:721–730.
12. Kubová H, Haugvicová R, Suchomelová L, Mareš P. Does status epilepticus influence the motor development of immature rats? *Epilepsia* 2000; 41 suppl. 6:S64–S69.
13. Lai MC, Liou CW, Yang SN, Wang CL, et al. Recurrent bicuculline-induced seizures in rat pups cause long-term motor deficits and increased vulnerability to a subsequent insult. *Epilepsy Behav* 2002; 3:60–66.
14. Huang LT, Yang SN, Liou CW, Hung PL, et al. Pentylenetetrazol-induced recurrent seizures in rat pups: time course on spatial learning and long-term effects. *Epilepsia* 2002; 43:567–573.
15. Wu CL, Huang LT, Liou CW, Wang TJ, et al. Lithium-pilocarpine-induced status epilepticus in immature rats results in long-term deficits in spatial learning and hippocampal cell loss. *Neurosci Lett* 2001; 312:113–117.
16. dos Santos NF, Arida MR, Trindade EM, Priel MR, et al. Epileptogenesis in immature rats following recurrent status epilepticus. *Brain Res Brain Res Rev* 2000; 32:269–276.
17. dos Santos NF, Marques RH, Correia L, Sinigaglia-Coimbra R, et al. Multiple pilocarpine-induced status epilepticus in developing rats: a long-term behavioral and electrophysiological study. *Epilepsia* 2000; 41 Suppl.6:S57–S63.
18. Stafstrom CE, Chronopoulos A, Thurber S, Thompson JL, et al. Age-dependent cognitive and behavioral deficits after kainic acid seizures. *Epilepsia* 1993; 34:420–432.
19. Liu Z, Holmes GL. Basic fibroblast growth factor is highly neuroprotective against seizure-induced long-term behavioural deficits. *Neuroscience* 1997; 76:1129–1138.
20. Mikati MA, Holmes GL, Werner S, Bakkar N, et al. Effects of nimodipine on the behavioral sequelae of experimental status epilepticus in prepubescent rats. *Epilepsy Behav* 2004; 5:168–174.
21. Sayin U, Sutula TP, Stafstrom CE. Seizures in the developing brain cause adverse long-term effects on spatial learning and anxiety. *Epilepsia* 2004; 45:1539–1548.

22. de Rogalski Landrot I, Minokoshi M, Silveira DC, Cha BH, et al. Recurrent neonatal seizures: relationship of pathology to the electroencephalogram and cognition. *Brain Res Dev Brain Res* 2001; 129:27–38.

23. Erdogan F, Golgeli A, Kucuk A, Arman F, et al. Effects of pentylenetetrazole-induced status epilepticus on behavior, emotional memory and learning in immature rats. *Epilepsy Behav* 2005; 6:537–542.

24. Holmes GL, Gaiarsa JL, Chevassus-Au-Lois N, Ben-Ari Y. Consequences of neonatal seizures in the rat: morphological and behavioral effects. *Ann Neurol* 1998; 44:845–857.

25. Thurber S, Chronopoulos A, Stafstrom CE, Holmes GL. Behavioral effects of continuous hippocampal stimulation in the developing rat. *Brain Res Dev Brain Res* 1992; 68:35–40.

26. Koh S, Storey TW, Santos TC, Mian AY, et al. Early-life seizures in rats increase susceptibility to seizure-induced brain injury in adulthood. *Neurology* 1999; 53:915–921.

27. Lynch M, Sayin U, Bownds J, Janumpalli S, et al. Long-term consequences of early postnatal seizures on hippocampal learning and plasticity. *Eur J Neurosci* 2000; 12:2252–2264.

28. de Feo MR, Mecarelli O, Palladini G, Ricci GF: Long-term effects of early status epilepticus on the acquisition of conditioned avoidance behavior in rats. *Epilepsia* 1986; 27:476–482.

29. Kubová H, Mikulecká A, Haugvicová R, Langmeier M, et al. Nonconvulsive seizures result in behavioral but not electrophysiological changes in developing rats. *Epilepsy Behav* 2001; 2:473–480.

30. Tandon P, Yang Y, Stafstrom CE, Holmes GL. Downregulation of kainate receptors in the hippocampus following repeated seizures in immature rats. *Brain Res Dev Brain Res* 2002; 136:145–150.

31. Sarkisian M, Tandon P, Liu Z, Yang Y, et al. Multiple kainic acid seizures in the immature and adult brain: ictal manifestations and long-term effects on learning and memory. *Epilepsia* 1997; 38:1157–1166.

32. Cilio MR, Bolanos AR, Liu Z, Schmid R, et al. Anticonvulsant action and long-term effects of gabapentin in the immature brain. *Neuropharmacology* 2001; 40:139–147.

33. Liu Z, Gatt A, Werner SJ, Mikati MA, et al. Long-term behavioral deficits following pilocarpine seizures in immature rats. *Epilepsy Res* 1994; 19:191–204.

34. Cilio MR, Sogawa Y, Cha BH, Liu X, et al. Long-term effects of status epilepticus in the immature brain are specific for age and model. *Epilepsia* 2003; 44:518–528.

35. Kubová H, Mareš P, Suchomelová L, Brožek G, et al. Status epilepticus in immature rats leads to behavioural and cognitive impairment and epileptogenesis. *Eur J Neurosci* 2004; 19:3255–3265.

36. Kubová H, Rejchrtová J, Redkozubova O, Mareš P. Outcome of status epilepticus in immature rats varies according to the paraldehyde treatment. *Epilepsia* 2005; 46 Suppl. 5:38–42.

37. Rutten A, von Albada M, Silveira DC, Cha BH, et al. Memory impairment following status epilepticus in immature rats: time-course and environmental effects. *Eur J Neurosci* 2002; 16:501–513.

38. Kostakos M, Persinger MA, Peredery O. Deficits in working but not reference memory in adult rats in which limbic seizures had been induced before weaning: implications for early brain injuries. *Neurosci Lett* 1993; 158:209–212.

39. Neill JC, Liu Z, Mikati M, Holmes GL. Pilocarpine seizures cause age dependent impairment in auditory location discrimination. *J Exp Anal Behav* 2005; 84:357–370.

40. Huang LT, Lai MC, Wang CL, Wang CA, et al. Long-term effects of early-life malnutrition and status epilepticus: assessment by spatial navigation and CREB$^{Serine-133}$ phosphorylation. *Brain Res Dev Brain Res* 2003; 145:213–218.

41. Akman C, Zhao Q, Liu X, Holmes GL. Effect of food deprivation during early development on cognition and neurogenesis in the rat. *Epilepsy Behav* 2004; 5:446–454.

42. Lai MC, Holmes GL, Lee KH, Yang SN, et al. Effect of neonatal isolation on outcome following neonatal seizures in rats: the role of corticosterone. *Epilepsy Res* 2006; 68:123–136.

43. Faverjon S, Silveira DC, Fu DD, Cha BH, et al. Beneficial effects of enriched environment following status epilepticus in immature rats. *Neurology* 2002; 59:1356–1364.

44. Yang Y, Liu Z, Cermak JM, Tandon P, et al. Protective effects of prenatal choline supplementatiom on seizure-induced memory impairment. *J Neurosci* 2000; 20:RC109 1–6.

45. Hung PL, Lai MC, Yang SN, Wang CL, et al. Aminophylline exacerbates status epilepticus-induced neuronal damages in immature rats: a morphological, motor and behavioral study. *Epilepsy Res* 2002; 49:218–225.

46. Huang LT, Liou CW, Yang SN, Lai MC, et al. Aminophylline aggravates long-term morphological and cognitive damages in status epilepticus in immature rats. *Neurosci Lett* 2002; 321:137–140.

47. Hoffman AF, Zhao Q, Holmes GL. Cognitive impairment following status epilepticus and recurrent seizures during early development support the "two-hit hypothesis." *Epilepsy Behav* 2004; 5:873–877.

48. Boukhezra O, Riviello P, Fu DD, Lui X, et al. Effect of the postictal state on visual-spatial memory in immature rats. *Epilepsy Res* 2003; 55:165–175.

49. Baram TZ, Schultz L. Corticotropin-releasing hormone is a rapid and potent convulsant in the infant rat. *Brain Res Dev Brain Res* 1991; 61:97–101.

50. Brunson KL, Eghbal-Ahmadi M, Bender R, Chen Y, et al. Long-term progressive hippocampal cell loss and dysfunction induced by early-life administration of corticotropin-releasing hormone reproduce the effects of early-life stress. *PNAS* 2001; 98:8856–8861.

51. Jensen FE, Holmes GL, Lombroso CT, Blume HK, et al. Age-dependent changes in long-term seizure susceptibility and behavior after hypoxia in rats. *Epilepsia* 1992; 33:971–980.

52. Mátéffyová A, Otáhal J, Tsenov G, Mareš P, et al. Intrahippocampal injection of endothelin-1 in immature rats results in neuronal death, development of epilepsy, and behavioral abnormalities later in life. *Eur J Neurosci* 2006; 24:351–360.

53. Lee CL, Hannay J, Hrachovy R, Rashid S, et al. Spatial learning deficits without hippocampal neuronal loss in a model of early-onset epilepsy. *Neuroscience* 2001; 107:71–84.

54. Stafstrom CE, Sasaki-Adams DM: NMDA-induced seizures in developing rats cause long-term learning impairment and increased seizure susceptibility. *Epilepsy Res* 2003; 53: 129–137.

55. Bo T, Jiang Y, Cao H, Wang J, et al. Long-term effects of seizures in neonatal rats on spatial learning and N-methyl-D-aspartate receptor expression in the brain. *Brain Res Dev Brain Res* 2004; 152:137–142.

56. Huang LT, Cilio MR, Silveira DC, McCabe BK, et al. Long-term effects of neonatal seizures: a behavioral, electrophysiological, and histological study. *Brain Res Dev Brain Res* 1999; 118:99–107.

57. Sogawa Y, Monokoshi M, Silveira DC, Cha BH, et al. Timing of cognitive deficits following neonatal seizures: relationship to histological changes in the hippocampus. *Brain Res Dev Brain Res* 2001; 131:73–83.

58. Neill JC, Liu Z, Sarkisian M, Tandon P, et al. Recurrent seizures in immature rats: effect on auditory and visual discrimination. *Brain Res Dev Brain Res* 1996; 95:283–292.

59. Zhao Q, Hu Y, Holmes GL. Effect of topiramate on cognitive function and activity level following neonatal seizures. *Epilepsy Behav* 2005; 6:529–536.

60. Cha BH, Silveira DC, Liu X, Hu Y, et al. Effect of topiramate following recurrent and prolonged seizures during early development. *Epilepsy Res* 2002; 51:217–232.

61. Chen CC, Chaung HC, Chung MY, Huang LT. Menhaden fish oil improves spatial memory in rat pups following recurrent pentylenetetrazole-induced seizures. *Epilepsy Behav* 2006; 8:516–521.

62. Mikulecká A, Kršek P, Mareš P. Nonconvulsive kainic acid-induced seizures elicit age-dependent impairment of memory for the elevated plus-maze. *Epilepsy Behav* 2000; 1:418–426.

63. Camfield PR. Recurrent seizures in the developing brain are not harmful. *Epilepsia* 1997; 38:735–737.

64. Wasterlain CG. Recurrent seizures in the developing brain are harmful. *Epilepsia* 1997; 38:728–734.

65. Galanopoulou AS, Vidaurre J, Moshé SL. Under what circumstances can seizures produce hippocampal injury: evidence for age-specific effect. *Dev Neurosci* 2002; 24:355–363.

66. Stafstrom CE. Assessing the behavioral and cognitive effects of seizures on the developing brain. *Prog Brain Res* 2002; 135:377–390.

67. Holmes GL. Effects of early seizures on later behavior and epileptogenicity. *Ment Retard Dev Disabil Res Rev* 2004; 10:101–105.

68. Holmes GL. Effects of seizures on brain development: lessons from the laboratory. *Pediatr Neurol* 2005; 33:1–11.

69. Haut SR, Velíšková J, Moshé SL. Susceptibility of immature and adult brains to seizure effects. *Lancet Neurol* 2004; 3:608–617.

5 Cognitive and Behavioral Effects of Seizures: Adult Animals

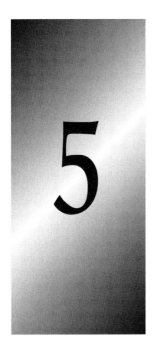

Gregory L. Holmes
Carl E. Stafstrom

The ultimate challenge to clinicians and scientists is to provide therapies that prevent any adverse effects associated with epileptic seizures. The first step in this quest is to understand the pathophysiological basis of such adverse effects. While the human condition clearly differs from that occurring in animals, human studies are often difficult to interpret because of the large number of variables associated with human epilepsy. Neuropsychologic outcome in individuals with epilepsy may be influenced by such factors as etiology; age of onset; duration of the disorder; seizure type, frequency, and severity; concomitant disorders; genetic background; and treatment. Animal studies allow investigators control over most of these variables. Indeed, a large number of investigators have utilized animal models, leading to many fundamental insights into seizure-induced changes in the brain.

As suggested by clinical studies, it is now recognized that the effects of seizures are influenced by the maturity of the neuronal circuitry; the effects of seizures in the immature brain with developing and plastic neuronal connections are quite different from those in the adult brain with relatively fixed neuronal circuits. Indeed, animal studies have demonstrated that the pathophysiological consequences of both status epilepticus (SE) and recurrent seizures in the developing brain differ considerably from those of the mature brain (1). In this chapter the effects of seizures on cognitive and affective function in the mature brain will be reviewed. Pavel Mareš (Chapter 4) reviews the topic in the immature brain.

ANIMAL MODELS

There are a large number of animal models employed in epilepsy research (2). A majority of the animal models have been used to induce a single seizure, usually prolonged (status epilepticus) or recurrent repetitive seizures. Chemoconvulsants and electrical stimulation have been most widely used in adult rodents, although recently a larger number of genetic models have been employed (3). Genetic models often are complex, with the animals having other structural, functional, or developmental issues (4). In addition, there may be considerable differences among strains in regards to seizure susceptibility and outcome (5).

Because of costs and convenience, most investigators have used rodent models. While these models provide considerable insight into pathophysiological mechanisms, they are limited in regards to the human condition. Subtle cognitive and behavioral changes are difficult to measure, and higher cortical function such as language and abstract thinking cannot be studied in rodents.

Another issue with animal studies is that they do not mimic epileptic syndromes well. For example, there are no animal models of disorders such as juvenile myoclonic epilepsy or Lennox-Gastaut syndrome. Likewise, complex electroencephalographic (EEG) patterns seen in humans cannot be mimicked in rodents. Nevertheless, the biological mechanisms responsible for seizures in humans and animals are similar, and rodent models have the potential to delineate mechanisms of behavioral changes associated with seizures, which, it is hoped, will lead to new therapeutic strategies.

Epilepsy is characterized by recurrent, unprovoked seizures. Some patients with epilepsy will have their onset of epilepsy with a bout of SE, defined as ongoing seizure activity lasting more than 30 minutes, or will have an episode of SE during the course of their illness. The cognitive and behavioral deficits occurring after SE may be quite different from those associated with chronic epilepsy. For that reason, in this chapter we consider the cognitive and behavioral deficits seen with SE and recurrent seizures separately.

EFFECTS OF STATUS EPILEPTICUS ON SPATIAL LEARNING AND MEMORY

Although a variety of tests can be used to assess learning and memory (6,7), one of the most popular is the Morris water maze (MWM), a measure of visual-spatial memory (8). In the water maze the animal uses visual clues to learn the location of a platform submerged below the water line in a tank of water. The primary outcome measure is the time it takes the rat to find the platform. Although rats swim well, they would prefer to be out of the water, so the water maze uses negative reinforcement.

As used in our laboratory, test animals are placed in a 2-meter-diameter tank filled with water. Four points on the rim of the pool are designated north (N), south (S), east (E), and west (W), thus dividing the pool into four quadrants (NW, NE, SE, SW). An 8 × 8-centimeter acrylic plastic platform, onto which the rat can escape, is positioned in the center of one of the quadrants, 1 centimeter below the water surface.

On day 1, each rat is placed in the pool for 60 seconds without the platform present; this free swim enables the rat to become habituated to the training environment. On days 2–5 rats are trained for 24 trials (six trials a day) to locate and escape onto the submerged platform. For each rat, the quadrant in which the platform is located remains constant, but the point of immersion into the pool is varied among N, E, S, and W in a quasi-random order for the 24 trials so that the rat is not able to predict the platform location from the point at which it is placed into the pool. The latency from immersion into the pool to escape onto the platform is recorded for each trial, and the observer also manually records the route taken by the rat to reach the platform. On mounting the platform, the rats are given a 30-second rest period, after which the next trial is started. If the rat does not find the platform in 120 seconds, it is manually placed on the platform for a 30-second rest. At the start of each trial, the rat is held facing the perimeter and dropped into the pool to ensure immersion.

One day after completion of the last latency trial (Day 6), the platform is removed and animals are placed in the water maze in the quadrant opposite to where the platform had previously been located. The path and time spent in the quadrant where the platform had been previously placed is recorded. In this part of the water maze, known as the probe test, normal animals typically spend more time in the quadrant where the platform had been previously located than in the other quadrants.

The MWM is a test of hippocampal-dependent spatial memory, which parallels episodic memory in humans. Although intact hippocampus function plays a major role in the test, lesions in other brain regions, including neocortex, retrosplenial cortex, striatum, basal forebrain, and cerebellum, can alter water maze performance (9). The testing procedure used during the four days of locating the hidden platform provides a measure of both working memory and reference memory. The animal uses working memory to know which areas of the tank have been visited while trying to find the platform, and it uses reference memory to know where the platform was previously placed. The probe test is a measure of the strength of reference memory.

There are many variations of the water maze used, including size of the tank and escape platform, number of trials per session, and duration of trials. The test procedure may vary depending on the type of memory studied. For example, to study working memory, the platform is changed every two trials so that the rat's performance is based solely on what is learned on the previous trial. The outcome measure is the length of time required to find the platform during the second trial (10). The MWM is a favorite test of many laboratories because food or water deprivation is not necessary. In addition, rats can learn to do the test shortly after weaning (11).

Many studies have examined the effect of seizures on water maze performance. In the adult rat, spatial learning is impaired following status epilepticus induced by kainic acid (12,13), pilocarpine (14–18), sarin (19), or electrical stimulation (20–22).

The radial arm maze is also widely used to test spatial memory in rodents. Unlike the water maze, the radial arm maze requires food deprivation to ensure motivation to search for food. In the radial arm maze using eight arms, the rat typically learns to go to four baited arms and not enter four unbaited arms. The test provides a measure of working errors (i.e., returning to a previously entered arm) and reference errors (entering an unbaited arm). Outcome measures include the number of trials to achieve a criterion performance, such as consumption of all bait without any errors (reentering an arm or going down an unbaited arm), or number of reference and working memory errors.

As with the water maze, the radial arm maze protocol can be varied to address specific hypotheses. The number of arms used can vary, as can the ratio of baited to nonbaited arms. The radial arm maze can also be placed in a tank of water with the animal required to learn which arm has the escape platform (23).

In the adult rat, status epilepticus results in long-term deficits in learning and memory (12, 14, 15, 22, 24–26). When studied weeks or months following SE, rats have longer latencies to the escape platform and spend less time in the target quadrant than non-SE rats (25). Both reference and working memory are impaired in these studies. The increased latency to the escape platform was not related to motor deficits or swimming speed. Rats subjected to SE and then tested after they developed spontaneous seizures had impaired function in the 8-arm radial maze (27). SE induced by electrical stimulation of the amygdala results in neuronal loss of the amygdala, the hippocampus, and surrounding cortical areas, along with mossy fiber sprouting in the dentate gyrus.

BEHAVIORAL DISORDERS FOLLOWING STATUS EPILEPTICUS

Changes in Anxiety

A variety of tests are available to measure anxiety in rodents. Anxiety levels are measured by exposing animals to an unfamiliar, aversive environment (28). The elevated plus maze consists of two elevated, open (brightly lit) arms perpendicular to two enclosed dark arms. In this test there are two forces driving behavior. Elevating the platform off the ground is frightening to the rodent. Rodents prefer dark, enclosed spaces rather than open, lit areas. At the same time, rodents are curious and like exploring. The elevated plus maze is an unconditioned spontaneous behavioral conflict test that measures the conflict between exploration of a novel environment and avoidance of a brightly lit, open area (29). The shorter the amount of time the animal spends in the open arms relative to total time, the greater the animal's anxiety.

Status epilepticus caused by pilocarpine or kainic acid results in increased anxiety in adult rats (30). On the other hand, SE induced by pentylenetetrazole (PTZ) does not result in increased anxiety (31).

Changes in Socialization

Tests of socialization include the home cage intruder test. Another animal of similar age, size, and gender is placed in the cage of the experimental animal. Aggressive, passive, and other interactive and noninteractive behaviors are recorded (32–34). A variation of the home cage intruder test is the social recognition task. In this test the experimental rat is exposed to another rat, usually a juvenile rat. It is expected that the two animals will explore each other actively on the initial encounter but that this exploration will decrease with repeated exposures. Outcome measures include time spent sniffing, grooming, and so forth. Following SE, animals are significantly more aggressive, irritable, and difficult to handle by experimenters; however, these animals often display increased passivity toward the intruder animal (32). Abnormalities in the home cage intruder tests have been documented after pilocarpine-induced nonconvulsive SE (35) and kainic acid–induced SE (36).

Changes in Response to Discomfort

The handling test is a measure of emotional response to graded amounts of discomfort, elicited by non-stressful handling (rubbing the fur along the grain), stressful handling (rubbing the fur against the grain), and graded tail pinch with a hemostat. Responses are graded on an ordinal scale from 1 to 4. Immature rats undergoing kainic acid–induced SE and tested as adults were notably more aggressive on the handling test (36). Following SE, adult animals become more irritable and aggressive in the handling test (12, 37) and become more hyperactive (12).

Mechanisms of SE-Induced Cognitive and Affective Disorders

The mechanisms of SE-induced cognitive and affective disorders remain unclear. A number of morphological and physiological changes occur as a result of SE. In the adult animal, status epilepticus causes neuronal loss in hippocampal fields CA1 and CA3 and in the dentate hilus (38, 39), with the pattern of cell loss dependent upon the agent used to induce the seizures (40, 41). In addition to cell death, prolonged seizures in the adult brain lead to synaptic reorganization, with aberrant growth (sprouting) of granule cell axons (the so-called mossy fibers) in the supragranular zone of the fascia and infrapyramidal region of CA3 (42, 43). Sprouting and new synapse formation occur in other brain regions—notably the CA1 pyramidal neurons, where it has been shown that newly formed synapses produce an enhanced frequency of glutamatergic spontaneous synaptic currents (44).

The relationship between cell loss, sprouting, and behavioral and cognitive dysfunction remains unclear. A relationship between cell loss and memory deficits following SE has been reported (26). Aggressive behavior in male rats subjected to lithium-pilocarpine status epilepticus was closely related to cell loss (45, 46).

Physiologic Effects of SE

To directly address the physiologic effects of SE, we recorded the activity of single hippocampal neurons in freely moving rats subjected to SE and compared this activity to that in control rats. Neurons in the hippocampus called place cells encode the animal's location within its environment. When a rat is exploring a given environment, hippocampal pyramidal neurons discharge when the animal enters certain locations of the environment, called the cells' firing field. Field location, size, and shape are specific to each cell and each environment, and fields cover the surface of the environment homogeneously. For a given environment, in normal rats, they remain unchanged, even between exposures separated by months (47–50). Since there is a relationship between place cells activity and the ongoing spatial behavior of rats (51, 52), it is believed that such signals provide the animal with a spatial representation in order to navigate efficiently within the environment. These cells provide a very useful single-cell measure of spatial memory.

We found that adult rats that experienced SE show deficient performance in two variants of a complex spatial task (the Morris swimming task) and, in parallel, have defective place cells, as expected from the spatial mapping theory. The place cells from the SE rats were defective in two ways: (1) Their firing fields were less orderly than those of normal rats, and (2) their firing fields were less stable than those of normal rats. Each of these defects provides a reasonable explanation of why water maze performance is deficient in SE rats and suggests that the cognitive impairment seen in our rats cannot be attributed to cell loss alone. However, the mechanisms responsible for the aberrant firing patterns remain unclear.

In summary, the majority of studies in the rat have shown deficits in behavior and memory following the SE. While there are some variations in the findings, the SE models appear to mimic the clinical situation well and serve as a useful tool in further understanding the pathophysiology of cognitive and behavioral deficits.

REPETITIVE SEIZURES

Somewhat surprisingly, there have been fewer studies examining the effects of recurrent seizures on cognitive and behavioral effects than following SE. As will be seen, in general the effects of recurrent seizures on cognition and behavior are less severe than those following SE.

Although there have been a variety of agents to induce recurrent seizures, kindling has been studied most extensively. Kindling is the process whereby repeated application of seizure-evoking stimulation produces neuronal changes that result in an enduring enhancement of susceptibility to seizure-evoking stimulation. Electrical kindling is most commonly used, although a variety of chemical agents have also been used. Recurrent generalized seizures can also result in a kindling effect. For example, repeated exposures to the volatile agent flurothyl (bis-2, 2, 2-trifluoroethyl ether), a potent and rapidly acting central nervous stimulant, produces seizures within minutes of exposure (53). With repeated exposures to flurothyl, rats have reduced latencies to seizure onset and longer duration of the seizures (54).

Since kindling is a gradually acquired process, behavioral tests can be done during the kindling or after the animal has fully kindled. If done during the acquisition of kindling, the investigator can assess behavior before or following each stimulation. If testing occurs after kindling, the investigator can manipulate the time of the testing to determine the duration of any postkindling effect.

Investigators have examined the effect of kindling on spatial memory with the animal being studied after or during kindling. Both the radial arm maze (55–57) and water maze (58–61) have been used. Leung and colleagues reported that hippocampal kindling produces deficits in working memory when the animals are tested later in the radial arm maze or water maze after the kindling (56, 57, 62). However, McNamara and coworkers (63, 64) reported that following full kindling in the perforant path, septum, or amygdala, spatial learning in the water maze was unimpaired when the animals were tested several days after the last seizure. Likewise, perirhinal cortex kindling had no effect on water maze performance (65). These results in the perirhinal cortex contrast with the selective disruption of spatial memory produced by dorsal hippocampal kindling. The site selectivity of the behavioral disruptions produced by kindling indicates that such effects are probably mediated by changes particular to the site of seizure initiation rather than to changes in the characteristic circuitry activated by limbic seizure generalization.

Rats partially kindled in the hippocampus after learning the radial arm maze showed deficits in retention (66). Lopes da Silva and coworkers (55) found that kindling of the hippocampus produced persistent deficits in reference memory and transient decreases in working memory when the rats were studied during the kindling phase. Robinson et al. (67) compared the transient and persistent effects of kindling the perforant path on acquisition in the radial arm task, finding learning impairment only in rats kindled 30–45 minutes prior to each learning trial. Animals that were fully kindled and then had a stimulation-free period prior to the testing had no deficits. Gilbert and coworkers [68] used two procedures to assess the spatial learning and memory of rats in the Morris water maze task subsequent to hippocampal kindling. Kindling was performed either before water maze testing or after the water maze task was learned. Generalized seizures elicited prior to water maze testing impaired acquisition of the task, whereas either partial or generalized seizures administered following kindling impaired retention. Even a few localized hippocampal stimulations delivered prior to the task can disrupt spatial cognition (69).

The effects of kindling on spatial memory are not confined solely to electrical kindling. With repetitive pentylenetetrazole-induced seizures given every other day for 28 days, rats made more reference errors in the radial arm water maze (70). Genetically epilepsy-prone rats (GEPRs) subjected to 66 audiogenic stimulations showed impairment in both the water maze and T-maze when compared to littermates that were handled and placed in the sound chamber but were not stimulated (71). Neonatal rats subjected to recurrent flurothyl-induced seizures also have impaired spatial memory when tested in the water maze (72, 73).

It is likely that the effects of kindling on cognition are dependent on the underlying condition. For example, Ihara epileptic rats (IER/F substrain) have neuropathologic abnormalities and develop generalized convulsive seizures when they reach the age of approximately 5 months. Okaichi et al. (74) tested nine IER/F rats that had not yet experienced seizures and older IER/F rats that had repeatedly experienced seizures with identical tasks. Both groups showed behaviors that were different from those of control rats in the water maze. Because young IER/F rats without prior seizures also showed severe learning impairments, the results suggested that recurrent seizures had no discernible effect on spatial learning and memory. Genetically programmed microdysgenesis in the hippocampus was suspected as a cause of the severe learning deficits of IER/Fs, rather than the seizures themselves.

It appears from the literature that kindling disrupts learning and memory, particularly when the kindling stimulations are administered shortly before training sessions. While hippocampal kindling can result in long-term impairment of spatial memory, nonhippocampal kindling effects on hippocampal function are substantially less prominent.

Amygdala-kindled animals also exhibit heightened anxiety (75). Kindling of the amygdaloid complex in rats results in an enhanced emotionality, frequently expressed by an elevated anxiety and defensive attitude toward other animals (76). Kalynchuk and coworkers (77) kindled the hippocampus, amydala, or caudate nucleus. Rats were then tested in the open field, in the elevated plus maze, and for resistance to capture. Rats kindled in the amygdala and hippocampus were less active in the open field, were more resistant to capture from the open field, and engaged in more open-arm activity in the elevated plus maze. The authors suggested that the reduced activity in the open field and the increased activity in the open arm in the elevated plus maze were signs of increased anxiety. Perirhinal cortex kindling also increased anxiety-related behavior in both the elevated plus and open field mazes and disrupted spontaneous object recognition (78). Pentylenetetrazole-treated rats have also been shown to have a higher anxiety levels in the open-field exploratory maze test (70).

Amygdala kindling also alters social attraction between rats in the open field test, with kindled rats showing a higher likelihood of remaining in close proximity to a partner rat (76). Partial kindling of the ventral perforant path in cats produced a lasting increase in defense response of cats to both rats and conspecific threat howls. In addition, there was a suppression of approach-attack behaviors directed toward rats (79). Pentylenetetrazole-treated rats also displayed decreased offensive behaviors in the home cage intruder test (80). GEPRs subjected to repetitive seizures were less active in the open field activity test, less aggressive in the home cage intruder test, and more irritable and aggressive in the handling test (71). In a test that mimics depression (the forced swim test), animals receiving repetitive pentylenetetrazole injections were immobile significantly longer than control rats (70).

In summary, most studies have demonstrated that rats subjected to recurrent seizures show deficits in learning, memory, and behavior. As such, these animals provide a useful model of postseizure dysfunction, which may serve as a screen for potential treatments for these cognitive, emotional, and neuropathological deficits that resemble those symptoms observed in human epilepsy. However, as in humans, there is considerable variation in outcome following repetitive seizures. Genetic background of the animals, as in humans, appears quite important.

MECHANISMS OF SE-INDUCED COGNITIVE AND AFFECTIVE DISORDERS

Kindling has been shown to produce sprouting of the mossy fiber axons of the dentate granule cells of the hippocampus (43), cell loss (81–83), enhanced function of N-methyl-D-aspartate receptors (84–86), reduction in intracellular calcium binding (86), and a myriad of synaptic changes (87, 88). In addition, recurrent flurothyl seizures in immature rats are associated with mossy fiber sprouting in CA3 (89). Which of these changes are associated with the cognitive and behavioral effects seen in rats following kindling or repetitive seizures is not yet known.

CONCLUDING REMARKS

There is now a substantial literature demonstrating that both SE and recurrent seizures result in cognitive

impairment and behavioral changes. These cognitive and behavioral changes mimic many of the problems faced by patients with seizures. The challenge for investigators now is to determine which of the seizure-induced changes in the brain lead to these adverse outcomes. Understanding the pathophysiology of these changes should lead to the development of novel therapeutics.

Acknowledgments

Supported by the Western Massachusetts Epilepsy Awareness Fund, Friends of Shannon McDermott, the Sara fund, and grants from NINDS (Grants: NS27984 and NS44295).

References

1. Haut SR, Velíšková J, Moshé SL. Susceptibility of immature and adult brains to seizure effects. *Lancet Neurol* 2004; 3:608–617.
2. Pitkänen A, Schwartzkroin PA, Moshé SL, eds. *Models of Seizures and Epilepsy*. San Diego: Elsevier; 2006.
3. Sarkisian MR. Overview of the current animal models for human seizure and epileptic disorders. *Epilepsy Behav* 2001; 2:201–216.
4. Cole AJ, Koh S, Zheng Y. Are seizures harmful: what can we learn from animal models? *Prog Brain Res* 2002; 135:13–23.
5. Schauwecker PE. Complications associated with genetic background effects in models of experimental epilepsy. *Prog Brain Res* 2002; 135:139–148.
6. Metz GA, Kolb B, Whishaw IQ. Neuropsychological tests. In: Whishaw IQ, Kolb B, eds. *The Behavior of the Laboratory Rat. A Handbook with Tests*. Oxford: Oxford University Press, 2005:475–498.
7. Heinrichs SC, Seyfried TN. Behavioral seizure correlates in animal models of epilepsy: a road map for assay selection, data interpretation, and the search for causal mechanisms. *Epilepsy Behav* 2006; 8:5–38.
8. Morris RGM, Garrud P, Rawlins JNP, O'Keefe J. Place navigation impaired in rats with hippocampal lesions. *Nature* 1982; 297:681–683.
9. Stafstrom CE. Behavioral and cognitive testing procedures in animal models of epilepsy. In: Pitkänen A, Schwartzkroin PA, Moshé S, eds. *Models of Seizures and Epilepsy*. Boston: Elsevier Academic Press, 2006:613–628.
10. Dudchenko PA. An overview of the tasks used to test working memory in rodents. *Neurosci Biobehav Rev* 2004 Nov; 28:699–709.
11. Rutten A, van Albada M, Silveira DC, Cha BH, et al. Memory impairment following status epilepticus in immature rats: time-course and environmental effects. *Eur J Neurosci* 2002; 16:501–513.
12. Stafstrom CE, Chronopoulos A, Thurber S, Thompson JL, et al. Age-dependent cognitive and behavioral deficits after kainic acid seizures. *Epilepsia* 1993; 34:420–432.
13. Holmes GL, Yang Y, Liu Z, Cermak JM, et al. Seizure-induced memory impairment is reduced by choline supplementation before or after status epilepticus. *Epilepsy Res* 2002; 48:3–13.
14. Zhou JL, Zhao Q, Holmes GL. Effect of levetiracetam on visual-spatial memory impairment following status epilepticus. *Epilepsy Res* 2007; 73:65–74.
15. Rice AC, Floyd CL, Lyeth BG, Hamm RJ, et al. Status epilepticus causes long-term NMDA receptor-dependent behavioral changes and cognitive deficits. *Epilepsia* 1998; 39:1148–1157.
16. Niessen HG, Angenstein F, Vielhaber S, Frisch C, et al. Volumetric magnetic resonance imaging of functionally relevant structural alterations in chronic epilepsy after pilocarpine-induced status epilepticus in rats. *Epilepsia* 2005; 46:1021–1026.
17. Hort J, Brozek G, Komarek V, Langmeier M, et al. Interstrain differences in cognitive functions in rats in relation to status epilepticus. *Behav Brain Res* 2000; 112:77–83.
18. McKay BE, Persinger MA. Normal spatial and contextual learning for ketamine-treated rats in the pilocarpine epilepsy model. *Pharmacol Biochem Behav* 2004; 78:111–119.
19. Gilat E, Kadar T, Levy A, Rabinovitz I, et al. Anticonvulsant treatment of sarin-induced seizures with nasal midazolam: an electrographic, behavioral, and histological study in freely moving rats. *Toxicol Appl Pharmacol* 2005; 209:74–85.
20. Halonen T, Nissinen J, Pitkanen A. Effect of lamotrigine treatment on status epilepticus-induced neuronal damage and memory impairment in rat. *Epilepsy Res* 2001; 46:205–223.
21. Halonen T, Nissinen J, Jansen JA, Pitkanen A. Tiagabine prevents seizures, neuronal damage and memory impairment in experimental status epilepticus. *Eur J Pharmacol* 1996; 299:69–81.
22. Nissinen J, Halonen T, Koivisto E, Pitkanen A. A new model of chronic temporal lobe epilepsy induced by electrical stimulation of the amygdala in rat. *Epilepsy Res* 2000; 38:177–205.
23. Huang LT, Lai MC, Wang CL, Wang CA, et al. Long-term effects of early-life malnutrition and status epilepticus: assessment by spatial navigation and CREB$^{Serine-133}$ phosphorylation. *Brain Res Dev Brain Res* 2003; 145:213–218.

24. Kelsey JE, Sanderson KL, Frye CA. Perforant path stimulation in rats produces seizures, loss of hippocampal neurons, and a deficit in spatial mapping which are reduced by prior MK-801. *Behav Brain Res* 2000; 107:59–69.
25. Liu X, Muller RU, Huang LT, Kubie JL, et al. Seizure-induced changes in place cell physiology: relationship to spatial memory. *J Neurosci* 2003; 23:11505–11515.
26. Letty S, Lerner-Natoli M, Rondouin G. Differential impairments of spatial memory and social behavior in two models of limbic epilepsy. *Epilepsia* 1995; 36:973–982.
27. Leite JP, Nakamura EM, Lemos T, Masur J, et al. Learning impairment in chronic epileptic rats following pilocarpine-induced status epilepticus. *Braz J Med Biol Res* 1990; 23:681–683.
28. Belzung C, Griebel G. Measuring normal and pathological anxiety-like behaviour in mice: a review. *Behav Brain Res* 2001; 125:141–149.
29. Crawley JN. Behavioral phenotyping of transgenic and knockout mice: experimental design and evaluation of general health, sensory functions, motor abilities, and specific behavioral tests. *Brain Res* 1999; 835:18–26.
30. Dos SJ, Jr., Longo BM, Blanco MM, Menezes de Oliveira MG, et al. Behavioral changes resulting from the administration of cycloheximide in the pilocarpine model of epilepsy. *Brain Res* 2005; 1066:37–48.
31. Erdogan F, Golgeli A, Kucuk A, Arman F, et al. Effects of pentylenetetrazole-induced status epilepticus on behavior, emotional memory and learning in immature rats. *Epilepsy Behav* 2005; 6:537–542.
32. Mellanby J, Strawbridge P, Collingridge GI, George G, et al. Behavioural correlates of an experimental hippocampal epileptiform syndrome in rats. *J Neurol Neurosurg Psychiatry* 1981; 44:1084–1093.
33. Thurmond JB. Technique for producing and measuring territorial aggression using laboratory mice. *Physiol Behav* 1975; 14:879–881.
34. Kaliste-Korhonen E, Eskola S. Fighting in NIH/S male mice: consequences for behaviour in resident-intruder tests and physiological parameters. *Lab Anim* 2000; 34:189–198.
35. Krsek P, Mikulecka A, Druga R, Kubova H, et al. Long-term behavioral and morphological consequences of nonconvulsive status epilepticus in rats. *Epilepsy Behav* 2004; 5:180–191.
36. Holmes GL, Thompson JL, Marchi T, Feldman DS. Behavioral effects of kainic acid administration on the immature brain. *Epilepsia* 1988; 29:721–730.
37. Mikati MA, Holmes GL, Chronopoulos A, Hyde P, et al. Phenobarbital modifies seizure-related brain injury in the developing brain. *Ann Neurol* 1994; 36:425–433.
38. Olney JW, Fuller T, De Gubareff T. Acute dendrotoxic changes in the hippocampus of kainate treated rats. *Brain Res* 1979; 176:91–100.
39. Ben-Ari Y. Limbic seizure and brain damage produced by kainic acid: mechanisms and relevance to human temporal lobe epilepsy. *Neuroscience* 1985; 14:375–403.
40. Nadler JV. Kainic acid as a tool for the study of temporal lobe epilepsy. *Life Sci* 1981; 29:2031–2042.
41. Ben-Ari Y. Cell death and synaptic reorganizations produced by seizures. *Epilepsia* 2001; 42 Suppl 3:5–7.
42. Represa A, Tremblay E, Ben-Ari Y. Kainate binding sites in the hippocampal mossy fibers: localization and plasticity. *Neuroscience* 1987; 20:739–748.
43. Sutula T, Xiao-Xian H, Cavazos J, Scott G. Synaptic reorganization in the hippocampus induced by abnormal functional activity. *Science* 1988; 239:1147–1150.
44. Esclapez M, Hirsch J, Ben-Ari Y, Bernard C. Newly formed excitatory pathways provide a substrate for hyperexcitablity in experimental temporal lobe epilepsy. *J Comp Neur* 1999; 408:449–460.
45. Desjardins D, Parker G, Cook LL, Persinger MA. Agonistic behavior in groups of limbic epileptic male rats: pattern of brain damage and moderating effects from normal rats. *Brain Res* 2001; 905:26–33.
46. Desjardins D, Persinger MA. Association between intermale social aggression and cellular density within the central amygdaloid nucleus in rats with lithium/pilocarpine-induced seizures. *Percept Mot Skills* 1995; 81:635–641.
47. Muller RU, Kubie JL, Ranck JB, Jr. Spatial firing patterns of hippocampal complex-spike cells in a fixed environment. *J Neurosci* 1987; 7:1935–1950.

48. Muller RU, Kubie JL. The effects of changes in the environment on the spatial firing patterns of hippocampal complex-spike cells. *J Neurosci* 1987; 7:1951–1968.

49. Thompson LT, Best PJ. Place cells and silent cells in the hippocampus of freely-behaving rats. *J Neurosci* 1989; 9:2382–2390.

50. Thompson LT, Best PJ. Long-term stability of the place-field activity of single units recorded from the dorsal hippocampus of freely behaving rats. *Brain Res* 1990; 509:299–308.

51. Lenck-Santini PP, Muller RU, Save E, Poucet B. Relationships between place cell firing fields and navigational decisions by rats. *J Neurosci* 2002; 22:9035–9047.

52. Lenck-Santini PP, Save E, Poucet B. Evidence for a relationship between place-cell spatial firing and spatial memory performance. *Hippocampus* 2001; 11:377–390.

53. Zhao Q, Holmes GL. Repetitive seizures in the immature brain. In: Pitkänen A, Schwartzkroin PA, Moshé S, eds. *Models of Seizures and Epilepsy.* San Diego: Elsevier Academic. 2006:341–350.

54. Liu Z, Yang Y, Silveira DC, Sarkisian MR, et al. Consequences of recurrent seizures during early brain development. *Neuroscience* 1999; 92:1443–1454.

55. Lopes da Silva FH, Gorter JA, Wadman WJ. Kindling of the hippocampus induces spatial memory deficits in the rat. *Neurosci Lett* 1986; 63:115–120.

56. Leung LS, Boon KA, Kaibara T, Innis NK. Radial maze performance following hippocampal kindling. *Behav Brain Res* 1990; 40:119–129.

57. Leung LS, Shen B. Hippocampal CA1 evoked response and radial 8-arm maze performance after hippocampal kindling. *Brain Res* 1991; 555:353–357.

58. Gilbert TH, Hannesson DK, Corcoran ME. Hippocampal kindled seizures impair spatial cognition in the Morris water maze. *Epilepsy Res* 2000; 38:115–125.

59. Holmes GL, Chronopoulos A, Stafstrom CE, Mikati MA, et al. Effects of kindling on subsequent learning, memory, behavior, and seizure susceptibility. *Brain Res Dev Brain Res* 1993; 73(1):71–77.

60. Hannesson DK, Howland J, Pollock M, Mohapel P, et al. Dorsal hippocampal kindling produces a selective and enduring disruption of hippocampally mediated behavior. *J Neurosci* 2001; 21:4443–4450.

61. Hannesson DK, Mohapel P, Corcoran ME. Dorsal hippocampal kindling selectively impairs spatial learning/short-term memory. *Hippocampus* 2001; 11:275–286.

62. Leung LS, Shen B. Hippocampal partial kindling decreased hippocampal GABA$_B$ receptor efficacy and wet dog shakes in rats. *Behav Brain Res* 2006; 173:274–281.

63. McNamara RK, Kirkby RD, dePace GE, Corcoran ME. Limbic seizures, but not kindling, reversibly impair place learning in the Morris water maze. *Behav Brain Res* 1992; 50:167–175.

64. McNamara RK, Kirkby RD, DePape GE, Skelton RW, et al. Differential effects of kindling and kindled seizures on place learning in the Morris water maze. *Hippocampus* 1993; 3:149–152.

65. Hannesson DK, Howland JG, Pollock M, Mohapel P, et al. Anterior perirhinal cortex kindling produces long-lasting effects on anxiety and object recognition memory. *Eur J Neurosci* 2005; 21:1081–1090.

66. Leung LS, Brzozowski D, Shen B. Partial hippocampal kindling affects retention but not acquisition and place but not cue tasks on the radial arm maze. *Behav Neurosci* 1996; 110:1017–1024.

67. Robinson GB, McNeill HA, Reed GD. Comparison of the short- and long-lasting effects of perforant path kindling on radial maze learning. *Behav Neurosci* 1993; 107:988–995.

68. Gilbert TH, McNamara RK, Corcoran ME. Kindling of hippocampal field CA1 impairs spatial learning and retention in the Morris water maze. *Behav Brain Res* 1996; 82:57–66.

69. Hannesson DK, Wallace AE, Pollock M, Corley S, et al. The relation between extent of dorsal hippocampal kindling and delayed-match-to-place performance in the Morris water maze. *Epilepsy Res* 2004; 58:145–154.

70. Mortazavi F, Ericson M, Story D, Hulce VD, et al. Spatial learning deficits and emotional impairments in pentylenetetrazole-kindled rats. *Epilepsy Behav* 2005; 7:629–638.

71. Holmes GL, Thompson JL, Marchi TA, Gabriel PS. Effects of seizures on learning, memory, and behavior in the genetically epilepsy-prone rat. *Ann Neurol* 1990; 27:24–32.

72. Holmes GL, Gairsa JL, Chevassus-Au-Louis N, Ben-Ari Y. Consequences of neonatal seizures in the rat: morphological and behavioral effects. *Ann Neurol* 1998; 44:845–857.

73. Huang L, Cilio MR, Silveira DC, McCabe BK, et al. Long-term effects of neonatal seizures: a behavioral, electrophysiological, and histological study. *Brain Res Dev Brain Res* 1999; 118:99–107.

74. Okaichi Y, Amano S, Ihara N, Hayase Y, et al. Open-field behaviors and water-maze learning in the F substrain of Ihara epileptic rats. *Epilepsia* 2006; 47:55–63.

75. Adamec RE, McKay D. Amygdala kindling, anxiety, and corticotrophin releasing factor (CRF). *Physiol Behav* 1993; 54:423–431.

76. Haimovici A, Wang Y, Cohen E, Mintz M. Social attraction between rats in open field: long-term consequences of kindled seizures. *Brain Res* 2001; 922:125–134.

77. Kalynchuk LE, Pinel JP, Treit D. Long-term kindling and interictal emotionality in rats: effect of stimulation site. *Brain Res* 1998; 779:149–157.

78. Hannesson DK, Howland JG, Pollock M, Mohapel P, et al. Anterior perirhinal cortex kindling produces long-lasting effects on anxiety and object recognition memory. *Eur J Neurosci* 2005; 21:1081–1090.

79. Adamec RE. Partial kindling of the ventral hippocampus: identification of changes in limbic physiology which accompany changes in feline aggression and defense. *Physiol Behav* 1991; 49:443–453.

80. Franke H, Kittner H. Morphological alterations of neurons and astrocytes and changes in emotional behavior in pentylenetetrazol-kindled rats. *Pharmacol Biochem Behav* 2001; 70:291–303.

81. Cavazos JE, Sutula TP. Progressive neuronal loss induced by kindling: a possible mechanism for mossy fiber synaptic reorganization and hippocampal sclerosis. *Brain Res* 1990; 527:1–6.

82. Cavazos JE, Golarai G, Sutula TP. Mossy fiber synaptic reorganization induced by kindling: time course of development, progression, and permanence. *J Neurosci* 1991; 11:2795–2803.

83. Cavazos JE, Das I, Sutula TP. Neuronal loss induced in limbic pathways by kindling: evidence for induction of hippocampal sclerosis by repeated brief seizures. *J Neurosci* 1994; 14:3106–3121.

84. McNamara JO. Cellular and molecular basis of epilepsy. *J Neurosci* 1994; 14:3413–3425.

85. Mody I, Stanton PK, Heinemann U. Activation of N-methyl-D-aspartate receptors parallels changes in cellular and synaptic properties of dentate gyrus granule cells after kindling. *J Neurophysiol* 1988; 59:1033–1054.

86. Mody I, Reynolds JN, Salter MW, Carlen PL, et al. Kindling-induced epilepsy alters calcium currents in granule cells of rat hippocampal slices. *Brain Res* 1990; 531:88–94.

87. Mody I. Synaptic plasticity in kindling. *Adv Neurol* 1999; 79:631–643.

88. Morimoto K, Fahnestock M, Racine RJ. Kindling and status epilepticus models of epilepsy: rewiring the brain. *Prog Neurobiol* 2004; 73:1–60.

89. Holmes GL, Sarkisian M, Ben-Ari Y, Chevassus-Au-Louis N. Mossy fiber sprouting after recurrent seizures during early development in rats. *J Comp Neurol* 1999; 404:537–353.

6 Cognitive Effects of Antiepileptic Drugs

Harlan E. Shannon

omplaints of impaired memory and/or cognition are not uncommon in patients with epilepsy (1). Many factors may contribute to these complaints, including the underlying pathophysiology of the disease state. However, antiepileptic drug (AED) therapy has the potential to contribute to cognitive impairments. For example, it is well established clinically that drugs that enhance gamma-aminobutyric acid (GABA)-mediated (GABAergic) inhibitory neurotransmission, such as barbiturates and benzodiazepines, can have marked negative effects on cognitive processes in normal volunteers (2). Since AEDs are the major therapeutic modality for control of seizures, being able to assess the potential impact of AEDs on cognitive processes is of particular importance. A growing body of literature has focused on evaluating the potential effects of AEDs on cognition in normal volunteers and patients with epilepsy (1–3). However, being able to assess the potential adverse effects of AEDs on cognition in animals would be of great benefit, not only in helping to delineate the effects of AEDs and possibly optimize current therapy, but also in the discovery of the next generation of AEDs with greater efficacy and no negative, and potentially positive, impact on cognition.

Cognition is not a unitary concept. Rather, cognition may be divided into multiple domains, including attention, working memory, and learning. A negative impact on any cognitive domain could give rise to a cognitive deficit that could very strongly impact quality of life. However, the extent to which AEDs impact any one domain, or whether different mechanistic classes impact different domains to different extents, is unclear. We (4–6) therefore undertook a series of experiments to evaluate the potential for a broad series of AEDs (Table 6-1) (7) to affect the cognitive domains of attention, working memory, and learning in rats.

The term *attention* refers to the selective aspects of perception which function so that at any particular moment an organism focuses on certain features of the environment to the relative exclusion of other features. An organism must, presumably, first "attend" to a stimulus before the stimulus can be cognitively processed, and it is therefore potentially the most basic of all cognitive processes. Attention tasks can be subdivided into vigilance (or sustained-attention), selective-attention, and divided-attention tasks, which are aimed at measuring the subject's ability to focus on one task for a sustained period of time, to resist distraction by irrelevant stimuli, and to perform more than one task at a time, respectively. Tasks used to evaluate attention in humans include variations of the continuous performance test, the Brief Test of Attention, and digit symbol substitution tests. In animals, an often-used attention test is the five-choice serial reaction

TABLE 6-1
Minimal Effective Doses of AEDs for Cognitive vs. Anticonvulsant Effects

Drug	Attention (5-CSRT)	Working Memory (Spatial Alternation)	Complex Learning (Repeated Acquisition)	Locomotor Activity Change[a]	Threshold Electroshock Test[a]	6-Hz Electroshock Test[a]
	MED, MG/KG	MED, MG/KG	MED, MG/KG	ED50, MG/KG	ED50, MG/KG	MED, MG/KG
Phenobarbital	56	30	56	30	5.6	5.8
Triazolam	1.0	0.1	nd	nd	nd	nd
Chlordiazepoxide	17.5	nd	17.8	>30	5.7	0.78
Tiagabine	nt	30	>30	nt	1.4	0.32
Valproate	>300	300	>300	>300	90	121
Gabapentin	>300	>300	nd	100	10.5	327[b]
Carbamazepine	56	30	56	30	5.5	12.5[b]
Phenytoin	>30	>30	30	>30	3.4	33[b]
Topiramate	>100	100	>100	>30	1.4	>30
Lamotrigine	>100	>100	100	30	1.7	30[b]
Levetiracetam	>200	>200	200	300	>300	6.0
Ethosuximide	nd	300	nd	>560	>560	179

Comparison of minimal effective doses for disrupting attention, working memory, and learning in rats with the minimal effective doses for decreasing locomotor activity in mice and the ED_{50} doses in the threshold electroshock (TES) and the 6-Hz electroshock tests in mice.
[a]From Shannon et al. (7).
[b]Maximum effect between 50 and 100%.
nd, not determined.

time (5CSRT) task developed and popularized by Robbins and coworkers (8). In this task, a stimulus is briefly presented at one of five locations, and a response at that location results in the presentation of a reinforcer. The 5CSRT task thus primarily assesses sustained attention.

Working memory is a theoretical concept that refers to a set of cognitive processes that provide temporary maintenance and manipulation of the information necessary for complex cognitive tasks (9). Tasks used to evaluate working memory in humans include various forms of the N-back test, digit span, and the Corsi test. In animals, working memory has often been operationally defined as the maintenance of information in memory and making a subsequent response based on, but in the absence of, that information or event. One approach to assessing working memory is a delayed spatial alternation task, in which an animal is required to respond alternately on left and right levers in order to obtain a reinforcer. Thus, in order to respond correctly during the current trial, an animal must remember where it had responded during the just preceding trial. By varying the interval between trials, time-dependent memory processes can be evaluated. Thus, spatial alternation behavior primarily assesses the time-related maintenance component of working memory.

Intact attention and working memory are necessary for higher cognitive processes such as learning. In humans, learning is often assessed by having subjects master lists of words, as in the Selective Reminding Test. Requiring an animal to master a sequence of behaviors, such as a sequence of lever press responses, is analogous to mastering a list of words in a particular order. In a repeated acquisition of response sequences task, animals are required to learn a sequence of behavioral responses (lever presses) that is constant during a given experimental session but is varied between experimental sessions (10). This general procedure has permitted the investigation of steady states of "rule" learning across experimental sessions and has been an important behavioral baseline for determining the effects of drugs on learning.

In order to assess the effects of AEDs on these cognitive domains of attention, working memory, and learning, we determined dose-response curves in each task for AEDs from multiple mechanistic classes, including the older AEDs phenobarbital, valproate, and carbamazepine and the newer AEDs lamotrigine, topiramate, gabapentin, levetiracetam, and tiagabine. For purposes of comparison, dose-response curves were also determined for the anticonvulsant benzodiazepines chlordiazepoxide or triazolam, as well as the muscarinic cholinergic receptor antagonist scopolamine, which are well known to disrupt cognition in both humans and rats.

ATTENTION: 5-CHOICE SERIAL REACTION TIME

Under baseline conditions, stimuli were presented for 0.5 seconds duration with equal probability above each of five response levers (5). The percentage of trials with an error of omission, a typical measure of a lapse of attention, was typically approximately 15–20%. Including only those trials during which an animal did respond, the percentage of correct responses was approximately 85–90%, and the percentage of incorrect responses was approximately 10–15%. The GABA-related AEDs phenobarbital, triazolam, and chlordiazepoxide significantly disrupted attention in that they produced dose-related increases in errors of omission. In fact, after a dose of 100 mg/kg of phenobarbital, the animals failed to respond on any trial, resulting in 100% omissions (Figure 6-1, upper left, and Table 6-1). In contrast, the GABA-related AEDs tiagabine and gabapentin did not increase errors of omission. The sodium channel blocker carbamazepine increased errors of omission, whereas the sodium channel blockers phenytoin, topiramate, and lamotrigine

(Figure 6-1, lower left) were without significant effect on performance. Similarly, levetiracetam had no effect on attention. The disruptions produced by phenobarbital, triazolam, chlordiazepoxide, and carbamazepine were similar in magnitude to those produced by scopolamine. These results demonstrated that the positive allosteric modulators of GABA receptors phenobarbital, triazolam, and chlordiazepoxide produced marked disruption of attention, but other GABA-related AEDs as well as sodium channel blockers (with the exception of carbamazepine) and levetiracetam had little or no effect on attention in nonepileptic rats.

WORKING MEMORY: SPATIAL ALTERNATION BEHAVIOR

In this task, animals were required to respond alternately on the left and right levers with a retention interval delay between trials, during which the chamber was dark, which varied from 2 to 32 seconds (4). Averaged across all retention intervals, the percentage of correct responses was

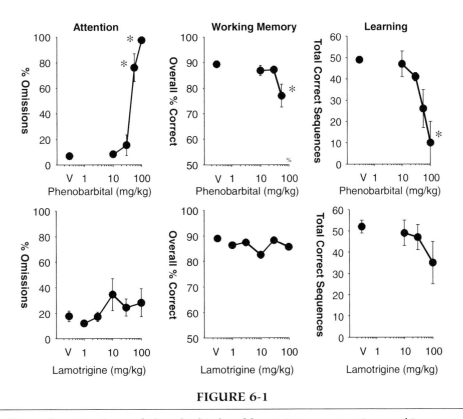

FIGURE 6-1

Comparison of the effects of varying doses of phenobarbital and lamotrigine on attention, working memory, and learning in nonepileptic rats. Each point represents the mean of six different animals. Vertical lines represent ± SEM and are absent when less than the size of the point. *, $p < .05$ versus vehicle, Dunnett's *t*-test. %, Animals failed to respond sufficiently after 100 mg/kg of phenobarbital to calculate a reliable value for percent correct.

II

MECHANISMS UNDERLYING EPILEPSY AND BEHAVIOR

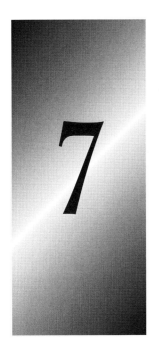

7

The Role of Sprouting and Plasticity in Epileptogenesis and Behavior

Devin J. Cross
Jose E. Cavazos

P harmacological therapy for intractable partial-onset epilepsy is aimed to symptomatically relieve seizure frequency and severity. Over the past 30 years, almost 30,000 compounds have been screened using two animal models of acute evoked convulsions for clinical trial development. Thus, it should not be surprising that this strategy has provided clinicians with excellent anticonvulsants, but that these compounds appear to be less effective against other seizure types, and ineffective in altering the development and natural history of the epilepsies. The development of therapies that alter the natural history of this condition has been hampered by our lack of understanding of the fundamental mechanisms of epileptogenesis, the pathophysiological process underlying the development of epilepsy. Understanding the mechanisms of epileptogenesis might lead to better experimental models for discovery of compounds that are disease modifying, altering the natural history of symptomatic partial-onset epilepsy. This chapter critically summarizes potential mechanisms for epileptogenesis, including synaptic reorganization in the hippocampal circuitry, aiming to characterize these mechanisms within the perspective of the most common pharmacologically intractable form of partial-onset epilepsy: mesial temporal lobe epilepsy. As synaptic reorganization of hippocampal structures appears to progressively enhance limbic hyperexcitability, it might also contribute toward pharmacological intractability in partial-onset epilepsy.

MESIAL TEMPORAL LOBE EPILEPSY

Mesial temporal lobe epilepsy (MTLE) is the most common epilepsy syndrome with pharmacologically intractable partial-onset seizures. This epileptic syndrome has a high association with a remote history of febrile seizures, particularly complex or prolonged febrile seizures, but has also been observed to be associated with other acute neurologic insults such as an episode of partial-onset status epilepticus, closed head injury, brain tumors, and stroke. However, many patients with MTLE have no obvious brain insult other than the cumulative effect of repeated brief partial-onset seizures. Typically, when there is a history of a prior neurologic injury, there is a latent period between the initial insult and the onset of MTLE that can span at least several weeks, but more commonly several years. Severe prolonged insults such as prolonged febrile convulsions and generalized convulsive status epilepticus appear to have a shorter latency to the onset of spontaneous partial-onset seizures, compared with other less severe precipitating events such as simple febrile seizures. The latent period between the precipitating event and the onset of epilepsy is one of the hallmarks of the pathophysiological process underlying the progression of epileptogenesis in MTLE.

Most of our understanding of the pathophysiology of MTLE derives from studies of brain tissue obtained surgically from patients with intractable and unilateral MTLE; typically, the tissue is examined after 20 or more years from the onset of their epilepsy. The majority of these highly selected patients dramatically improve after an anterior temporal lobectomy, which includes resection of the hippocampus, amygdala, and adjacent temporal neocortex (1). Thus, it has been presumed that the mechanisms underlying the development and intractability of MTLE must lie within the resected tissue.

Neurophysiologic studies have shown that most patients with intractable MTLE have seizure onset within the hippocampal formation (1), which has led to the study of hippocampal slices from the resected hippocampus obtained during resective surgery in these epileptic patients. The neurophysiologic studies demonstrate evidence of cellular hyperexcitability in granule cells and hippocampal pyramidal neuron, but only under certain conditions that impair inhibitory mechanisms (2). In addition, investigators found a general correlation between the degree of cellular hyperexcitability of granule cells under these conditions and the degree of synaptic reorganization of the mossy fiber pathway, a form of morphological plasticity observed in patients with MTLE and in experimental models of MTLE. This study suggests that the neurophysiologic abnormalities can be associated with neuropathological alterations in patients with MTLE. However, causative relationships between these phenomena cannot be established with this approach, which examines only the late stage of these phenomena many years after the onset of partial seizures.

Studies of the resected tissue from patients with intractable MTLE have shown several neuropathological abnormalities, including (1) a pattern of hippocampal neuronal loss known as mesial hippocampal sclerosis, (2) sprouting and reorganization of the mossy fibers in the dentate gyrus (DG), (3) hippocampal gliosis, and (4) dispersion of granule cells with ectopic locations. These neuropathological abnormalities might be consequences of repeated seizures or the result of the initial precipitating brain insult that led to repeated seizures. However, each of them might be a potential mechanism that contributes toward the pathophysiological process of epileptogenesis that resulted in pharmacologically intractable MTLE. Understanding the relative contribution of these neuropathological abnormalities in epileptogenesis has been considerably improved by multiple experimental models of MTLE, where the relationships between these phenomena and other potential mechanisms can be systematically tested.

EXPERIMENTAL MODELS OF MTLE

Several strategies are used to study the process of epileptogenesis in experimental models of MTLE. One strategy utilizes chemoconvulsants to produce an acute excitotoxic insult that results in status epilepticus, which later results in the development of spontaneous brief seizures. This strategy demonstrates a latency of several days between the insult and the development of seizures, but it is unclear how representative it is of the majority of patients with intractable MTLE who have no identifiable insult earlier in life. Two frequently used models that employ this approach are the kainic acid and pilocarpine models of MTLE. Rats that have experienced convulsive status epilepticus induced with these chemo-convulsants exhibit neuropathological and neurophysiologic abnormalities similar to those observed in intractable MTLE. Adult rats that have experienced kainic acid–induced status epilepticus demonstrate prominent neuronal damage and gliosis in hippocampal pyramidal neurons and the hilar polymorphic neurons of the DG. After hippocampal neuronal loss, these regions demonstrate morphological plasticity, with sprouting of the mossy fiber pathway into the inner molecular layer of the DG. Synaptic reorganization induced by seizures has been studied extensively in the mossy fiber pathway because of the ease of detecting changes in the laminar pattern of this pathway using Timm histochemistry or dynorphin-A immunocytochemistry (3). Most studies in experimental models of MTLE have shown sprouting in the mossy fiber pathway into the inner molecular layer of the DG and sprouting of the distal mossy fiber projection to the CA3 region.

Another strategy utilizes repeated exposure to seizures, using chemo-convulsants or electrical stimulation of limbic pathways (i.e., kindling) to produce frequent small insults that lead only to brief repeated seizures. In general, these chronic models of MTLE exhibit considerably less injury compared with the acute models that require an initial episode of status epilepticus. Furthermore, the neuropathological and neurophysiologic abnormalities evoked in the chronic models are less severe than those evoked in the acute models. Although the chronic models more appropriately mimic the seizure burden and frequency of patients with intractable MTLE, they also lead to apparently less frequent late spontaneous seizures than the kainic acid or pilocarpine model of MTLE.

Sprouting and synaptic reorganization have been investigated only in hippocampal pathways; however, neuronal loss has been demonstrated in multiple limbic areas. Experimental models that evoke a more limited degree of hippocampal injury, such as electrical kindling, demonstrate a lesser degree of synaptic reorganization, compared with the acute models of status

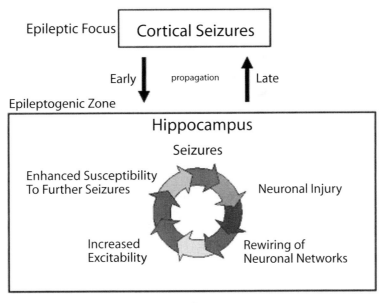

FIGURE 7-1

Mechanisms of epileptogenesis. The schematic diagram describes the relationships between pathophysiological phenomena and brain location during epileptogenesis in mesial temporal lobe epilepsy. Partial-onset seizures might initially originate in neocortical areas, but after the establishment of intractability, there is a vicious circle of interrelated pathophysiological phenomena within the hippocampal circuitry that self-sustains intractable seizures with propagation to neocortical structures.

epilepticus (4). An advantage of the acute models of MTLE is that the time course of progression of the neuropathological and neurophysiologic abnormalities can be studied in relation to the development of spontaneous partial-onset seizures. Following an acute excitotoxic insult, several of these neuropathological phenomena develop during the latency period for several days, before the emergence of cellular hyperexcitability and the onset of spontaneous seizures (5). During the latency period, there are transitory functional impairments of inhibitory control that recover during the chronic state; whereas other neuropathological abnormalities are permanent. It has been hypothesized that the permanent neuropathological alterations might underlie the mechanisms of epileptogenesis in intractable MTLE that lead to late intractable spontaneous seizures (Figure 7-1); in particular, several investigators have shown that the progressive development of synaptic reorganization parallels the increased cellular excitability in the DG (6) preceding spontaneous seizures. This type of synaptic reorganization of the mossy fiber has been observed in essentially all acute and chronic adult models of MTLE and in pathological specimens of humans with MTLE. Thus, synaptic reorganization of hippocampal structures is a potential mechanism explaining hippocampal hyperexcitability in patients with intractable MTLE.

SPROUTING AND SYNAPTIC REORGANIZATION OF THE MOSSY FIBERS

Mossy fiber sprouting can be examined using Timm histochemistry, which depicts the projection pattern of the mossy fibers in the hippocampus by means of the high zinc content of their synaptic terminals. In normal rats and humans there are few Timm granules in the inner molecular layer of the dentate gyrus. However, after many repeated seizures or status epilepticus, a dense band of Timm granules is present in the inner molecular layer (Figure 7-2). Granule cell axons—the mossy fibers—reorganize and sprout axons into the inner molecular layer to form new synaptic terminals with the dendrites of interneurons, but primarily on spines and dendrites of granule cells. Timm histochemistry has been used at the light and ultrastructural levels to assess the time course of development and permanence of the reorganized projection pattern. Small amounts of mossy fiber sprouting into the inner molecular layer can be recognized as early as 5 days; sprouting peaks at 3 weeks and has been observed to last as long as 18 months (1). After an excitotoxic insult, neuronal degeneration in the hilus can be recognized as early as 6 hours, and at 24 hours terminal degeneration in the inner molecular layer can be detected prior to the development of mossy fiber sprouting. Neuronal loss of the hilar polymorphic neurons is considered to be

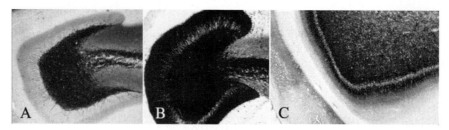

FIGURE 7-2

Mossy fiber sprouting. These are three photomicrographs from histological sections of the dentate gyrus (DG) stained with Timm histochemistry. Dark punctate granules depict the projection pattern of mossy fiber terminals that originate from granule cell axons. (A) The DG from a normal rat shows dense staining in the hilus (area within the U-shape of the DG) and in the CA3 region, with an absence of dark punctate granules in the molecular layer of the DG (arrow). (B) The DG from a rat that experienced status epilepticus induced with kainic acid demonstrates prominent staining in the molecular layer. (C) Human DG obtained surgically during a standard anterior temporal lobectomy for the treatment of pharmacologically intractable mesial temporal lobe epilepsy. Note that the molecular layer of the DG has prominent staining, demonstrating mossy fiber sprouting into that region. See color section following page 266.

the mechanism that triggers mossy fiber sprouting into the inner molecular region of the DG. Ultrastructural experiments with acute lesions of pathways projecting to the molecular layer of the DG have taught us that the synaptic densities in the molecular layer are restored by 21 days after the lesion (7). In the kainic acid and pilocarpine models, most of the newly formed synaptic terminals in the inner molecular layer of the DG are on granule cell spines, creating primarily a recurrent excitatory collateral circuit. It has been estimated that a sprouted granule cell develops about 500 newly formed synaptic contacts with granule cells and fewer than 25 contacts on interneurons (8). The chronic model of repeated kindling seizures to limbic structures was also used to demonstrate that the early stages of mossy fiber sprouting consist of the development of punctate granules that formed "strings" in the inner molecular layer before spreading to the rest of the layer (1). These strings were subsequently identified as collections of synaptic contacts on interneurons including basket cells (9). Thus, it is likely that mossy fiber sprouting, early on, is a homeostatic compensatory mechanism to restore inhibitory control by providing feedback synaptic connections on basket cell interneurons. However, as the repeated seizures continue, the terminal degeneration in the inner molecular layer may become overwhelming from the death of hilar polymorphic neurons, and the newly formed synaptic contacts develop primarily on granule cell spines, dendrites, and soma.

Seizure-induced plasticity of the mossy fibers is not limited to the formation of aberrant recurrent collaterals into the inner molecular layer of the DG. Other alterations of the normal terminal field of the mossy fibers include (1) increased branching within the hilus of the DG, (2) development of abnormal connectivity between the two blades of the DG, (3) increased connectivity to granule cells and hilar region along the septotemporal axis of the hippocampus, and (4) formation of aberrant recurrent collaterals into the stratum oriens of CA3, where the pyramidal neurons extend their basal dendrites.

To summarize, the latency to the development of morphological plasticity matches the time course of development of spontaneous seizures in acute and chronic experimental models of MTLE. Neuronal loss and terminal degeneration precede the development of mossy fiber sprouting into the inner molecular layer in acute models of MTLE, and in addition, there is a direct correlation between degree of neuronal cell loss, mossy fiber sprouting into the inner molecular layer, and granule cell hyperexcitability. However, the physiological consequences of hilar polymorphic neuronal loss and mossy fiber sprouting remain a controversial subject.

SYNAPTIC REORGANIZATION BEYOND THE MOSSY FIBERS

In humans and experimental models of MTLE, CA1 pyramidal neurons also demonstrate persistent cellular hyperexcitability and a pattern of neuronal loss that is similar to the epileptic DG. Examination of the time course to formation of sprouted CA1 recurrent collaterals in acute models of MTLE suggests that seizure-induced CA1 hyperexcitability is due to the formation of recurrent excitatory collaterals in the CA1 region (10). Prolonged excitatory postsynaptic potential (EPSP) bursts observed in bicuculline-treated hippocampal slices from kainic acid–treated rats showed an all-or-none behavior (11). The all-or-none behavior cannot be explained by changes in the intrinsic properties of CA1 pyramidal neurons because the EPSP bursts would then be graded. Thus, the prolonged EPSP bursts are mediated by synaptic transmission reflecting a network-driven hyperexcitability, suggesting a role for synaptic reorganization and sprouting in the CA1. However, the prolonged EPSP bursts were only seen in 28% of the isolated CA1 transverse slices spontaneously (11). Although this may be due to a sampling error, one possibility is that the critical recurrent CA1 collaterals are cut away from the hippocampal slice because of the variability in the plane of cutting slices. Subsequently, Smith and Dudek (10), using isolated CA1 transverse slices, demonstrated that glutamate microapplication to the CA1 pyramidal cell layer increased excitatory postsynaptic current frequency only in slices of kainic acid–treated rats but not in control slices. These results support the hypothesis that the increased recurrent excitatory connections between CA1 pyramidal cells after kainic acid–induced status epilepticus are functional connections that increase the excitatory drive of the hippocampal circuitry.

Hyperexcitability in CA1 neurons has been proposed to result from sprouting of recurrent CA1 axon collaterals; however, all of these results were demonstrated in hippocampal slice preparations, which have limited depiction of the axonal projection perpendicular to the plane of the hippocampal slice and do not articulate the complexity of the anatomical topography of the CA1 projection to the subiculum. A recent study examined the possibility that the distal axonal projection of the epileptic CA1 pyramidal neurons reorganizes outside of its normal laminar boundaries within the subiculum and CA1 hippocampal region (Figure 7-3) (12). Sprouting of the CA1 projection to its primary output, the subiculum, might provide a mechanism for the enhanced and persistent cellular hyperexcitability in this region that has been observed using a variety of techniques. The major finding of this study was synaptic reorganization in the terminal field (distal axonal branches) of the CA1 axonal projection to the subiculum, demonstrated in five animal models of MTLE. Tracing experiments showed that the retrograde labeling extended 42–67% beyond the normal lamellar organization to include lamellae above and below the injection site. This is a demonstration of substantial plasticity of the CA1 projection to the subiculum along the septo-temporal axis of the hippocampus, allowing for increased transverse connectivity among hippocampal lamellae above and below the normal circuitry. The reorganized circuitry might allow epileptic activity in a hippocampal lamella to recruit and synchronize activity in additional hippocampal lamellae, amplifying the epileptic response and playing a role in the persistent hyperexcitability observed in intractable partial-onset epilepsy (Figure 7-4).

Synaptic reorganization of the CA1 axons projecting to the subiculum might have a major role in explaining the persistent cellular hyperexcitability in the epileptic hippocampal circuitry. In the pilocarpine and kainic acid models of MTLE, there is some degree of neuronal degeneration

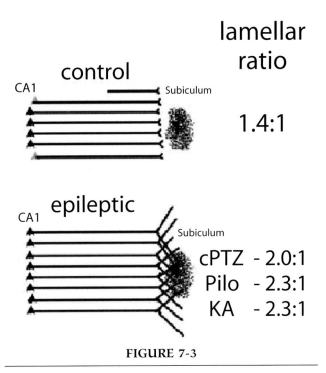

FIGURE 7-3

Synaptic reorganization in the CA1 projection to subiculum. There is prominent reorganization of the lamellar projection of the CA1 axonal pathway to the subiculum in several animal models of mesial temporal lobe epilepsy using retrograde tracers. In control rats, the extent of CA1 retrograde labeling from an injection site is limited to a couple of lamellae above and below the injection site in subiculum. In contrast, in epileptic rats, the retrograde labeling extends beyond several CA1 lamellae above and below the normal projection. This is direct evidence that axonal terminals from neurons in those layers extend their axons into the area of injection. Modified, with permission, from Cavazos et al. (4).

in the subiculum that is less than that in CA1 or the hilus of the DG. In a study using the pilocarpine model, there was only 30% neuronal loss in the subiculum, whereas more than 60% of CA1 pyramidal and hilar polymorphic neurons degenerated (13). This selective vulnerability has also been observed in patients with MTLE (14). The principal neurons in the subiculum are electrophysiologically characterized by their firing properties: regular spiking or bursting action potentials. Neuronal loss results in a change in the relative ratio of bursting pyramidal neurons in the subiculum. After induction of status epilepticus with pilocarpine, there is a prominent increase in the number of bursting neurons in the subiculum, from 40% in normal rats to 82% (15), perhaps due to selective vulnerability of the nonbursting pyramidal neurons in the subiculum. Nevertheless, the presence of increased numbers of intrinsically bursting neurons in the output gate of the hippocampus may allow the reorganized subiculum to play a potentially critical role in modulating the transition between interictal and ictal events.

Control   Latent   Epileptic

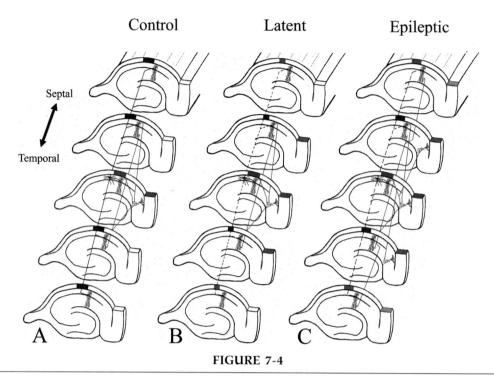

FIGURE 7-4

Synaptic reorganization in CA1 projection to the subiculum results in translamellar hyperexcitability in the hippocampal formation. The schematic drawings illustrate normal hippocampal circuitry and abnormal circuitry during the latent state and after development of spontaneous seizures in the kainic acid model of mesial temporal lobe epilepsy. The red neurons and axons are excitatory neurons; the blue neurons are inhibitory interneurons. (A) In the normal hippocampus, activation of the CA1 pyramidal neurons in a lamella results in limited activation of subicular neurons shown also in red, and the CA1 interneurons inhibit CA1 pyramidal neurons from lamellae above and below the activated lamella (shown as a blue block over those lamellae). (B) During the latent state, inhibitory mechanisms are functionally impaired, with slow improvement in the inhibitory tone (perhaps, in part, due to synaptic reorganization of inhibitory pathways). There is a mild degree of disinhibition in lamellae above and below the activated lamella (shown as smaller blue block in those lamellae). Furthermore, mild disinhibition results in a greater degree of activation in subiculum (shown as a greater number of activated subiculum sections). (C) Once spontaneous seizures develop in epilepsy models, there is prominent synaptic reorganization of the CA1 pyramidal axons, making synaptic contacts with additional CA1 pyramidal neurons and subicular neurons in sections (lamellae) above and below their normal projection pattern. The resulting increased recurrent excitatory connectivity between principal neurons in the hippocampus and within hippocampal lamellae results in translamellar sprouting. See color section following page 266.

TRANSLAMELLAR HYPEREXCITABILITY

The observation of synaptic reorganization in the CA1 projection to subiculum with an increased lamellar ratio might be better understood in the context of the lamellar hypothesis of hippocampal organization. The lamellar hypothesis proposes that the hippocampal formation consists of a stack of hippocampal slices that are functionally connected unidirectionally along the rostrocaudal axis. In this manner, the entorhinal cortex projects to the DG via the perforant pathway. The granule cells of the DG then project to the CA3 pyramidal region via the mossy fiber pathway. The CA3 region projects to the CA1 pyramidal region through the Schaffer collaterals and the CA1 region projects to the subiculum. Principal neurons of the subiculum then project back to the entorhinal cortex, completing the loop within the hippocampal formation. The myelinated fibers of these synaptic pathways project in the rostrocaudal

axis following the alveolar surface of the hippocampus. In essence, the function of the structure is organized primarily topographically into hippocampal slices or lamellae, and interconnections with lamellae above or below have no significance with respect to its primary function. However, there is some divergence of the projections within lamellae. For example, experiments have shown that injection of 10% of the ventrodorsal axis of the entorhinal cortex projected to about 25% of the DG (16). Furthermore, some types of hilar polymorphic neurons give rise to highly dense projections to the DG for almost two-thirds of the entire ventrodorsal axis. Even though the presence, density, and extent of these associational interconnections seem to invalidate the lamellar hypothesis, detailed functional studies are lacking. Some of the hilar polymorphic neurons could be activating local inhibitory circuits tuning out lamellae above or below the activated lamella (17). Nevertheless, the projections in the hippocampal formation clearly follow a topographical organization that is reorganized in experimental models of MTLE, providing additional pathways for further activation of hippocampal circuitry that do not normally receive these projections. The functional consequences of these alterations are not completely understood, but might contribute to the state of hypersynchrony and hyperexcitability observed in epilepsy.

A revision of the lamellar hypothesis using extracellular field potentials in vivo showed that it still "remains a useful concept for understanding of hippocampal connectivity." Andersen et al. (18) showed that the amplitude of the compound action potential was largest in a slightly oblique transverse band across the CA1 toward the subiculum, with decreasing activation in the lamellae above and below the activated lamella despite the larger dorsoventral extent of the neuroanatomical projection. Recent experiments (17, 19) have also shown that the larger extent of dorsoventral projections actually serves to inhibit the surrounding lamellae to limit the spread of activation. In the DG, the excitatory associational projections play a major role in activating inhibitory hilar circuits in lamellae away from the source of the associational projection. This pattern of organization strengthens the lamellar hypothesis by fine-tuning the activation to the "on lamella" while there is an increase in inhibition in the "off lamella" (Figure 7-4). Furthermore, Zappone and Sloviter (17) suggest that hilar neuronal loss in epilepsy models leads to translamellar disinhibition in the DG. Although the functional consequences of remodeling of the CA1 projection to the subiculum are not known, it is possible that the enhanced excitatory spread of CA1 axonal collaterals that make contact with spine profiles would enhance translamellar hyperexcitability in the subiculum (Figure 7-4), the output gate of the hippocampal formation. Early during the process of epileptogenesis it is likely that the primary effect of translamellar sprouting is to restore inhibitory tone. However, as the number of potential targets for the sprouted fibers decreases, translamellar sprouting results in primarily recurrent excitatory collaterals with cellular hyperexcitability. There are many unanswered questions deserving further investigation.

CONCLUSIONS

Synaptic reorganization of hippocampal pathways induced by excitotoxicity or repeated seizures is not limited to the mossy fiber pathway. Increased connectivity of the epileptic hippocampal network allows for increased synchrony and faster propagation of epileptic discharges within the structure. Synaptic reorganization of mossy fiber projections of the DG has been shown to play a significant role underlying persistent cellular hyperexcitability in the epileptic circuitry of the hippocampal formation. As the subiculum is the output gate of the hippocampus, its critical location in the limbic pathways, the presence of intrinsically bursting neurons, and the increased lamellar interconnectivity in epilepsy models may also explain the persistent cellular hypersynchrony and hyperexcitability in the limbic system observed in humans with intractable MTLE. Although synaptic reorganization of limbic pathways is not a necessary precondition for the occurrence of partial-onset seizures, it might be the cellular mechanism underlying the pharmacological intractability of human MTLE.

Acknowledgments

This review was supported by a grant from NINDS (NS02078) to J.E.C. We appreciate the administrative assistance of Laura Moreno.

References

1. Engel J Jr. Update on surgical treatment of the epilepsies. *Clin Exp Neurol* 1992; 29: 32–48.
2. Franck JE, Pokorny J, Kunkel DD, Schwartzkroin PA. Physiologic and morphologic characteristics of granule cell circuitry in human epileptic hippocampus. *Epilepsia* 1995; 36:543–558.
3. Sutula T, He XX, Cavazos J, Scott G. Synaptic reorganization in the hippocampus induced by abnormal functional activity. *Science* 1988; 239:1147–1150.
4. Cavazos JE, Golarai G, Sutula TP. Mossy fiber synaptic reorganization induced by kindling: time course of development, progression, and permanence. *J Neurosci* 1991; 11:2795–2803.
5. Hellier JL, Patrylo PR, Buckmaster PS, Dudek FE. Recurrent spontaneous motor seizures after repeated low-dose systemic treatment with kainate: assessment of a rat model of temporal lobe epilepsy. *Epilepsy Res* 1998; 31:73–84.
6. Wuarin JP, Dudek FE. Excitatory synaptic input to granule cells increases with time after kainate treatment. *J Neurophysiol* 2001; 85:1067–1077.
7. Laurberg S, Zimmer J. Lesion-induced sprouting of hippocampal mossy fiber collaterals to the fascia dentata in developing and adult rats. *J Comp Neurol* 1981; 200:433–459.
8. Boyett JM, Buckmaster PS. Somatostatin-immunoreactive interneurons contribute to lateral inhibitory circuits in the dentate gyrus of control and epileptic rats. *Hippocampus* 2001; 11:418–422.
9. Ribak CE, Peterson GM. Intragranular mossy fibers in rats and gerbils form synapses with the somata and proximal dendrites of basket cells in the dentate gyrus. *Hippocampus* 1991; 1:355–364.
10. Smith BN, Dudek FE. Network interactions mediated by new excitatory connections between CA1 pyramidal cells in rats with kainate-induce epilepsy. *J Neurophysiol* 2002; 87:1655–1658.
11. Meier CL, Dudek FE. Spontaneous and stimulation-induced synchronized bursts afterdischarges in the isolated CA1 of kainate-treated rats. *J Neurophysiol* 1996; 76: 2231–2239.
12. Cavazos JE, Jones SM, Cross DJ. Sprouting and synaptic reorganization in the subiculum and CA1 region of the hippocampus in acute and chronic models of partial-onset epilepsy. *Neuroscience* 2004; 126:677–688.
13. Knopp A, Kivi A, Wozny C, Heinemann U, et al. Cellular and network properties of the subiculum in the pilocarpine model of temporal lobe epilepsy. *J Comp Neurol* 2005; 483:476–488.
14. Cohen I, Navarro V, Clemenceau S, Baulac M, et al. On the origin of interictal activity in human temporal lobe epilepsy in vitro. *Science* 2002; 298:1418–1421.
15. Wellmer J, Su H, Beck H, Yaari Y. Long-lasting modification of intrinsic discharge properties in subicular neurons following status epilepticus. *Eur J Neurosci* 2002; 16: 259–266.
16. Amaral DG, Witter M. The three-dimensional organization of the hippocampal formation: a review of anatomical data. *Neuroscience* 1989; 31:571–591.
17. Zappone CA, Sloviter RS. Translamellar disinhibition in the rat hippocampal dentate gyrus after seizure-induced degeneration of vulnerable hilar neurons. *J Neurosci* 2004; 24:853–864.
18. Andersen P, Soleng AF, Raastad M. The hippocampal lamella hypothesis revisited. *Brain Res* 2000; 886:165–171.
19. Buckmaster PS, Dudek FE. Neuron loss, granule cell axon reorganization, and functional changes in the dentate gyrus of epileptic kainate-treated rats. *J Comp Neurol* 1997; 385:385–404.

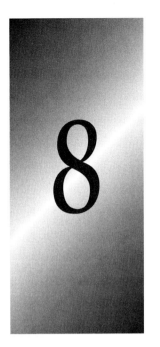

8 Regulation of Neuronal Excitability in the Amygdala and Disturbances in Emotional Behavior

N. Bradley Keele
Cathryn Rene Hughes
Hillary J. Blakeley
David H. Herman

The amygdala, a collection of nuclei located in the temporal lobe, is a key structure of the limbic system with well-defined roles in both emotion and epilepsy. Normal learning and memory, motivation and reward, and the regulation of mood and affective states are all dependent on amygdala activity (1). However, the amygdala is also a common locus of abnormal synchronous neuronal hyperexcitability in temporal lobe (complex partial) epilepsy. Amygdala dysfunction is also implicated in some psychiatric conditions such as anxiety and mood disorders, and people with temporal lobe epilepsy may experience psychiatric symptoms.

In a very general sense, the amygdala functions by sampling sensory input and directing behavioral output based on the emotional salience of the input. Behavioral output contingent on reward or punishment requires sufficient affective input to direct the most advantageous course of action. To be adaptive, the neural processing in the amygdala must be extremely rapid, not relying on highly processed, detailed sensory information to guide behavior. Thus, neuroanatomical and neurophysiologic mechanisms have evolved that provide a rapid "all-or-none" type of response to environmental danger. This functional organization of the amygdala may predispose this nucleus to abnormal neuronal excitability. In its most severe form,

neuronal hyperexcitability is expressed as seizure activity. In this chapter, we discuss the relationship between emotion and epilepsy in terms of the cellular and molecular mechanisms of neuronal excitability in the amygdala. Whereas extreme excessive activity results in epileptic seizures, subseizure levels of neuronal hyperexcitability may underlie the abnormal biological processes that contribute to emotional dysfunction. That is, the seemingly unrelated functional roles of the amygdala in epilepsy and emotion may share a common set of biological underpinnings. The synapses and circuits that normally operate to coordinate adaptive emotional responses may become overly sensitized, resulting in an epilepsy-like state of hyperexcitability associated with emotional disorders (2, 3). Conversely, during the interictal period, patients with temporal lobe epilepsy may experience altered mood states because of heightened neural activity in the amygdala.

In this chapter, we begin with a brief description of the biology of the amygdala before discussing the role of the amygdala in producing normal emotional experience, focusing on the critical role of the amygdala in fear learning. We also describe some changes in amygdala neurons that follow experimental induction of epilepsy in animals (i.e., kindling), and also address cellular and molecular mechanisms of excitability (transmitter receptors and ion channels) in the amygdala. These mechanisms can contribute to changes in excitability that may be associated with disturbed emotional behavior occurring between seizures, and to psychiatric symptoms in people without epilepsy.

ANATOMY AND PHYSIOLOGY OF AMYGDALA NEURONS

The amygdaloid complex is composed of thirteen nuclei, which are divided into three groups that are highly interconnected: the basolateral complex, the cortical nuclei, and the centromedial nuclei. The basolateral complex of the amygdala consists of the basolateral amygdala (BLA) and lateral amygdala (LA) nuclei. The LA is the primary target of sensory input from the thalamus and cortex to the amygdala. The central amygdala (CeA) functions as the main output nucleus of the amygdala. From the CeA, information is projected to many areas of the brain, including the hypothalamic-pituitary axis (HPA), the bed nucleus of the stria terminalis (BNST), and the reticular formation. Because of these connections, the amygdala has the ability to control the HPA and consequent stress-related emotional reactions.

The morphology and physiology of the basolateral complex has been investigated in detail; see Sah et al. (4) for a thorough review. There are two main cell types found in the basolateral nuclei: pyramidal neurons and smaller stellate neurons. Pyramidal neurons have several dendrites originating from the soma that give rise to spiny dendritic trees and are recognized physiologically by action potential accommodation (i.e., cessation of firing) in the continued presence of a depolarizing stimulus. Efferent pathways from the basolateral complex consist of axons of pyramidal neurons, which release glutamate onto their synaptic targets. In contrast stellate cells are spine-sparse, or aspiny, and can be recognized physiologically by the absence of action potential accommodation during depolarization. Stellate cells in the basolateral complex are GABAergic interneurons, making local circuit connections within the basolateral complex and among other amygdala nuclei.

Afferent input to the basolateral complex arises from sensory relay nuclei of the thalamus, as well as sensory and association cortices. Thalamic and cortical inputs are glutamatergic, and ionotropic glutamate (iGlu) receptors are expressed on the somata and dendrites of both pyramidal and stellate neurons in the basolateral complex; however, they are differentially distributed. Pyramidal neurons express both N-methyl-D-aspartate (NMDA) and non-NMDA subtypes of glutamate receptors; whereas stellate interneurons have non-NMDA receptors but very few or no NMDA receptors. There is also substantive monoamine input from the brainstem that supplies the amygdala with serotonin

(5-hydroxytryptamine, or 5-HT), norepinephrine (NE), and dopamine (DA). The rich aminergic input is important in regulating neuronal excitability and, thus, in controlling amygdala-dependent behavior.

THE ROLE OF THE AMYGDALA IN EMOTIONAL BEHAVIOR

Studies in humans have revealed the functional role of the amygdala in human emotion, especially fear (1, 5). In humans, electrical stimulation of the amygdala produces subjective feelings of fear, apprehension, and rage. Functional magnetic resonance imaging (fMRI) studies show that the amygdala is activated during the acquisition of learned (conditioned) fear, and that amygdala activation is greater when viewing masked fearful faces than when viewing masked happy faces, even when subjects are not consciously aware of the facial expressions. This suggests that substantial subcortical input reaches the amygdala and is processed quickly to control behavior. Damage to the amygdala or areas of the temporal lobe including the amygdala produce deficits in fear conditioning. In humans, amygdala lesions are associated with deficiencies in emotional processing, including dysfunctional fear learning and impaired recognition of emotional facial expression. Nonhuman primate studies further support a critical role of the amygdala in emotional behavior. In monkeys, bilateral destruction of the temporal lobes produces a state of emotional dysfunction, including significant changes in social behavior and the absence of emotional motor and vocal reactions usually associated with emotional states. The emotional deficits are mimicked by discrete amygdala lesions. Amygdala-lesioned monkeys become socially isolated from the troupe, they are no longer able to maintain their position in the dominance hierarchy, and mothers do not adequately nurture their offspring. The severe emotional processing deficit that results from amygdala lesions makes both human and nonhuman primates especially poorly suited to compete in a complex environment.

Fear Conditioning as a Model of Human Emotional Disturbance

Since Pavlov, it has been known that an initially neutral stimulus (the conditioned stimulus, or CS) can acquire affective properties when paired with a biologically significant event (the unconditioned stimulus, or US). As the CS–US association is learned, the innate physiologic and behavioral responses elicited by the US come under the control of the CS. For example, after several pairings of a visual CS with an electric shock US, an experimental subject will show defensive responses when exposed to only the CS. Specific defensive behaviors include freezing and potentiated startle reflex, as well as changes in autonomic (heart rate and blood pressure) and endocrine (hormone release) activity. The association between CS and US is quite adaptive and can be observed in several species at many levels of phylogenetic complexity. Every species that has been examined is capable of learned fear responses.

Research from several laboratories has combined to provide a remarkably clear picture of the neuroanatomy of conditioned fear in mammals (5, 6). Conditioned fear is mediated by the transmission of information about the CS and US to the amygdala, which initiates a constellation of fear reactions via projections to behavioral, autonomic, and endocrine response control centers located in the brainstem. The input and output pathways, as well as internuclear connections, have been elucidated. The critical nuclei mediating fear conditioning are the lateral (LA), basolateral (BLA), and central (CeA) nuclei, and the connections between these.

CS sensory inputs to the amygdala terminate mainly in the LA, and damage to the LA interferes with fear conditioning. Sensory inputs to the LA come from both the thalamus and the cortex, and fear conditioning to a simple CS can be mediated by either of these pathways. Thalamic input is involved in rapid conditioning to simple CSs, and the slower corticoamygdalar pathway appears to be involved in conditioning to more complex stimulus patterns (e.g., vocalizations or speech). Sensory information about the US reaches the amygdala through several pathways, including spinothalamic input from the thalamus to both the LA and the BLA, and nociceptive input from the medullary parabrachial nucleus to the CeA. Evidence from both humans and animals suggests that neuronal plasticity in the LA underlies at least part of the CS–US association that occurs in fear conditioning.

The CeA projects to hypothalamic and brainstem areas that mediate the autonomic and behavioral responses to feared stimuli. Although damage to CeA interferes with the expression of an array of fear responses, damage to areas to which CeA projects selectively disrupts the expression of individual fear responses. For example, damage to the lateral hypothalamus affects blood pressure responses, and damage to the bed nucleus of the stria terminalis disrupts the conditioned release of stress hormones. Projections to the brainstem are to three main areas: the periaqueductal gray (PAG), which controls vocalization, potentiated startle, freezing, analgesia, and cardiovascular changes; the nucleus of the solitary tract (NTS), which is connected with the vagal system; and the parabrachial nucleus, which is involved in pain pathways.

Mechanisms of Conditioned Fear

CS–US convergence is thought to occur primarily in the LA during fear conditioning, and the LA is the primary site of neuronal plasticity associated with fear conditioning (7). There is evidence that some LA neurons respond to both auditory and nociceptive stimulation and that conditioning induces plasticity in CS-elicited responses in this area. The strength of thalamoamygdalar synapses are increased following fear conditioning, a physiologic measure shown both in vivo and in vitro. However, plasticity in the auditory thalamus may contribute to LA plasticity. Plasticity has also been observed in the auditory cortex and in the BLA and CeA nuclei during aversive conditioning. However, the acoustic response latencies in the LA within trials (<20 msec) and the rate of acquisition of learned fear (one to three trials) are best explained by changes in direct thalamoamygdalar neurotransmission. Thus, the LA seems to be at least the initial site of plasticity in the amygdala. Furthermore, cellular mechanisms controlling excitability of the amygdala are able to strongly impact the distributed fear circuitry.

Long-term potentiation of neurotransmission (LTP) is an experimentally advantageous, but artificial, form of plasticity that was first pioneered in studies of the hippocampus. Much evidence suggests that LTP engages cellular mechanisms similar to those that underlie natural learning. Extensive studies of the CA1 region of the hippocampus have outlined one form of LTP in great detail. In short, glutamate binds to alpha-amino-5-hydroxy-3-methyl-4-isoxazole propionic acid (AMPA) receptors. The AMPA receptor–mediated postsynaptic depolarization allows activation of glutamate and voltage-gated NMDA receptors. Calcium then enters the cell through the channel complex of the NMDA receptor and initiates a cascade of intracellular signaling events, resulting in long-term changes in synaptic plasticity through altered gene expression and the synthesis of new proteins. Cellular mechanisms that promote prolonged depolarization impact the biological mechanisms underlying fear learning.

LTP-like mechanisms have been investigated in the amygdala both in vitro and in vivo. Fear conditioning enhances synaptic responses recorded subsequently in vitro from amygdala slices. However, the receptor mechanisms underlying this form of plasticity are not completely understood. In vitro studies suggest that LTP in the thalamoamygdalar pathway also involves calcium influx into the postsynaptic cell, but that the calcium enters through L-type voltage-gated calcium channels rather than through NMDA channels. L-type calcium channels have also been implicated in hippocampal LTP.

In vivo studies of LTP in the thalamoamygdalar pathway have relied on the use of extracellular field potential recordings. These studies have shown that LTP occurs in fear-processing pathways and that fear conditioning and LTP induction produce similar changes in the processing of CS-like stimuli. LTP has also been found in vivo in the hippocampal-amygdalar pathway thought to mediate contextual conditioning. However, in vivo studies provide some of the strongest evidence to date of the link between natural learning and LTP.

Drugs that block LTP have been infused into amygdala areas where LTP is thought to occur, and effects on the acquisition and expression of conditioned fear behavior assessed. Infusion of NMDA receptor antagonists, such as 2-amino-5-phosphonovalerate (APV), into the amygdala prevents the acquisition but not the expression of conditioned fear. This suggests that NMDA receptors are involved mainly in the plasticity underlying learning rather than the transmission of signals through the amygdala. However, later studies have shown that NMDA receptors contribute significantly to synaptic transmission in the amygdala and that blockade of NMDA receptors with APV may affect both the acquisition and expression of contextual and cue-specific fear learning in vivo. One proposed explanation of these findings is that NMDA receptors have different expression patterns or different functional roles in the thalamoamygdalar and corticoamygdalar plasticity pathways. For example, NMDA receptors contribute less to synaptic responses in the cortical input pathway than they do in the thalamic input pathway. Thus, infusion of APV would block both transmission and plasticity in the thalamic pathway, but only plasticity in the cortical pathway. Another, but not necessarily exclusive, possibility is that behaviorally significant plasticity occurs downstream of LA, and that APV infusions affect this plasticity rather than plasticity at the input synapses of the LA.

The plastic mechanisms in the amygdala are likely a key contributor to adaptive fear learning. One possibility is that CS–US associations are stored in the LA as enhanced synaptic strength of thalamoamygdalar synapses. The gain of this synapse is regulated by LTP-like processes. The adaptive nature of this phenomenon lies in the brain's ability to make selective associations about specific stimuli (i.e., cued CSs). However, dysfunctional emotional behaviors may result when this system becomes supersensitized such that the CS–US associations become more generalized. In this supersensitized state, the organism may have exaggerated reactions to fearful stimuli, or conversely, pathological emotional behavior may be evoked by low-intensity stimuli. In the next section, we consider the receptor changes that accompany amygdala kindling–induced epilepsy, a clinically relevant model of temporal lobe epilepsy, and then discuss how kindling-like changes in cell excitability in the amygdala may affect mechanisms of emotion.

CELLULAR MECHANISMS OF EXCITABILITY IN THE AMYGDALA AFFECTING BEHAVIOR

The cellular and molecular mechanisms of excitability in the amygdala involve many ion channels and neurotransmitter systems, and the ensuing intracellular signal transduction cascades. Much of what is known about the role of glutamate in amygdala excitability stems from experiments using the kindling model of epilepsy. These studies implicate important roles for the amino acid transmitters glutamate and gamma-aminobutyric acid (GABA) in controlling excitability. However, the amygdala is also richly innervated by amine transmitters such as 5-HT and DA. Investigating the cellular physiologic mechanisms mediated by these transmitters in the amygdala leads to interesting hypotheses of how 5-HT and DA can affect cellular excitability. Calcium-activated potassium channels and hyperpolarization-activated, cyclic nucleotide–activated, nonselective cationic (HCN) channels also have important roles in controlling cellular excitability. Last, growth factors such as brain-derived growth factor (BDNF) are known to affect fear behaviors and cellular excitability. Although this list of chemical correlates is by no means exhaustive, consideration of these specific systems can yield important insight into basic cellular and molecular mechanisms of amygdala-dependent behavior, as well as suggest biologically valid targets for development of newer, safer anticonvulsant and mood-stabilizing compounds.

Receptor-Mediated Mechanisms

Glutamate Receptors.   Glutamate receptors have an essential role in normal neurotransmission and are also important regulators of cellular excitability and synaptic plasticity in many brain areas, including the amygdala. Glutamate receptors, especially ionotropic receptors, are responsible for the majority of fast excitatory neurotransmission in the brain. Release of glutamate from presynaptic nerve terminals activates NDMA and non-NMDA receptors that underlie excitatory postsynaptic potentials (EPSPs).

Normal neuronal plasticity in the amygdala, which uses LTP-like mechanisms, promotes associative fear learning. In learning to fear environmental dangers, the mechanisms underlying LTP are adaptive, promoting survival of the organism. The learning mechanisms involve strengthening synapses through up-regulation of glutamate receptors, thereby sensitizing amygdala synapses and increasing neuronal excitability in the amygdala. However, in pathological conditions such as epilepsy, circuits involving the amygdala become hyperexcitable and lead to seizure behavior. Additionally, cellular hyperexcitability in the amygdala may lead not only to seizure activity, but also up-regulate activity in fear circuits and contribute to many of the psychiatric symptoms sometimes seen in temporal lobe epilepsy. Since the amygdala has one of the lowest seizure thresholds in the brain and is a common focus of abnormal synchronous firing of temporal lobe epilepsy, the amygdala is often used for experimental induction of epilepsy by the kindling method. Amygdala-kindling experiments have revealed much about the cellular mechanisms controlling excitability in the amygdala.

Kindling is a well-established animal model of temporal lobe epilepsy. In vivo electrical stimulation of the amygdala (or hippocampus), which is initially delivered at a subconvulsive intensity, eventually leads to spontaneous seizures when stimulations are repeated daily. Following the induction of "fully kindled" seizures, there are long-term changes in receptor function. Amygdala neurons become hyperexcitable. In vitro, epilepsy-like bursting is evident in BLA neurons from amygdala-kindled rats. Both spontaneous bursting and synaptically evoked bursting elicited by stimulation of afferent fibers to the amygdala are recorded from amygdala-kindled neurons. Synaptic bursting activity is elicited by activating afferent input at low stimulation intensity, much lower intensity than that needed to evoke single-action-potential firing from control neurons. In BLA neurons from amygdala-kindled rats, NMDA receptor antagonists attenuate burst firing in kindled neurons whereas non-NMDA receptor antagonists block all synaptically mediated firing activity. This suggests a critical role for NMDA and non-NMDA glutamate receptors not only in the physiologic changes necessary to support LTP and fear learning, but also in the receptor changes that follow kindling-induced epilepsy.

Metabotropic glutamate (mGlu) receptors in the amygdala also undergo functional changes following kindling-induced epilepsy. In control BLA neurons, activation of mGlu receptors produces a hyperpolarization followed by depolarization. The hyperpolarization is mediated by a calcium-activated potassium current, whereas several mechanisms contribute to the depolarization (e.g., inhibition of leak potassium conductance and activation of electrogenic sodium-calcium exchange). mGlu receptors classified as group 2 receptors (mGlu2 and mGlu3) mediate the inhibitory hyperpolarization, whereas group 1 receptors (mGlu1 or mGlu5) are involved in the depolarization. Following kindling, the mGlu-mediated hyperpolarization is lost and the depolarization is increased in BLA neurons. Together, these kindling-induced changes in mGlu receptor function further promote pathological changes in amygdala excitability that likely contributes to seizure activity.

Although excessive hyperexcitability of amygdala neurons may lead to seizures and temporal lobe epilepsy, we and others suggest that there may be a subseizure level of hyperexcitability that underlies maladaptive emotional behaviors. That is, some degree of excitability is adaptive and underlies normal fear-learning mechanisms. On the other end of the spectrum is pathological excitability associated with seizure activity and epilepsy. But in a supersensitized state, the circuitry in the amygdala may produce disturbances in mood, anxiety, and aggression even in the absence of overt seizure activity. This is one hypothesis for the pathophysiology of interictal violence and aggression, fear and anxiety disorders, and impulsive or aggressive behavior. This hypothesis is further supported by the finding that many antiepileptic drugs are also mood stabilizers, thus suggesting related mechanisms in neuronal hyperexcitability and emotional disturbances (8), and that amygdala kindling increases fearful and defensive behaviors in rats (9).

The majority of excitatory transmission in the amygdala is mediated by glutamate receptors, whereas GABA receptors are important for controlling inhibitory tone. In addition to these important chemical transmitters, biogenic amine transmitters such as serotonin and dopamine act as modulatory transmitters to influence the relative tone of excitatory transmission in the amygdala. In a very simplistic view, serotonin acts to dampen amygdala excitability whereas dopamine acts to increase excitability. The loss of adequate serotonergic input to the amygdala, or excessive dopaminergic transmission, can both tip the balance of excitation to maladaptive levels that may in part underlie psychiatric symptoms. The roles of these transmitters are considered next.

Serotonin Receptors. Serotonin is implicated in modulating emotional behaviors, and serotonergic activity can modulate the excitability of amygdala neurons. Release of 5-HT can activate several subtypes of 5-HT receptors. There are at least 14 different 5-HT receptors, which can be grouped into seven classes, named 5-HT1 to 5-HT7. Activation of any of these receptors may be involved in modulating cellular properties of neurons and thus change behavioral output. Serotonin modulates neuronal excitability in many brain areas. In hippocampus, postsynaptic 5-HT1A receptors may have either excitatory or inhibitory effects on the neuronal membrane by modulating potassium conductances underlying membrane hyperpolarization. 5-HT2 receptors enhance both excitatory and inhibitory synaptic transmission in cortex. In neurons from the nucleus of the solitary tract (NTS), the 5-HT2 agonist 1-(2,5-dimethoxy-4-iodophenyl)-2-aminopropane (DOI) inhibits single-neuron activity that is mimicked by the 5-HT2C–selective agonist MK-212. Moreover, the selective 5-HT2C antagonist RS-102221 inhibits the activity of both DOI and MK-212, showing that 2C receptors are important for inhibitory action in NTS cells. Therefore, the role of 5-HT on neuronal excitability depends on many factors, including the native receptors at a given synapse, the synaptic locus of those receptors, and the excitatory or inhibitory function of the neuron modulated by serotonin.

Many areas of the amygdala, including the basolateral complex, receive dense serotonergic projections. Receptor protein expression and mRNA studies show that many 5-HT receptors are found in the amygdala, especially

accommodation is dependent on the size of I_{sAHP}. Neurons that show complete accommodation have larger amplitude I_{sAHP} than neurons that do not completely accommodate. In an elegant series of experiments (11), it was shown that the slow AHP (mediated by I_{sAHP}) in amygdala projection neurons is mediated by a calcium-activated current that is not mediated by either SK or BK channels. Blockade of SK channels reduces the amplitude of the medium AHP (I_{AHP}) with no effect on accommodation.

By controlling the shape, frequency, and number of action potentials fired during a prolonged depolarization, calcium-activated potassium channel activity is involved in neuronal excitability. Pharmacological substances that affect these channels and the currents they carry can have profound effects on excitability. Cholinergic, adrenergic, and serotonergic agonists that block the slow AHP decrease the degree of action potential accommodation in amygdala neurons (11). Thus, calcium-activated potassium channels represent another physiologic mechanism whereby neurotransmitter receptors can affect cellular excitability. However, the behavioral consequences of action potential accommodation in amygdala neurons are not well understood. Furthermore, it is likely there are other, as yet unidentified, currents that also contribute to accommodation properties of amygdala neurons.

HCN Channels. The hyperpolarization-activated current (I_H) is a depolarizing, mixed cationic current that is activated by membrane hyperpolarization. The channels that underlie I_H constitute a family of membrane proteins that are sensitive to membrane hyperpolarization and intracellular accumulation of cyclic adenosine $3',5'$-monophosphate (cAMP). Cloning of the hyperpolarization-activated, cyclic nucleotide–gated, nonselective cation channel subunits 1–4 (HCN1–4) reveals the molecular basis of I_H function. These subunits can assemble as homo- or heterodimers, to yield channels with diverse physiologic properties. The voltage dependence and the activation kinetics are both influenced by channel subunit composition. For example, the hyperpolarization-activated current mediated by homomeric HCN1 channels occurs at a more depolarized membrane potential and shows faster kinetics than currents mediated by heteromeric HCN1–HCN2 subunits. The diversity of channel subunit composition imparts a wide range of physiologic characteristics that result in HCN channels having sometimes different activities in different brain areas. In thalamic relay neurons, I_H is active at rest and contributes to passive and active membrane properties. In hippocampus, HCN channels are expressed more abundantly with greater distance from the soma and make substantial contributions to synaptic integration. Thus, the nature of I_H is dependent on the native subunits expressed in specific brain areas.

Recent studies show that I_H is an important molecular determinant in the physiologic processes that contribute to epilepsy-like states of hyperexcitability. However, it is unclear whether activation of HCN channels is anticonvulsant or proconvulsant. For example, I_H prevents low-threshold calcium channel activity that leads to absence seizure–like bursting activity in the thalamus. Therefore, in thalamus, activation of I_H could be anticonvulsant. In the hippocampus, I_H is activated by increased inhibitory tone brought on by hyperthermia-induced febrile seizures. In this case, activation of I_H is proconvulsant. Although these results further suggest there are regional specificities to H-current activation, there are certain perturbations that consistently cause up- or down-regulation of H-current. Manipulations that increase neuronal activity are generally associated with increased I_H, such as LTP-inducing tetanic stimulation, febrile seizures, and neuropathic pain. Inhibiting neuronal activity is generally associated with decreased I_H, as is found following loss of cortical input to the hippocampus. Altogether, these data suggest there is a relationship between neuronal activity and I_H and that I_H is an important determinant in seizure-related hyperexcitability. Currently, the behavioral consequences of activation or inhibition of I_H on amygdala-dependent behavior are unknown.

SUMMARY

We conceptualize the effect of cellular excitability in the amygdala on emotional behavior as existing on a continuum. At the low end of the excitability continuum, neuronal firing activity is kept in check by a predominance of inhibitory mechanisms. 5-HT levels in the amygdala are sufficient to inhibit excessive excitability. In this state, the amygdala functions to monitor internal and external stimuli, waiting for an emotionally salient event. In the presence of an environmental danger, fear-learning processes are engaged. These LTP-like mechanisms allow emotionally relevant stimuli to increase the level of amygdala excitability in an adaptive, survival-promoting manner. Dopamine release during stress releases the inhibitory brake to facilitate cellular mechanisms of associative learning. At the top end of the excitability continuum, seizure mechanisms are engaged. However, we propose there is a hyperexcited state that is subthreshold for activating overt seizures. This hyperexcited state may result by many interacting receptor- and ion channel–mediated mechanisms. For example, reducing 5-HT input may promote a tendency toward hyperexcitability by diminishing important braking mechanisms on amygdala neurons. This perhaps results in a state of disinhibition in which epilepsy-like neuronal activity is easily evoked. Similarly, excessive dopaminergic transmission may promote amygdala hyperexcitability, since DA suppresses important inhibitory drive (i.e., disinhibition) mediated by GABAergic interneurons. Although the behavioral correlates of calcium-activated potassium channels and HCN channels are currently unknown, future investigation may reveal similar relationships between cellular mechanisms of excitability controlled by these channels and changes in fear and seizure behavior.

In the subseizure state of cellular disinhibition, amygdala activity may resemble an interictal state that perhaps underlies the psychiatric symptoms associated with temporal lobe epilepsy. Controlling neuronal hyperexcitability may account for the mood-stabilizing properties of anticonvulsant medications. Further understanding of the cellular and molecular mechanisms that control excitability in the amygdala may promote the development of more efficacious treatments of temporal lobe epilepsy and the associated emotional difficulties sometimes faced by these patients.

References

1. Aggleton JP. The amygdala: a functional analysis. 2nd ed. New York: Oxford University Press, 2001.
2. Keele NB. The role of serotonin in impulsive and aggressive behaviors associated with epilepsy-like neuronal hyperexcitability in the amygdala. *Epilepsy Behav* 2005; 7: 325–335.
3. Rosen JB, Schulkin J. From normal fear to pathological anxiety. *Psychol Rev* 1998; 105:325–350.
4. Sah P, Faber ES, Lopez dA, Power J. The amygdaloid complex: anatomy and physiology. *Physiol Rev* 2003; 83:803–834.
5. Maren S. Neurobiology of Pavlovian fear conditioning. *Annu Rev Neurosci* 2001; 24: 897–931.
6. LeDoux JE. Emotion circuits in the brain. *Annu Rev Neurosci* 2000; 23:155–184.
7. Rodrigues SM, Schafe GE, LeDoux JE. Molecular mechanisms underlying emotional learning and memory in the lateral amygdala. *Neuron* 2004; 44:75–91.
8. Rogawski MA, Loscher W. The neurobiology of antiepileptic drugs for the treatment of nonepileptic conditions. *Nat Med* 2004; 10:685–692.
9. Kalynchuk LE. Long-term amygdala kindling in rats as a model for the study of interictal emotionality in temporal lobe epilepsy. *Neurosci Biobehav Rev* 2000; 24:691–704.
10. Marowsky A, Yanagawa Y, Obata K, Vogt KE. A specialized subclass of interneurons mediates dopaminergic facilitation of amygdala function. *Neuron* 2005; 48:1025–1037.
11. Faber ES, Sah P. Physiological role of calcium-activated potassium currents in the rat lateral amygdala. *J Neurosci* 2002; 22:1618–1628.

9

Computer Simulation of Epilepsy: Implications for Seizure Spread and Behavioral Dysfunction

Mark Stewart
Rena Orman
Karen Fernandez
William W. Lytton

Mesiotemporal lobe epilepsy (MTLE), with or without hippocampal sclerosis, has been reported to be associated with memory, emotional, behavioral, and cognitive anomalies, which many would expect based on our current understanding of hippocampal formation function; but the role of seizures in altering cells and circuits has been difficult to define. Other reported behavioral or psychiatric alterations, including depression, schizophreniform disorders, and personality anomalies, may arise by the same mechanisms, but the biological bases for these manifestations have been even more difficult to define, in part due to limitations with regard to animal models.

The hippocampal formation, comprising the hippocampus, entorhinal cortex, and subicular areas, is a collection of cortical brain regions with a variety of cell types and circuits (1). Two allocortical regions, the dentate gyrus and Ammon's horn (CA1–CA3), commonly referred to as the hippocampus, are characterized by a single layer of principal neurons. The neighboring parahippocampal region incorporates entorhinal cortex, parasubiculum, presubiculum, and subiculum (2). These periallocortical structures form the anatomical transition between the hippocampus and the six-layered isocortex (or neocortex; see Figures 9-1 and 9-2). The entorhinal cortex, parasubiculum, and presubiculum crudely resemble isocortex, having multiple distinct cell layers with stellate and pyramidal cells. The subiculum is morphologically intermediate between the single-layered hippocampus and multilayered presubiculum with a single broad layer of pyramidal cells.

Studies of the various hippocampal regions have led to the widely held view that the combination of a critical density of recurrent excitatory connectivity and spontaneous activity in some of the cells (pacemaker cells) is required for a brain region to generate seizure activity. The excitatory connectivity is both intra-regional (intrinsic) and inter-regional.

Several hippocampal formation regions possess substantial intrinsic connectivity. The pyramidal cells of CA3 are relatively heavily interconnected (1, 3), and the parahippocampal regions all have some degree of intrinsic connectivity (1). Even area CA1, discussed in more detail later, has an intrinsic connectivity that cannot be overlooked. The hippocampal formation is also rich with inter-regional connectivity, from the long circuit that begins with the trisynaptic pathway and serially connects entorhinal cortex with every element of the hippocampal formation, to much smaller two-region circuits such as the reentrant subiculum–presubiculum circuitry.

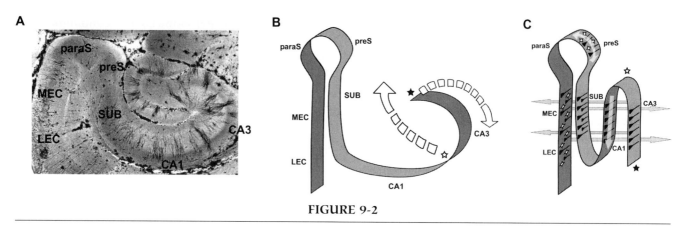

FIGURE 9-2

Refolding hippocampus simplifies the topology of inter-regional connectivity and suggests that the entire hippocampus might function as a single laminar unit. (A) Horizontal section of rat ventral hippocampus stained with rapid Golgi techniques and counterstained with thionine to highlight the cell layers of hippocampus. Major regions are labeled: LEC, lateral entorhinal cortex; MEC, medial entorhinal cortex; paraS, parasubiculum; preS, presubiculum; SUB, subiculum; CA1 and CA3, Ammon's horn; dentate gyrus is not labeled. (B) Regions (excluding dentate gyrus) are schematized as a ribbon. Broken arrows indicate the directions that the cortical sheet will be moved to achieve the refolded configuration in C. Open and closed stars mark points in the normal (panel B) and refolded (panel C) configurations. (C) After refolding, the "close-to-close" and "far-to-far" topography of CA3-to-CA1 and CA1-to-subiculum connections are simplified. The topography of MEC-to–distal subiculum and LEC-to–proximal subiculum/distal CA1 connectivity is clear from the natural folding of subicular and entorhinal areas. Light double- or single-headed arrows in each region indicate known symmetrical or asymmetrical intrinsic collateral systems for seizure spread. The refolding suggests that the entire hippocampus might function as a single multilaminar unit, where the laminae are distinct regions (e.g., CA1 or subiculum). In this view, the inter-regional connectivity is analogous to the columnar organization of isocortical structures, and the intrinsic (intra-regional) connectivity is analogous to the intralaminar circuitry of isocortex (19). See color section following page 266.

A combination of biological experimentation and computer simulations has been used to define the cellular and synaptic basis for epileptiform activity in CA3, as reviewed by Traub et al. (3). These are unstructured, hence topologically zero-dimensional networks. Two major conditions have been identified as important in the formation of epileptiform activity in CA3. First, there are relatively dense recurrent excitatory connections. Second, depolarization of apical dendrites can drive repetitive dendritic calcium spiking at rates up to 10 Hz. An epileptiform burst event is terminated as the after-hyperpolarizing conductance (a slowly activating and inactivating calcium-dependent potassium conductance) grows to offset the intrinsic calcium current and the sustained NMDA receptor–mediated synaptic excitation. GABA-mediated conductances (in particular GABA$_B$, especially if the convulsant is a GABA$_A$ antagonist) can also shape the duration of the event.

In this scenario, the primary epileptiform burst and any subsequent afterdischarges are the result of sustained depolarization of the dendrites. This depolarization causes calcium spiking and subsequent after-hyperpolarization due to potassium conductances. The result is repetitive dendritic calcium spiking. Each dendritic burst triggers a somatic burst that, through axon collaterals and AMPA receptors, keeps the whole network synchronous. The string of afterdischarges stops as the after-hyperpolarization grows. Blockade of NMDA receptors shortens the primary burst and eliminates the afterdischarges, so it is thought that the NMDA receptor activation is the sustained depolarizing stimulus that drives afterdischarges.

Whereas the basic elements for seizure generation seem to be in place for CA3, dentate gyrus and CA1 are normally resistant to seizure generation. Pacemaker activity does not seem to differ significantly between CA3 and CA1 (10), so the lack of a critical density of recurrent excitatory connectivity is the preferred explanation for why CA1 does not produce spontaneous epileptiform activity in response to bicuculline (3). In our studies of the ability of CA1 to relay population discharges from CA3 toward the subiculum, we discovered that the intrinsic connectivity of CA1 was asymmetric (Figure 9-3), unlike that described for CA3, entorhinal cortex, subiculum, presubiculum, and parasubiculum.

How does the asymmetric spread in CA1 arise? One possibility is that the asymmetry results from differences in the numbers of collaterals from each cell on its subicular side compared with the number on its CA3 side. A weak

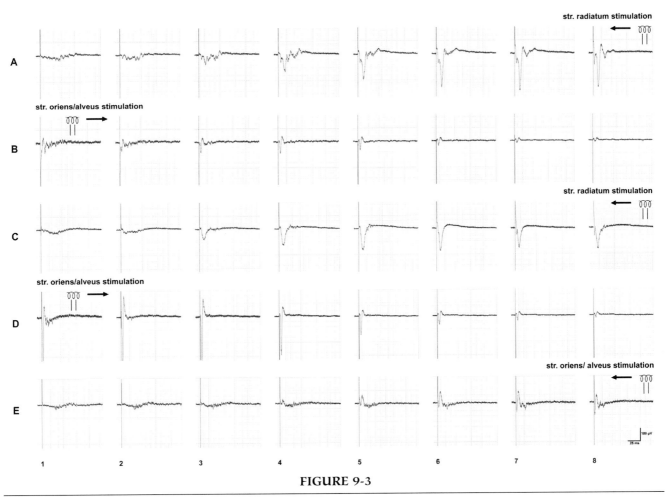

FIGURE 9-3

Spread and broadening of evoked population discharges in rat area CA1. Population discharges evoked in the presence of bicuculline (50 μM). (A–E) Spread with broadening of event duration when stimuli are applied on the CA3 side of CA1 (stratum oriens/alveus or radiatum; column 8), but not when stimuli are applied on the subicular side of CA1 (column 1). Ventral hippocampal brain slices were cut from Sprague-Dawley rats and maintained in a recording chamber that permitted 64 simultaneous extracellular recordings. In each row, the set of eight electrodes that followed the cell layer are shown. Brief single stimulus pulses were applied with bipolar electrodes to the CA3 side or the subicular side of CA1.

argument can be made in favor of this notion from the anatomical evidence for a strong projection by CA1 to subiculum (1), and evidence that collaterals can emerge from projection axons. Alternatively, we have seen weak evidence for more extensive local axonal arbors on CA1 cells close to CA3. This is clearly a quantitative issue that none of the anatomical data will settle. Simulations will be necessary to test whether these anatomical differences are plausible for controlling activity spread, but the definitive answers will necessarily await data from more experiments.

Uniformly connected cells in a distributed network model show features of the forward spreading in CA1 or activity seen in other hippocampal formation areas whose intrinsic connectivity appears symmetrical. Figure 9-4 shows the two main features of activity spreading through such a network. First, there is a threshold to activate the cells of a cluster that is associated with a rate for the propagation of the population event (10, 11). Second, as a cluster of neurons excites an adjacent cluster, the duration of activity increases, a process we refer to as broadening.

What functional purpose would the asymmetric intrinsic connectivity serve? One possibility derives from the inter-regional connectivity (Figure 9-2). Given the inter-regional connectivity of areas CA3, CA1, and subiculum, there exists the possibility of an unusual and dangerous reverberant activity. A normal event such as a sharp wave spreading from the dentate side of CA3 toward CA1 will activate CA1 near subiculum and successively back toward CA3 (enhanced by intrinsic connectivity). Reverberations of activity going toward and away from the CA1/CA3 border can be started. Changing the intrinsic connectivity to favor spreading only in the

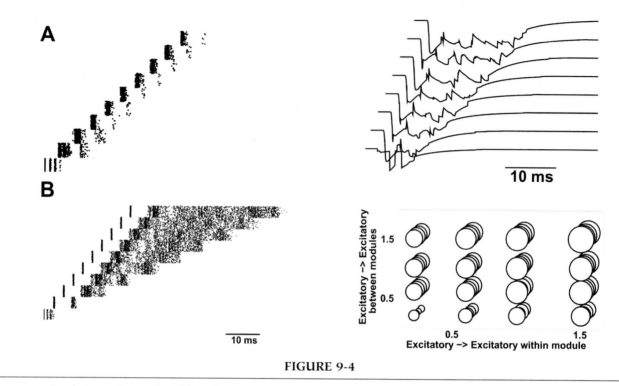

FIGURE 9-4

Computer simulations of spread and broadening in a model with uniform intra- and intercluster connectivity. Activity spread in different activity-chain models. (Left) Raster plots show time of spiking with sequential activation of modules after initial triggering (lower left in each). Weak connectivity (A) shows minimal broadening. Strong connectivity (B) shows pronounced broadening. (Right, top) Simulated field potentials show broadening and amplitude reduction as spikes desynchronize. (Right, bottom) Duration of activity (circle size) in most distant module from stimulus as a function of excitatory–excitatory connectivity strength within each module (x-axis), between modules (y-axis). Strength of excitatory–inhibitory connections between modules (z-axis). Increasing inhibition (diagonal up to the right) has relatively smaller impact on broadening.

direction from CA3 toward the subiculum reduces the chances of reverberation.

The subiculum, anatomically a transition zone, can generate epileptiform activity similar to CA3 (12), but it also participates in a variety of more complex seizures involving neighboring structures. The subiculum is a target of projections from CA1, which can relay epileptiform activity that originates in area CA3 (13). The subiculum is also the target of inputs from entorhinal cortex and presubiculum. Single subicular neurons can follow activity originating in CA3 or entorhinal cortex (13). Reciprocal connections between subiculum and presubiculum lead to complex reentrant seizure activity (14). Intracellular and field potential recordings revealed two reentrant paths for the interaction of presubicular and subicular neurons. We demonstrated a deep presubicular input to the subiculum and separate return paths from subicular bursting neurons onto deep and superficial layer pre- or parasubicular neurons. Recordings from subicular cell apical dendrites showed repetitive burst firing during sustained depolarizing current injection.

Reentrant activity in this presubiculum–subiculum circuit generated epileptiform activity in both regions that was more complex than activity seen in either region when it was isolated from surrounding areas. It appeared that the presubicular inputs to subiculum depolarized apical dendrites, which caused them to burst repetitively. These bursts were transmitted back to the presubiculum. Iterations on this circuit acted to prolong the dendritic depolarization of subicular bursting neurons and to entrain the activity across subicular cells, resulting in multiple afterdischarges (Figure 9-5).

Interlaminar circuits in the multilayered cortices can also generate seizure activity (15). These circuits can generate more complex patterns of activity such as epileptiform spikes with multiple afterdischarges. In disinhibited brain slices, epileptiform events from entorhinal cortex and the associated parahippocampal cortices contained many more afterdischarges compared with the simpler events seen in disinhibited slices of CA3. Similarly, individual isolated parahippocampal regions (subiculum, presubiculum, or parasubiculum) produce limited epileptiform

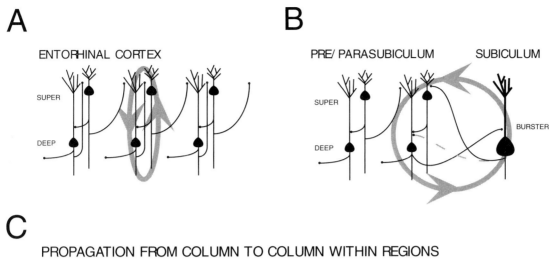

A

ENTORHINAL CORTEX

B

PRE/ PARASUBICULUM   SUBICULUM

C

PROPAGATION FROM COLUMN TO COLUMN WITHIN REGIONS

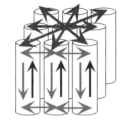

ENTORHINAL CORTEX

Columnar activity supports propagation
in any direction.

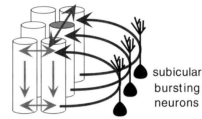

PRE/ PARASUBICULUM   SUBICULUM

subicular
bursting
neurons

A circuit involving subicular bursting neurons
can mimic columnar activity. Propagation requires
subiculo-presubicular interaction, restricting propagation.

FIGURE 9-5

Circuits involving parahippocampal cortices with different structural complexity. (A) An interlaminar circuit involving layer III (superficial) pyramidal cells and layer V (deep) pyramidal cells in entorhinal cortex is capable of generating complex seizure activity patterns and providing multiple pathways for spread within entorhinal cortex. (B) An incomplete interlaminar circuit exists in pre- and parasubiculum. Superficial to deep connections exist, but the return connections do not. Interconnections with the adjacent subiculum provide a full circuit capable of generating complex seizure activity patterns. (C) Multiple schematic columns and circuits are drawn to illustrate pathways for spread in the parahippocampal areas.

activity: simple population spikes with no afterdischarges. Interlaminar and inter-regional circuits will also be critical for seizure spread. Models of cortical columns are starting to appear in the literature (16).

IMPLICATIONS FOR BEHAVIOR

An enormous amount of biological detail, acquired over decades, has caused computer simulations to mature at an extraordinary pace. Perhaps the best demonstration of this maturity is the recent work by Traub and colleagues in which they found that their detailed models of CA3 could not replicate high-frequency oscillations seen in biological experimentation unless gap junctions between axons were

added. This addition was the only modification necessary to extend the model's capabilities (3). This is an extraordinary accomplishment of modeling. This is also likely to be an uncommon event, because the dramatic mismatch between the biological activity and the performance of the model was cleared up by adding a single new element. More commonly, there will be subtle differences between the biology and the modeling, or multiple missing parameters in the model resulting from an incomplete understanding of the biology. Glial–neuron interactions, extracellular chemistry, changes in cell and synapse physiology with activity, roles of modulatory neurotransmitters, and the distributed nature of intra-regional and inter-regional networks—these are some features of the biology that are very poorly understood.

The more interesting area is to use simulations for the development of tools to define population events or activity based on samples of cells. We need to develop an entirely new set of tools to describe and study population phenomena. Whereas we have long been able to witness population-based phenomena (e.g., seizure discharges), it is only recently that we have the tools to record a number of single cells at a time. We will develop tools once we develop concepts to describe. Such concepts may include firing rate spaces (J. B. Ranck, Jr., unpublished data) and ideas about determining the dimensionality of the rate space for sets of neurons encoding a particular thing (e.g., the set of neurons that forms the cognitive map of a particular environment, or the set of neurons whose activity generates a seizure discharge). The use of principal component analysis to define an activity "fingerprint" or "signature" for a neuronal ensemble during a task (17) may also be a useful concept. Simulations can be used to formulate and test the relations between the activity of cellular elements and the resulting population activity.

The activity of individual regions changes throughout a seizure and, more significantly, over time as a result of repeated seizures. Neuronal loss is an established consequence of repeated seizures in the hippocampal formation. Neuronal loss concentrated in a particular region such as CA3 will disrupt major interregional circuits. Scattered neuronal loss will impact intrinsic and inter-regional circuitry. Surviving neurons remain connected to the rest of the brain. It is generally uncertain how these neurons' firing patterns relate to firing in the normal brain. We propose four alternative hypotheses for the interictal activity of these neurons: (1) They produce normal patterns of activity, perhaps changing their individual roles to accommodate the neuronal losses. (2) Surviving neurons in epileptic brain regions are actively walled off from the rest of the brain by inhibitory neuronal circuits or some non-epileptiform abnormal oscillation that prevents their normal functional interactions with other brain areas. The functional effect would be comparable to that of an ablation. (3) Surviving neurons remain active and involved in brain function but are unable to fully produce the signals or oscillations that are required for normal brain function because of lost neighbors and/or inputs. (4) The worst alternative is that the activity of surviving neurons and circuits is altered to confer seizure-generating capabilities on regions that previously subserved follower roles. Repeated seizures leading to massive neuronal loss (e.g., in CA3) do not impair seizure generation, but rather transform the remaining hippocampal circuitry such that other regions (e.g., subiculum) become new seizure foci.

The alternatives suggested in our first three hypotheses will most likely be associated with milder forms of brain damage. Sublethal cellular consequences of seizures are likely to include aberrant changes in synaptic strength, disrupting memories or the ability to learn, which, together with circuit alterations, will likely have major effects on behaviors that depend on normal hippocampal formation activity. With regard to the origins of behavioral disturbances, the third hypothesis from our list—that brain areas are "active but abnormal"—would appear to best explain positive symptoms such as those seen in the personality disorders or psychoses associated with MTLE. Additional support for this hypothesis comes from nonlinear analyses of the preictal electroencephalogram (EEG). These analyses suggest that the area surrounding the epileptic focus produces normal synchronization and phase-locking with the rest of the brain up until a period several hours before the seizure. At this time the epileptiform area appears to "unlink" from the rest of the brain (phase scattering) before relinking at the pathological frequencies just before the onset of the clinical seizure. One can extrapolate from this to suggest that the unlinking is the initial pathophysiological phase. This unlinking would presumably produce mild brain dysfunctions. Such a propensity to unlinking would be a candidate cause for interictal disturbances of behavior and cognitive and emotional function even under circumstances where progression to seizure did not occur.

CA3 models have demonstrated the basic properties necessary for a seizure, but therapeutically they have led to only relatively obvious suggestions such as GABA potentiation. There is still little known about seizure initiation and spread in intermediate and complex cortical circuits. The emergent properties of these circuits will determine how pharmacologically mediated channel or receptor alterations, or specific surgical disconnections, will affect abnormal and normal dynamics. Studies of hippocampal formation circuits and dynamics will offer new possibilities for drug and surgical intervention, so that a pattern of activity becomes the therapeutic target rather than a class of cells or receptors. This will extend the concept of rational pharmacotherapeutics from strictly biochemical computer modeling to a broader model effort leading from pathophysiological dynamics to drug choice (18).

OTHER RESOURCES

Many simulations are available via the NEURON ModelDB database (http://senselab.med.yale.edu/senselab/ModelDB/default.asp). This resource permits the reader of a study to obtain all of the files needed to generate one or more figures of that study. This allows researchers to build directly on the work of other researchers, providing a complete and fully verifiable methods section.

References

1. Witter MP, Amaral DG. Hippocampal formation. In: Paxinos G, ed. *The Rat Nervous System*. 3rd ed. San Diego: Elsevier Academic Press, 2004:635–704.
2. Harris E, Witter MP, Weinstein G, Stewart M. Intrinsic connectivity of the rat subiculum: I. Dendritic morphology and patterns of axonal arborization by pyramidal neurons. *J Comp Neurol* 2001; 435:490–505.
3. Traub RD, Jefferys JGR, Whittington MA. Fast oscillations in cortical circuits. Cambridge, MA: MIT Press, 1999.
4. Lytton WW. From computer to brain: foundations of computational neuroscience. New York: Springer, 2002.
5. Rall W. Core conductor theory and cable properties of neurons. In: Kandel ER, Brookhart JM, Mountcastle VB, eds. *Handbook of Physiology, Section 1: The Nervous System*. Baltimore: Williams & Wilkins, 1977:39–97.
6. Pinsky PF, Rinzel J. Intrinsic and network rhythmogenesis in a reduced Traub model for CA3 neurons. *J Comput Neurosci* 1994; 1(1-2):39–60.
7. Lytton WW, Hellman KM, Sutula TP. Computer models of hippocampal circuit changes of the kindling model of epilepsy. *Artif Intell Med* 1998; 13(1-2):81–97.
8. Pytte E, Grinstein G, Traub RD. Cellular automaton models of the CA3 region of the hippocampus. *Network* 1991; 2:149–167.
9. Lytton WW, Hines M. Hybrid neural networks—combining abstract and realistic neural units. In: Hudson DL, Liang Z-P, Dumont G, IEEE Engineering in Medicine and Biology Society, eds. *EMBC 2004: 26th Annual International Conference of the IEEE Engineering in Medicine and Biology Society: Conference Proceedings: Linkages for Innovation in Biomedicine*. September 1–5, 2004, San Francisco, Calif. Piscataway, NJ: IEEE, 2004:3996–3998.
10. Lytton WW, Orman R, Stewart M. Computer simulation of epilepsy: implications for seizure spread and behavioral dysfunction. *Epilepsy Behav* 2005; 7:336–344.
11. Beggs JM, Plenz D. Neuronal avalanches in neocortical circuits. *J Neurosci* 2003; 23:11167–11177.
12. Harris E, Stewart M. Intrinsic connectivity of the rat subiculum: II. Properties of synchronous spontaneous activity and a demonstration of multiple generator regions. *J Comp Neurol* 2001; 435:506–518.
13. Stewart M. Intrinsic properties and evoked responses of guinea pig subicular neurons in vitro. *J Neurophysiol* 1993; 70:232–245.
14. Funahashi M, Harris E, Stewart M. Re-entrant activity in a presubiculum-subiculum circuit generates epileptiform activity in vitro. *Brain Res* 1999; 849(1-2):139–146.
15. Funahashi M, Stewart M. Presubicular and parasubicular cortical neurons of the rat: functional separation of deep and superficial neurons in vitro. *J Physiol* 1997; 501(Pt 2):387–403.
16. Traub RD, Contreras D, Cunningham MO, Murray H, et al. Single-column thalamo-cortical network model exhibiting gamma oscillations, sleep spindles, and epileptogenic bursts. *J Neurophysiol* 2005; 93:2194–2232.
17. Chapin JK, Nicolelis MA. Principal component analysis of neuronal ensemble activity reveals multidimensional somatosensory representations. *J Neurosci Methods* 1999; 94:121–140.
18. Lytton WW, Contreras D, Destexhe A, Steriade M. Dynamic interactions determine partial thalamic quiescence in a computer network model of spike-and-wave seizures. *J Neurophysiol* 1997; 77:1679–1696.
19. Douglas RJ, Martin KA. Neuronal circuits of the neocortex. *Annu Rev Neurosci* 2004; 27:419–451.

III

SEIZURES AND BEHAVIOR

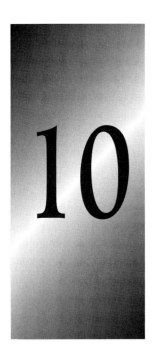

10 Neuroethology and Semiology of Seizures

Norberto Garcia-Cairasco

When the Commission of the International League Against Epilepsy (ILAE) published their proposal for revised classification of epileptic seizures (1) and proposal for revised classification of epilepsies and epileptic syndromes (2), they proposed a framework to which epileptologists could look for objective orientations for diagnosis, treatment, or research. However, when we talk about ictal semiology of seizures and epilepsies, we need to point out the most precise term that defines *semiology*. Therefore, in a recent report from the ILAE Task Force on Classification and Terminology (3), it is said that semiology is "the branch of linguistics concerned with signs and symptoms."

Furthermore, following a recent discussion on epilepsy semiology Wolf (4) says: "when neurologists analyze seizures, as they develop in time, we try to understand what brain phenomena are reflected in the development of the seizures. The more we understand, the more we move from a mere semiological approach to true semiology: an understanding of the significance of signs and symptoms. . . . This should be the ultimate scientific aim at our efforts at classifying seizures."

Engel (3) follows:

The description of the ictal event, without reference to etiology, anatomy, or mechanisms, can be very brief *or extremely detailed* as required for clinical or research purposes. *Although detailed descriptions of the onset and evolution of localized ictal phenomena often are not necessary, they can be useful: for instance, in patients who are candidates for surgical treatment or for research designed to elucidate the anatomic substrates or pathophysiologic mechanism underlying specific clinical behaviors. Communication among clinicians, and among researchers, will be greatly enhanced by the establishment of standardized terminology for describing ictal semiology. . . .* (emphasis added).

The ILAE developed the *diagnostic axes scheme* (3), where "Axis 1 consists of a description of ictal phenomenology using a standardized Glossary of Descriptive Terminology." (see this glossary in Blume et al. [5]). Moreover, as an alternative approach, and analogous to the ILAE axes, researchers at the Cleveland Clinic proposed the so-called *dimensions scheme* (6–8), where dimension 2 corresponds to ictal semiology. Furthermore, Loddenkemper and Kotagal (8) state "semiology can reflect only the symptomatogenic zone and, therefore, can give only indirect information about the seizure onset zone or the epileptogenic zone, as the epileptic activity may have spread from a 'silent' cortical area into a different cortical area that actually produces symptoms."

In fact, the discussion on seizures and epileptic syndromes classification versus what some have called "diagnostic manuals" is currently a more complicated one (see a recent debate [4,9,10–13]). For example, Engel et al. (9) state that "at the present time the designation of specific epilepsy syndromes and epileptic seizure types are [sic] based more on clinical experience and expert opinion than on scientific principles. . . . The ILAE Commission on Classification is beginning to develop scientific and evidence based approaches to defining and recognizing these diagnostic entities as distinct conditions. . . . Any classification must be constantly reevaluated, challenged, and revised as necessary, and clinical care must always be based on features of individual patients, whether or not a specific diagnosis can be made. . . ."

In the same controversy, Lüders et al. (10) mention that most epileptic syndromes were never defined scientifically. Furthermore, Avanzini (14) comments on how the sequence of events characterizing some partial seizures is not easily incorporated into the International Commission on Epileptic Syndromes 1981 definitions (1). Following on that discussion, Bauer and Trinka (13) believe that the Cleveland Clinic seizure system, based upon *five-dimensional patient-oriented epilepsy classification*, documents the sequence of seizure symptoms, but that, analogously to the *diagnostic axes* of the ILAE, the system represents a checklist for symptoms and signs but not a classification of seizures; for recent data on this matter see (7, 8). Moreover, Bauer and Trinka (13) consider the mathematical or statistical (cluster analysis) approach to the sequence of seizure symptoms (15, 16) to be difficult to use.

We strongly believe that—independently of which is the most suitable scheme, either diagnostic axes or dimensions—it is obvious that for the purpose of knowledge of (1) the basic mechanisms and (2) the neural substrates associated with the origin and spreading of seizures, or (1) for diagnostic purposes and (2) for presurgical evaluations, detailed descriptions of ictal semiology will be always desirable.

Thus, one of the main purposes of the current chapter is to demonstrate that *ethology* and particularly *neuroethology* will be adequate to any attempt to approach quantitative semiology of seizures and epilepsy. In other words, we will present data from animal models and clinical setups showing how appropriate the use of neuroethological approaches is for quantitative semiological studies of epilepsy.

ETHOLOGY: A SYSTEMATIC STUDY OF BEHAVIOR

Ethology is the systematic study of animal behavior. Most of the studies on animal and human behavior have oscillated between descriptions of innate behaviors and reactions to a given stimulus. Although pioneering research—such as that of Konrad Lorenz (17), the father of ethology—was mostly descriptive, it would not be fair to call it superficial or innocuous in terms of its contribution to the knowledge of the physiologic mechanism of behaviors, both in animal and in humans, either in nature,

in urban conditions, in clinical setups, or in laboratories. Indeed, a great deal of contemporary behavioral research is based, for example, on the concepts of innate behaviors, fixed-action patterns, *imprinting*, among others—all of them derived from these original ethological studies and observations. Recent studies call attention to the fact that stereotyped action patterns of seizure repertoire can be found even in invertebrates such as *Drosophila* (18), with great similarity to other animals (19) and obviously to humans (20). Furthermore, it is also clear that much information from those ethology pioneers was linked to the seminal interpretation of Darwin, who, in his magnificent *On the Origin of Species* (21) and in his further *The Expression of Emotions in Man and Animals* (22), built the bases for a phylogenetic evaluation of behaviors. Describing emotions and facial expressions, Darwin, for example, wrote that "the young and the old of widely different races, both with man and animals, express the same state of mind by the same movements."

NEUROETHOLOGY: LOOKING FOR NEURAL BASIS OF BEHAVIOR

The more recent concept of neuroethology (23, 24) is defined as the search for neural substrates of behavior. Curiously, and in spite of the current advance in molecular techniques, we know that the return to the fundamental questions in ethology is desirable, particularly when we are trying to characterize new phenotypes or constructs, such as the protocols of transfer and removal of selective genetic information, the so-called transgenics and knockouts (25).

In what manner could the more conventional ethological studies contribute (1) to the evaluation of normal but complex motor patterns such as postural patterns and (2) to the evaluation of alterations in motor control systems? Old and new developments in behavioral neuroscience have shown that, for example, the control of posture and movement evolved with a phylogenetic progression of competent circuits that can be studied in natural, clinical, or laboratory conditions.

One can make, then, the following assumption: If neuroethological interpretation of the physiology of the normal movement is clear, its impact in the evaluation of motor pathologies should be also evident. But how, for example, can exuberant alterations, such as epilepsies with motor manifestations, be evaluated under a neuroethological approach? What would be the advantages or disadvantages of using clinical or experimental approaches? Why not compare both of them? Would it be possible to use the very same approach for sensory, autonomic, or even cognitive alterations?

It is evident that the progressive knowledge we have obtained over the last decades on the neural substrates that control behaviors has allowed a stepwise construction of a model of fine correlation between ethological expression and corresponding neural mechanisms. Some examples can be seen in recent discussions on brainstem-dependent versus limbic system–dependent seizures (26–29) and on participation of basal ganglia and limbic circuits in the expression of neurologic and neuropsychiatric disorders (30, 31).

This development gave rise to the concept of neuroethology, because on the one hand, it facilitated the understanding of the adaptive values of behaviors or sequences of behaviors associated with the activation of specific circuits in the encephalon, and on the other hand, it provided multidisciplinary tools for behavioral evaluation. The contrast between the evaluation of behavioral components of seizures and epilepsy, for example, by means of seizure severity indexes, behavioral scores, or scales (generally arbitrary and linear), and the evaluation of behavioral sequences (flowcharts) and even behavioral clusters (correlations) associated with their neural substrates, is greatly illustrative.

In the case of clinical epileptology, the research usually has been based on qualitative descriptions of either seizures or epileptic syndromes and, in the case of animal models of epilepsy, very limited methods, supported by seizure severity indexes. Most of them, unfortunately, do not utilize quantitative protocols to show behavioral sequences that could be associated with the activation of their control by fine neural circuits.

In fact, when research on the models of repetitive, generally electrical subthreshold stimulation of limbic regions—which has since become known worldwide as kindling—was still in its beginning stage (32), some attempts to quantify seizure behavior were done by means of seizure severity indexes such as the Racine (33) limbic seizures scale. Racine established a behavioral hierarchy, or seizure classes (from 0 to 5), which corresponded to the sequence of behaviors and the severity of the limbic seizures. Further stimulation showed more severe seizures with brainstem components (wild running and tonic-clonic seizures) and even spontaneous recurrent seizures (SRS). This gave support to the Pinel and Rovner (34) seizure severity scale (from 0 to 8). Situations such as those involved in models of status epilepticus (SE) and their consequent SRS have also been mostly described by these severity indexes or scores; for a review, see Leite et al. (35). The so-called brainstem seizures have also been evaluated through severity indexes (28, 29).

To some extent, the importance of the use of ethological evaluations in epilepsy was further evidenced in several experimental models that considered the necessity to discriminate between, for example, mood disorders as a consequence of repeated ictal phenomena and ictal anxiety or ictal fear (36). Furthermore, the pioneering work by Stevens and Livermore (37) in the development of kindling of the mesolimbic system, as a model of psychosis, was supported by the acceptance that, analogously

to kindling of epileptic seizures, anxiety, panic disorders, obsessive-compulsive disorders, pain disorders and depression, follow kindling-like progression processes (31).

Historically, attempts to evaluate seizure semiology over the decades have been, in general, frustrating. One of the main reasons has been that more than a quantitative endeavor, this has been a very descriptive task (nonetheless, extremely elegant and thoughtful descriptions were present in the times of Jackson, Jasper, and Penfield and followers), because most of the time there were no clear and operational definitions of an ethogram, or glossary of behaviors that could be used extensively anywhere, anytime, whenever the ictal phenomenology was depicted. As pointed out in the beginning of the chapter, the need for this glossary is fundamental not only for classification purposes but for neuroethological research on seizures and epilepsy. Furthermore, once the glossary has been built and validated, the next logical question should be: how to depict the seizure sequence reliably. Ultimately, the question is whether the behavioral sequence helps to predict the underlying neural substrates, which is the primary goal of neuroethology.

TOWARD A QUANTITATIVE CLINICAL ICTAL SEMIOLOGY

Some historical approaches that have had great value to the study of semiology of seizures are those of Jackson, Jasper, and Penfield; see recent comments by Wolf (4).

More recently a pioneering study in which statistical tools were used in the characterization of ictal semiology, in this case in temporal lobe epilepsy (TLE), was published by Wieser (15). This author used cluster analysis to correlate groups of signs and symptoms and to verify the sequence of behaviors occurring during complex partial seizures. Two strategies were used in presurgical monitoring of TLE patients by Wieser (15). One of them was a precisely guided deep-brain stimulation that allowed the expression of specific sequences of behaviors, coupled to video-electroencephalographic (EEG) recordings. The other was the capturing of SRS through video-EEG.

Subsequently, Kotagal et al. (16, 38) applied a simplified version of the method developed by Wieser (15) and detected the predominant sequences of seizure behaviors to characterize temporal and frontal lobe epileptic seizures throughout analysis of only SRS. The studies by Kotagal's group are of great importance in seizure semiology, and although they did not incorporate any analysis of ictal EEG, obviously the latter was used as a criterion for a patient's inclusion in the studied groups. The consequent work on the proposition of a semiological classification of seizures performed by Lüders et al. (39) was certainly supported by those quantitative studies developed by Kotagal et al. (16). In substantiation of those efforts, Loddemkemper and Kotagal (8) emphasize that the ILAE recognizes the importance of seizure semiology and clinical lateralizing information. These authors also emphasize that terminology based on semiology (6, 39) has been used to characterize semiological patterns with potential localizing or lateralizing value (3, 5) with clear impact to new proposals for epilepsy classification (5, 7, 11).

In an additional effort to contribute to the differential semiological characterization of patients with TLE and frontal lobe seizures, Manford et al. (40) published their own study using video-EEG. This study was based on the premise that clinical-EEG seizures (semiology-EEG coupling) could be important for the discrimination of seizure etiology and helpful for diagnosis and treatment. The main result of this study was expressed as a combination of cluster analysis and flowchart representation to differentiate TLE from frontal lobe epilepsy and to correlate magnetic resonance imaging (MRI) data with ictal behaviors. Representation of ictal behaviors was made in the form of flowcharts, with temporal progression of seizures as arrows connecting pairs of behaviors. Manford et al. (40) concluded that few seizures could have their origin reliably localized by using this methodology, but unfortunately their criteria for patient selection were very broad, including distinct epileptic syndromes, and they applied nonstatistical criteria to exclude patients.

Another study by Fong et al. (41) emphasized the clinical importance of identifying body asymmetry in patients with seizure disorders, because that could provide strong clinical evidence for the diagnosis of localization-related seizures, particularly because of the known associations between body asymmetry, localization-related seizures, and brain lesions.

Furthermore, the studies by Meletti et al. (42) and Tassinari et al. (20) are based on the neuroethological supposition that there are connections between the behaviors expressed by patients and the phylogenetic roots to which we all, as animals, are attached. Specifically, Meletti et al. (42) describe a group of behaviors collectively named *face wiping,* which includes nose wiping. According to these authors an ethological and phylogenetic interpretation of this motor behavior confirms its presence from rodents to primates, and they suggest that the postictal emergence with greater frequency than ictally or preictally could be an innate action pattern modulated by external emotional cognitive stimuli. This concept was already discussed by Gloor (43), who evaluated olfactory system neuroethology in reference to the association between limbic activity of the old "rhinencephalon" and behavioral alterations of TLE.

When referring to emotional expressions, Darwin's seminal contribution was recently celebrated in Volume 1000 of the *Annals of the New York Academy of Sciences* (44). In that issue, the role of the right hippocampal-amygdalar formation in the recognition of fearful faces (45), in a group of patients with TLE, is described. Additionally, Tassinari et al. (46) compared the expression of emotions in human TLE and frontal seizures.

Recently we hypothesized that neuroethological analysis, successfully applied and validated for various experimental models of epilepsy (see details herein), could also be useful in the analysis of human seizure semiology. In fact, the main objectives of such studies were to apply and validate neuroethological methods and flowchart representation for the analysis of preictal, ictal, and postictal signs and symptoms of patients with TLE (47).

Thus, in the following sections we will show how we proceeded from the neuroethological evaluation of experimentally induced seizures to the characterization of seizures in presurgical patients with TLE. Most of the work was initiated in our Neurophysiology and Experimental Neuroethology Laboratory (LNNE), beginning with animals selected nongenetically for audiogenic seizures and continued with studies using selective brain lesions and drug treatments. Further studies were performed with a special audiogenic strain genetically selected in our laboratory (see further discussion herein). More recently, we used neuroethological tools to compare spider venoms having convulsant properties with the widely known convulsant kainic acid (48). Finally we applied this methodology to the study of human epilepsies, the latter in collaboration with our Epilepsy Surgery Center (CIREP) at the Neurology, Psychiatry and Medical Psychology Department.

NEUROETHOLOGY OF EXPERIMENTAL GENERALIZED TONIC-CLONIC SEIZURES

The first attempts to correlate semiology with brain substrates, by means of actual neuroethological methods, were by Garcia-Cairasco's group (49, 50), who studied audiogenic seizures in rats, a known model of generalized tonic-clonic seizures. These pioneering studies were followed by neuroethological characterization of TLE models such as audiogenic kindling (51), genetic selection of the Wistar audiogenic rat (WAR) strain (52), and the induction of SE by systemic pilocarpine (53).

In the previously mentioned studies, behaviors were recorded according to a behavioral dictionary. Sequences observed on video analysis were codified and inserted into specially developed statistics software called ETHOMATIC (50). All data were then displayed in flowcharts depicting frequency, duration, and sequential interactions between pairs of behaviors (dyads). This method has been validated for comparisons of behavioral sequences in distinct experimental situations, such as audiogenic susceptible versus audiogenic resistant animals, acute versus chronic seizures, and comparison of pre- and post-drug effects (for a recent review, see Garcia-Cairasco [29]).

In Figure 10-1A we can see the flowchart highlighting the various phases of a typical audiogenic seizure in

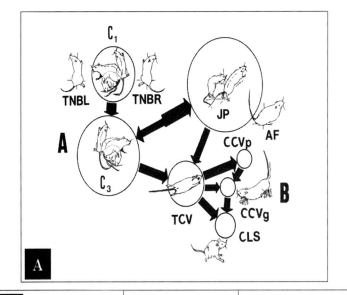

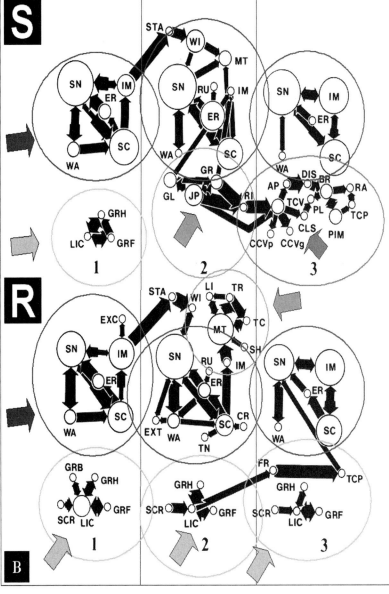

FIGURE 10-1

Neuroethological studies of audiogenic seizures in Wistar rats from the main vivarium of the Ribeirão Preto Campus of the University of São Paulo, before any genetic selection of an audiogenic strain. **(A)** Flowchart that illustrates a typical audiogenic seizure. Susceptible animals (10% of the whole Wistar population in the outbred conditions of the vivarium) begin their seizures with a phase of postural asymmetries (TNBL; TNBR), running (C3), followed by jumping (JP) and atonic falling (AF), a group of behaviors known as *wild running*. A further tonic-clonic phase (TCV, CCVp, CCVg, CLS) of generalized seizures finishes with postical immobility. **(B)** Flowcharts that depict behavioral sequences of audiogenic resistant (R; controls) and audiogenic susceptible (S) animals. The circles represent behaviors, and the arrows, with variable widths, represent statistically significant associations between pairs of behaviors. The ellipses and colored large arrows highlight behavioral categories: Exploration (dark blue); grooming (clear blue); orofacial automatisms (green); *wild running* (orange); generalized tonic-clonic seizures (red). **Abbreviations:** AF, atonic falling; AP, apnea; BR, bradypnea; CCVg, clonic convulsion (generalized); CCVp,clonic convulsion (partial); CLS, clonic spasms; CR, crawling; DIS, dyspnea; ER, erect posture; EXC, excretion of feces and urine; EXT, extended posture; FR, freezing of posture; GL, gyrating-left; GR, gyrating-right; GRB, grooming of body; GRF, grooming of face; GRH, grooming of head; IM, immobile; JP, jumping, LI, licking; LIC, licking of claws; MT, masticatory movements; PIM, postical immobility; PL, piloerection; RA, raising of body; RI, tonic rigidity; RU, running; SC, scanning; SCR, scratching of body; SH, head shaking; SN, sniffing; STA, startle; TC, teeth chattering; TCP, tachypnea; TCV, tonic convulsions; TNBL, tonic neck and body turning-left; TNBR,tonic neck and body turning-right; TR, trembling; WA, walking; WI, withdrawing. See details in **(A)** Garcia-Cairasco and Sabbatini, 1989 (54) and **(B)** Garcia-Cairasco and Sabbatini, 1983 (49). With permission from Elsevier **(A)** and *Brazilian Journal of Medical and Biological Research* **(B)**. See color section following page 266.

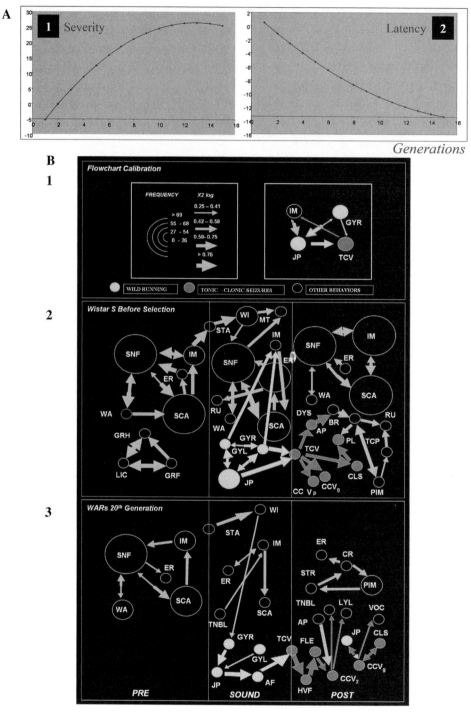

FIGURE 10-2

Development of the *Wistar audiogenic rat* (WAR) strain. **(A)** Through endogamous mating (brothers × sisters) a strain of animals with high seizure severity **(1)** and low latency **(2)** was produced. Although only 17 generations of the genetic selection process are illustrated in this figure, we are currently in the 43rd generation of the WAR selection, with maintenance of the same behavioral patterns. **(B) (1)** Calibration scales for flowchart construction. **(2)** Flowcharts that illustrate audiogenic seizures before the genetic selection. **(3)** After the genetic selection (20 generations), animals present faster audiogenic seizures that pass rapidly from acoustic startle to *wild running* and high-severity generalized tonic-clonic seizures. The flowchart data are coincident with those from seizure severity **(A1)** and seizure latency **(A2)**, parameters that were used as phenotypic markers for the genetic selection **(A)**. See Figure 10-1 for abbreviations. See details in **(A, B)** Doretto et al., 2003 (52). With permission from Springer-Plenum Publishing Corporation. See color section following page 266.

susceptible animals (54) from a nongenetically selected population of rats (Wistars). Figure 10-1B(S) shows flowcharts of audiogenic-susceptible Wistars showing exploratory and grooming behavioral clusters, before the acoustic stimulation, the development of wild running during the sound stimulation, and the strong expression of tonic-clonic seizures after the sound stimulation has been removed (once the tonic seizures begins, the sound is off). For comparison with the Wistar audiogenic resistant rat (control), see Figure 10-1B(R), which shows behavioral clusters of exploration and grooming, before the sound is applied, and orofacial automatisms, exploration and grooming clusters during the sound phase, followed by freezing behavior and exploration after the sound is removed. In summary, this group of animals does not develop any seizure pattern.

Several studies were done subsequently with success, using the very same methodology for comparison of audiogenic-resistant animals that became susceptible after electrolytical lesions or drug microinjections in their brains (55, 56).

A very important step in our research activities was the development of the Wistar Audiogenic Rat (WAR) strain by quantitative genetic selection (52). In addition to the regular program needed for the genetic selection of the strain, we characterized the animals in a clear-cut manner, before and after the genetic selection, using the neuroethological tools. Figure 10-2 presents some details of this procedure.

NEUROETHOLOGY OF EXPERIMENTAL TEMPORAL LOBE SEIZURES: SE INDUCED BY SYSTEMIC PILOCARPINE IN WARS

Although in previous studies we had demonstrated, by means of neuroethological approaches, video-EEG, and structural evaluations, the usefulness of chronic audiogenic seizures (audiogenic kindling) as a model of TLE (51, 57–59), we were also interested in showing the interaction between an epilepsy genetic background (or predisposition) and the experience of seizures. Therefore, we developed a protocol to apply systemic pilocarpine to WARs (53). Then we induced SE after pilocarpine injection in WARs; a sample of the behavioral effects is shown in Figures 10-3 and 10-4.

To reinforce the need for objective behavioral studies correlated to EEG studies or to neuroanatomical ones, we recently demonstrated that SE severity, even when measured with less sophisticated behavioral approaches such as seizure severity scales, is associated with lesion size in a model of SE induced by 30 minutes of electrical stimulation of the amygdala (60). We emphasized that usually in this kind of protocol SE duration and SE latency are considered, but SE intensity is erroneously neglected.

NEUROETHOLOGY OF HUMAN TEMPORAL LOBE SEIZURES

Our neuroethological method was first applied to patient semiology in 1998 (V. C. Terra et al., unpublished data), and later the adaptation of the method to human TLE was completed (47) (Figure 10-5A). Neuroethology was developed in individual seizures of a patient, in the sum of seizures of a patient, and in the group of seizures of a group of patients. The analysis of the flowchart of a group of seizures of one patient provides a pattern of behavioral sequences that occur during the seizure, and it may suggest a preferential propagation circuit for this patient (Figure 10-5B1). Figure 10-5B1 shows an example of the analysis of seven seizures of the same patient and shows a pattern of pressing the alarm button (focal seizure) followed by leg automatisms and later oroalimentary automatisms (temporal lobe activation) and dystonias that begin in the right hand and are followed by left hand dystonia (left and later right basal ganglia activation). The sum of seizures of a group of patients (for example, left and right temporal lobe patients) provides information about differences in behavioral patterns that may have a value in determining the side of the brain from which the seizure originates (47, 61).

CONCLUSIONS AND FUTURE PERSPECTIVES

Definitions and glossary of behaviors are built to help recognize ictal semiology. They are very important for the clinical neurologist interested in the diagnosis and treatment of epilepsy and for the basic scientist interested in understanding the brain mechanisms or selective circuits involved in the expression of specific seizure patterns. Current controversies on semiology, linked or not to classifications of seizures, epilepsies, and epileptic syndromes, are in some way polarized between a diagnostic axes scheme (ILAE) and a semiological or dimensional scheme (Cleveland Clinic). However, both of them, or even future mixed or new alternatives, depend on the development of accurate and detailed methods for seizure sequence descriptions.

When we decided to study ictal semiology, we began characterizing different experimental models such as regular Wistar rats (49) and those derived from the genetically developed WAR strain (52). Later we studied other models in which natural convulsants (48), known synthetic convulsant drugs (53), or electrical stimulation (61) was given to the animals. Finally we decided to apply all these methodological tools to TLE patients from a

References

1. Commission on Classification and Terminology of the International League Against Epilepsy. Proposal for revised clinical and electroencephalographic classification of epileptic seizures. *Epilepsia* 1981; 22:489–501.
2. Commission on Classification and Terminology of the International League Against Epilepsy. Proposal for revised classification of epilepsies and epileptic syndromes. *Epilepsia* 1989; 30:389–399.
3. Engel J Jr. A proposed diagnostic scheme for people with epileptic seizures and with epilepsy: report of the ILAE Task Force on Classification and Terminology. *Epilepsia* 2001; 42:796–803.
4. Wolf P. Of cabbages and kings: some considerations on classifications, diagnostic schemes, semiology, and concepts. *Epilepsia* 2003; 44:1–4.
5. Blume WT, Lüders HO, Mizrahi E, Tassinari C, et al. Glossary of descriptive terminology for ictal semiology: report of the ILAE Task Force on Classification and Terminology. *Epilepsia* 2001; 42:1212–1218.
6. Lüders HO, Noachtar S, Burgess RC. Semiologic classification of epileptic seizures. In: Lüders HO, Noachtar S, eds. *Epileptic Seizures: Pathophysiology and Clinical Semiology.* New York: Churchill Livingstone, 2000:263–285.
7. Kellinghaus C, Loddenkemper T, Najm IM, et al. Specific epileptic syndromes are rare even in tertiary epilepsy centers: a patient-oriented approach to epilepsy classification. *Epilepsia* 2004; 45:268–275.
8. Loddenkemper T, Kotagal P. Lateralizing signs during seizures in focal epilepsy. *Epilepsy Behav* 2005; 7:1–17
9. Engel J Jr. Reply to "Of cabbages and kings: some considerations on classifications, diagnostic schemes, semiology, and concepts." *Epilepsia* 2003; 44:4–6.
10. Lüders H, Njam I, Willey E. Reply to "Of cabbages and kings: Some considerations on classifications, diagnostic schemes, semiology, and concepts." *Epilepsia* 2003; 44:6–8.
11. Engel J Jr, Berg A, Andermann F, Avanzini G, et al. Debate on the classification of epileptic seizures and syndromes. Are epilepsy classifications based on epileptic syndromes and seizure types outdated? *Epileptic Disord* 2006; 8:159–163.
12. Lüders HO, Acharya J, Alexopoulos A, Baumgartner C, et al. Are epileptic classifications based on epileptic syndromes and seizure types outdated? *Epileptic Disord* 2006; 8:81–85.
13. Bauer G, Trinka E. Debate on the classification of epileptic seizures and syndromes. Seizures, syndromes and classifications. *Epileptic Disord* 2006; 8:162–163.
14. Avanzini G. Of cabbages and kings: Do we really need a systematic classification of epilepsies? *Epilepsia* 2003; 44:12–13.
15. Wieser HG. Electroclinical features of the psychomotor seizure. London: Fischer G; Stuttgart: Butterworths, 1983.
16. Kotagal P, Lüders HO, Williams G, Nichols TR, et al. Psychomotor seizures of temporal lobe onset: Analysis of symptom clusters and sequences. *Epilepsy Res* 1995; 20:49–67.
17. Lorenz K. The evolution of behavior. *Sci Am* 1958; 199:67–78.
18. Lee J, Wu C. Electroconvulsive seizure behavior in *Drosophila*: analysis of the physiological repertoire underlying a stereotyped action pattern in bang-sensitive mutants. *J Neurosci* 2002; 22:11065–11079.
19. Reichert H, Wine JJ. Neural mechanism for serial order in a stereotyped behavior sequence. *Nature* 1982; 296:86–87.
20. Tassinari CA, Rubboli G, Gardella E, Cantalupo G, et al. Central pattern generators for a common semiology in fronto-limbic seizures and in parasomnias. A neuroethologic approach. *Neurol Sci* 2005; 26:s225–s232.
21. Darwin C. The origin of species by means of natural selection. The preservation of favoured races in the struggle for life. London: John Murray, 1859.
22. Darwin C. The expression of emotions in man and animals. London: John Murray, 1881.
23. Fentress JC. History of developmental neuroethology: early contributions from ethology. *J Neurobiol* 1992; 23:1355–1369.
24. Pfluger H-J, Menzel R. Neuroethology, its roots and future. *J Comp Physiol A* 1999; 185: 389–392.
25. Gerlai R, Clayton NS. Analysing hippocampal function in transgenic mice: an ethological perspective. *Trends Neurosci* 1999; 22:47–51.
26. Faingold CL. Emergent properties of CNS neuronal networks as targets for pharmacology: application to anticonvulsant drug action. *Prog Neurobiol* 2004; 72:55–85.
27. Garcia Cairasco N. A critical review on the participation of inferior colliculus in acoustic-motor and acoustic-limbic networks involved in the expression of acute and kindled audiogenic seizures. *Hear Res* 2002; 168:208–222.
28. Jobe PC, Browning R. From brainstem to forebrain in generalized models of seizures and epilepsies. In: Hirsch E, Andermann F, Chauvel P, Engel J, et al, eds. *Generalized Seizures: From Clinical Phenomenology to Underlying Systems and Networks. Progress in Epileptic Disorders.* Vol 2. Esher, Surrey, UK: John Libbey-Eurotext, 2006:33–52.
29. Garcia-Cairasco N. Behavior, neural circuits and plasticity in acute and chronic models of generalized tonic-clonic seizures. In: Hirsch E, Andermann F, Chauvel P, Engel J, et al, eds. *Generalized Seizures: From Clinical Phenomenology to Underlying Systems and Networks.* Progress in Epileptic Disorders 2. Esher, Surrey, UK: John Libbey-Eurotext, 2006:197–228.
30. Garcia-Cairasco N, Miguel EC, Rauch S, Leckman J. Current controversies and future directions on basal ganglia research: integrating basic neuroscience and clinical investigation. In: Miguel EC, Rauch SC, Leckman JF, eds. *Neuropsychiatry of Basal Ganglia. Psychiatric Clinics of North America* 20. Philadelphia: USA Sinauer Associates, 1997:945–962.
31. Post RM. Do the epilepsies, pain syndromes, and affective disorders share common kindling-like mechanisms? *Epilepsy Res* 2002; 50:203–219.
32. Goddard GV, McIntyre DC, Leech CK. A permanent change in brain function resulting from daily electrical stimulation. *Exp Neurol* 1969; 25:295–330.
33. Racine RJ. Modification of seizure activity by electrical stimulation: II. Motor seizure. *Electroencephalogr Clin Neurophysiol* 1972; 32:281–294.
34. Pinel JP, Rovner LI. Experimental epileptogenesis: kindling-induced epilepsy in rats. *Exp Neurol* 1978; 58:190–202.
35. Leite JP, Garcia-Cairasco N, Cavalheiro EA. New insights from the use of pilocarpine and kainate models. *Epilepsy Res* 2002; 50:93–103.
36. Griffith N, Engel J Jr, Bandler R. Ictal and enduring interictal disturbances in emotional behaviour in an animal model of temporal lobe epilepsy. *Brain Res* 1987; 400:360–364.
37. Stevens JR, Livermore A Jr. Kindling of the mesolimbic dopamine system: animal model of psychosis. *Neurology* 1978; 28:36–46.
38. Kotagal P, Arunkumar G, Hammel J, Mascha E. Complex partial seizures of frontal lobe onset statistical analysis of ictal semiology. *Seizure* 2003; 12:268–281.
39. Lüders H, Acharya J, Baumgartner C, Benbadis S, et al. Semiological seizure classification. *Epilepsia* 1998; 39:1006–1013.
40. Manford M, Fish DR, Shorvon SD. An analysis of clinical seizure patterns and their localizing value in frontal and temporal lobe epilepsies. *Brain* 1996; 119:17–40.
41. Fong GCY, Mak YF, Swartz BE, Walsh GO, et al. Body part asymmetry in partial seizure. *Seizure* 2003; 12:606–612.
42. Meletti S, Cantalupo G, Stanzani-Miserati M, Rubolli G, et al. The expression of interictal, preictal, and postictal facial-wiping behavior in temporal lobe epilepsy: a neuro-ethological analysis and interpretation. *Epilepsy Behav* 2003; 4:635–643.
43. Gloor P. The temporal lobe and limbic system. New York: Oxford University Press, 1997:865.
44. Eckman P, Campos JJ, Davidson RJ, De Waal FBM, eds. Emotions inside out: 130 years after Darwin's *The Expression of Emotions in Man and Animals.* Ann N Y Acad Sci 2003;1000 (special volume).
45. Meletti S, Benuzzi F, Nichelli P, Tassinari CA. Damage to the right hippocampal-amygdala formation during early infancy and recognition of fearful faces. Neuropsychological and fMRI evidence in subjects with temporal lobe epilepsy. *Ann N Y Acad Sci* 2003; 1000:385–388.
46. Tassinari CA, Gardella E, Rubboli G, Meletti S, et al. Facial expression emotion in temporal and frontal lobe epileptic seizures. *Ann N Y Acad Sci* 2003; 1000:393–394.
47. Dal-Cól MLC, Terra-Bustamante VC, Velasco TR, Oliveira JAC, et al. Neuroethology application for the study of human temporal lobe epilepsy: from basic to applied sciences. *Epilepsy Behav* 2006; 8:149–160.
48. Rodrigues MCA, Guizzo R, Santos WF, Garcia-Cairasco N. A comparative neuroethological study of limbic seizures induced by *P. bistriata* venom and kainic acid injections in rats. *Brain Res Bull* 2001; 55:79–86.
49. Garcia-Cairasco N, Sabbatini RM. Role of substantia nigra in audiogenic seizures: a neuroethological analysis in the rat. *Braz J Med Biol Res* 1983; 16:171–183.
50. Garcia-Cairasco N, Doretto MC, Prado P, Jorge BPD, et al. New insights into behavioral evaluation of audiogenic seizures: a comparison of two ethological methods. *Behav Brain Res* 1992; 48:49–56.
51. Garcia-Cairasco N, Wakamatsu H, Oliveira JAC, Gomes ELT, et al. Neuroethological and morphological (Neo-Timm staining) correlates of limbic recruitment during the development of audiogenic kindling in seizure susceptible Wistar rats. *Epilepsy Res* 1996; 26:177–192.
52. Doretto MC, Fonseca CG, Lobo RB, Terra VC, et al. Quantitative study of the response to genetic selection of the Wistar audiogenic rat strain (WAR). *Behav Genet* 2003; 33:33–42.
53. Garcia-Cairasco N, Rossetti F, Oliveira JAC, Furtado MA. Neuroethological study of status epilepticus induced by systemic pilocarpine in Wistar audiogenic rats (WAR strain). *Epilepsy Behav* 2004; 5:455–463.
54. Garcia-Cairasco N, Sabbatini, RM. Neuroethological evaluation of audiogenic seizures in hemidetelencephalated rats. *Behav Brain Res* 1989; 33:65–77.
55. Tsutsui J, Terra VC, Oliveira JAC, Garcia-Cairasco N. Neuroethological evaluation of audiogenic seizures and audiogenic-like seizures induced by microinjection of bicuculline into the inferior colliculus. I. Effects of midcollicular knife cuts. *Behav Brain Res* 1992; 52:7–17.
56. Doretto MC, Garcia-Cairasco N. Differential audiogenic seizure sensitization by selective unilateral substantia nigra lesions in resistant Wistar rats. *Physiol Behav* 1995; 58:273–282.
57. Dutra Moraes MFD, Galvis-Alonso OY, Garcia-Cairasco N. Wistar audiogenic rat kindling: an epilepsy model for secondary limbic structures recruitment. *Epilepsy Res* 2000; 39:251–259.
58. Romcy-Pereira RN, Garcia-Cairasco N. Hippocampal cell proliferation and epileptogenesis after audiogenic kindling are not accompanied by mossy fiber sprouting or fluoro-jade staining. *Neuroscience* 2003; 119:533–546.
59. Galvis-Alonso OY, Cortes de Oliveira JA, Garcia-Cairasco N. Limbic epileptogenicity, cell loss and axonal reorganization induced by audiogenic and amygdala kindling in Wistar Audiogenic Rats (WAR strain). *Neuroscience* 2004; 125:787–802.
60. Tilelli CQ, Del Vecchio F, Fernandes A, Garcia-Cairasco N. Different types of status epilepticus lead to different levels of brain damage in rats. *Epilepsy Behav* 2005; 7:401–410.
61. Dal-Cól ML, Terra-Bustamante VC, Velasco TR, Oliveira JAC, et al. Neuroethological comparison between human left and right temporal lobe epilepsy. Proceedings of American Epilepsy Society and American Clinical Neurophysiology Society Joint Annual Meeting, Washington, DC, 2005.
62. Engel J Jr. Classifications of the International League Against Epilepsy: time for reappraisal. *Epilepsia* 1998; 39:1014–1017.

11 Neuropsychologic Effects of Seizures

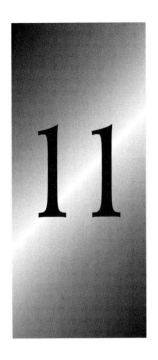

Gus A. Baker
Joanne Taylor

Although a significant proportion of people report cognitive impairments, in particular memory problems, as a consequence of their epilepsy and its treatment (1, 2), there is a continuous debate as to what factors may be important in understanding the development and course of these neuropsychologic impairments. The main culprits, as shown in Figure 11-1, appear to be the effects of continuous seizures and subclinical epileptiform activity, neuronal dysfunction, the side effects of antiepileptic medication and psychosocial problems (3–5).

In this chapter we will discuss specifically the effects of seizures on neuropsychologic functioning but will also address the other potential factors explaining the development and maintenance of neuropsychologic problems related to epilepsy and its treatment.

EFFECTS OF UNDERLYING LESION

Recent evidence has highlighted the role of the underlying lesion as a significant factor in explaining the development of neuropsychologic impairment. Äikiä and colleagues investigated verbal memory functioning in untreated adult patients with newly diagnosed partial epilepsy compared to a sample of volunteer controls. Patients with newly diagnosed epilepsy demonstrated verbal memory impairments, particularly in delayed recall of unrelated words at the time of diagnosis (6, 7). Similarly, impairments were in seen in a large sample of adults with recent onset epilepsy prior to the administration of antiepileptic medication compared to a sample of neurologically normal controls. The controls performed better than the patients with epilepsy across a number of neuropsychologic tasks; however, it was the measures of verbal memory and motor speed that reached statistical significance (8). Deficits in motor and cognitive functions have been further evaluated in a study of 59 newly diagnosed patients with epilepsy and 26 controls. Prior to the administration of antiepileptic drugs (AEDs), participants were assessed on measures of motor functioning, attention and concentration, mental flexibility, and memory. After adjusting for multiple comparisons and covarying for intellectual functioning, controls performed better on 16 of the 20 measures, although these did not always reach statistical significance (9). Several authors have shown that people with epilepsy already demonstrate subtle impairments of motor coordination, attention, concentration, mental flexibility, and memory at the time of diagnosis.

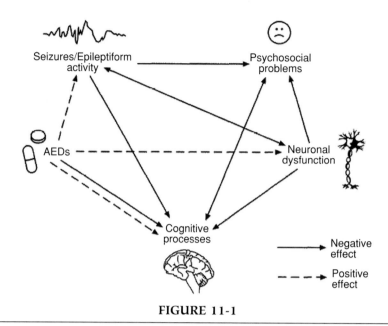

FIGURE 11-1

Nonindependent contributory factors for cognitive dysfunction in epilepsy (4).

EFFECTS OF ANTIEPILEPTIC MEDICATION

There has been a wealth of literature over the last 25–30 years documenting the effects of antiepileptic medication. Older drugs such as phenytoin and phenobarbital are associated with adverse cognitive effects, whereas newer drugs such as oxcarbazepine and lamotrigine appear to exert a less negative influence on cognition (10–17). However, in those patients taking topiramate, language dysfunction, problems with executive function, and attention have been noted (18–24).

EFFECTS OF SEIZURES

In contrast relatively little is known about the effects of recurrent seizures on neuropsychologic functioning. This is partly due to the methodological difficulties in conducting studies that are able to determine and estimate the individual role of these variables (25–27).

In his recent review, Vingerhoets described how cross-sectional studies appear to overestimate seizure effects because they cannot disentangle the effects of epilepsy from the underlying lesion (25). Many studies fail to document the type and number of seizures that have occurred during the study period (26). Although prospective longitudinal studies are preferable, they also suffer from confounding variables, such as the highly interrelated variables of duration of epilepsy, number of seizures, exposure to AEDs, age of onset, and number of seizure-related head injuries, that make interpretation uncertain (25, 26).

The issue is further complicated because seizures seem to have different effects in adults and children as a result of the structural and functional development of the human brain (26, 28, 29). However, in this chapter the authors will consider only the neuropsychologic effects of seizures in adults.

Two recent reviews that have investigated the neuropsychologic effects of seizures have reported mixed findings (25, 26), and the effect of seizures on neuropsychologic functioning remains unclear. Many studies have shown that people with epilepsy seem to deteriorate in different aspects of their cognitive functioning over time, which is often correlated with duration of epilepsy (27, 30–33). However, duration is a composite factor, which reflects the lifetime number of seizures, number of AEDs, and age of onset, and appears to be modified by education, as a measure of cerebral reserve (25, 26, 30, 31). In contrast, other studies have failed to find deteriorations over time (7, 34, 35).

Some deteriorations in functioning have been found to be significantly correlated with frequency of seizures (32, 33, 36). Frequency of tonic-clonic seizures was the most significant predictor of decreases in verbal IQ and performance IQ in a sample of 136 adults with epilepsy (32), and generalized tonic-clonic seizures are thought to have a greater cognitive impact than partial seizures (37). Further support for the detrimental impact of recurrent seizures on neuropsychologic functioning comes from several studies that have shown that following successful epilepsy surgery, patients have postsurgical improvements in cognitive functioning, and that seizure-free patients after surgery perform better than those who continue to experience seizures (30, 33, 34).

However, Kramer and colleagues correlated neuropsychologic test scores of 44 patients with epilepsy with clinical and demographic variables such as side of epileptic focus, age of onset, duration, and estimated number of complex partial and generalized seizures. No significant correlations were found, leading the authors to conclude that these findings support the notion that a multifactorial model is responsible for cognitive dysfunction (38). Similarly, despite finding that approximately 25% of 46 patients with temporal lobe epilepsy exhibited adverse cognitive changes on measures of intellectual ability, language, visuoperceptual/spatial ability, memory, executive functions, speeded psychomotor processing, and fine motor dexterity, number of seizures was not associated with these adverse changes. Those patients who experienced adverse cognitive changes were older, had a longer duration of epilepsy, lower baseline full-scale IQ, and abnormalities of quantitative volumes on magnetic resonance imaging (MRI) (39).

EFFECTS OF SUBCLINICAL SEIZURE ACTIVITY

Despite the mixed findings regarding the effects of ictal events, interictal subclinical activity may also lead to transitory cognitive impairment (TCI) that alters neuropsychologic functioning. However, neuropsychologic tests and cognitive activity can also elicit electroencephalographic (EEG) discharges that lead to a complex interaction (40, 41). TCI can have adverse effects on formal neuropsychological tests, such as tests of intellectual functioning or educational tasks, which may be material and site specific (41–44), as well as effects on daily living skills, such as driving (45), avoiding everyday hazards, and social interaction skills (40).

RECENT RESEARCH INTO THE NEUROPSYCHOLOGIC CONSEQUENCES OF EPILEPSY

It is clear from the previous reviews (25, 26) that prospective studies with newly diagnosed patients in whom information is collected on seizure type, seizure frequency, and AED treatment are going to be important in the determination of the differential factors associated with neuropsychologic impairment. One prospective study that clearly has the advantage of achieving this is a recent trial comparing Standard and New Antiepileptic Drugs (SANAD) (Baker GA, Taylor J, Aldenkamp AP, Smith D, et al., submitted). In this trial newly diagnosed patients, who have yet to establish a seizure history and have not yet started AED treatment, provide a unique opportunity to study the natural history of neuropsychologic functioning in epilepsy. Further, they allow us to give consideration to the effect of continuous seizures on neuropsychologic functioning.

RESULTS FROM THE NEUROPSYCHOLOGY ARM OF THE SANAD TRIAL

As part of the SANAD trial, patients were randomized to one of two arms: Arm A recruited patients for whom the clinician thought carbamazepine was the standard treatment and compared carbamazepine, gabapentin, lamotrigine, oxcarbazepine, and topiramate, and Arm B recruited patients for whom the clinician thought valproate was the standard treatment and compared valproate, lamotrigine, and topiramate (46, 47). The clinician prescribed according to their usual practice, using the dose and titration they thought most appropriate to the patient. At time of randomization into the SANAD trial, newly diagnosed participants from seven hospital centers in the United Kingdom were invited to take part in the neuropsychology add-on study (Baker et al., submitted).

Before the start of antiepileptic medication, 257 patients completed a comprehensive battery of neuropsychologic tests that assessed many aspects of cognitive functioning, as can be seen in Table 11-1. These 257 patients had an average age of 38.9 years; 52% were males; 72% had partial epilepsy, 13% had generalized epilepsy, and in 15% their epilepsy syndrome was unknown. Those patients recruited to Arm A of the study had a median number of 11 seizures at baseline and in Arm B had a median number of 9 seizures at baseline. They were comparable to the 740 SANAD patients from the same hospital centers who did not take part in the neuropsychology add-on study.

A total of 180 participants were retested at 3 months and 149 were followed up at 12 months. Patients dropped out for several reasons including withdrawing due to family pressures, relocation to another country, and being lost to follow-up. However, there was no evidence of any differences among those who responded at 1 year and those who did not, in terms of cognitive performance at baseline, randomized drug, or whether they achieved a 12-month remission immediately or not. However, there was a significant association for response at 1 year and drug withdrawal before 1 year, with a bias toward those who had changed their medication during the 12-month period not returning for neuropsychologic assessment.

Based on analysis of a final group of 223 patients who fulfilled the inclusion and exclusion criteria, analyses have been carried out that look at cognitive change

unexpected recurrent seizures (49, 50). Therefore, research that tries to resolve this debate and isolate and assess the relative effects of epilepsy and its treatment on neuropsychologic functioning is important to help us have a greater understanding of the factors involved in the development and course of neuropsychologic impairment.

The authors are now looking at the longer term effects of seizures and treatment on cognition; future results of the SANAD study may help to shed some light on their cognitive effects and tell us more about the natural history of cognitive impairment in people with epilepsy. However, it is clear that understanding the relationship between epilepsy and cognition requires a multidisciplinary approach. Input on the structural effects of seizures (by considering, for example, both human and animal models on the developed and developing brain) is necessary to understand the mechanisms by which functional consequences may arise. Further, considering the huge impact epilepsy has on psychosocial functioning and quality of life for the patient, we should consider both ictal and interictal epileptiform activity on not just cognitive performance, using traditional standardized neuropsychologic tests, but on day-to-day functioning of the patient as well.

References

1. Baxendale SA, van Paesschen W, Thompson PJ, Connelly A, et al. The relationship between qualitative MRI and neuropsychological functioning in temporal lobe epilepsy. *Epilepsia* 1998; 39:158–166.
2. Hermann BP, Seidenberg M, Schoenfeld J, Davies K. Neuropsychological characteristics of the syndrome of mesial temporal lobe epilepsy. *Arch Neurol* 1997; 54:369–376.
3. Aldenkamp AP, Baker GA, Meador KJ. The neuropsychology of epilepsy: what are the factors involved? *Epilepsy Behav* 2004; 5:S1–S2.
4. Aldenkamp AP. Cognitive impairment in epilepsy: state of affairs and clinical relevance. *Seizure* 2006; 15:219–220.
5. Hirsch E, Schmitz B, Carreño M. Epilepsy, antiepileptic drugs and cognition. *Acta Neurol Scand* 2003; 108(S180):23–32.
6. Äikiä M, Kälviäinen J, Riekkinen PJ. Verbal learning and memory in newly diagnosed partial epilepsy. *Epilepsy Res* 1995; 22:157–164.
7. Äikiä M, Salmenpera T, Partanen K, Kälviäinen J. Verbal memory in newly diagnosed patients and patients with chronic left temporal lobe epilepsy. *Epilepsy Behav* 2001; 2:20–27.
8. Prevey ML, Delaney RC, Cramer JA, Mattson RH. VA Epilepsy Cooperative Study 264 Group. Complex partial and secondarily generalised seizure patients: cognitive functioning prior to treatment with antiepileptic medication. *Epilepsy Res* 1998; 30:1–9.
9. Pulliainen V, Kuikka P, Jokelainen M. Motor and cognitive functions in newly diagnosed adult seizure patients before antiepileptic medication. *Acta Neurol Scand* 2000; 101:73–78.
10. Smith DB, Baker GA, Davies G, Dewey M, et al. Outcomes of add-on treatment with lamotrigine in partial epilepsy. *Epilepsia* 1993; 34:312–322.
11. Salinsky MC, Spencer DC, Oken BS, Storzbach D. Effects of oxcarbazepine and phenytoin on the EEG and cognition in healthy volunteers. *Epilepsy Behav* 2004; 5:894–902.
12. Meador KJ, Loring DW, Huh K, Gallagher BB, et al. Comparative cognitive effects of anticonvulsants. *Neurology* 1990; 40:391–394.
13. Meador KJ, Loring DW, Moore EE, Thompson WO, et al. Comparative cognitive effects of phenobarbital, phenytoin and valproate in healthy adults. *Neurology* 1995; 45:1494–1499.
14. Kalviainen R, Aikia M, Saukkonen AM, Mervaala E, et al. Vigabatrin vs carbamazepine monotherapy in patients with newly diagnosed epilepsy. *Arch Neurol* 1995; 52:989–996.
15. Coenen AML, Konings GMLG, Aldenkamp AP, Renier WO, et al. Effects of chronic use of carbamazepine and valproate on cognitive processes. *J Epilepsy* 1995; 8:250–254.
16. Meador KJ. Cognitive and memory effects of the new antiepileptic drugs. *Epilepsy Res* 2006; 68:63–67.
17. Äikiä M, Kälviäinen J, Sivenius J, Halonen T, et al. Cognitive effects of oxcarbazepine and phenytoin monotherapy in newly diagnosed epilepsy: one year follow-up. *Epilepsy Res* 1992; 11:199–203.
18. Fritz N, Glogau S, Hoffman J, Rademacher M, et al. Efficacy and cognitive side effects of tiagabine and topiramate in patients with epilepsy. *Epilepsy Behav* 2005; 6:373–381.
19. Thompson PJ, Baxendale SA, Duncan JS, Sander JW. Effects of topiramate on cognitive function. *J Neurol Neurosurg Psychiatry* 2000; 69:636–641.
20. Ojemann LM, Ojemann GA, Dodrill CB, Crawford CA, et al. Language disturbances as side effects of topiramate and zonisamide therapy. *Epilepsy Behav* 2001; 2:579–584.
21. Aldenkamp AP, Baker GA, Mulder OG, Chadwick DW, et al. A multicenter, randomized clinical study to evaluate the effect on cognitive function of topiramate compared with valproate as add-on therapy to carbamazepine in patients with partial-onset seizures. *Epilepsia* 2000; 41:1167–1178.
22. Kockelmann E, Elger CE, Helmstaedter C. Cognitive profile of topiramate as compared with lamotrigine in epilepsy patients on antiepileptic drug therapy polytherapy: relationships to blood serum levels and comedication. *Epilepsy Behav* 2004; 5:716–721.
23. Burton LA, Harden C. Effect of topiramate on attention. *Epilepsy Res* 1997; 27:29–32.
24. Martin R, Kuzniecky R, Ho S, Hetherington H, et al. Cognitive effects of topiramate, gabapentin and lamotrigine in healthy young adults. *Neurology* 1999; 52:321–327.
25. Vingerhoets G. Cognitive effects of seizures. *Seizure* 2006; 15:221–226.
26. Dodrill CB. Neuropsychological effects of seizures. *Epilepsy Behav* 2004; 5:S21–S24.
27. Andersson-Roswall L, Engman E, Samuelsson H, Sjöberg-Larsson C, et al. Verbal memory decline and adverse effects on cognition in adult patients wih pharmacoresistant partial epilepsy: a longitudinal controlled study of 36 patients. *Epilepsy Behav* 2004; 5:677–686.
28. Bjørnæs H, Stabell K, Henriksen O, Løyning Y. The effects of refractory epilepsy on intellectual functioning in children and adults. A longitudinal study. *Seizure* 2001; 10:250–259.
29. Bjørnæs H, Stabell K, Henriksen O, Røste G, et al. Surgical versus medical treatment for severe epilepsy: consequences for intellectual functioning in children and adults: A follow-up study. *Seizure* 2002; 11:473–482.
30. Jokeit H, Ebner A. Long term effects of refractory temporal lobe epilepsy on cognitive abilities: a cross-sectional study. *J Neurol Neurosurg Psychiatry* 1999; 67:44–50.
31. Oyegbile TO, Dow C, Jones J, Bell B, et al. The nature and course of neuropsychological morbidity in chronic temporal lobe epilepsy. *Neurology* 2004; 62:1736–1742.
32. Thompson PJ, Duncan JS. Cognitive decline in severe intractable epilepsy. *Epilepsia* 2005; 46:1780–1787.
33. Helmstaedter C, Kurthen M, Lux S, Reuber M, et al. Chronic epilepsy and cognition: A longitudinal study in temporal lobe epilepsy. *Ann Neurol* 2003; 54:425–432.
34. Selwa LM, Berent S, Giordani B, Henry TR, et al. Serial cognitive testing in temporal lobe epilepsy: longitudinal changes with medical and surgical therapies. *Epilepsia* 1994; 35:743–749.
35. Holmes MD, Dodrill CB, Wilkus RJ, Ojemann LM, et al. Is partial epilepsy progressive? Ten-year follow-up of EEG and neuropsychological changes in adults with partial seizures. *Epilepsia* 1998; 39:1189–1193.
36. Upton D, Thompson PJ. Neuropsychological test performance in frontal-lobe epilepsy: the influence of aetiology, seizure type, seizure frequency and duration of disorder. *Seizure* 1997; 6:443–447.
37. Aldenkamp AP, Bodde N. Behaviour, cognition and epilepsy. *Acta Neurol Scand Suppl* 2005; 182:19–25.
38. Kramer U, Kipervasser S, Neufeld MY, Fried I, et al. Is there any correlation between severity of epilepsy and cognitive abilities in patients with temporal lobe epilepsy? *Eur J Neurol* 2006; 13:130–134.
39. Hermann BP, Seidenberg M, Dow C, Jones J, et al. Cognitive prognosis in chronic temporal lobe epilepsy. *Ann Neurol* 2006; 60:80–87.
40. Binnie CD. Cognitive performance, subtle seizures and the EEG. *Epilepsia* 2001; 42(S1):16–18.
41. Binnie CD, Kasteleijn-Nolst Trenite DGA, Smit AM, Wilkins AJ. Interactions of epileptiform EEG discharges and cognition. *Epilepsy Res* 1987; 1:239–245.
42. Kasteleijn-Nolst Trenite DGA, Bakker DJ, Binnie CD, van Raaij M. Psychological effects of subclinical epileptiform discharges: scholastic skills. *Epilepsy Res* 1988; 2:111–116.
43. Siebelink BM, Bakker DJ, Binnie CD, Kasteleijn-Nolst Trenite DGA. Psychological effects of subclinical epileptiform EEG discharges in children: general intelligence tests. *Epilepsy Res* 1988; 2:117–121.
44. Aarts JH, Binnie CD, Smit AM, Wilkins AJ. Selective cognitive impairment during focal and generalized epileptiform EEG activity. *Brain* 1984; 107:293–308.
45. Kasteleijn-Nolst Trenite DGA, Riemersma JBJ, Binnie CD, Smit AM, et al. The influence of subclinical epileptiform EEG discharges on driving behaviour. *Electroencephalogr Clin Neurophysiol* 1987; 67:167–170.
46. Marson AG, Al-Kharusi AM, Alwaidh M, Appleton R, et al. The SANAD study of effectiveness of carbamazepine, gabapentin, lamotrigine, oxcarbazepine, or topiramate for treatment of partial epilepsy: an unblinded randomised controlled trial. *Lancet.* 2007; 369(9566):1000–15.
47. Marson AG, Al-Kharusi AM, Alwaidh M, Appleton R, et al. The SANAD study of effectiveness of valproate, lamotrigine, or topiramate for generalised and unclassifiable epilepsy: an unblinded randomised controlled trial. *Lancet.* 2007; 369(9566): 1016–26.
48. Binnie CD. Cognitive impairment during epileptiform discharges: is it ever justifiable to treat the EEG? *Lancet* 2003; 2:725–730.
49. Shackleton DP, Kasteleijn-Nolst Trenite DGA, de Craen AJ, Vandenbroucke JP, et al. Living with epilepsy: long term prognosis and psychosocial outcomes. *Neurology* 2003; 61:64–70.
50. Swinkels WA, Shackleton DP, Trenite DG. Psychosocial impact of epileptic seizures in a Dutch epilepsy population: a comparative Washington Psychosocial Inventory study. *Epilepsia* 2000; 41:1335–1341.

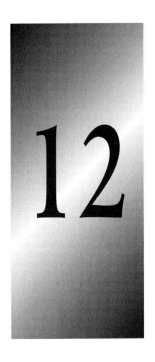

12 Seizures and Consciousness

Andrea Eugenio Cavanna

His sensation of being alive and his awareness increased tenfold . . . his mind and heart were flooded by a dazzling light . . . culminating in a great calm, full of serene and harmonious joy and hope, full of understanding and the knowledge of the final cause.

Prince Myshkin's seizure in Fyodor Dostoyevsky's *The Idiot* (1868)

Epilepsy has long been associated with alterations in consciousness. Not surprisingly, altered conscious states are thought to represent a touchstone for the recognition of seizure activity (1). This was formalized in 1981, when the revised classification of epileptic seizures recommended that impairment of consciousness be used as the criterion for differentiating simple from complex partial seizures (2). Since then, the evaluation of consciousness has been essential to the phenomenological description, diagnosis, and classification of epilepsy (3).

In addition to complex partial seizures, two other types of seizures are classically known as causing impairment of consciousness: generalized tonic-clonic and absence seizures. The difficulties surrounding the criteria for determining impairment of consciousness were partly resolved by operationally defining consciousness as the patient's responsiveness during the ictal state. However,

it has been shown that ictal disturbances of sensory processes, speech, memory, or attention, resulting in transient unresponsiveness, are easily misinterpreted as impaired consciousness (3). Furthermore, such a use of the concept of consciousness can be misleading, because both generalized and complex partial seizures entail unresponsiveness during the epileptic discharge, but their effects on the patient's ictal conscious state show significant differences, as a consequence of the different involvement of the neurologic substrates (4, 5).

Despite well-recognized difficulties in formulating an unequivocal definition of the concept of consciousness, converging evidence from neurophysiologic and neuroimaging studies suggests a fundamental distinction between the quantitative (level) and qualitative (content) features of consciousness (6). The level of consciousness is the degree of wakefulness or arousal, ranging from alertness through drowsiness to coma. It depends on the integrity of the ascending pontomesodiencephalic reticular pathways and the widespread thalamocortical projections, and it can be quantified by analyzing the behavioral responses that are constituent functions of consciousness as general awareness (i.e., motor and verbal responses to external stimuli). The level of consciousness is what clinical neurologists usually refer to when reporting "impairment" or "loss" of consciousness in the phenomenological description of epileptic seizures (3).

Video monitoring has long been used to document the full extent of ictal unresponsiveness in clinical settings.

The second major dimension of consciousness is the content of subjective experience: sensations, emotions, memories, intentions, and all the feelings that color our inner world. This feature is determined by the interaction between exogenous factors derived from our environment and endogenous factors such as attention. The "vividness" and the emotional significance associated with such experiences seem to be modulated by temporolimbic activity and show a remarkable variability, ranging from "peripheral consciousness" phenomena to highly intense experiences (7). Although the subjective dimension of the ictal conscious state characterizes most complex partial seizures of temporal lobe origin, it is often neglected in clinical practice, partly because of definitional problems and related miscommunication between patients with epilepsy and their physicians.

It has been pointed out that the assessment of both the level and the contents of conscious states is crucial for an in-depth understanding of the clinical alterations of consciousness occurring during the various kinds of epileptic seizures (8). Monaco et al. (9) stressed the conceptual usefulness of plotting the level and contents of consciousness in a biaxial diagram that indicates the possible conscious states of a subject according to these features. For instance, in the normal waking state the level of consciousness is almost constantly elevated, whereas the contents of subjective experience show a greater variability, depending on the environmental stimuli and the internal focus of the individual (Figure 12-1A).

In epileptology, the overall assessment of the ictal conscious state has been left so far to the observer's interpretation and personal vocabulary, often with poor inter-rater and intra-rater reliability, especially in the absence of standardized tools to perform a quantitative analysis of each dimension. The Ictal Consciousness Inventory (ICI) is a self-report twenty-item instrument specifically developed by the author to quantify the level of general awareness/responsiveness (items 1–10) and the "vividness" of ictal experiential phenomena (items 11–20) during epileptic seizures (see Appendix). Such an instrument should guide the standard representation of the ictal conscious state through the outlined bidimensional model (level vs. contents of consciousness). Moreover, the ICI helps to dissect the exact nature of the impairment of consciousness, thus leading to a clear-cut differentiation between seizures that primarily affect the level of awareness (generalized seizures) and seizures that specifically alter the contents of the ictal conscious state (focal seizures). The following paragraphs provide an up-to-date review of the neurologic literature on the relationship between epilepsy and consciousness, in light of the level-versus-content dichotomy about the description of seizure-induced alterations of conscious states.

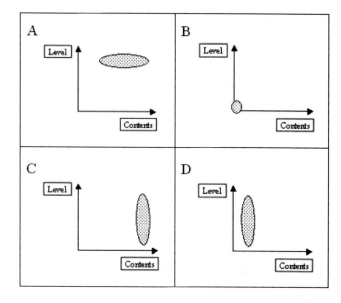

FIGURE 12-1

Bidimensional model of consciousness (level vs. contents). Dots indicate possible conscious states in different conditions. (A) Healthy subject during wakefulness. Unlike the level of arousal, which is almost constantly high, the vividness of the contents of consciousness experienced in the wakeful state shows a wide degree of variability. (B) Generalized seizure. Both the level of arousal and the contents of conscious experience are virtually absent. (C) Focal seizure with experiential symptoms. The level of arousal displays a wide range of degrees, and the contents of consciousness are almost constantly vivid. (D) Limbic status epilepticus. The level of arousal and responsiveness can vary, but no subjective experiences are present ("zombie-like behavior"). Reprinted from Monaco F, Mula M, Cavanna AE. Consciousness, epilepsy, and emotional qualia. *Epilepsy Behav* 2005;7:150–160, with permission from Elsevier.

ICTAL CONSCIOUSNESS IN GENERALIZED SEIZURES

Both primary and secondary generalized seizures are associated with a transient disappearance of both level and contents of consciousness. Consequently, generalized tonic-clonic seizures ("grand mal" epilepsy) and typical childhood absences ("petit mal" epilepsy) are the most common causes of epileptically induced loss of consciousness (5). The bidimensional model of complete loss of consciousness during a generalized tonic-clonic or absence seizure is shown in Figure 12-1B.

The dramatic alteration of consciousness observed during the course of a generalized convulsive seizure can persist up to minutes and is invariably accompanied by rigid stiffening of the limbs followed by violent bilateral spasms. Profound lethargy and confusion (i.e., decreased level of general awareness) typically last for a variable period after the main episode ends. Several studies based on electrophysiological, blood flow, and metabolic mapping suggested that the entire brain could be homogeneously involved in primary generalized tonic-clonic seizures. However, a recent single-photon emission computed tomography (SPECT) ictal-interictal imaging study reported that the regions most intensely involved by cerebral blood flow (CBF) increase were bilateral frontal and parietal association cortices, together with thalamus and upper brainstem (10). The transient disruption of the functional connectivity between bilateral cortical regions, and between thalamus and cortex, seems to be the main mechanism accounting for the loss of consciousness.

Absence seizures are characterized by rather stereotyped phenomenological features, consisting of a brisk interruption of the patient's behavior, with staring, unresponsiveness, and possible eyelid fluttering or mild myoclonic spasms. No subjective experience accompanies these relatively frequent seizures, as they entail a sudden blackout of both level of awareness and conscious contents. Several human and animal studies have suggested that absence seizures are generated through abnormal network oscillations involving the cortex of the two hemispheres and the thalamic nuclei, which represent the target of the brainstem reticular activating projections (11). These oscillations result in the classical electroencephalographic (EEG) pattern of large amplitude, bilateral, 3- to 4-Hz spike-wave discharges, usually lasting less than 10 seconds. Human imaging studies have yielded more controversial results, with some studies showing global increases in CBF and others showing variable patterns of increased or decreased brain metabolism; for a comprehensive review, see the study by Blumenfeld (12). By combining these data with the results of their studies in animal models, Blumenfeld and Taylor (5) formulated the hypothesis that loss of consciousness in absence seizures is due to a disruption of the normal information processing at the level of bilateral frontal and parietal association cortices and related subcortical structures.

More recently, studies of patients with generalized spike-wave activity have achieved excellent standards of spatial and temporal resolution by coupling functional magnetic resonance imaging (fMRI) with simultaneous EEG recordings (13, 14). Interestingly, preliminary EEG-fMRI findings confirmed that generalized seizures may selectively involve certain networks while sparing others. In particular, they demonstrated bilateral thalamic activation and cortical signal decrease in a characteristic distribution of association areas that are most active during conscious rest, that is, prefrontal, lateral parietal, and midline precuneus/posterior cingulate cortex. According to the "default mode of brain function" hypothesis, these areas show transient deactivations whenever healthy subjects are engaged in non-self-referential cognitive tasks and in conditions of strongly reduced vigilance, such as deep sleep, coma or vegetative states, and drug-induced general anesthesia (15). EEG-fMRI studies of impaired consciousness in generalized seizures provide further evidence that default mode areas likely represent a key part of the neural network subserving the level of general awareness.

ICTAL CONSCIOUSNESS IN FOCAL SEIZURES

Focal epileptic seizures originate in specific parts of the cortex and either remain confined to those areas or spread to other parts of the brain. The clinical manifestations are related to the area of the cortex in which the seizures start, how widely they are propagated, and how long they last. Since the early observations by Hughlings-Jackson on "psychical states which are much more elaborate than crude sensations" (16), it is clear that local epileptic activity arising from the temporal lobe often creates experiential events in the patient's mind. Such manifestations of temporal lobe epilepsy are among the most fascinating and poorly understood neurologic phenomena.

Experiential phenomena are usually brief and coincide with the onset of a complex partial seizure or with psychic epileptic auras (17). Sometimes they are followed by automatisms, stereotyped behavioral patterns (e.g., lip smacking, chewing) that occur with altered responsiveness, and amnesia for the activity. Both experiential sensory seizures and auras can include affective, mnemonic, or composite perceptual phenomena, such as complex illusions and hallucinations involving any sensory system, but most commonly the visual or auditory modalities. The affective components of experiential phenomena include unpleasant (fear, guilt, sadness) or pleasant (euphoria, joy, excitement) subjective feelings, along with symptoms of depersonalization (altered sense of self) and derealization (altered experience of the external world) (18). Mystical and ecstatic feelings have been occasionally reported—and beautifully described by one of the most talented and prolific authors affected by epilepsy, Fyodor Dostoyevsky (Figure 12-2) (19).

In addition to their clinical significance, these psychic phenomena raise interesting questions concerning brain mechanisms involved in the production of some the most elusive, yet familiar, human experiences, which the current philosophical jargon refers to as phenomenal *qualia* (9). Roughly speaking, a quale (singular of qualia) is the "what it is like" character of a mental state: the way it feels to have a mental state such as feeling pain, seeing red, smelling a rose, and so forth. Therefore, qualia are the subjective texture of experience, which is the essence of the qualitative dimension of consciousness. The detailed investigation of the neural processes taking place at the level of the limbic structures of the medial temporal lobe during complex partial seizures will likely result in useful insights for the ultimate search for the neural correlates of these subjective experiences.

Psychic or experiential phenomena that involve perceptual, mnemonic, and affective processes have been elicited by medial temporal lobe seizures, discharges, and stimulation. For example, it has been proposed that the activation of the amygdala and other limbic structures is responsible for the affective component of experiential phenomena (20). Consequently, focal seizures are thought to modulate the contents of the ictal conscious state in medial temporal lobe epilepsy. Figure 12-1C shows the bidimensional model of altered conscious states during a focal seizure or aura with experiential symptoms, characterized by the dissociation between vivid contents (qualia) and unstable level of arousal.

Another set of peculiar alterations of ictal consciousness occur during limbic status epilepticus, formerly called "psychomotor status." Penfield (21) described patients with epilepsy who were "totally unconscious," but nonetheless continued their activities of walking in a crowded street or driving home or playing a piano piece even for hours, but in a sort of inflexible and uncreative way. They seemed capable of sidestepping obstacles in the environment, grasping objects, and sometimes responding to movement and speech—yet, they were not aware of their purposeful actions. More recently Koch and Crick (22) called these seemingly automatic activities "zombie modes." In philosophy of mind, zombies are conceived as beings whose behavior is utterly indistinguishable from that of normal humans, but who have no "inner life" at all. In other words, philosophical zombies lack phenomenal qualia and therefore do not experience subjective contents of consciousness. This scenario is represented in Figure 12-1D.

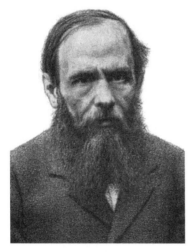

FIGURE 12-2

Fyodor Dostoyevsky (1821–1881).

The neurobiological changes associated with complex partial seizures have also been recently addressed by functional imaging studies. Interictal and ictal SPECT with early injection during complex partial seizures in patients with hippocampal sclerosis showed ictal hyperperfusion in the temporal lobe ipsilateral to the seizure focus, along with ipsilateral middle frontal and precentral gyrus and both occipital lobes. Conversely, the frontal lobes, contralateral posterior cerebellum, and ipsilateral precuneus showed hypoperfusion (23). In another SPECT ictal-interictal study in patients with surgically confirmed mesial temporal sclerosis, Blumenfeld et al. (24) analyzed ictal CBF changes while performing continuous video-EEG monitoring. They found that temporal lobe seizures associated with loss of consciousness (complex partial seizures) produced CBF increases in the temporal lobe, followed by increases in bilateral midline subcortical structures, including the mediodorsal thalamus and upper brainstem. These changes were accompanied by marked bilateral hypometabolism in the frontal and parietal association cortices (lateral prefrontal, anterior cingulate, orbital frontal, and lateral parietal cortex). In contrast, temporal lobe seizures in which consciousness was spared (simple partial seizures) were associated with more limited changes, mainly confined to the temporal lobe, and were not accompanied by such widespread impaired function of the frontoparietal association cortices. Intracranial EEG recordings from temporal lobe seizures accompanied by impaired responsiveness confirmed the profound slowing in bilateral frontal and parietal association cortices, which is particularly severe in the late ictal phase and extends to the early postictal period (25).

These findings are consistent with Norden and Blumenfeld's "network inhibition hypothesis," according to which focal seizures arising in the medial temporal lobe spread to subcortical structures (medial diencephalon and pontomesencephalic reticular formation) and disrupt their activating function, secondarily leading to widespread inhibition of nonseizing regions of the frontal and parietal association cortex (26). The frontoparietal network inhibition may ultimately be responsible for the impaired level of consciousness reported in the late ictal and immediate postictal phase of some complex partial seizures. Such an intriguing, yet sophisticated, model of selective association cortex inhibition by a focal cortical seizure is gradually replacing the long-lasting concept of critical mass of cerebral tissue involved in seizure spread to cause impairment of consciousness.

CONCLUDING REMARKS

The concept of consciousness is central in epileptology, despite the methodological difficulties concerning its application to the multifaced ictal phenomenology. The different epileptic ictal semiologies offer unique avenues for the understanding of the relationship between pathological brain function and altered conscious states. Both the level of awareness and the contents of conscious states are affected by epileptic seizures. Generalized tonic-clonic and absence seizures primarily impair the level of consciousness ("blackout"), whereas focal seizures mainly alter the patient's private experiences. Sometimes the changes in the conscious state encompass both the level and the contents, in a very articulate and entangled way, as in complex partial seizures of temporal lobe origin. In this respect, a bidimensional model displaying the level and the contents of consciousness in two separate axes could prove to be highly valuable in assessing both the quantitative and qualitative changes that characterize the ictal conscious state. Table 12-1 summarizes the pattern of alterations of the level and contents of consciousness in the ictal semiologies described in this chapter. Neurophysiologic and imaging findings provide a sound basis for the development of such a model, because different neural mechanisms have been shown to underlie the level and the content of consciousness. As for determining the level of awareness, a crucial role seems to be played by either primitive (in generalized seizures) or secondary (in focal seizures) involvement of subcortical structures, thus leading to disrupted activity in frontoparietal and midline (precuneus/posterior cingulate cortex) associative networks. On the other hand, the qualitative features of experiential phenomena—arguably the most precise neurobiological correlate of the philosophical concept of qualia—are mainly the expression of the activity of limbic

TABLE 12-1

Summary of the Possible Alterations in the Cardinal Parameters of the Bidimensional Model (Level and Contents of the Ictal Conscious State) in the Main Seizure Types Affecting Consciousness*

SEIZURE	LEVEL OF CONSCIOUSNESS	CONTENTS OF CONSCIOUSNESS
Generalized tonic-clonic	↓	↓
Absence	↓	↓
Focal, experiential type	↓↑	↑
Limbic status	↓↑	↓

*Reprinted from Monaco F, Mula M, Cavanna AE. Consciousness, epilepsy, and emotional qualia. *Epilepsy Behav* 2005;7:150–160, with permission from Elsevier.

components of the temporal lobe. A systematic analysis of such experiential phenomena should be included in a complete diagnostic protocol for epilepsy, to achieve a better understanding of the patient's subjective ictal experience. Conversely, further investigations of the neural correlates of seizure-induced alterations of consciousness may contribute to shed light on some of the unanswered questions concerning the brain mechanisms involved in the production of human conscious experiences.

References

1. Zappulla RA. Epilepsy and consciousness. *Semin Neurol* 1997; 17:113–119.
2. Commission on Classification and Terminology of the International League Against Epilepsy. Proposal for revised clinical and electroencephalographic classification of seizures. *Epilepsia* 1981; 22:489–501.
3. Gloor P. Consciousness as a neurological concept in epileptology: a critical review. *Epilepsia* 1986; 27(Suppl 2):14–26.
4. Kalamangalam GP. Epilepsy and the physical basis of consciousness. *Seizure* 2001; 10:484–491.
5. Blumenfeld H, Taylor J. Why do seizures cause loss of consciousness? *Neuroscientist* 2003; 9:1–10.
6. Zeman A. Consciousness. *Brain* 2001; 124:1263–1289.
7. Johanson M, Revonsuo A, Chaplin J, et al. Level and contents of consciousness in connection with partial epileptic seizures. *Epilepsy Behav* 2003; 4:279–285.
8. Gloor P. Experiential phenomena of temporal lobe epilepsy: facts and hypotheses. *Brain* 1990; 113:1673–1694.
9. Monaco F, Mula M, Cavanna AE. Consciousness, epilepsy, and emotional qualia. *Epilepsy Behav* 2005; 7:150–160.
10. Blumenfeld H, Westerveld M, Ostroff RB, et al. Selective frontal, parietal, and temporal networks in generalized seizures. *Neuroimage* 2003; 19:1556–1566.
11. Kostopoulos GK. Involvement of the thalamocortical system in epileptic loss of consciousness. *Epilepsia* 2001; 42:13–19.
12. Blumenfeld H. Consciousness and epilepsy: why are patients with absence seizures absent? *Prog Brain Res* 2005; 150:271–286.
13. Gotman J, Grova C, Bagshaw A, et al. Generalized epileptic discharges show thalamo-cortical activation and suspension of the default state of the brain. *Proc Natl Acad Sci U S A* 2006; 102:15236–15240.
14. Laufs H, Lengler U, Hamandi K, et al. Linking generalized spike-and-wave discharges and resting state brain activity by using EEG/fMRI in a patient with absence seizures. *Epilepsia* 2006; 47:444–448.
15. Cavanna AE, Trimble MR. The precuneus: a review of its functional anatomy and behavioural correlates. *Brain* 2006; 129:564–583.
16. Hogan RE, Kaiboriboon K. The "dreamy state": John Hughlings-Jackson's ideas of epilepsy and consciousness. *Am J Psychiatry* 2003; 160:1740–1747.
17. Alvarez-Silva S, Alvarez-Silva I, Alvarez-Rodriguez J, et al. Epileptic consciousness: concept and meaning of aura. *Epilepsy Behav* 2006; 8:527–533.
18. Mula M, Cavanna A, Collimedaglia L, et al. The role of aura in psychopathology and dissociative experiences in epilepsy. *J Neuropsychiatry Clin Neurosci* 2006; 18:536–542.
19. Hughes JR. The idiosyncratic aspects of the epilepsy of Fyodor Dostoevsky. *Epilepsy Behav* 2005; 7:531–538.
20. Fried I. Auras and experiential responses arising in the temporal lobe. *J Neuropsychiatry Clin Neurosci* 1997; 9:420–428.
21. Penfield W. The mystery of the mind: a critical study of consciousness and the human brain. Princeton, NJ: Princeton University Press, 1975.
22. Koch C, Crick FC. The zombie within. *Nature* 2001; 411:893.
23. Van Paesschen W, Dupont P, Van Driel G, et al. SPECT perfusion changes during complex partial seizures in patients with hippocampal sclerosis. *Epilepsia* 2003; 42:857–862.
24. Blumenfeld H, McNally KA, Vanderhill SD, et al. Positive and negative network correlations in temporal lobe epilepsy. *Cereb Cortex* 2004; 14:892–902.
25. Blumenfeld H, Rivera M, McNally KA, et al. Ictal neocortical slowing in temporal lobe epilepsy. *Neurology* 2004; 63:1015–1021.
26. Norden AD, Blumenfeld H. The role of subcortical structures in human epilepsy. *Epilepsy Behav* 2002; 3:219–231.

APPENDIX: MEASURING ICTAL BEHAVIORS

ICI (Ictal Consciousness Inventory)

Please answer the following questions by referring to a single seizure, witnessed by another person. Answers: 0 = no; 1 = yes, a bit (yes, vaguely); 2 = yes, much (yes, clearly).

DURING THE SEIZURE WERE YOU . . .			
1. aware of what was happening to you?	0	1	2
2. aware of your surroundings?	0	1	2
3. aware of the time passing by?	0	1	2
4. aware of the presence of anyone around you?	0	1	2
5. able to understand other people's words?	0	1	2
6. able to reply to other people's words (e.g., *What's wrong with you?*)?	0	1	2
7. able to obey other people's commands (e.g., *Sit down!*)?	0	1	2
8. able to control the direction of your gaze?	0	1	2
9. able to focus your attention?	0	1	2
10. able to take any initiative?	0	1	2
DURING THE SEIZURE DID YOU . . .			
11. feel like you were in a dream?	0	1	2
12. feel like you were in an unusually familiar place?	0	1	2
13. feel that things around you were unknown?	0	1	2
14. feel that everything was in slow motion or sped up?	0	1	2
15. feel the presence of another person who was not there?	0	1	2
16. see or hear things that were not real?	0	1	2
17. see people/objects changing shape?	0	1	2
18. experience flashbacks or memories of past events (as though you were reliving the past)?	0	1	2
19. experience unpleasant emotions (e.g., fear, sadness, anger)?	0	1	2
20. experience pleasant emotions (e.g. joy, happiness, pleasure)?	0	1	2

13 Postictal Phenomena in Epilepsy

Andres M. Kanner

n a review article published in 2000 in the journal *Epilepsy & Behavior*, Fisher and Schachter observed that "some of the disability deriving from epilepsy derives from the postictal state. The postictal state may be complicated by impaired cognition, headache, injuries, or secondary medical conditions. Postictal depression is common, postictal psychosis relatively rare, but both add to the morbidity of seizures." They concluded that "the mechanisms of the postictal state are poorly understood" (1). Indeed, the postictal state has multiple clinical expressions, which include cognitive deficits, psychiatric symptoms or episodes, neurologic disturbances in the form of positive symptoms such as headaches, or deficits such as paralysis or hypoesthesia. Often, postictal symptoms may help localize (i.e., suggest the ictogenic lobe) or lateralize the site of the seizure focus, or they may be a window to an underlying neurologic deficit that may be subtle or inconspicuous in its presentation interictally. Furthermore, as shown subsequently, postictal psychiatric symptoms may serve as a red flag of potential interictal psychiatric disorder. The aim of this chapter is to review the most frequent clinical expressions of the postictal state (PS) along with their implications for an underlying pathologic state and implications for localization of the ictal focus.

The PS comprises clinical, electrical, and neurochemical changes that occur after a seizure. Yet these changes can occur at different times. For example, the most obvious clinical change is the confusional state displayed by patients *immediately* after a seizure (i.e., within the first 20 minutes of a seizure). Immediate postictal neurochemical changes yield significant serum elevation of prolactin and cortisol levels that peak 10 to 20 minutes after the ictus and return to baseline levels within 60 to 90 minutes (2, 3). On the other hand, postictal symptoms can occur following a "symptom-free" period that can range from several hours to up to five days, as is the case of postictal psychiatric symptoms or episodes. We refer to this PS as "delayed" PS. Failure to recognize it leads to the frequent misdiagnosis of postictal psychiatric episodes as interictal episodes. This topic is discussed in great detail in this chapter. Accordingly, PS should be divided into the *immediate* and *delayed* states.

ENDOGENOUS CHANGES DURING THE PS

The classic electrographic evidence of the PS is represented by a focal or generalized slowing of the background activity, the duration of which may be related to the duration of the ictus, its extent of propagation, and the "seizure density" preceding the recorded slow-wave activity. Such electrographic changes have led to the suggestion that the PS reflects a state of "exhaustion" of the brain. Fisher and Prince, however, refuted such hypotheses, as they demonstrated in animal models that "neurons can be made to fire after a seizure when properly stimulated after a seizure" (4).

Neuronal cells hyperpolarize after a seizure. Three mechanisms have been identified: (i) fast inhibitory postsynaptic potentials (IPSP) that act at the gamma-aminobutyric acid-$_A$ receptor (GABA$_A$); (ii) late hyperpolarizing potentials mediated at the GABA$_B$ receptors; and (iii) calcium-activated potassium currents resulting in after-hyperpolarization (AHP) (1, 5). Fisher and Schachter, however, noted that these mechanisms are too short in duration to explain the PS. Instead, they suggested the role of hyperpolarizing pumps that yield a neuronal inactivation long enough to correlate with clinical phenomena of the PS (1). Such pumps are mediated through mechanisms mediated by ATP.

Several neurotransmitters have been involved in the PS, including adenosine, opiates, acetylcholine, catecholamines, serotonin, and, finally, nitrous oxide, though the actual mechanisms by which they are operant in the PS are yet to be clearly established. Fisher and Schachter suggested that nitrous oxide may mediate its impact on PS through an effect on cerebral flow. Disturbance of the cerebral circulation in the PS is supported by recent studies of Perfenova et al. (6). Indeed, in animal seizure models carried out in piglets, these investigators demonstrated severe postictal cerebral vascular dysfunction after sustained seizures that was evident at least two days after the seizure. In addition, they showed a marked reduction of cerebral vascular responses to both endothelium-dependent and -independent, physiologically relevant vasodilators (hypercapnia, bradykinin, isoproterenol, and sodium nitroprusside) during the extended postictal period. These investigators attributed these vascular disturbances to an inhibition of the antioxidative enzyme heme oxygenase (HO), which is necessary for increased cerebral blood flow during the ictal episode and for normal cerebral vascular functioning during the immediate postictal period.

For its part, adenosine is a known powerful suppressor of synaptic activity, which increases severalfold during a seizure (7). It is a potent inhibitory neuromodulator and has been proposed as an endogenous anticonvulsant. Adenosine receptor densities increase after repeated seizures in young rats, and its inhibitory effect in humans has also been demonstrated. For example, During and Spencer implanted depth electrodes in the hippocampi of four patients with intractable temporal lobe epilepsy (TLE) (8). The probes were modified to include a microdialysis and were kept for periods of 10 to 16 days. Extracellular adenosine samples were collected bilaterally at 3-minute intervals before, during, and after a single, spontaneous-onset seizure in each patient. All seizures commenced in one hippocampus and propagated to the contralateral hippocampus. Extracellular adenosine levels increased by 6- to 31-fold, with the increase significantly greater in the epileptogenic hippocampus. Adenosine levels remained elevated above basal values for the entire 18-minute postictal period. Furthermore, animal models have shown that adenosine agonists prolong the PS, while antagonists block it. Also, adenosine has been found to play a role in the cerebral regulation during and following a seizure. Indeed, DiGeronimo et al. demonstrated that postictal administration of adenosine restores hypoxia-induced cerebral vasodilation in piglets, even when a nondilating concentration is employed (9). This suggests that depletion of adenosine with seizure activity is a mechanism for the loss of postictal cerebral vasodilatation to hypoxia.

Opiates play important but very complex pathogenic roles in epilepsy. For example, a high density of opiate mu receptors has been identified in the vicinity of ictal foci in TLE (1). This finding has been interpreted to imply a role of these opiate receptors in limiting the spread of the epileptic activity. Furthermore, administration of the opiate antagonist naloxone was found to yield an increase of close to 40% of postictal epileptiform discharges in patients undergoing a prolonged video-EEG (v-EEG) monitoring study (10). See also the section on postictal psychiatric phenomena.

POSTICTAL NEUROLOGIC PHENOMENA

The most frequent include cognitive disturbances, focal motor and sensory deficits, postictal headaches and migraines, and postictal automatisms. These will be briefly reviewed in the following subsections.

Postictal Cognitive Deficits

In a study of 100 consecutive patients with refractory epilepsy, Kanner et al. identified postictal cognitive and psychiatric symptoms occurring after more than 50% of seizures during a three-month period (see Table 13-1) (11). Among the 100 patients, they identified a mean of 8.8 ± 6.5 habitual postictal symptoms (range: 0 to 25; median = 8) corresponding to 2.8 ± 1.8 postictal cognitive symptoms (range: 0 to 5; median = 3). Sixty-eight patients experienced postictal cognitive and psychiatric symptoms, and 14 experienced only postictal cognitive symptoms; 12 patients failed to experience any postictal symptom.

These data clearly demonstrate the relatively long duration of postictal cognitive symptoms. The wide ranges in the duration of these symptoms are the reflection of the interplay of several variables. These include the duration of the ictus, the location of the seizure focus, and the existence of underlying specific deficits (e.g., verbal

TABLE 13-1
Prevalence of Postictal Cognitive Symptoms

TYPE OF COGNITIVE DEFICIT	PREVALENCE, N = 100	DURATION IN HRS, MEAN ± S.D. [MEDIAN IN HRS] (RANGE)
Cognitive symptoms, total	82	
Difficulty in concentration	71	16.2 ± 22.6 [6] (10 min–108 hr)
Problems with memory	66	18.2 ± 23.6 [6] (10 min.–108 hr)
Confusion	65	10.6 ± 14.6 [2] (10 min–72 hr.)
Disorientation	46	2.6 ± 5.5 [1] (5 min–24 hr.)
Thought blockage	42	16.7 ± 21.2 [6] (10 min–98 hr)
Only cognitive symptoms, total	14	

memory disturbances in left TLE). For example, a patient with a seizure disorder that resulted from a stroke in the territory of the middle cerebral artery of the dominant hemisphere, which resulted in a residual mild dysphasia, may experience a global aphasia of several hours duration following a seizure. Likewise, it is not unusual for patients with TLE to notice a marked deterioration of an underlying memory deficit during the PS. Some of the cognitive disturbances deserve closer scrutiny, as they may help lateralize the ictal focus. Such is the case of postictal language disturbances.

Postictal Aphasia

A review of the literature associates postictal language disturbances with a temporal lobe seizure focus in the dominant hemisphere (12). For example, Adam et al. analyzed the semiology of epileptic seizures on the v-EEG of 35 patients (26 temporal, 8 frontal, 1 parietal) with a good postsurgical outcome (Engel's class I and II) (13). Language dominance had been established with the intracarotid amobarbital test. In 15 cases (29 seizures), postictal language manifestations were analyzed in relation with the propagation of the epileptic activity recorded by intracerebral EEG. They found that postictal aphasia was observed only when seizures originated in the dominant hemisphere and ictal activity spread to Wernicke and/or Broca language areas. They noted that no postictal aphasia was observed when the epileptic focus was in the nondominant hemisphere, even if there was secondary generalization of ictal activity affecting the language areas of the dominant hemisphere. The data of Williamson et al. support these findings, as they found that postictal aphasia and prolonged recovery time were characteristic of seizure origin in the language-dominant hemisphere (14). Privitera et al. performed a prospective study of ictal and postictal language function after 105 temporal lobe complex partial seizures (CPSs) in 26 patients (15). At the time of the seizure, the patients were asked to read a test phrase aloud until it was read

correctly and clearly. In all 62 seizures originating from the left temporal lobe, the patients took more than 68 seconds to read the test phrase correctly (mean, 321.9 seconds); in 42 of 43 seizures from the right temporal lobe, the patients read the test phrase in less than 54 seconds (mean, 19.7 seconds). Postictal paraphasias occurred in 46 of 62 seizures from the left temporal lobe in 11 of 14 patients.

Other studies, however, have found that propagation of ictal activity from the nondominant to the dominant temporal lobe can account as well for postictal language disturbances. For example, Ficker et al. found that patients whose seizures began in the nondominant temporal lobe and propagated to the contralateral temporal lobe had a prolonged postictal language delay with paraphasic errors compared with seizures that did not spread (16). Shorter propagation time was also associated with longer postictal language disturbances. The findings of a study by Devinsky et al. tend to support the lack of specificity in the localization of ictal foci with postictal language disturbances (17). These investigators studied postictal behavior following 65 CPSs in 18 patients with left-hemisphere language dominance using subdural electrode recordings. The mean interval for a first correct verbal response did not differ significantly between patients with right and left ictal foci (left foci, 275 seconds; right foci, 167 seconds). Impaired comprehension with fluent but unintelligible speech, as well as anomia, occurred after seizures arising from either temporal lobe. On the other hand, all nine seizures followed by global or nonfluent aphasia originated on the left side, and the researchers found that paraphasic errors were significantly more common after left temporal CPSs.

Several studies have demonstrated that postictal aphasia appears to be significantly more common among patients with TLE than among patients with frontal lobe seizures. For example, Goldberg-Stern et al. studied postictal language disturbances in 118 frontal lobe CPSs recorded in 24 patients (18). Prolonged postictal disturbances occurred in only 7% of CPSs confined to the dominant frontal lobe, compared with 91% of CPSs that started as frontal and spread to the dominant temporal lobe.

Postictal Memory Disturbances

Postictal memory disturbances are relatively frequent and can last several days. Postictal memory disturbances are more particularly frequent in TLE, given the pivotal role of the mesial temporal structures in memory processing. In fact, Helmstaedter et al. found no effect on postictal memory performances in frontal lobe seizures, whereas verbal and visual recognition memory were significantly decreased after temporal lobe seizures (19). Decrease in either verbal or visual memory and time of recovery were related to lateralization of seizure onset.

The severity of postictal memory disturbances are a function of the damage to mesial temporal structures. This was illustrated in animal models of postictal memory disturbances carried out by Boukhezra et al., who compared the behavioral features of seizures with postictal memory impairment in young seizure-naïve rats and rats with a prior history of status epilepticus (SE) (20). In addition, they also examined the relationship between postictal EEG changes and cognitive recovery. Following generalized seizures, rats had impaired performance in the water maze, a measure of visual spatial memory processing in these animals. The duration of their inability to find a platform exceeded the length of the seizure, and there was not a close relationship between duration of cognitive impairment and either latency to onset of seizure or duration. The animal's neurologic status (i.e., having had SE) was a factor in the duration of the inability to find the platform following seizures, as animals with a prior history of SE had a longer period of impairment following a seizure than animals without such a history. Postictal cognitive impairment was associated with changes in theta activity in animals with a prior history of SE but not in seizure-naïve animals.

Postictal Motor and Sensory Deficits

Postictal motor deficits, also referred to as Todd's paralysis, is defined as a prolonged focal loss of function or weakness lasting from two minutes up to two days after a seizure. Such hemiparesis may represent a new hemiparesis or an accentuation of a previous interictal deficit related to structural pathology. In fact, in a study of 14 patients with transient postictal hemiparesis, Rolak et al. found a contralateral structural abnormality in eight patients (21).

The presence of a postictal motor deficit is suggestive of an extratemporal seizure focus, though it is not specific for frontal, parietal, or occipital foci. Of note, postictal

paresis has been reported as well in eight of 70 children with benign rolandic epilepsy of childhood (22).

Postictal sensory deficits include somatosensory abnormalities, hemineglect, and visual deficits. Somatosensory deficits have not been identified in isolation. Rather, they have always been reported in conjunction with motor deficits.

In contrast to the lack of specificity of postictal motor deficits in the localization of the seizure focus, postictal visual deficits, in the form of homonymous hemi- or quadrantanopsia, have been identified in seizure foci in occipital-parietal epilepsy, contralateral to the seizure focus.

Postictal Headaches

Postictal headaches (PHA) and migraines are among the more common postictal occurrences. For example, Yankovsky et al. studied 100 consecutive patients undergoing presurgical evaluation for pharmacologically intractable partial epilepsy (23). For each PHA type, they characterized the lateralization, localization, quality of pain, and results of treatment. They found that periictal HAs were reported by 47 patients. Of those, 11 had preictal HA (PIHA) and 44 had PHA. Eight patients had both PIHA and PHA. Interictal HA was reported by 31 patients. Twenty-nine (62%) of 47 patients had frontotemporal PHA. Twenty-five patients had migraine-like HA without aura: 18 (60%) of 30 patients with TLE and seven (41%) of 17 with extratemporal epilepsy. No correlation between pathology and presence of HA was found in 59 pathologically verified patients, except in four who had arteriovenous malformations (AVMs): three had, and one did not have, PHA. Similar findings were reported by Ito et al. in a study of 77 patients with TLE, 34 patients with occipital lobe epilepsy (OLE), and 50 with frontal lobe epilepsy (FLE) (24). They found an incidence of PHA of 23% for TLE, 62% for OLE, and 42%, for FLE. The risk of PHA was significantly higher for OLE than for TLE or FLE and for patients with generalized tonic-clonic (GTC) seizures. Younger age at onset of epilepsy was also a risk factor for PHA.

In a study of 110 consecutive patients with epilepsy, Förderreuther et al. found seizure-associated HA in 47 patients (43%) (25). Forty-three patients had exclusively PHA. One patient had exclusively preictal headaches. Three patients had both pre- and PHA. The duration of PHA was longer than 4 hours in 62.5% of the patients. In the majority of patients, PHA occurred in more than 50% of the seizures. Postictal HAs were associated with focal seizures in 23 patients and/or with generalized seizures in 54 patients. According to the headache classification of the International Headache Society, HAs were classified as migraine-type in 34% of patients and as tension-type headache in 34% of patients; they could not be classified in 21% of patients.

In a separate study, Ito et al. compared patients with different types of epilepsy to investigate the association between migraine-like HA and seizure type in 364 patients with partial epilepsy (26). TLE was found in 177 patients, FLE in 116, and OLE in 71. Forty percent had postictal HA, and 26% of these patients had migraine-like HA. Migraine-like postictal HA occurred significantly more often in cases of TLE and OLE than in cases of FLE. In addition, the incidence of interictal migraine headache was significantly higher in patients with migraine-like postictal HA.

Postictal Automatisms

Persistence of ictal automatisms into the PS or development of de-novo postictal automatisms have been described in the literature. Some of these postictal automatisms have been shown to have a localizing value of the ictal focus. For example, Leutmezer et al. carried out a retrospective study with videotapes of 160 patients with focal epilepsy who underwent presurgical evaluation, with the aim of identifying postictal symptoms that may have any localizing or lateralizing value in defining the seizure onset zone (27). Automatisms that started during the ictus and continued in the postictal period occurred in 25.2% of 135 patients with TLE but not in patients with FLE. Postictal "nose wiping" was evident in 51.3% of 76 TLE patients but only in 12.0% of 25 extratemporal lobe epilepsy patients, and it was performed with the hand ipsilateral to the hemisphere of seizure onset in 86.5% of all temporal lobe seizures. Rasonyi et al. reviewed 193 videotaped seizures of 55 consecutive patients with refractory TLE who became seizure-free after surgery (28). Thirty-four (62%) of the 55 patients showed postictal automatisms at least once during their seizures. They were identified in 70 (36%) seizures as manual (21%), oral (13%), or speech (9%) automatisms. Fifteen seizures contained a combination of two different postictal automatisms. The presence of postictal oral automatisms did not lateralize the seizure onset zone. Speech automatisms (repetitive verbal behavior) occurred more frequently after left-sided seizures ($p = 0.002$). Postictal unilateral manual automatism showed no lateralizing value.

A review of the literature suggests that among the postictal hand automatisms, nose wiping is more likely to occur in TLE, but it is not specific to this type of partial epilepsy. For example, Hirsch et al. conducted a retrospective study of 319 videotaped CPSs of 87 patients: 47 with unilateral TLE defined by successful surgical outcome with medial TLE (MTLE) and 17 with neocortical TLE; and 40 with extratemporal epilepsy (29). Postictal nose wiping was significantly more common in patients with unilateral TLE (60%) than in those with extratemporal epilepsy (33%). With regard to lateralizing potential, in the TLE group, unilateral postictal nose wiping (performed with a single hand only) within 60 seconds of seizure offset was observed in 53% of patients (25 of 47) and was performed with the hand ipsilateral to the seizure focus in 92% (23 of 25). Thirteen patients (9 with TLE) wiped their nose more than once with the same hand in a single seizure within 60 seconds of offset in 18 seizures; this was done with the hand ipsilateral to the seizure focus in all 18 instances (predictive value = 100%).

POSTICTAL PSYCHIATRIC PHENOMENA

Postictal psychiatric symptoms (PPS) have been recognized for a long time but, in general, remain poorly understood, particularly with respect to their prevalence, clinical characteristics, and pathogenic mechanisms. They may present as individual symptoms or as a cluster of symptoms, mimicking any type of psychiatric disorder (e.g., anxiety, depression, or psychosis). The vast majority of articles on postictal psychiatric symptoms have revolved around postictal psychotic symptoms and episodes that have been encountered in the course of v-EEG.

Experimental Perspective on Postictal Psychiatric Phenomena

Engel et al. (30) studied behavioral changes during the PS, specifically, postictal aggression that presents as reactive biting in amygdaloid-kindled seizures in rats. Caldecott-Hazard et al. (31, 32) identified the role of opioid involvement in postictal explosive motor behavior, noting that pretreatment with naloxone can exacerbate it, whereas pretreatment with morphine can suppress it. Engel et al. suggested that this hyperreactivity could reflect endogenous-opioid withdrawal phenomena. Indeed, endogenous opioids usually are released during seizures; therefore, the animal is exposed repeatedly to transient increments, creating a state of dependency.

Engel et al. (30) suggested that this model may reflect the pathogenic mechanisms mediating *interictal* depression, as endogenous opioids also may play the role of natural mood elevators and have been thought to mediate, at least in part, the therapeutic effects of electroconvulsive therapy (ECT) (33, 34). They support this hypothesis with data from positron emission tomographic studies that used the mu opioid receptor ligand [^{11}C] carfentanil. These studies revealed that temporal lobe hypometabolism is associated with enhanced opioid receptor binding (35, 36). In support of a pathogenic role of endogenous opioids in postictal affective disturbances, Engel et al. cite the transient suppression of the multiple-squeak response in the rat, the duration of which can be shortened by pretreatment with naloxone. This reaction to pain has been considered to reflect a measure of affective function (37). Whether these theories are applicable to the occurrence of postictal depressive episodes in humans is yet to be established. Engel et al. (30) also reviewed the potential role of dopamine changes in mediating psychotic processes in epilepsy. They point out how amygdaloid kindling in cats can induce enhanced sensitivity of dopamine receptors. Because psychotic symptoms are dopamine mediated, postictal and interictal psychotic processes conceivably could result from such changes.

Postictal Psychiatric Episodes

Postictal psychiatric symptoms may cluster and mimic discrete psychiatric episodes such as major depressive episodes of short duration or postictal psychotic episodes (PIPE). The prevalence of postictal psychiatric episodes in the general population of patients with epilepsy is yet to be established. The reported postictal psychiatric episodes have focused almost exclusively on postictal psychotic episodes identified in the course of v-EEG. This is not surprising, because the circumstances around v-EEG are optimal to facilitate the occurrence of PIPE. These include the occurrence of frequent seizures over a short time period, following the discontinuation or dose reduction of antiepileptic drugs (AEDs). In a study published in 1996, Kanner et al. estimated the yearly incidence of postictal episodes during v-EEG to be 7.9% among patients with partial epilepsy (38). The majority, or 6.4%, presented as PIPE. While patients may experience postictal psychiatric episodes mimicking any type of psychiatric disorders, here data only for postictal depressive and psychotic episodes will be reviewed.

Postictal Depressive Episodes

Postictal depressive episodes (PIDE) remain practically unexplored. In a study by Kanner et al., 18 of 100 patients experienced a cluster of at least five symptoms of depression that mimicked a major depression disorder with a duration exceeding 24 hours but significantly shorter than the 2 weeks required by the *Diagnostic and Statistical Manual of Mental Disorders, Fourth Edition* (DSM-IV) criteria (39). A comparison of seizure-related variables between the 18 patients with PIDE and 23 patients without any postictal psychiatric symptom failed to reveal any differences between the two groups. However, patients with PIDE were more likely to have a psychiatric history than controls were (Kanner, unpublished data). Isolated reports of PIDE have been published. For example, Fincham et al. described the case of a woman with stereotypic recurrent episodes of severe depression with suicidal ideation that followed clusters of simple partial seizures that

went unrecognized for a long time (40). The successful treatment of these seizures resulted in remission of her depressive episodes.

Postictal Psychotic Episodes

Several case series of PIPE have been published (38, 41–47). The following clinical characteristics of PIPE were identified in all the series: (i) delay between the onset of psychiatric symptoms and the time of the last seizure; (ii) relatively short duration; (iii) affect-laden symptomatology; (iv) clustering of symptoms into delusional and affective-like psychosis; (v) increase in the frequency of secondarily generalized tonic-clonic seizures preceding the onset of PIPE; (vi) onset of PIPE after having seizures for a mean period of more than 10 years.

In the study cited, Kanner et al. identified psychiatric symptomatology that mimicked a psychotic episode in ten of 13 patients (38). It presented as a delusional psychosis in four patients; and it mimicked a mixed manic-depressive–like psychosis in one patient, a psychotic depression-like disorder in two, a hypomanic-like psychosis in one, and a manic-like psychosis in one. The tenth patient presented with bizarre behavior associated with a thought disorder. In every case, the onset of symptoms lagged by a mean period of 24 hours (range 12 to 72 hours) relative to the time of the last seizure. The mean duration of the PIPE was 69.6 hours (range 24 to 144 hours). The psychotic episode remitted with low doses of neuroleptic medication (2 to 5 mg per day of haloperidol) in five patients; one patient required high doses (40 mg per day of haloperidol); and remission occurred without pharmacotherapy in four patients. Six of these ten patients had experienced an average of 2.4 PIPE prior to v-EEG; in the remaining four patients, the PIPE was the first one ever experienced. Other authors have reported similar findings with respect to response to pharmacotherapy (41–46).

Kanemoto et al. (47) studied the clinical differences between PIPE and acute and chronic interictal psychosis of epilepsy. They noted that patients with PIPE are more likely to experience grandiose and religious delusions in the presence of elevated moods and a feeling of mystic fusion of the body with the universe. On the other hand, perceptual delusions or voices commenting were less frequent, and feelings of impending death were common among patients with PIPE.

Clinical phenomena during PIPE have included cases of manic symptoms following complex partial seizures (48). Directed aggression has been reported to occur significantly more frequently during PIPE than during interictal psychosis or during the postictal confusional state following complex partial seizures (49). Gerard et al. reported six patients with subacute postictal aggression following a cluster of seizures (50). The episodes of postictal aggression were not isolated events but recurred repeatedly; the behaviors were uniquely stereotyped in each patient. All patients had medically intractable epilepsy and were remorseful in the interictal period.

Postictal psychotic episodes have also been reported with unusual presentations, including cases of Capgras' syndrome (51, 52) and a case mimicking a Klüver-Bucy syndrome reported in a patient with persistent seizures following a left temporal lobectomy (53). In children, cases of PIPE have been reported *only* following status epilepticus by two groups (54, 55). One was a case of a 9-year-old boy; the other was a case of a 12-year-old boy. In both children, EEG recordings were obtained during the psychotic episode, documenting that the seizure activity had remitted. Thus, although PIPE is unlikely to occur in children, the exception is status epilepticus.

Postictal psychotic episodes have also been described in the context of a "forced normalization phenomenon." Akanuma et al. reported two patients with TLE who developed PIPE that lasted 12 weeks (56). Repeated EEGs during the period of psychosis showed that their habitual focal epileptiform abnormalities had disappeared. Responses to neuroleptic treatments were not remarkable. Their psychotic symptoms gradually dispelled after their epileptiform abnormalities reappeared.

Various investigators have attempted to identify potential pathogenic mechanisms of PIPE. Thus, Kanner et al. compared magnetic resonance imaging (MRI), interictal and ictal EEG data derived from v-EEG, and past psychiatric history from 18 patients with PIPE and 36 controls (Kanner et al., submitted). A logistic regression model clearly demonstrated that bilateral independent ictal foci and secondarily generalized tonic-clonic seizures were strong predictors of PIPE. By the same token, the presence of PIPE predicted the existence of bilateral ictal foci with a probability of 89%. Umbricht et al. (45) reported similar findings in a study comparing eight patients with PIPE, seven patients with interictal psychosis, and 29 controls. In addition, they found that patients with PIPE and interictal psychosis had a lower verbal IQ and the absence of mesial temporal sclerosis. Devinsky et al. (44) reported a higher frequency of bilateral independent interictal foci in 20 patients with PIPE compared to 150 controls.

The pathogenic role of bilateral ictal foci in PIPE in patients with TLE was further suggested by Christodoulou et al., who reported three patients with postictal psychosis after a temporal lobectomy. All patients had persistent seizures originating from the side contralateral to the resection (57). In addition, Mathern et al. reported a patient with TLE who developed a PIPE during a v-EEG and died of unknown reasons four weeks after temporal lobectomy (58); pathological examination of surgical and autopsy hippocampal specimens revealed bilateral asymmetric neuron losses.

Among other potential risk factors, Alper et al. suggested that mood disorders among first- and second-degree relatives could be a predictor of PIPE (59). Briellmann et al. found that dysplasias in temporal lobe structures were associated with a higher risk of developing PIPE in a study that compared findings from high-resolution MRI and histopathologic studies between six patients who experienced PIPE and 45 controls. Of note, in the patients with PIPE the volume of hippocampal formations was normal (60). Kanemoto et al., on the other hand, found that hippocampal atrophy was significantly associated with the development of PIPE in a study of 111 patients with TLE (61).

PIPE and Electroshock Therapy

The development of de-novo PIPE has been reported. Zwil and Pomerantz described the case of a patient who developed delusional and hallucinatory psychosis following a course of ECT (62). Sackeim et al. reported the development of excitement in two patients following bilateral and/or right-unilateral ECT but not following left-unilateral ECT (63). On the other hand, ECT has been also used as a treatment for PIPE. Pascual-Aranda et al. reported the case of a 23-year-old woman who developed a postictal catatonic-like psychosis after a cluster of partial complex seizures; ECT resulted in complete recovery (64).

Postictal Psychiatric Symptoms

The only systematic investigation of the prevalence and clinical characteristics of postictal psychiatric symptoms (PPS) published to date was carried out by Kanner et al. and hence will be reviewed in some detail. This study was conducted at the Rush Epilepsy Center with 100 consecutive patients who suffered from pharmacoresistant partial epilepsy (11). Every patient was asked to complete a 42-item questionnaire (The Rush Postictal Psychiatric Questionnaire) (11) designed to identify the frequency of 26 PPS and five cognitive symptoms during a three-month period. These included symptoms of depression and of various anxiety disorders (i.e., general anxiety, panic attacks, agoraphobia, obsessions, and compulsions), hypomanic and psychotic symptoms, and neurovegetative and physical symptoms. These latter two types of symptoms are common in seizures as well as in depressive and anxiety disorders. Accordingly, they were recorded as separate symptom categories, so as not to erroneously increase the number of postictal symptoms of depression and anxiety. The postictal period was defined as the 72 hours that followed a seizure. The questionnaire was also developed to discriminate between interictal and postictal symptoms and to identify interictal symptoms that worsened in severity during the postictal period. Each question inquired about the frequency of occurrence of the symptom, and only symptoms identified after more than 50% of seizures were included in this study, so as to reflect a "habitual" phenomenon.

Among the 100 patients, the authors identified a lifetime prevalence of psychiatric disorders in 54 patients, which consisted of mood disorders in 33, anxiety disorder in 16 (12 of whom also had a mood disorder), and attention deficit hyperactivity disorder in five. No patient had experienced a history of a psychotic disorder. Eleven patients reported one or more psychiatric hospitalizations.

A median of eight postictal symptoms were identified (range: 0 to 25) corresponding to a median of three cognitive symptoms (range: 0 to 5) and 5 PPS (range 0 to 22); 74 patients experienced at least one type of PPS, 68 experienced both PPS and cognitive symptoms, and six reported only PPS. The prevalence of the different types of PPS and their median duration appear in Table 13-2.

Among the 74 patients with PPS, 60 (81%) experienced PPS belonging to more than one psychiatric disorder. The most frequent combination included postictal symptoms of anxiety, depression, and

TABLE 13-2
Prevalence of Postictal Psychiatric Symptoms in 100 Consecutive Patients with Pharmacoresistant Epilepsy

POSTICTAL SYMPTOM	PREVALENCE	MEDIAN DURATION IN HOURS (RANGE)
Symptoms of depression, total	43	
Irritability	30	24 (0.5–108)
Poor frustration tolerance	36	24 (0.1–108)
Anhedonia	32	24 (0.1–148)
Hopelessness	25	24 (1.0–108)
Helplessness	31	24 (1.0–108)
Crying bouts	26	6 (0.1–108)
Suicide ideation	13	24 (1.0–240)
Active suicidal thoughts	8	
Passive suicidal thoughts	13	
Feelings of self deprecation	27	24 (1.0–120)
Feelings of guilt	23	24 (0.1–240)
Neurovegetative symptoms, total	62	
Early night insomnia	11	–
Middle night awakening	13	–
Early morning awakening	11	–
Excessive somnolence	43	24 (2–72)
Loss of appetite	36	24 (2–148)
Excessive appetite	10	15 (0.5–48)
Loss of sexual interest (not related to fatigue)	26	39 (6–148)
Symptoms of anxiety, total	45	
Constant worrying	33	24 (0.5–108)
Panicky feelings	10	6 (0.1–148)
Agoraphobic symptoms	29	24 (0.5–296)
Due to fear of seizure recurrence	20	-
Compulsions	10	15 (0.1–72)
Self consciousness	26	6 (0.05–108)
Psychotic symptoms, total	7	
Referential thinking	5	15 (0.1–108)
Auditory hallucinations	2	6.0 (0.1–108)
Paranoid delusions	4	0.2 (0.1–0.25)
Religious delusions	3	6.0 (0.1–108)
Visual hallucinations	1	36 (6–48)
Hypomanic Symptoms, total	22	
Excessive energy	9	2 (0.15–48)
Thought racing	15	2 (0.1–24)
Fatigue	37	24 (0.1–108)

neurovegetative symptoms. Of note, the existence of PPS had been investigated only in seven patients prior to this study, and only one was offered treatment specifically directed to the remission of habitual postictal symptoms of depression.

Clinical Characteristics of PPS and Relation to Past Psychiatric History

Postictal Symptoms of Depression. Forty-three patients reported a median of five postictal symptoms of depression (range: 2 to 9). The median duration of each symptom was 24 hours (0.1–240 hours), with the exception of postictal crying, which had a median duration of six hours (0.1–108 hours). Thirty-two patients experienced postictal symptoms of depression of *at least* 24 hours duration (18 experienced a minimum of six symptoms lasting 24 hours or longer), five reported symptoms of 1 to 23 hours duration, and only three patients had symptoms lasting less than one hour. Thirteen patients reported habitual postictal suicidal ideation; eight experienced passive and active suicidal thoughts, while five reported only passive suicidal ideation. No patient ever acted on these symptoms. Postictal symptoms of depression *always* occurred in combination with other PPS categories, though correlations were only identified with postictal symptoms of anxiety, psychotic symptoms, and neurovegetative symptoms.

Among these 43 patients, 25 had a history of a mood disorder and 11 of an anxiety disorder. There was a significant association between a history of depression and the postictal symptoms of self-deprecation and guilt, while a significant association with a history of anxiety and postictal guilt was identified. Furthermore, the number of postictal symptoms of depression was higher in patients with a prior history of depression and anxiety. Of note, 10 of the 13 (77%) patients with postictal suicidal ideation had a history of either major depression or bipolar disorder. Also, postictal suicidal ideation was an indicator of previous severe psychiatric disorders, as it was significantly associated with previous psychiatric hospitalization.

Postictal Symptoms of Anxiety. Forty-five patients reported a median of 2 (range: 1 to 5) postictal symptoms of anxiety. The median duration of individual symptoms ranged from six to 24 hours (0.1 to 296 hours). In 30 patients at least one symptom lasted 24 hours or longer (15 patients [33%] reported a cluster of four postictal symptoms of anxiety of at least 24 hours); ten patients reported at least one symptom of 1 to 23 hours duration, and five patients had symptoms lasting less than one hour. Twenty-nine patients experienced symptoms of postictal agoraphobia; 18 (62%) attributed these symptoms to the fear of seizure recurrence. Nevertheless, the presence of this fear was *not*

related to the actual occurrence of seizures in clusters. A prior history of anxiety disorder was identified in 15 patients (33%). There was an association between a history of anxiety disorder and the occurrence of postictal symptoms of constant worrying and panicky feelings.

Postictal Psychotic Symptoms. Seven patients experienced a median of two postictal psychotic symptoms (range: 1 to 5). Five patients reported referential thinking ("people are staring and talking about me"); two, auditory hallucinations; four, paranoid delusions; three, religious delusions; and one, visual hallucinations. The duration of individual symptoms ranged from 0.2 to 36 hours (0.1–108 hours). In four of these patients, at least one psychotic symptom lasted a minimum of 24 hours, two patients experienced symptoms lasting between 1 and 23 hours, and one patient reported symptoms of less than one hour duration. These seven patients also experienced postictal symptoms of anxiety and depression, and five patients reported postictal hypomanic symptoms. No patient had experienced a history of interictal psychosis. A psychiatric history was not significantly associated with the development of postictal psychotic symptoms, but a history of anxiety disorder was associated with a greater number of psychotic symptoms.

Postictal Hypomanic Symptoms. Postictal hypomanic symptoms included excessive energy and racing thoughts, which were identified in 22 patients: 15 patients reported racing thoughts, nine reported increased energy, but only two reported both symptoms. The median duration of both symptoms was 2 hours (0.1–48 hours). Six patients experienced hypomanic symptoms lasting 24 hours or longer. There was no significant association between a psychiatric history and the development of hypomanic symptoms.

Postictal Neurovegetative Symptoms. Postictal neurovegetative symptoms were among the most commonly reported postictal symptoms—above all, postictal somnolence and loss of appetite. Sixty-two patients experienced a median of two symptoms (range: 1 to 5), and in 12 they were the only PPS category reported. In addition, early night insomnia was reported by 11% of patients, middle night awakening by 13%, early morning awakening by 11%, and excessive appetite by 10%. These are four symptoms not typically associated with the postictal state. The median durations of individual symptoms ranged from 15 to 39 hours (0.5 to 148 hours). A psychiatric history did not worsen or act as a risk factor of these postictal symptoms.

Postictal Fatigue. Thirty-seven patients reported postictal fatigue with a median duration of 24 hours (0.1 to 108 hours).

Relation between Postictal Cognitive and Psychiatric Symptoms. Eighty-two patients experienced a median of four postictal cognitive symptoms (range: 1 to 5). Fourteen patients reported only postictal cognitive symptoms, while the other 68 experienced postictal cognitive and psychiatric symptoms. The median duration of individual cognitive symptoms ranged from 1 to 9 hours (0.05 to 108 hours). In general, the "estimated" duration of PPS was significantly longer than that of cognitive symptoms. The presence of postictal symptoms of depression was associated with the worst postictal cognitive disturbances, as evidenced by a greater number of postictal cognitive symptoms.

Interictal Psychiatric Symptoms with Postictal Exacerbation. Thirty-eight patients experienced a median of three (range: 1–15) psychiatric symptoms during the interictal period, 34 of whom had symptoms of depression ($n = 24$), anxiety ($n = 3$) or mixed anxiety/depression ($n = 6$), and four only neurovegetative symptoms. Thirty-six of these 38 patients (94%) experienced interictal symptoms with postictal exacerbation in severity as well, and in 19, all interictal recorded symptoms were only coded as such. Furthermore, among these 36 patients, 30 (83%) also experienced de-novo PPS. Among 20 patients with interictal fatigue, eighteen reported significant worsening during the postictal period. Finally, 37 patients reported interictal cognitive symptoms that worsened postictally; all of these patients also experienced de-novo postictal cognitive symptoms.

Thirteen patients were taking antidepressant medications at the time of the study: 10 for the treatment of an interictal depressive disorder, two for an anxiety disorder, and one for the treatment of irritability. Being on antidepressants, however, did not prevent the development of postictal symptoms ($n = 3$) or the postictal exacerbation of interictal symptoms of depression and/or anxiety ($n = 10$), despite a significant improvement of the interictal disorder.

There was no significant association between the development of PPS and the location of the seizure focus, the type of seizures, or the occurrence of seizures in clusters. On the other hand, taking AEDs with negative psychotropic properties (barbiturates and benzodiazepines) yielded a trend toward a greater likelihood of developing postictal psychotic symptoms.

Clearly, these data illustrate the relatively high prevalence of PPS and the *very tight* relationship between interictal and postictal symptomatology and between a prior psychiatric history and the development of PPS. Without a doubt, recognition of PPS is of the essence in the understanding of psychiatric symptomatology in patients with epilepsy, including as it pertains to the interpretation of its response to treatment.

Relationship between Ictal, Postictal, and Interictal Psychiatric Symptomatology

As shown by the foregoing results, postictal and interictal psychiatric symptomatology are closely related, implying common pathogenic mechanisms. Further evidence of such a relationship is supported by the following data.

Mintzer and Lopez compared interictal psychiatric disorders between 12 patients with TLE and ictal fear and 12 matched controls without ictal fear (65). Patients with ictal fear were significantly more likely to suffer from interictal panic disorders and other anxiety disorders than the control group.

Kohler et al. compared presurgical and postsurgical psychiatric disorders among 22 patients with ictal fear, 22 patients with auras of a different type (nonfear aura), and 15 patients without auras, all of whom underwent an anterotemporal lobectomy (ATL) (66). Pre-operatively, 68% of patients with ictal fear, 55% of those with nonfear aura, and 57% of those without aura had a history of mood and/or anxiety disorders. Although fewer patients experienced mood and anxiety disorders after surgery (nonfear aura group, 37%; group without aura, 21%), patients with ictal fear experienced a significant increase in mood and anxiety disorders (86%), independently of the persistence of auras. Although mood and anxiety disorders were more prevalent postsurgically among patients with persistent seizures, mood and anxiety disorders were more frequent in the seizure-free patients with presurgical fear aura than in the other two groups. As expected, patients in the fear aura group were on psychotropic medication with a significantly higher frequency than patients from the other two groups.

By the same token, the occurrence of PIPE was associated with an increased risk of postsurgical mood disorders. Thus, in a study of 52 patients who underwent an ATL, Kanemoto et al. also found that PIPE was associated with postsurgical mood disorders, presenting as manic and depressive episodes during the first 2 postsurgical years (67).

The evolution of PIPE unto interictal psychotic episodes has also been recognized by several investigators. Tarulli et al. found that six out of 43 (13.9%) patients with a history of PIPE went on to develop interictal psychosis (68). Adachi et al. identified patients with both interictal psychotic episodes and PIPE (69); 10 initially experienced PIPE and went on to develop interictal psychosis, while four patients experienced an interictal psychotic disorder that remitted and later on developed PIPE. The mean age was 10.8 ± 4.3 years at the onset of the epilepsy, 24.4 ± 6.1 years for interictal psychosis, and 33.8 ± 4.5 years for PIPE. Furthermore, these patients did not differ with respect to the epilepsy-related characteristics found in patients with only PIPE, as the four patients had bilateral EEG abnormalities and borderline (or decreased) intellectual functioning. Kanner et al. compared the development of interictal psychosis between 18 patients with PIPE and 36 controls. Six of the patients with PIPE developed an interictal psychosis, while none of the controls did (Kanner et al., submitted). Finally, Devinsky et al. reported the case of a 49-year-old man who experienced partial seizures with unpleasant olfactory hallucinations. Following the remission of his ictal symptoms he developed a disabling delusional syndrome consisting of a delusional belief that his body was emitting foul odors (70).

CONCLUDING REMARKS

Postictal phenomena are relatively frequent and account to a great degree for the poor quality of life of patients with epilepsy. Despite their high prevalence, postictal symptoms—particularly, psychiatric symptoms—remain unrecognized and, not surprisingly, have been poorly studied. Future research will need to focus on the pathogenic mechanisms mediating postictal symptomatology and to identify ways of minimizing its occurrence when seizure remission is not possible.

References

1. Fisher RS, Schachter SC. The postictal state: a neglected entity in the management of epilepsy. *Epilepsy Behav* 2000; 1:52–59.
2. Trimble M. Serum prolactin in epilepsy and hysteria. *BMJ* 1978; 2:1682.
3. Pritchard PB III, Wannamaker BB, Sagel J, et al. Serum prolactin and cortisol levels in the evaluation of pseudoepileptic seizures. *Ann Neurol* 1985; 18:87–89.
4. Fisher RS, Prince DA. Spike-wave rhythms in cat cortex induced by parenteral penicillin. II. Cellular features. *Electroencephalogr Clin Neurophysiol* 1977; 42:625–639.
5. Haglund MM, Schwartzkroin PA. Role of Na–K pump potassium regulation and IPSPs in seizures and spreading depression in immature rabbit hippocampal slices. *J Neurophysiol* 1990; 63:225–239.
6. Parfenova H, Carratu P, Tcheranova D, Fedinec A, et al. Epileptic seizures cause extended postictal cerebral vascular dysfunction that is prevented by HO-1 overexpression. *Am J Physiol Heart Circ Physiol* 2005; 288(6):2843–2850.
7. Kostopoulos G, Drapeau C, Avoli M, Olivier A, et al. Endogenous adenosine can reduce epileptiform activity in the human epileptogenic cortex maintained in vitro. *Neurosci Lett* 106; 1989:119–124.
8. During MJ, Spencer DD. Adenosine: a potential mediator of seizure arrest and postictal refractoriness. *Ann Neurol* 1992; 32(5):618–624.
9. DiGeronimo RJ, Gegg CA, Zuckerman SL. Adenosine depletion alters postictal hypoxic cerebral vasodilation in the newborn pig. *Am J Physiol* 1998; 274(5 Pt 2):495–501.
10. Linseman MA, Corrigall WA. Effects of naloxone on hippocampal seizure activity. *Behav Neural Biol* 1987; 48:159–164.
11. Kanner AM, Soto A, Gross-Kanner H. Prevalence and clinical characteristics of postictal psychiatric symptoms in partial epilepsy. *Neurology* 2004; 62:708–713.
12. Luders HO, Szabo A. Todd's paralysis and postictal aphasia. In: Luders HO, Noachtar S, eds. *Epileptic Seizures: Pathophysiology and Clinical Semiology.* Philadelphia: Churchill Livingstone, 2000:652–657.
13. Adam C, Adam C, Rouleau I, Saint-Hilaire JM. Postictal aphasia and paresis: a clinical and intracerebral EEG study. *Can J Neurol Sci* 2000; 27(1):49–54.
14. Williamson PD, Thadani VM, French JA, Darcey TM, et al. Medial temporal lobe epilepsy: videotape analysis of objective clinical seizure characteristics. *Epilepsia* 1998; 39(11):1182–1188.
15. Privitera MD, Morris GL, Gilliam F. Postictal language assessment and lateralization of complex partial seizures. *Ann Neurol* 1991; 30:391–396.
16. Ficker DM, Shukla R, Privitera MD. Postictal language dysfunction in complex partial seizures: effect of contralateral ictal spread. *Neurology* 2001; 56(11):1590–1592.
17. Devinsky O, Kelley K, Yacubian EM, Sato S, et al. Postictal behavior. a clinical and subdural electroencephalographic study. *Arch Neurol* 1994; 51(3):254–259.
18. Goldberg-Stern H, Gadoth N, Ficker D, Privitera M. The effect of age and structural lesions on postictal language impairment. *Seizure* 2005; 14(1):62–65.
19. Helmstaedter C, Elger CE, Lendt M. Postictal courses of cognitive deficits in focal epilepsies. *Epilepsia* 1994; 35:1073–1078.
20. Boukhezra O, Riviello P, Fu DD, Lui X, et al. Effect of the postictal state on visual-spatial memory in immature rats. *Epilepsy Res* 2003; 55(3):165–175.
21. Rolak LA, Rutecki P, Ashizawa T, Harati Y. Clinical features of Todd's post-epileptic paralysis. *J Neurol Neurosurg Psychiatry* 1992; 55:63–64.
22. Dai AI, Weinstock A. Postictal paresis in children with benign rolandic epilepsy. *J Child Neurol* 2005; 20(10):834–836.
23. Yankovsky AE, Andermann F, Bernasconi A. Characteristics of headache associated with intractable partial epilepsy. *Epilepsia* 2005; 46(8):1241–1245.
24. Ito M, Adachi N, Nakamura F, et al. Characteristics of postictal headache in patients with partial epilepsy. *Cephalalgia* 2004; 24(1):23–28.
25. Förderreuther S, Henkel A, Noachtar S, Straube A. Headache associated with epileptic seizures: epidemiology and clinical characteristics. *Headache* 2002; 42(7):649.
26. Ito M, Adachi N, Nakamura F, et al. Multi-center study on post-ictal headache in patients with localization-related epilepsy. *Psychiatry Clin Neurosci* 2003; 57(4):385–389.
27. Leutmezer F, Serles W, Pataraia E, Olbrich A, et al. The postictal state: a clinically oriented observation of patients with epilepsy. *Wien Klin Wochenschr* 1998 Jun 5; 110(11):401–407.
28. Rasonyi G, Fogarasi A, Kelemen A, Janszky J, et al. Lateralizing value of postictal automatisms in temporal lobe epilepsy. *Epilepsy Res* 2006; 70(2–3):239–243.
29. Hirsch LJ, Lain AH, Walczak TS. Postictal nosewiping lateralizes and localizes to the ipsilateral temporal lobe. *Epilepsia* 1998; 39:991–997.
30. Engel J Jr, Bandler R, Griffith NC, et al. Neurobiological evidence for epilepsy induced interictal disturbances. *Adv Neurol* 1991; 55:97–111.
31. Caldecott-Hazard S, Ackermann RF, Engel J Jr. Opioid involvement in postictal and interictal changes in behavior. In: Fariello RG, Morselli PL, Lloyd K, et al., eds. *Neurotransmitters, Seizures and Epilepsy II.* New York: Raven Press 1984:305–314.
32. Caldecott-Hazard S, Engel J Jr. Limbic postictal events: anatomical substrates and opioid receptor involvement. *Prog Neuropsychopharmacol Biol Psychiatry* 1987; 11:389–418.
33. Holladay JW, Tortella FC, Long JB, et al. Endogenous opioids and their receptors: evidence for the involvement in the postictal effects of electroconvulsive shock. *Ann N Y Acad Sci* 1986; 462:124–139.
34. Tortella FC, Long JB. Characterization of opioid peptide-like anticonvulsant activity in rat cerebrospinal fluid. *Brain Res* 1988; 426:139–146.
35. Frost JJ, Mayberg HS, Fisher RS, et al. Mu-opiate receptors measured by positron emission tomography are increased in temporal lobe epilepsy. *Ann Neurol* 1988; 23:231–237.
36. Hitzemann JR, Hitzemann BA, Blatt S, et al. Repeated electroconvulsive shock: effect on sodium dependency and regional distribution of opioid-binding sites. *Mol Pharmacol* 1987; 31:562–566.
37. Carroll MN, Lim RKS. Observations on the neuropharmacology of morphine and morphine-like analgesia. *Arch Int Pharmacodyn Ther* 1960; 125:383–403.
38. Kanner AM, Stagno S, Kotagal P, et al. Postictal psychiatric events during prolonged video-electroencephalographic monitoring studies. *Arch Neurol* 1996; 53:258–263.
39. American Psychiatric Association. Diagnostic and statistical manual of mental disorders, 4th ed. Washington, DC: American Psychiatric Press, 1994.
40. Fincham R, Anderson S. Postictal depression following subtle seizures. *Epilepsy Behav* 2000; 1(4):278–280.
41. Logsdail SJ, Toone BK. Postictal psychosis. A clinical and phenomenological description. *Br J Psychiatry* 1988; 152:246–252.
42. Savard G, Andermann F, Olivier A, et al. Postictal psychosis after complex partial seizures: a multiple case study. *Epilepsia* 1991; 32:225–231.
43. Lancman ME, Craven WJ, Asconape JJ, et al. Clinical management of recurrent postictal psychosis. *J Epilepsy* 1994; 7:47–51.
44. Devinsky O, Abrahmson H, Alper K, et al. Postictal psychosis: a case control study of 20 patients and 150 controls. *Epilepsy Res* 1995; 20:247–253.
45. Umbricht D, Degreef G, Barr WB, et al. Postictal and chronic psychosis in patients with temporal lobe epilepsy. *Am J Psychiatry* 1995; 152:224–231.
46. Szabo CA, Lancman M, Stagno S. Postictal psychosis: a review. *Neuropsychiatry Neurosurg Behav Neurol* 1996; 9:258–264.
47. Kanemoto K, Kawasaki J, Kawai I. Postictal psychosis: a comparison with acute interictal and chronic psychoses. *Epilepsia* 1996; 37:551–556.
48. Barczak P, Edmunds E, Bettes T. Hypomania following complex partial seizures: a report of three cases. *Br J Psychiatry* 1988; 152:137–139.
49. Steinert T, Froscher W. Differential diagnosis of aggressive behavior in epilepsy. *Psychiatr Prax* 1995; 22:15–18.
50. Gerard ME, Spitz MC, Towbin JA, Shantz D. Subacute postictal aggression. *Neurology* 1998; 50:384–388.
51. Drake ME. Postictal Capgras syndrome. *Clin Neurol Neurosurg* 1987; 89:271–274.
52. Kim E. A postictal variant of Capgras' syndrome in a patient with a frontal meningioma: a case report. *Psychosomatics* 1991; 32:448–451.
53. Anson JA, Kuhlman DT. Postictal Kluver-Bucy syndrome after temporal lobectomy. *J Neurol Neurosurg Psychiatry* 1993; 56:311–313.
54. Nissenkorn A, Moldavsky M, Lorberboym M, Raucher A, et al. Postictal psychosis in a child. *J Child Neurol* 1999; 14(12):818–819.
55. Joshi CN, Booth FA, Sigurdson ES, Bolton JM, et al. Postictal psychosis in a child. *Pediatr Neurol* 2006; 34(5):388–391.

56. Akanuma N, Kanemoto K, Adachi N, Kawasaki J, et al. Prolonged postictal psychosis with forced normalization (Landolt) in temporal lobe epilepsy. *Epilepsy Behav* 2005; 6(3):456–459.

57. Christodoulou C, Koutroumanidis M, Hennessy MJ, Elwes RD, et al. Postictal psychosis after temporal lobectomy. *Neurology* 2002; 59(9):1432–1435.

58. Mathern GW, Pretorius JK, Babb TL, Quinn B. Unilateral hippocampal mossy fiber sprouting and bilateral asymmetric neuron loss with episodic postictal psychosis. *J Neurosurg* 1995; 82(2):228–233.

59. Alper K, Devinsky O, Westbrook L, Luciano D, et al. Premorbid psychiatric risk factors for postictal psychosis. *J Neuropsychiatry Clin Neurosci* 2001; 13(4):492–499.

60. Briellmann RS, Kalnins RM, Hopwood MJ, Ward C, et al. TLE patients with postictal psychosis: mesial dysplasia and anterior hippocampal preservation. *Neurology* 2000; 55(7):1027–1030.

61. Kanemoto K, Takeuchi J, Kawasaki J, Kawai I. Characteristics of temporal lobe epilepsy with mesial temporal sclerosis, with special reference to psychotic episodes. *Neurology* 1996; 47(5):1199–1203.

62. Zwil AS, Pomerantz A. Transient postictal psychosis associated with a course of ECT. *Convuls Ther* 1997; 13(1):32–36.

63. Sackeim HA, Decina P, Malitz S, Hopkins N, et al. Postictal excitement following bilateral and right-unilateral ECT. *Am J Psychiatry* 1983; 140(10):1367–1368.

64. Pascual-Aranda A, Garcia-Morales I, Sanz-Fuentenebro J. Postictal psychosis: resolution after electroconvulsive therapy. *Epilepsy Behav* 2001; 2(4):363–366.

65. Mintzer S, Lopez F: Comorbidity of ictal fear and panic disorder. *Epilepsy Behav* 2002; 3(4):330–337.

66. Kohler CG, Carran MA, Bilker W et al. Association of fear auras with mood and anxiety disorders after temporal lobectomy. *Epilepsia* 2001; 42(5):674–681.

67. Kanemoto K, Kawasaki J, Mori E. Postictal psychosis as a risk factor for mood disorders after temporal lobe surgery. *J Neurol Neurosurg Psychiatry* 1998; 65(4): 587–589.

68. Tarulli A, Devinsky O, and Alper K. Progression of postictal to interictal psychosis. *Epilepsia* 2001; 42:1468.

69. Adachi N, Kato M, Sekimoto M, Ichikawa I, et al. Recurrent postictal psychosis after remission of interictal psychosis: further evidence of bimodal psychosis. *Epilepsia* 2003; 44:1218.

70. Devinsky O, Khan S, Alper K.Olfactory reference syndrome in a patient with partial epilepsy. *Neuropsychiatry Neuropsychol Behav Neurol* 1998; 11(2):103–105.

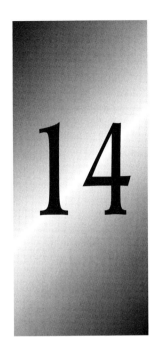

14 Behavioral Aspects of Nonconvulsive Status Epilepticus

Thien Nguyen
Peter W. Kaplan

INTRODUCTION

Nonconvulsive status epilepticus (NCSE) is a condition of continuous or intermittent epileptic activity without convulsions associated with electroencephalographic (EEG) evidence of seizure. NCSE encompasses a number of clinically distinct groups: (1) complex partial status epilepticus (CPSE), (2) typical absence (a rare subtype), and (3) status epilepticus (SE) in comatose patients. It may occur in about 8% of all comatose patients without evidence of significant motor signs and may persist in 14% of patients following generalized convulsive status epilepticus. NCSE is underrecognized and underdiagnosed. However, with the increasing awareness of varying clinical presentations of NCSE and access to EEG testing, clinicians should be better able to identify and manage this challenging group of disorders.

DIFFERENTIAL DIAGNOSIS AND CLASSIFICATION

The diagnosis of NCSE traditionally entails the clinical picture of abnormal mental status with diminished responsiveness, a confirmatory epileptic pattern on EEG, and, often, an improvement with antiepileptic drugs (AEDs). Several classification systems have been developed. Older classifications categorize NCSE into two groups based on EEG findings: (1) absence status epilepticus (ASE) and (2) localization-related NSCE or complex partial status epilepticus. However, since morbidity and mortality in NCSE stems from the underlying cause of NCSE rather than clinical or EEG type, an emerging unifying approach is to divide NCSE based on whether it is due to a primary epileptic encephalopathy or due to some other brain pathology. Kaplan developed a detailed classification using clinical characteristics and EEG findings to categorize patients (1). This classification system includes (1) localization-related NCSE, (2) generalized NCSE (GNSE), and (3) indeterminate or intermediate NCSE. GNSE is further divided as described in Table 14-1.

Classification of NCSE based on clinical presentations using exclusion criteria can be problematic. This difficulty is due to significant overlap among clinical characteristics of different types of NCSE. EEG patterns such as paroxysmal lateralized epileptiform discharges (PLEDs) may present in patients with facial twitching, subtle limb jerks, and an altered level of consciousness; however, these clinical signs can occur with SE. Infectious, toxic, or metabolic encephalopathy as well as psychogenic states with staring, mutism, or increased body tone (such as with benzodiazepine withdrawal encephalopathy, lithium toxicity, serotonin syndrome, and neuroleptic

such as writing on the wall. Therefore, TAS typically presents with inappropriate rather than retrogressive or deteriorating behaviors.

Even with some amnesia depending on the severity of confusion and stupor, patients may remember some events and be able to perform some quite complex activities. One patient was able to write thoughts and feelings and the sequence of ictal events as the attack progressed. Patients sometimes described seeing the world differently, "not being there," having uncontrollable pressured thoughts, or concern for losing their mind. In one case, a patient reportedly stared at a poem by Walter Scott, and the following day—surprisingly—retained the entire poem without having read it previously (2).

In contrast to CPSE, TAS has no postictal confusion or cycling in levels of responsiveness. Neuroimaging is normal. Cognitive compromise is mild compared to the severity of psychic symptoms.

Atypical Absence Status Epilepticus (AASE)

Atypical absence status usually occurs in patients with mental retardation or Lennox-Gastaut syndrome (LGS). The onset of status is often unclear, and interictal states may be hard to differentiate from ictal ones. AASE is typified by the relative alteration in attention, behavior, and reactivity. Cognitive impairment is most often exhibited during AASE. Unlike TAS, tonic-clonic convulsions may trigger or terminate SE, though this is rare. About 50% of patients with AASE have perioral, facial, or limb myoclonus. Additional discussions are described in the sections on NCSE in Children and Adolescents with Delayed Development and NCSE in Adults with Mental Retardation.

Simple Partial Nonconvulsive Status Epilepticus

Nonconvulsive simple partial status epilepticus may be difficult to demonstrate because of the usually normal surface EEG. There may be ictal fear and bizarre abdominal symptoms with depression, mild confusion, and resistive or even suicidal behavior. Occipital simple partial status may show adversive eye movements with nystagmus, amaurosis, motor paralysis (somatoinhibitory status), and impairment of spatial perception that may be demonstrated only on neuropsychologic testing. Simple partial status is often assumed even in the absence of any EEG correlate.

Complex Partial Status Epilepticus (CPSE)

Originally described by Gastaut et al. in 1956, CPSE remained scantly reported, with less than 20 well-documented cases by the 1980s (3). Several hundred cases have now been described. It is now widely

agreed that CPSE is not a rare condition but is probably underrecognized.

Video EEG has demonstrated both cyclic and continuous varieties, with some patients evolving from one type to the other. Cyclic and continuous clinical patterns have also been noted in ASE, making differentiation between these two "types" of SE problematic (4).

CPSE almost always presents with an impairment of consciousness. Hippocampal, amygdalar, or amygdalohippocampal origin may produce a cycling in clinical behavioral correlates. When hippocampus and amygdala are involved, lip smacking, chewing, and gesticulatory automatism are typical. Patients are also noted to have an ongoing twilight state with impaired consciousness and some amnesia, motionless staring, and partial or arrested speech. Sometimes there are borborygmi, vocalizations, and perseveration.

When the seizure arises from extratemporal loci, visual illusion and hallucination, dizziness, or unilateral arm movements can appear. There may be a perception of warm feeling, nausea, somesthetic hallucination, facial pallor or suffusion, auditory hallucination, and jerks and tonic posturing of the arm. With seizures in the temporo-parieto-occipital region, alterations of vision and eye deviation with nystagmus can occur. Spreading to the temporal lobe could produce postural changes with peculiar limb automatisms, head turnings, or "wandering or fencing" posture. In contrast to generalized absence status, patients with temporal lobe CPSE often are markedly unresponsive with strikingly abnormal behavior.

Thomas et al. differentiated two varieties of frontal NCSE. Type I had mood disturbances, affective disinhibition or indifference, and mild involvement of cognitive function, but without overt confusion. EEG revealed unilateral frontal seizure activity. In contrast, the less frequent Type II exhibited marked impairment of consciousness, and the EEG showed bilateral asymmetric frontal foci on an abnormal background.

The unilateral frontal focus (Type I) was seen in patients who could perform daily tasks including dressing, eating, and washing and could follow simple commands. Conversely, complex tasks, such as subtracting serial 7s or copying simple patterns, could not be performed. Perseveration and slowing of motor activity also occurred. Mood was often hypomanic with affective disinhibition or pressured speech. Some patients manifested indifference with a blank facial expression, mutism, or blunt emotion. Amnesia was typically very mild. A few patients had cyclic fluctuations, with forced thinking, head or eye deviation, and, rarely, facial myoclonus. Automatisms including picking at clothes, rubbing, or scratching were seen. Complex bipedal or bimanual automatism and oro-alimentary automatism were never observed.

Type II frontal lobe NCSE with bilateral ictal foci manifested as marked behavioral disturbances, temporospatial confusion, perseveration, distractibility, and agitation. Behavior was cyclic. Some postictal patients had catatonia with simple gestural automatisms. Amnesia was present in all patients.

NCSE PRESENTING ACCORDING TO AGE OF EXPRESSION

Neonatal Nonconvulsive Status Epilepticus

In general, neonatal status presents differently from that seen at other ages. Nonconvulsive seizures may occur in premature and term infants with slight jerking, eye deviation, eyelid fluttering, orofacial movement, autonomic changes, apnea, and limb movements including boxing, pedaling, or swimming movements. Seizures may persist for days, often without clear epileptiform morphologies on EEG, which may reveal high-voltage slow activity, burst suppression, or rhythmic activity. Electrographic seizures may occur without clinical correlate in many neonates.

NCSE in Infants

In patients with West syndrome, diagnosis is often problematic, as variability in attention can be difficult to recognize. Developmentally delayed infants may exhibit decreased affective and visual interaction when there is hypsarrhythmia. They often present with apathy, stupor, eye blinking, and salivation.

Primary generalized myoclonic-astatic epilepsy manifests as NCSE in 30% to 40% of patients. It is characterized by impairment of consciousness, varying from apathy to stupor, associated with facial and limb myoclonus, which is more apparent by palpation than by visual inspection.

In secondary generalized myoclonic-astatic epilepsy or LGS, there can be atonia, head nodding, facial myoclonia, obtundation, and developmental delay. These features will normalize with AEDs.

NCSE in Children with Normal Intelligence

Benign rolandic epilepsy rarely manifests as status epilepticus. There have been only a handful of documented cases to date. This condition is characterized by facial weakness, speech arrest, drooling, swallowing difficulties, tonic head deviation, and confusion, with some EEG resemblance to ESES. Benign occipital nonconvulsive status can cause nausea, anorexia, and visual hallucination.

Syndromes with NCSE During Childhood

Electrical Status Epilepticus During Slow-wave Sleep (ESES). Electrical status epilepticus during slow-wave sleep (ESES) usually occurs in mentally retarded children with speech disturbance with nighttime seizures or as an AASE. More than 60 cases have been published, with the typical spike-wave discharges occurring during non-REM sleep. Onset is between 1 and 14 years of age. Patients' IQs vary between 45 and 80. Clinical presentation manifests as hyperkinetic and aggressive behavior, psychosis, memory impairment, and spatial disorientation associated with progressive language deterioration. ESES resembles Landau-Kleffner syndrome, although in the latter non-REM spike waves are rare, and there is a different psychologic clinical evolution. It is not clear whether the EEG findings are an encephalopathic epiphenomenon or whether they are the cause.

Landau-Kleffner Syndrome (Acquired Epileptic Aphasia). Although Landau-Kleffner syndrome is rare, some 200 cases have been reported, often in normally developing children between 3 and 7 years of age. Patients decline clinically over weeks to years with increasing receptive and expressive aphasia, word agnosia (an inability to understand the meaning of sound), and decreased speech output or mutism. The EEG focus does not necessarily correspond to the hemisphere of language dominance. There may be hyperkinetic activity, personality changes, and intellectual decline.

Minor Epileptic Status of Brett. A particular syndrome of minor motor status epilepticus (myoclonic encephalopathy) was delineated by Brett in 1966, with obtundation, head atonia, drooling, and mutism. There were asymmetric eye, limb, and trunk myoclonus with a lurching gait (pseudoataxia). Many cases resembled Lennox-Gastaut syndrome.

NCSE in Children and Adolescents with Delayed Development

NCSE may be difficult to delineate in children and adolescents with learning difficulties because it is often difficult to differentiate between changes caused by seizures and baseline cognitive and behavioral function. Patients may appear less talkative, cooperative, or attentive. Most patients have Lennox-Gastaut syndrome (LGS), but a rare case with Landau-Kleffner syndrome has been reported. Although clinicians are now more aware of the diagnostic challenges of making the diagnosis of NCSE in LGS patients, few specific characteristics are available to warn clinicians about the presence of NCSE.

Additionally, NCSE in later childhood may include ASE, AASE, and CPSE. Reported findings include "some days he switches off"; "stares vacantly ahead, dribbling, answers questions very slowly, speech very slow and deliberate"; "sluggish, uncooperative and drowsy"; and "has periods of appearing deaf and blind"—referred to as a pseudodementia (5). Patients have been noted to have "pseudoataxia" with impaired balance, bumping into objects, or walking into doors.

NCSE in Adults with Mental Retardation

As in children, it may be very difficult to recognize ictal behavioral abnormalities in adult patients with mental retardation. Frequently, it is also impossible to differentiate continuous lateralized seizure activity (complex partial seizures) from atypical absences. Most patients are moderately to profoundly mentally retarded, often with lifelong epilepsy. In one series, observers describing NCSE behavioral changes noted "apathy for days; staring vacantly into the air, appeared almost comatose"; that patient(s) were "extremely stubborn and would not eat or find the toilet"; that patient(s) "responded after a considerable delay"; "appeared anxious and insecure"; "had episodes of faintness with empty staring and perioral movements"; "shut eyes while short lasting jerks or shivering affected the shoulders for hours"; "were restless and aggressive" during which time the patient(s) "could run straight against the wall"; or exhibited "unintelligible verbal outbursts"; "perseverative answering of 'yes' to all questions"; "absent mindedness and clumsiness"; and "eye blinking with generalized shivering." Patients universally had Lennox-Gastaut syndrome (6).

In conclusion, diagnosing NCSE in this patient population is more difficult, simply because it is harder to recognize deviations from ordinary behaviors in these patients than in higher-functioning patients. Often, impressive psychiatric features suggest a psychiatric problem rather than NCSE, as there may be only subtle changes in attentiveness. There may be a gradual start and stop to these periods. A typical feature, however, is "regressive behavior" from the patient's behavioral baseline.

NCSE in the Elderly

Diagnosis of NCSE in patients over 65 years of age is often missed or delayed, with the confusional state attributed to other disorders. Thomas et al. noted that a diagnosis of status could be delayed for eight hours to five days (7). The condition presented with clinical features such as "interrupted speech, catatonia, or slow and ataxic gait." In this population of *de novo* late-onset reactive absence status, daily activities could still be performed by many patients, but decision making was impaired. Sometimes, automatisms such as chewing or compulsive handling of objects occurred with clinical evidence of frontal release signs and a Babinski reflex.

A review of patients seen at Johns Hopkins Bayview Medical Center and a literature review showed that almost 75% of patients over 40 years of age were women, with typical triggers being toxic/metabolic dysfunction, drug withdrawal, or the use of neuroleptic and psychotropic medications (8). Although one-fifth of those patients showed minimal obtundation, two thirds had some impairment of consciousness, with staring, unresponsiveness, and catalepsy (waxy rigidity), severe language dysfunction, mutism, and verbal perseveration. There often were bizarre behaviors, agitation, aggressiveness, emotional lability, and hallucinations. Minor features were eyelid twitching or facial and limb myoclonus. There often was marked clinical variability from patient to patient.

EEG EVIDENCE OF SEIZURE ACTIVITY

The diagnosis of NCSE requires EEG evidence of seizure. Without EEG, the diagnosis remains questionable, and the etiology of behavioral or cognitive change can only be speculated. Some EEG findings have been discussed in the preceding section.

In brief, absence SE demonstrates a continuous or discontinuous 3-Hz spike-and-wave pattern on EEG. In addition, irregular spike and wave, prolonged bursts of spike activity, sharp wave, or polyspike wave patterns may occur. Complex partial status epilepticus may show focal epileptiform discharges that may be continuous or cyclical, with failure to regain consciousness between seizures.

The diagnosis of NCSE is straightforward when the EEG demonstrates typical ictal patterns. However, in many circumstances, EEG findings are difficult to differentiate from other encephalopathic patterns. Differentiation between NCSE and encephalopathies can be made by unequivocal electrographic seizure activity with typical evolution of EEG changes with a buildup of rhythmic activity, periodic epileptiform discharges or rhythmic discharges with clinical seizure activity, and rhythmic discharges with either clinical or electrographic response to antiepileptic medication.

PROGNOSIS

Prognosis of NCSE patients usually depends on the underlying etiology of NCSE (Tables 14-4, 14-5). CPSE in patients with epilepsy often recurs but responds to oral benzodiazepines. However, with systemic illness such as hypoxia and ischemic injury, head injury, stroke, infection, metabolic disorders, or dementia, the prognosis of CPSE largely depends on the underlying illness. Prognosis is poor with anoxic insult. Patients with nonconvulsive status epilepticus in coma may require intensive treatment.

Typical absence SE often ends with a tonic-clonic seizure and rarely causes neuronal damage. Though oral benzodiazepines are usually effective, oral or IV sodium valproate are alternatives in cases where respiratory

TABLE 14-4
Prognosis of NCSE

TYPES	PROGNOSIS	RESPONSE TO AEDs	RECURRENCE	OUTCOME
Ia. Absence status epilepticus (ASE)				
i. Typical absence SE (TAS)	Excellent	Excellent	Frequent	Excellent without comorbidity
ii. "De novo" absence status in the elderly	Excellent	Good, but may be delayed	Dependent on trigger	Excellent
iii. Absence status with degenerative generalized epilepsies; progressive myoclonic epilepsies	Guarded to fair	Variable	Frequent	Variable; occasional cognitive decline
Ib. Atypical absence status epilepsy (AASE)	Fair to poor	Relatively refractory	Frequent	Frequent cognitive morbidity, difficult to distinguish from the effects of disease progression
IIa. Simple partial nonconvulsive status epilepticus (SPSE)	Good to excellent in most cases	Excellent	Frequent	Excellent without comorbidity and mortality
IIb. Complex partial status epilepticus (CPSE)				
i. Complex partial SE of frontal lobe origin (FCPSE)	When not associated with comorbid insults, good to excellent	Good to very good, but often delayed	Frequent	Rare cognitive sequelae in < 1% of patients
ii. Complex partial SE of temporal lobe origin (TCPSE)	When not associated with comorbid insults, good to excellent	Good to very good, but often delayed	Frequent	Rare cognitive sequelae in < 1% of patients
III. NCSE Presentation by Age				
Electrical status epilepticus during slow sleep (ESES)	Fair to poor	Relatively refractory	Frequent	Frequent cognitive morbidity, difficult to distinguish from the effects of disease progression
Landau-Kleffner syndrome				
Minor epileptic status of Brett				
IV. Electrographic Seizures and Coma				
i. Subtle status usually postconvulsive status epilepticus (CSE)	Poor	Poor	Few	High morbidity and mortality
ii. With major CNS damage, but without apparent preceding CSE, often with multi-organ failure and/or myoclonias	Poor	Poor	Few	High morbidity and mortality

Adapted from Kaplan PW. Behavioral manifestations of non-convulsive status epilepticus. *Epilepsy & Behavior* 2002; 3:122–39.

TABLE 14-5
Recommended Treatment for NCSE

TYPE OF SEIZURE	TREATMENT CHOICE	ALTERNATIVE
Typical absence SE (TAS)	Oral or IV benzodiazepines	Acetazolamide or valproic acid
Atypical absence SE (AASE)	Oral or IV valproic acid	Oral or IV benzodiazepines (with caution), lamotrigine, or topiramate
Complex partial SE	Oral, rectal, or IV benzodiazepines	IV lorazepam and phenytoin (fosphenytoin) or phenobarbital
Electrical SE during sleep	Oral clobazam	Other benzodiazepines, corticosteroids, or subpial transection
Nonconvulsive SE in coma	IV benzodiazepines and phenytoin (fosphenytoin) or phenobarbital	Concomitant anesthesia with thiopental sodium, pentobarbital, propofol, or midazolam

IV = intravenous
Adapted from Wallace MC. Diagnosis and treatment of nonconvulsive status epilepticus. *CNS Drugs* 2001;15(12):931–939. With permission from Adis International.

depression is a concern. In *de novo* absence status, ongoing AED treatment is usually not needed.

CONCLUSION

The management of elderly patients experiencing SE presents many challenges to clinicians. Diagnosis and treatment are often complicated by comorbidities or age-related physiologic changes. The severity of SE and increased mortality of elderly patients experiencing SE magnify these difficulties. Treatment options may have different efficacies in older versus younger patients. There are few available data that are directly applicable to the elderly. Further studies on diagnosis and treatment options are needed.

*R*eferences

1. Kaplan PW. Behavioral manifestations of nonconvulsive status epilepticus. *Epilepsy Behav* 2002; 3:122–139.
2. Agathonikou A, Panayiotopoulos CP, Giannakodimos S, and Koutroumanidis M. Typical absence status in adults: diagnostic and syndromic considerations. *Epilepsia* 1988; 39:1265–1276.
3. Ballenger CE, King DW, Gallagher BB. Partial complex status epilepticus. *Neurology* 1983; 33:1545–1552.
4. Thomas P, Zifkin B, Migneco O, Lebrun C, et al. Nonconvulsive status epilepticus of frontal origin. *Neurology* 1999b; 52:1174–1183.
5. Stores G. Nonconvulsive status epilepticus in children. In: Pedley TA and Meldrum BS (eds). *Recent Advances in Epilepsy 3*. New York: Churchill Livingstone, 1986: 295–310.
6. Brodtkorb E, Sand T, Kristiansen A, Torbergsen T. Non-convulsive status epilepticus in the adult mentally retarded. *Seizure* 1993; 2:115–129.
7. Thomas P, Beaumanoir A, Genton P, et al. "De novo" absence status of late onset: report of 11 cases. *Neurology* 1992; 42:104–110.
8. Kaplan PW. Nonconvulsive status in the elderly. *Epilepsia* 1998:39(Suppl 6):122.

15 Reflex Epilepsies

Dorothée G.A. Kasteleijn-Nolst Trenité

It is a well-known fact that seizures can be provoked in general by both physical and mental stress. Physical stress includes fever, sleep deprivation, hyperventilation, drug or alcohol withdrawal, menstruation, and physical exercise. Mental or emotional stress is less clearly demonstrable and can be due to either happy occasions (birthdays, holiday celebrations, or the like), or more negative ones (problems at work, major life events such as death or divorce) (1).

In a recent prospective questionnaire survey among 1677 patients in Denmark, Norway, and the United States with a mixed epilepsy background, emotional stress (21%), sleep deprivation (12%), and tiredness (10%) were the most cited provocative factors (2).

About 6% of epilepsy patients recognize specific factors as their only or predominant precipitant of seizures. Usually the triggers are brief and sudden such as flashing lights, sudden noises, and tapping, provoking myoclonic jerks especially; they can also be more complex and gradual such as reading, thinking, listening to music, also with less sudden seizure expressions (temporal lobe type of seizures). All these patients have so-called reflex seizures and reflex epilepsies. If the trigger is exceptionally specific or exotic, the epilepsy is even named after the provocative factor such as mah-jong epilepsy, telephone epilepsy, vacuum cleaner epilepsy, and tooth brushing epilepsy (3–6).

Overall, the following types of provocative stimuli have repeatedly been reported in the literature: visual stimuli, startle, reading, speaking, tactile or somatosensory stimulation, drawing, praxis, listening to music (auditory), eating, bathing, arithmetic, thinking, decision making, and gaming (see for reviews 7, 8). Especially in the more complex type of reflex epilepsies, a general underlying provocative factor such as stress and emotion might play an important role: One patient with musicogenic epilepsy, for example, mentioned that seizures occurred exclusively when a specific part of an organ recital was played. That piece had been played in the church during the funeral of his father.

Most commonly, stimuli leading to seizures are sensory and external; others are internal triggers such as arithmetic, thinking, and decision making. This difference in trigger type must undoubtedly have impact on the behaviors and attitudes toward epilepsy of the respective patients, although no studies or reports have been made on this topic.

No patients have been reported in the literature with a history of more than one type of sensory or motor stimulus; whether it does not exist or simply is not detected as such is unclear. In this regard, in a recent case a 57-year-old man with temporal lobe epilepsy had 40% of his seizures provoked by tooth brushing, looking at the toothbrush, or even thinking about the brush (9). A somewhat wider epileptogenic network seemed to be involved than usually is considered in the reflex epilepsies.

Apart from the fact that reflex epilepsies are characterized by seizures consistently related to specific modes of precipitation either with or without spontaneous seizures, specific syndromes among the reflex epilepsies also have recently been recognized: idiopathic photosensitive occipital lobe epilepsy, other visual sensitive epilepsies, primary reading epilepsy, language-induced epilepsy, seizures induced by thinking, eating epilepsy, and musicogenic epilepsy (10).

The most common provocative factor (5%), well described (11) and by far the best-studied (12–14), is visual stimulation in its various forms (flickering sunlight, television, video games, and striped patterns). There are several reasons for this:

1. Flickering lights are rhythmic and are therefore more likely to lead to synchronization and thus to epileptic seizures than are, for example, music and bathing.
2. Flickering light is a relative simple and strong sensory stimulus, which can be detected easily in daily life (flickering sunlight).
3. Epileptic sensitivity to visual stimuli starts usually around 8 years of age and is at a maximum in adolescence. Lifestyle (disco, TV viewing at close distances) often leads to the first seizure, with a large impact as a result.
4. There is a simple equivalent, in the form of Intermittent Photic Stimulation (IPS), that can be applied during an electroencephalographic (EEG) recording and easily repeated.
5. Modern daily life is increasingly full of strong, repetitive visual stimuli, both at work and school (computer, TV) and during recreation (disco, video games).

This reflex phenomenon has fascinated clinicians for ages, and many case reports have been written.

The counterpart of provocation of seizures—reflex inhibition of seizures by specific actions, such as rubbing the skin or singing, as described by Vizioli in 1962 (15)—is rarely mentioned but must exist in a less conspicuous form in many patients (see also Matsuoka, Chapter 16, this volume). Vizioli described a boy who could suppress the generalization of his temporal onset seizures by singing any melody during his aura.

Reflex epilepsies have mainly been studied to learn more about the neuro- and pathophysiology of epilepsy. Behavior is a subject that has not been much touched upon. Only the self-inducing patients are known to have behavioral problems, which is not surprising, since it is rather strange that anyone would want to evoke seizures instead of suppressing them. Because of the difficulty in treating these patients, some behavioral intervention techniques have been described. Nevertheless, in this chapter an attempt will be made to highlight the issue of behavior in patients with reflex epilepsy, since it might help understand and treat epilepsy patients more effectively.

REFLEX SEIZURES AND BEHAVIOR

Psychosocial problems are more common among children with epilepsy than among controls (odds ratio five to nine) and are significantly related to epilepsy syndrome, main seizure type, age at onset, and seizure frequency (16).

No studies have been performed in patients with reflex epilepsies regarding these aspects. It has been hypothesized that the unpredictability of the occurrence of seizures especially causes feelings of anxiety and low-self esteem (17). Patients with reflex seizures do not have these problems, since there is a clear "explanation" for the seizures and seizures can be prevented by avoidance of the stimulus. Many of them are very creative in this respect; for example, a mother with a baby with hot-water epilepsy stopped bathing her child and wiped the baby clean with moist towelettes. A computer specialist figured out which screens were "safe" to use. A photosensitive patient found out that, for him, green glasses were the most effective measure to prevent visually triggered seizures, and this was later confirmed during an EEG with IPS.

The provocation of seizures by visual stimuli such as TV and flickering sunlight is rather well recognized nowadays, thanks to many publications in this field and dissemination of this knowledge to a broad public. Especially, outbreaks of photically induced seizures, such as by the video game Nintendo Super Mario World in 1992 or by the cartoon Pokémon shown in Japan on December 16,1997 (18, 19), have made the general public aware of the possibility that visual stimuli can provoke seizures in susceptible persons. Furthermore, inserts in manuals for video games, for liability purposes, remind the individual buyers of the possibility that playing video games can provoke epileptic seizures.

Other, more exotic stimuli are definitely less recognized by patients, family members, and physicians. Therefore, reflex epilepsy patients are seen by psychiatrists and psychologists—having a story about a specific trigger leading to seizures is considered abnormal behavior, and psychiatric consultation is the result. This was the case with a 30-year-old Dutch male patient complaining about simple and complex partial seizures and secondarily generalized tonic-clonic seizures (GTCS), all after answering a telephone, including his mobile phone, during both working hours and a holiday. The seizures started as follows: He could hear and recognize the voice through the phone but could not understand the meaning of the spoken words (described as "hearing out of phase"; "as if a strange language is spoken"). When he tried to answer, his words did not make sense, and further loss of contact with the surroundings followed (4). His general neurologist sent him immediately to the psychiatrist, but all neuropsychologic and psychiatric tests were normal. Later EEGs confirmed the reflex epilepsy nature of the complaints, and carbamazepine treatment was successful.

SELF-INDUCTION OR AUTO-INDUCTION

In General

Very few patients provoke seizures themselves by applying their reflex mechanism. They are called self-inducing patients. There is surprisingly little data about the reason why patients self-induce, apart from about 250 case reports that have been published so far. The vast majority are children using a visual stimulus. Most parents recognize the behavior as abnormal. Therapy resistance to antiepileptic drugs (AEDs) and to attempts to persuade and re-educate the child is characteristic. Although mentally retarded patients are mentioned often, by no means are they the majority; mentally retarded patients show the self-inducing behavior more bluntly, and it is also more accepted as such.

Fabisch and Darbyshire investigated a two-year-old boy who overbreathed regularly and increasingly in his bed, evoking a dazed state with eyes upwards and loss of consciousness. When the hyperventilation-induced attacks started to become longer, the absences ended in vomiting and incontinence. Treatment with ethosuximide (ESM) and primidone (PRM) did not help, but aversion techniques with drug-induced vomiting did for at least six months (20).

Voluntary bilateral compression of the carotid arteries, with jerks and loss of consciousness, has also been reported in a mentally retarded patient (21). Bebek et al. described self-induction in 9 out of 34 adolescents with hot water epilepsy. They poured water over their heads repeatedly while increasing the temperature of the water (22).

Other types of reflex mechanisms to self-induce seizures seem not to have been reported, but most likely they are not (yet?) recognized as such, since self-induced seizures are rare and often misdiagnosed as some sort of tic or strange behavior.

Self-Induction with Visual Stimuli

Radovici described in 1932 the first recognized self-inducing patient, who used bright sunlight (23). Patients generally wave hands in front of their eyes or blink with their heads turned toward the sun (sunflower syndrome).

Rhythmic rubbing of the forehead is another way of producing intermittent flicker, and maybe a somatosensory component adds to the effect. A strong artificial light can also be used. With the introduction of the TV in the 1960s, use of the screen as a means to self-induction became relatively popular: Several cases have been described with children being "drawn like a magnet" to the screen and being in trance, sometimes in combination with hand waving and blinking (4). Diagnosis can be very difficult, since many children are fascinated and attracted by the TV and therefore go closer and closer, absorbed in the program. Furthermore, in photo- and TV-sensitive patients the screen by itself evokes staring and loss of consciousness. Compulsive behavior and inability to change the behavior of the child to stay at a greater distance and use the remote control are strong indicators of self-induction.

Self-induction with striped and checkerboard patterns with high contrast are even rarer. Circular black-and-white patterns have also been described recently (24). The behavior of the child, seeking for patterns and being absorbed while looking at them, is in these cases very bizarre and thus easily recognized as self-induction. The combination of sunlight and curtains and fences can produce strong stimuli. One patient, an adolescent farmer boy, discovered that he could obtain certain sensations from standing in front of a snow fence when the sun was low and rocking back and forth so as to produce a flicker. He could also run back and forth under trees, using the interruption of the sunlight by the branches (25). Most patients, however, use more convenient methods such as eye blinking (14), and a change from hand waving to blinking is often noticed when the child gets older.

Until now the debate continues about whether the blinking and hand waving should be considered as part of the seizure itself (26, 27; eyelid movement with absences) or as the preceding act to evoke epileptiform discharges. The discrimination between the two is easy when the child or adult admits that he evokes the discharges and seizures deliberately. However, many persons feel ashamed of doing this, have developed a reflex type of more or less unconscious behavior, and thus will not or cannot tell the doctor.

Sparse EEG studies showed self-induction varying from 0.01 % (28) to 35% (14) of the 5% of all epilepsy patients who are photosensitive. Long term video-EEG monitoring increases the likelihood of finding self-inducers. In addition to observation of the patient, typical slow eye closures can be recorded (29).

Psychiatric Evaluation

In the literature there is mention of several reasons to self-induce: pleasure comparable to masturbation, compulsive behavior, reduction of irritability and anxiety, as well as a method to escape difficult situations (4, 25, 30, 31). Some authors have described in more detail the psychologic backgrounds, searching for reasons for the self-inducing behavior. Although it is difficult to generalize about motivational factors, all describe psychosocial problems, especially in relationship with the parents. Harley et al. considered them all as sensitive children who felt "different," inadequate, and unloved in families with little warmth (25).

A detailed report of psychoanalysis was given by Gottschalk of a 10-year-old only child, a boy with "screen spells" who underwent psychoanalysis for a period of 28 months with follow-up for another five years (32). This boy looked out the window into bright lights, looked occasionally at checkered or striped patterns on clothes, tablecloths, or drapery, with expression ranging from staring spells and jerks in the upper arms up to "grand mal" seizures. The onset of his stereotyped behavior occurred at the time his father left home to enter active duty in the army and his mother treated him as a man. He was adjudged by the psychiatrist as a very immature boy with whom it was difficult to establish close rapport. The boy explained his screen spells as "hypnotic powers, a habit, very silly." He considered these also as "uncontrollable attacks of rage," precipitated by seemingly trivial frustrating events. It gave him control and protection. AED treatment with bromides and phenytoin helped only partially. He felt also a terrible fear of punishment and abandonment for his forbidden impulses and primitive tensions. Becoming more aware of the mechanisms of his behavior, he started to feel ashamed and guilty and also recognized that he tried not to do it, but could not help it. After he left home at age 13 and learned how to handle his tensions, the spells gradually disappeared. Gottschalk considered the episodes as a kind of hysterical conversion, without a clear explanation of it.

No mention has ever been made of psychotic or manic episodes in patients with self-induced reflex epilepsies. Whether depression is an important reason to self induce is uncertain.

In the experience of the author, patients (children and adults) seem to have found a way to cope with daily life problems by using their escape mechanism. Nearly always there are problems between parents and children. Close collaboration with a psychiatrist knowledgeable in epilepsy is important to help the family (33).

Treatment

Preventive measures such as dark brown- or blue-colored glasses in photosensitive patients do not seem to work in self inducing patients; they manage to look around them or simply lose them. Prospective studies of pharmacological therapy are lacking. However, the scarce available clinical data suggest that patients respond best to immediate high dosages of the drugs that prevent the sensitivity to visual stimuli, such as valproate, in combination with psychologic treatment and, if necessary, such drugs as fenfluramine (34) and the dopamine-blocking agent pimozide (35). A prospective trial with pimozide at low doses of 2 mg was performed in 8 of the 37 invited self-inducing patients. Most patients were not interested in a trial, since the self-induction did not bother them; only teenagers wanted to get rid of their habit because they were nagged by their peers (35). The last-mentioned trial was performed based on the assumption that self-induction can be considered equivalent to self-stimulation in animals. In four patients a considerable decrease in self-induction rate was registered in the long-term video EEG recording; in two an increase was found. It appeared that although a slight increase in photosensitivity was found in the EEG, psychiatrists should not worry too much about antipsychotic treatment worsening the seizures. Increased fatigability and dystonia, however, were indeed found. Most remarkable was the complete lack of interest of the participating patients in the outcome of the trial. It was clear that they liked the attention they received during the trial very much but did not bother about its

---

TABLE 15-1

Issues to Consider in the Evaluation of Self-Inducing Patients

History
- Short-lasting seizures are repeatedly evoked by waving or blinking in bright sunlight or by looking at a close distance at the TV or at patterns.
- Episodes have a very high frequency; although GTCS might occur, usually the seizures are of very short duration, such as absences and jerks in the arms.
- During these episodes the self-inducer is lost in himself, and attention can be gained only by shouting or by touching.
- Compulsive stimulus-seeking behavior is exhibited.
- Psychosocial and learning problems are common.
- Intelligence can be normal or (slightly) abnormal.

Investigations
- EEG: Long-term video EEG recording with periods of inactivity and lack of attention, preferably in a sunny environment
- Psychiatric evaluation
- Ophthalmologic evaluation

Treatment
- High-dosage AEDs from the start, and dark glasses in addition
- Psychosocial support
- Neuropsychiatry drugs such as pimozide and fenfluramine if nothing seems to help

outcome. They all lost the diary. Noncompliance is a well-known problem in self-inducers.

SUMMARY AND CONCLUSIONS

Behavioral and psychiatric disorders are very little studied or described in patients with reflex epilepsy. No epidemiological, controlled, or prospective studies exist, possibly not only because a minority (6%) of epilepsy patients have a diversity of reflex seizures, but also because behavioral problems seem uncommon. On the other hand, the behavioral component in the self-inducing patients is recognized at large, albeit hardly studied, let alone treated as such. In many cases, the relationship between parents and child is disturbed

and intervention is necessary. The age and intelligence of the patient should especially be taken into account when considering psychosocial intervention therapy. The younger the patient, the greater the effect; most likely this is due to environmental factors such as peer pressure and to a lesser degree of imprinting and conditioning of the reflex behavior.

The diagnosis of reflex seizures depends highly on accurate and experienced history taking, capacity for observation of the patient inside and outside the hospital, and, above all, an open mind on the part of the neurologist. The self-inducing patients need neuropsychologic evaluation and involvement of a child psychiatrist knowledgeable in the field of epilepsy. Table 15-1 summarizes the issues to consider in the evaluation of self-inducing patients.

References

1. Webster A, Mawer GE. Seizure frequency and major life events in epilepsy. *Epilepsia* 1989; 30(2):162–167.
2. Nakken KO, Solaas MH, Kjeldsen MJ, Friis ML, et al. Which seizure-precipitating factors do patients with epilepsy most frequently report? *Epilepsy Behav* 2005; 6:85–189.
3. Kwan SY, Su MS. Mah-jong epilepsy: a new reflex epilepsy. *Zhonghua Yi Xue Za Zhi* 2000; 63(4):316–321.
4. Michelucci R, Gardella E, De Haan GJ, Bisulli F, et al. Telephone-induced seizures: a new type of reflex epilepsy. *Epilepsia* 2004; 45(3):280–283.
5. Carlson C, St Louis EK. Vacuum cleaner epilepsy. *Neurology* 2004; 63(1):190–191.
6. Holmes GL, Blair S, Eisenberg E, Scheebaum R, Margraf J, Zimmerman AW. Tooth-brushing-induced epilepsy. *Epilepsia* 1982; 23(6):657–661.
7. Wieser HG. Seizure induction in reflex seizures and reflex epilepsy. *Adv Neurol* 1998; 75:69–85.
8. Ng BY. Psychiatric aspects of self-induced epileptic seizures. *Aust N Z J Psychiatry* 2002 Aug; 36(4):534–543.
9. Navarro V, Adam C, Petitmengin C, Baulac M. Toothbrush-thinking seizures. *Epilepsia* 2006; 47(11):1971–1973.
10. Engel J Jr, International League Against Epilepsy (ILAE). A proposed diagnostic scheme for people with epileptic seizures and with epilepsy: report of the ILAE Task Force on Classification and Terminology. *Epilepsia* 2001; 42(6):796–803.
11. Gowers WR. Epilepsy and other chronic convulsive diseases: their causes, symptoms and treatment. New York: William Wood, 1885.
12. Harding GFA, Jeavons M. Photosensitive epilepsy. London: MacKeith Press, 1994.
13. Kasteleijn-Nolst Trenité DG. Reflex seizures induced by intermittent light stimulation. *Adv Neurol* 1998; 75:99–121.
14. Kasteleijn-Nolst Trenité DGA. Photosensitivity in epilepsy: electrophysiological and clinical correlates. *Acta Neurol Scand* 1989; 80 Suppl 25:1–150.
15. Vizioli R. The problem of human reflex epilepsy and the possible role of masked epileptogenic factors. *Epilepsia* 1962; 3:293–302.
16. Hoie B, Sommerfelt K, Waaler PE, Alsaker FD, et al. Psychosocial problems and seizure-related factors in children with epilepsy. *Dev Med Child Neurol* 2006; 48(3):213–219.
17. Ryan BL, Speechley KN, Levin SD, Stewart M. Parents' and physicians' perceptions of childhood epilepsy. *Seizure* 2003; 12(6):359–368.
18. Furusho J, Suzuki M, Tazaki I, Satoh H, et al. A comparison survey of seizures and other symptoms of Pokemon phenomenon. *Pediatr Neurol* 2002; 27:350–355.
19. Kasteleijn-Nolst Trenité DG, Van Der Beld G, Heynderickx I, Groen P. Visual stimuli in daily life. *Epilepsia* 2004; 45 Suppl 1:2–6.
20. Fabisch W, Darbyshire R. Report on an unusual case of self-induced epilepsy with comments on some psychological and therapeutic aspects. *Epilepsia* 1965; 6:335–340.
21. Lai C, Ziegler DK. Repeated self-induced syncope and subsequent seizures. *Arch Neurol* 1983; 40: 820–823.
22. Bebek N, Baykan B, Gurses C, Emir O, et al. Self-induction behavior in patients with photosensitive and hot water epilepsy: a comparative study from a tertiary epilepsy center in Turkey. *Epilepsy Behav* 2006; 9(2):317–326.
23. Radovici A, Mirsiliou V, Gluckman M. Épilepsie reflexe provoqueé par excitations optiques des rayons solaires. *Rev Neurol* 1932; 1:1305–1308.
24. Brockmann K, Huppke P, Karenfort M, Gartner J, et al. Visually self-induced seizures sensitive to round objects. *Epilepsia* 2005; 46(5):786–789.
25. Harley RD, Baird HW, Freeman RD. Self-induced photogenic epilepsy. *Arch Ophthal* 1967; 78:730–737.
26. Livingston S, Torres IC. Photic epilepsy: report of an unusual case and review of the literature. *Clin Pediatr (Phila)* 1964; 3:304–307.
27. Covanis A. Eyelid myoclonia and absence. *Adv Neurol* 2005; 95:185–96.
28. Wadlington WB, Riley HD. Light-induced seizures. *J Pediatr* 1965; 66:300–311.
29. Binnie CD, Kasteleijn-Nolst Trenité, DGA, De Korte RA, Overweg J. Self-induction of epileptic seizures: incidence, clinical features and treatment. *Electroencephalogr Clin Neurophysiol* 1981; 52(3):58–59.
30. Kasteleijn-Nolst Trenité DGA. Dostoevsky's epilepsy induced by television. *J Neurol Neurosurg Psychiatry* 1997; 63/2:273.
31. Rabending G, Klepel H, Krell D, Rehbein D. Selbstreizung bei photogener Epilepsie. *Psychiatrie, Neurologie und medizinische Psychologie* 1969,11:427–434.
32. Gottschalk LA. The relationship of psychologic state and epileptic activity: psychoanalytic observations on an epileptic child. Lecture given at the Psychoanalytic Society, March 1956.
33. Kanner AM. When did neurologists and psychiatrists stop talking to each other? *Epilepsy Behav* 2003; 4:597–601.
34. Aicardi J, Gastaut H. Treatment of self induced photosensitive epilepsy with fenfluramine. *N Engl J Med* 1985; 313:1419.
35. Kasteleijn-Nolst Trenité, DGA, Binnie, CD, Overweg J, Oosting J, et al. Treatment of self-induction in epileptic patients: who wants it? In: Beaumanoir A, Gastaut H, Naquet R, eds. *Reflex Seizures and Reflex Epilepsies.* Geneva: Editions Médecine & Hygiéne, 1989:439–445.

16 Behavioral Precipitants of Seizures

Hiroo Matsuoka

Behavior is the manifest aspect of mental activity. It remains unclear how much mental activities have an impact on each epilepsy or seizure, since standard electroencephalographic (EEG) examination usually includes only sleep, hyperventilation, photic stimulation, and opening and closing of the eyes, but not systematic mental tasks. Reflex epilepsies induced by daily behaviors such as movement, tapping, toothbrushing, eating, bathing, reading, singing, calculating, speaking, writing, drawing, game playing, and thinking have been described in the literature, but such triggers are considered to be uncommon. For example, standard EEG recordings at the Mayo Clinic in the United States included a mental arithmetic calculation task, but only 1 patient showed an EEG effect out of patients screened in over 100,000 recordings (1).

On the other hand, it has been pointed out that various daily mental activities can facilitate or inhibit seizure occurrence beyond expectation in patients with epilepsy (2).

REFLEX EPILEPSY INDUCED BY BEHAVIORS

Special EEG Activation Method ("Routine NPA")

To examine how much behavioral activities influence epileptic EEG discharges, we devised a particular EEG activation protocol, which we call neuropsychologic EEG activation (NPA), that tests for various mental activities (3–5). "Routine NPA" comprises reading silently and aloud, speaking, mental calculation, written calculation, writing, and spatial construction. Detailed descriptions of these activities were as follows.

1. Reading silently: Subjects silently read three Japanese sentences that were printed on a sheet of paper and were quoted from the Japanese version of the Binet test.
2. Reading aloud: Subjects read the same sentences out loud that they had read silently.
3. Speaking: Subjects described from memory what they had read silently and aloud.
4. Mental calculation: Subjects responded aloud with answers to four arithmetic problems. When a calculation was difficult for the subject, an easier problem was presented.
5. Written calculation: Subjects responded in writing to one arithmetic problem.
6. Writing: Subjects were asked to write out two Japanese sentences in phonograms (*kana*) and three Japanese phrases in ideograms (*kanji*).
7. Spatial construction: Subjects were instructed to draw a fish, a human face, and a clock, and they performed the block design test using 9 blocks of the Wechsler Adult Intelligence Scale-Revised (WAIS-R) (see Table 16-1 for more details).

TABLE 16-1
Routine Neuropsychologic EEG Activation

(1) Reading silently
Last night a fire broke out about 10 o'clock at Asakusa in Tokyo. The fire was put under control for an hour, in which 17 houses were destroyed. When a fireman rescued a girl who was sleeping soundly on the second floor, his face was burned.

(2) Reading aloud
(use the same sentences as (1))

(3) Speaking
(use the same sentences as (1))

(4) Mental arithmetic calculation
$18 - 7$, $23 + 48$, 11×11, $125 \div 5$

(5) Written arithmetic calculation
$15 \times 67 \times 23 \times 48$

(6) Writing
There is a large tree on the top of a mountain.
The sun rises in the east.
The 4 cardinal points
The 4 seasons
The Prime Minister

(7) Spatial construction
Drawing figures
Block design test

It took 10–20 minutes for each patient to accomplish the routine NPA. A surface electromyogram was often monitored to detect myoclonic seizures. Simultaneous video-EEG monitoring during the routine and detail NPA was utilized for later analysis.

Influence of Behavior on Epileptic Discharge

We studied 480 patients with epilepsy (247 males and 233 females), after obtaining each participant's informed consent (5, 6). All but 18 patients were treated with antiepileptic drugs (AEDs), and 25 patients were also given neuroleptics for psychiatric disturbances. At the time of EEG examination, mean age and standard deviation of the sample was 26.3 ± 10.8 years (range 10–66 years). The mean duration of illness was 10.8 ± 9.5 years (range 1–59 years). Criteria for sample selection and classification of epilepsies and epileptic syndromes have been shown in detail elsewhere (5).

To exclude the contamination of incidental discharges unrelated to activation, we defined the NPA effect operationally, based on the EEG in a state of relaxed wakefulness (including opening and closing of the eyes), known as the awake EEG.

When no discharge was found on the awake EEG, "an NPA provocation effect" meant that one or more tasks induced paroxysmal discharges and that its reproducibility was confirmed by retrial. No discharge in the awake or NPA condition was judged as "no NPA provocation effect."

When epileptic discharges were found on the awake EEG, the activation rate was calculated for each task as follows. The number of discharges per recording time (number per minute) in each task condition that induced paroxysms was divided by the frequency (number per minute) in the awake condition. We tentatively defined the "provocative NPA effect" as above 2.0, "inhibitory NPA effect" as below 0.5, and "zero NPA effect" as between 0.5 and 2.0, according to the activation rate.

NPA showed an inhibitory effect in 133 (63.9%) out of 208 patients with paroxysms in the awake EEG. On the other hand, the provocative effect of NPA tasking was observed in a total of 38 (7.9%) out of 480 patients, comprising 18 patients without paroxysms and 20 patients with paroxysms in the awake EEG.

Triggers identified by NPA were writing in 26 patients, spatial construction in 24, written calculation in 21, mental calculation in 3, and reading aloud or silently in 2. One patient with temporal lobe epilepsy among 38 patients sensitive to NPA showed nonspecific psychic tension, unrelated to the NPA tasks, to be a trigger. These triggers were almost the same as those identified by the previous history in these patients.

Epilepsy and Seizure Type Related to Behavioral Precipitants

The patients who were examined in our study showed a wide distribution of epilepsies and epileptic syndromes (5), with 36 out of the 38 patients showing provocative NPA effects being classified as having idiopathic generalized epilepsy (IGE). The remaining 2 patients were classified as having temporal lobe epilepsy (cryptogenic localization-related epilepsy). The percentage of patients with provocative NPA effect was 24.7% in IGE, and 1.0% in cryptogenic localization-related epilepsy.

Among IGE patients, NPA provocative effects were found in 22 (46.7%) with juvenile myoclonic epilepsy (JME); 6 (15.8%) with grand mal seizures on awakening (GMA); 3 (16.7%) with juvenile absence epilepsy (JAE); 1 (7.1%) patient with childhood absence epilepsy (CAE); and 4 (12.9%) with other generalized idiopathic epilepsies not defined above. Since four epileptic syndromes (JME, GMA, JAE, and CAE) overlap in their manifestations and the boundaries between them are obscure, there may be a nosologic relationship between these IGE subtypes (7, 8). Seizure susceptibility to mental activities

TABLE 16-2
Seizure Types in 146 Patients with Idiopathic Generalized Epilepsy

Combination Seizures	Total Number of Patients	Number (%) of Patients with Provocative Effect of NPA
MS only	12	6 (50.0%)
MS with GTCS	21	9 (42.9%)
MS with AS and GTCS	25	10 (40.0%)
MS with AS	19	7 (36.8%)
GTCS only	26	2 (7.7%)
AS with GTCS	34	2 (5.9%)
AS only	9	0 (0.0%)
(total)	146	36 (24.6%)

NPA: neuropsychologic EEG activation; MS: myoclonic seizure; GTCS: generalized tonic-clonic seizure; AS: absence seizure

in IGE suggests a pathophysiological similarity between syndromes.

According to the combinations of myoclonic seizure, absence seizure, and generalized tonic-clonic seizure, the IGE patients were divided into 7 groups as shown in Table 16-2. The groups comprising patients with myoclonic seizure showed higher provocative NPA effect rates (minimum; 36.8%, maximum 50.0%) than the others (minimum; 0.0%, maximum 7.7%).

MECHANISM OF BEHAVIORAL PRECIPITANTS

We conclude that certain behaviors such as reading, speaking, calculating, writing, drawing, and thinking inhibit and provoke seizure activity of the patients with epilepsy in 63.9% and 7.9%, respectively, and that the provocative effects were closely related to the epilepsy subtype (JME among IGE) and seizure type (myoclonic seizures). Such relevance may be linked to the pathophysiology of seizure-induction mechanism by behavioral activity (5, 6, 9).

Special EEG Activation Method ("Detail NPA")

When the routine NPA induced epileptic discharges in our study, a "detail NPA" was conducted to identify the precipitating factor precisely [3–5]. Table 16-3 outlines the detail NPA tasks and their respective cognitive categories, which are number-coded.

Neuropsychologic Evaluation

From the detailed NPA findings, we identified three activity types related to seizure induction (Figure 16-1): (1)

hand movement independent of higher mental activity (motor activity), (2) higher mental activity not requiring hand movement (thinking activity), and (3) higher mental activity requiring hand movement (action-programming activity).

To isolate motor activity as the seizure-inducing factor, we employed detailed NPA tasks requiring no higher mental activity (i.e., finger tapping, fine finger movement, and drawing meaningless lines). If a patient showed provocation of epileptic discharges during these tasks comparable to the provocation observed with writing, written calculation, or spatial construction, we judged the precipitating factor to be motor activity.

When motor activity was negligible, we further explored whether epileptic discharges would be triggered by thinking activity or action-programming activity. We carefully analyzed the video-EEG data and employed detail NPA tasks that did not require hand movement (i.e., visualizing letters and constructing sentences in the mind relative to writing, mental calculation relative to written calculation, and mental construction of a block design illustrated in the block design test of WAIS-R relative to spatial construction).

We judged the associated trigger to be thinking activity when epileptic discharges were induced by the tasks without hand movement, and we judged the trigger to be action-programming activity when epileptic discharges were induced only by tasks requiring hand movement. We excluded from this analysis any epileptic discharges that were induced during the testing if a subject was perplexed or embarrassed, since this made it difficult to identify the precipitating factor precisely. Based on the task demands of NPA, we carefully analyzed two activity types related to seizure induction: linguistic (or verbal) activity and praxic activity.

TABLE 16-3
Detail Neuropsychologic EEG Activation

(1) Writing
 1. Spontaneous writing
 2. Dictation
 3. Copying
 4. Spontaneous writing blindfolded
 5. Dictation blindfolded
 6. Dictation by foot
Each was examined for Japanese letters (Hiragana, Katakana, Kanji), Roman letters, and English letters.

(2) Speaking
 1. Spontaneous speaking
 2. Reading aloud
 3. Repeating
Each was examined in Japanese and English.

(3) Other verbal activities
 1. Reading silently
 2. Visualizing letters
 3. Constructing sentences in the mind

(4) Calculation
 1. Written arithmetic calculation
 2. Mental arithmetic calculation
 3. Calculation using an abacus
 4. Calculation using an electronic calculator
Each was examined for subtraction, addition, multiplication, and division.
 5. Uchida-Kraepelin's psychodiagnostic test

(5) Spatial construction
 1. Spontaneous drawing
 2. Sketching maps
 3. Copying figures
 4. Matchstick pattern reproduction
 5. Block design test of WAIS-R*
 6. Making plastic models
 7. Mental construction of block design (using illustrations of block design test of WAIS-R*)

(6) Other tests
 1. Finger tapping
 2. Fine finger movement (tremolo)
 3. Drawing meaningless lines
 4. Using a screwdriver
 5. Bourdon cancellation test
 6. Undoing puzzle rings
 7. Hand, eye, and ear tests
 8. Finger agnosia tests
 9. Color classification
 10. Humming
 11. Singing

WAIS-R: * Wechsler Adult Intelligence Scale—Revised.

CLASSIFICATION OF BEHAVIORAL PRECIPITANTS

Two Dimension Hypothesis of Reflex Epilepsy

We propose a hypothesis for the seizure-induction mechanism in IGE patients sensitive to mental activity (5, 6, 9). Reading epilepsy is excluded in this hypothesis because we had no patients with reading epilepsy. Precipitating factors were divided into two dimensions: action-programming vs. thinking activity, and linguistic vs. praxic activity (Figure 16-2). Planned multiple tasking, such as NPA, is necessary to analyze precipitating factors as mentioned above. The necessity of hand movements in the seizure-inducing tasks differentiates the action-programming activity from the thinking activity. The necessity of language in the seizure-inducing tasks differentiates the linguistic activity from the praxic activity.

There was no patient in whom the precipitating factor was judged to be motor activity rather than mental activity. Action-programming was critical for the induction of epileptic discharges in 32 out of the 36 IGE patients with provocative NPA effects. Among 32 patients, 5 patients showed the precipitating factor to be restricted to linguistic activity, that is, writing. The remaining 27 patients were affected by varying action-programming factors including both linguistic and praxic activities. In the remaining 4 out of 36 IGE patients, the precipitating factor was thinking, predominantly the linguistic task in 1 patient and the spatial task in 3 patients.

Reflex Epilepsies Induced by Thinking and Action-Programming

From the point of view of the two-dimension hypothesis, reflex epilepsies reported previously may overlap or interrelate with each other.

Epilepsy induced by thinking and spatial tasks (10, 11) has been described as a rather homogeneous IGE syndrome. Generalized seizures in this syndrome are activated by thinking or decision making, which is common to calculation, card and board games, and spatial tasks, and neuropsychologic analysis of the stimuli points to parietal cortical participation in seizure induction. The clinical profile of the condition is suggestive of JME or JAE. Writing has not been identified as a trigger in the form of reflex epilepsy, and action-programming activity associated with use of the hands is little emphasized (11). In our study, 4 IGE patients (3 JME and 1 GMA) showed susceptibility to thinking activity without action-programming activity and may have a pathophysiology similar to the reflex epilepsy induced by thinking and spatial tasks. Therefore, it is likely that

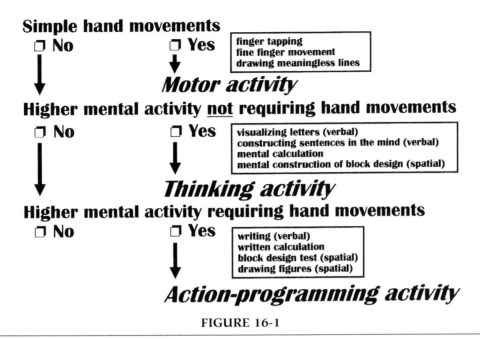

FIGURE 16-1

Decision process to identify the three precipitants. Motor activity, thinking activity, and action-programming activity are identified by the detail neuropsychologic EEG activation.

IGE seizures induced by mental activity consist of at least two forms: seizures induced by thinking and spatial tasks, and seizures induced by writing, written calculation, or drawing requiring action-programming activity. These two forms would either show distinct mechanisms of seizure induction or represent two ends of a pathophysiological continuum.

Inoue et al. (12, 13) reported patients with reflex epilepsy in whom myoclonic seizures mainly involving the arms were precipitated by a nonlinguistic praxic activity accompanied by calculation, game playing, writing, drawing, construction, or copying. They stressed "a combination of complicated process

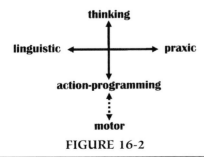

FIGURE 16-2

Two-dimension hypothesis. Reflex epilepsy in idiopathic generalized epilepsy would be sorted by the two dimensions: thinking vs. action-programming activity, and linguistic vs. praxic activity.

of thinking (decision-making) along with voluntary motor activities (including ideation of voluntary acts) involving the fingers and arms" as the seizure induction mechanism. In contrast with the reflex epilepsy induced by thinking and spatial tasks (10, 11), Inoue et al. (12, 13) listed writing as one of the major precipitating factors and emphasized requisite hand movement in seizure induction, factors that were quite similar to our action-programming activity provocations. Based on the NPA tasking results and detail analysis of habitual seizures, we confirmed precipitating factors to be action-programming activity in 32 out of the 36 patients with IGE; linguistic activity alone in 5, both linguistic and nonlinguistic activity in 20, and nonlinguistic activity alone in 7. Therefore, the mechanism of action-programming seizure induction would have two forms related to linguistic and nonlinguistic activities as the endpoints on a pathophysiological continuum. This is supported by the induced spike activity in a patient reported by Hasegawa et al. (14), which predominated over the dominant central EEG site with letter writing and over the nondominant parietocentral EEG site with spatial construction.

Figure 16-3 summarizes the position of reflex epilepsy induced by various mental activities. Decision-making epilepsy (4, 15) is characterized as the thinking activity at the interface between linguistic and praxic activities. Epilepsy induced by thinking and spatial tasks (10, 11) is classified as a praxic thinking activity. Epilepsy

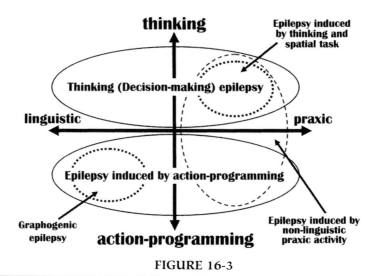

FIGURE 16-3

Two-dimension hypothesis and various reflex epilepsies. Various reflex epilepsies induced by mental activities are positioned based on the two dimensions. Reading epilepsy and language-induced epilepsy are excluded.

induced by nonlinguistic praxic activity (12, 13) would be classified as the praxic activity interfaced between thinking and action-programming activities. Graphogenic epilepsy (16) is classified as linguistic action-programming activity. Epilepsy induced by action-programming (4–6), observed in 27 out of 36 IGE patients with provocative NPA effects in our study, is classified as the action-programming activity interfaced between linguistic and praxic activities.

Language-Induced Epilepsy and Reading Epilepsy

Geschwind and Sherwin (17) described a case of language-induced epilepsy, in which seizures were precipitated by three language functions: speaking, writing, and reading. These observations made us expect reading to trigger seizure activity in our patients with epilepsy. However, reading aloud and silently were less provocative, and none of our patients were diagnosed with reading epilepsy (18) or language-induced epilepsy. Therefore, these types of reflex epilepsies may not be sorted in terms of the two-dimension hypothesis.

Since prolonged reading is usually necessary to induce seizures in reading epilepsy (19), the rarity of "reading" as a precipitating factor in the present study might stem simply from the activation method. However, we failed to find any suggestion of reading epilepsy in our series, despite our great interest in reflex epilepsy. This rarity might be characteristic of Japanese patients. We must consider ethnic variation, as noted in the genetic study of JME, or linguistic features specific to the Japanese written

languages. To clarify this question, NPA tasking should be applied in other languages to different sample groups of different racial backgrounds.

CONCLUSION

In the management of epilepsy, not only antiepileptic drug therapy but also identification and regulation of seizure-precipitating or -inhibiting factors are important for achieving successful treatment. Seizure-precipitating or -inhibiting factors have varying influences upon the diverse epilepsies and epileptic syndromes because of close relationships between these factors and the underlying pathophysiologic characteristics that differentiate the various forms of epilepsies. For elucidating the pathophysiology of epilepsy in any patient, it is important to know the relationship between seizure-precipitating or -inhibiting factors and the epilepsy subtype or seizure type. Neuropsychologic EEG activation confirmed the notion that various daily mental activities can facilitate or inhibit seizure occurrence beyond expectation in patients with epilepsy. We believe the two-dimension hypothesis in reflex epilepsy has heuristic value for future research into the mechanisms behind seizures induced by behavioral activities.

Acknowledgments

We thank T. Okuma, M. Sasaki, T. Hasegawa, T. Takahashi, and M. Sato for their help in various aspects of this research.

References

1. Wiebers DO, Westmoreland BF, Klass DW. EEG activation and mathematical calculation. *Neurology* 1979; 29:1499–1503.

2. Fenwick PBC. Self-generation of seizure by an action of mind. In: Zifkin BG, Andermann F, Beaumanoir A, Rowan AJ, eds. *Reflex Epilepsies and Reflex Seizures*. Advances in Neurology 75. Philadelphia: Lippincott-Raven, 1998:87–92.

3. Okuma T, Takahashi T, Hasegawa K, Wagatsuma S, et al. Neuropsychological EEG activation in epileptic patients. In: Ito M, ed. *Integrative Control Functions of the Brain*, vol. III. Tokyo: Kohdansha Scientific, 1980:103–104.

4. Matsuoka H, Hasegawa T, Takahashi T, Okuma T. Myoclonic seizures induced by decision making and psychic tension; with special reference to the findings obtained by neuropsychological EEG activation. *Psychiatr Neurol Jpn* 1981; 83:211–221.

5. Matsuoka H, Takahashi T, Sasaki M, et al. Neuropsychological EEG activation in patients with epilepsy. *Brain* 2000; 123:318–330.

6. Matsuoka H, Nakamura M, Ohno T, et al. The role of cognitive-motor function in precipitation and inhibition of epileptic seizures. *Epilepsia* 2005;46 Suppl. 1:17–20.

7. Janz D. Juvenile myoclonic epilepsy. In: Dam M, Gram L, eds. *Comprehensive Epileptology*. New York: Raven Press, 1990:171–85.

8. Reutens DC, Berkovic SF. Idiopathic generalized epilepsy of adolescence: are the syndromes clinically distinct? *Neurology* 1995; 45:1469–1476.

9. Matsuoka H. Neuropsychology of epilepsy. *Epilepsia* 2001; 42 Suppl. 6:42–46.

10. Wilkins A, Zifkin B, Andermann F, McGovern E. Seizures induced by thinking. *Ann Neurol* 1982; 11:608–612.

11. Andermann F, Zifkin BG, Andermann E. Epilepsy induced by thinking and spatial tasks. In: Zifkin BG, Andermann F, Beaumanoir A, Rowan AJ, eds. *Reflex Epilepsies and Reflex Seizures*. Advances in Neurology 75. Philadelphia: Lippincott-Raven; 1998:263–272.

12. Inoue Y, Suzuki S, Watanabe Y, Yagi K, et al. Non-lesional reflex epilepsy evoked by non-verbal higher cerebral activities. *J Jpn Epilepsy Soc* 1992; 10:1–9.

13. Inoue Y, Seino M, Tanaka M, et al. Epilepsy with praxis-induced epilepsy. In: Wolf P, ed. *Epileptic Seizures and Syndromes*. London: John Libbey, 1994:81–91.

14. Hasegawa T, Matsuoka H, Takahashi T, Okuma T. Myoclonic seizures induced by writing, calculation with figures and constructive acts: with special reference to neuropsychological EEG activation. *Psychiatr Neurol Jpn* 1981; 83:199–210.

15. Forster FM. Reflex epilepsy, behavioral therapy and conditional reflexes. Springfield: Charles C Thomas, 1977.

16. Ashbury AK, Prensky AL. Graphogenic epilepsy. *Trans Am Neurol Assoc* 1963; 88:193–194.

17. Geschwind N, Sherwin I. Language-induced epilepsy. *Arch Neurol* 1967; 16:25–31.

18. Bickford RG, Whelan JL, Klass DW, Corbin KB. Reading epilepsy; clinical and electroencephalographic studies of a new syndrome. *Trans Am Neurol Assoc* 1956; 81:100–102.

19. Ramani V. Reading epilepsy. In: Zifkin BG, Andermann F, Beaumanoir A, Rowan AJ, eds. *Reflex Epilepsies and Reflex Seizures*. Advances in Neurology 75. Philadelphia: Lippincott-Raven, 1998:241–262.

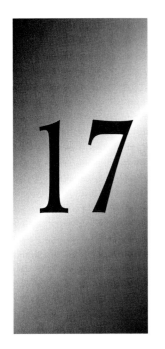

17

Behaviors Mimicking Seizures in Institutionalized Persons with Epilepsy

John C. DeToledo

Epilepsy and behaviors that mimic epilepsy are both common in the institutionalized patient with developmental disabilities (DD). Any physician caring for these patients in the institutions knows how much diligence and time it takes to separate one from the other. This diagnostic challenge increases substantially when these patients are seen in the community, where the consultant rarely has access to the entire medical history, and what is available is often incomplete and inaccurate.

The classic teaching on the semiology of epileptic seizures is that seizures are "stereotypic" events and that there is a correlation between some of these manifestations and the area of the brain where they are likely to originate (1). These diagnostic principles were generally based on, and are applicable to, older children and adults with otherwise reasonably intact CNS function. The semiology of seizures in other age groups including neonates, various idiopathic and cryptogenic early childhood epilepsy syndromes (2), and seizures in the elderly has proven more difficult to diagnose and classify (3). The same is true for epilepsy in individuals with multiple handicaps. The presence of diffuse CNS pathology occurring early in development and the coexistence of complex musculoskeletal deformities can result in atypical presentations of otherwise typical epileptic seizures. The presence of

various repetitive behaviors and the decreased ability to communicate further contribute to the difficulty. This chapter, therefore, reviews the characteristics of epileptic and nonepileptic behaviors in patients with DD.

EPILEPTIC EVENTS

The diagnostic challenges in reference to the diagnosis of epileptic seizures in the DD population fall basically in one of two groups: (i) new onset of events in patients without a previous history of epilepsy, (ii) new type of events in a patient with previously diagnosed epileptic seizures. In contrast to the general population, the prevalence of patients with multiple seizure types is relatively high in institutions (4). The physician caring for the DD patient with mixed seizure types, who feels constantly perplexed by the protean clinical manifestations of these seizures, should not feel alone. Multiple panels of epilepsy experts have spent years trying to describe the clinical manifestations and classify these seizures, not always with the greatest success (5). The International Classification of Epilepsies and Epileptic Syndromes resorted to terms such as "cryptogenic (presumed to be symptomatic but with unknown etiology)," "other symptomatic generalized epilepsies not defined above," and "epilepsies and syndromes undetermined as to whether focal or

TABLE 17-1

Behaviors Mimicking Epilepsy in Institutionalized Patients with Multiple Disabilities

STAFF DIAGNOSIS	TYPE OF BEHAVIOR	NUMBER OF PATIENTS	REMARKS
Absence seizures, petit mal seizures	Periods of decreased responsiveness	8	Chronic sleep deprivation, patients appeared to be taking "naps"
Buccolingual automatisms due to complex partial seizures	Chewing, lip smacking	6	(a) Tardive dyskinesia; (b) mouth breathers seemingly attempting to wet their tongues
Rule out seizures	Self-stimulation	5	Very difficult patients with self-stimulation and abuse; staff "grasping at straws" trying to find a treatable cause
	Self-abuse	2	
Temporal lobe seizures	Disruptive, aggressive behaviors	5	Difficult behavior patients; staff "grasping at straws" trying to find a treatable cause
"Petit mal" seizures	Behavioral "pauses"	5	Fatigue, boredom, medication effect
Absence seizures	Repeated eye blinking	4	
Petit mal seizures, laughing seizures	Spontaneous smiling	4	Profoundly retarded
"Petit mal" seizures	Spontaneous grimacing	3	Profoundly retarded
Tonic seizures	Dystonic posturing	3	Patients with spasticity and severe contractures of the extremities; posturing triggered by being startled (e.g., bath)
Seizures	Simulation of seizures	3	Higher-functioning patients, often to be excused from chores (i.e., work)
Drop attacks	Unexplained falls	3	Medication-induced ataxia
"Withdrawal seizures"	Increased alertness (more impatient)	2	
Eye deviation due to seizures	Roving eye movements	2	Roving eye movements in blind patients
Clonic seizures	Clonus of extremities	2	Patients with spasticity and severe contractures of the extremities
Rule out seizures	Tics	2	

Source: Adapted with permission from DeToledo JC, Lowe MR, Haddad H. Behaviors mimicking seizures in institutionalized individuals with multiple disabilities and epilepsy: a video-EEG study. *Epilepsy Behav* 2002;3(3):242–244.

generalized" to classify some of the seizure types seen in the DD population (2).

Seizures in these cases tend to be more refractory to medical treatment and more frequently result in status epilepticus and injuries. The possibility that an unusual behavior represents seizures is often cause for great concern and anxiety to caregivers, families, and institutional physicians, and an immediate diagnosis and treatment are often expected. These pressures can lead to the premature labeling of nonepileptic events as "epileptic" in the DD patient.

In those individuals with an established diagnosis of epilepsy, an occasional cause for confusion arises when someone, usually a teacher or caregiver, identifies a "new seizure type" in that person. Fortunately, the development of a new seizure type in institutionalized patients with a well-established seizure pattern is not common, and the majority of the newly identified episodes turn out to be nonepileptic in nature (Table 17-1) (6). Another cause of confusion in regard to the DD patient with an established diagnosis of epilepsy is the fact that, over time, there is some degree of variability in the severity and duration of a given seizure type in a given patient. Shorter episodes of the same seizure may contain only fragments of the whole episode, and staff may identify the fragments as a "new seizure type." Medication changes or concurrent systemic illnesses are common causes of changes in seizures in the DD patient.

Generalized convulsions may present very asymmetrically, resembling partial seizures, in patients with fixed neurologic deficits such as infantile hemiplegia, and the diagnosis of a partial seizure can be erroneously made.

Staff is sometimes confused by the fact that patients with a previous history of generalized convulsions seem to have developed a new seizure type after having an orthopedic or respiratory problem that requires forced lateral decubiti. Generalized seizures in these cases are almost always asymmetric, because only two of the extremities exhibit the tonic-clonic movements, the other two being now under the body.

NONEPILEPTIC EVENTS

Reaching the correct diagnosis of nonepileptic events in the outpatient setting is seldom a straightforward proposition. Parental anxiety, poor training of staff, and poor communication with and between caregivers are common problems.

Medication Changes

Episodes occurring during reduction of antiepileptic drugs (AEDs) can be misdiagnosed by the staff as representing seizures. A patient's complacent behavior may be due to sedation. As barbiturates or benzodiazepines are tapered and sedation subsides, the underlying personality emerges. It might be a pleasant one, but it often is not. Caregivers may mistake the less agreeable personality as representing seizures or "drug withdrawal." The new, more demanding personality often entails more work and is not necessarily welcome news to overworked staff.

Eye Movements

There are a number of eye movement abnormalities that can be confused with the manifestations of seizures. This occurs most often in patients with impaired visual fixation, as may be seen with amblyopia, congenital cataract, and congenital retinal degenerations. Perinatal anoxia, postmeningitic encephalopathies, and congenital rubella are common etiologies. The nature of the movements usually varies according to the position of the eyes. When the gaze is directed forward, the movement is largely pendular; with lateral gaze there may be a period of conjugate deviation of gaze accompanied by jerky nystagmus. These episodes can be differentiated from epileptic tonic deviation of gaze by the fact that the latter can be broken by rotation of the head in the horizontal plane. Other elements that help the diagnosis is the fact that these patients are blind or nearly so and that the nystagmus has been present for years.

Buccolingual Movements

These types of movements become a concern when staff is partially educated about seizures and fear the movements may represent epileptic automatisms. Causes for these movements are many, but most often cases are due to medication side effects or anatomic restrictions for nasal breathing. Buccolingual dyskinesias consisting of chewing, swallowing, smacking of lips, and protrusions of the tongue are a common complication of the long-term use of various antipsychotics. These movements occur intermittently during the day and vary in intensity with levels of anxiety. Facial tics, usually affecting the eyes and both side of the face, are frequently seen in the same individual. The correct diagnosis is established by the previous history of exposure to these drugs, the fact that awareness is preserved during the episodes, and the bilateral occurrence of tics in the same patient.

In a smaller group of patients, mouth breathing seems to be the reason for the buccolingual movements. Individuals with shallow nasal cavities and high palates seem to be at greater risk. This combination is often present in individuals with Down syndrome, and the lingual movements may be related to the dryness of the mouth.

Rumination can have a similar presentation. Rumination usually occurs shortly after feedings and presents as a hyperextension of the neck, with repetitive tongue thrusting and swallowing. As with the previously described episodes, the patient is alert as the movements occur.

Nonepileptic Head Drops

Isolated head drops are seldom the only manifestation of epileptic seizures in DD patients but are a common source of diagnostic confusion. They are more often reported by staff who interact with the patient during activities that require sustained levels of attention, such as the workshop or school. Epileptic head drops (or head nods, as they are more commonly referred to) are usually one of several seizure types seen in a given patient. They can be seen in patients with infantile spasms, atypical absences, atonic seizures, and complex partial seizures. The coexistence of head drops with other seizure types should raise the level of suspicion for an epileptic etiology.

A common cause of head drops in the institutionalized DD patient is drowsiness. Chronic sleep deprivation, boredom, and high doses of AEDs are the usual causes. Allowing patients to sleep longer hours and reducing AEDs rather than increasing AEDs is the treatment in these cases.

Daydreaming and "Absences"

Episodes of decreased alertness during the day are occasionally reported by workshop and school, with the concern that they may represent "absences or subclinical seizures." In a series of 8 cases in whom medication side effects were ruled out, video electroencephalographic

(EEG) evaluation showed no evidence of subclinical seizures (7). Erratic nocturnal sleep was again the likely explanation. These individuals were found to have repeated awakenings during the night for medications, repositioning to avoid skin breakdown, and diaper changing. The fact that a given patient did not sleep during the night might have been known to the night staff but not communicated to daytime staff or the physician. These patients improved as every-6-h medication schedules changed to "while awake" schedules and sleep was no longer interrupted. Excessive somnolence in some cases appeared to be secondary to prolonged periods of "forced" wakefulness. These patients were expected to stay awake for long periods during school or work and were probably chronically sleep deprived (4). Somnolence and behavior problems improved after daytime naps were "prescribed."

Migraine and Head Pains

Earaches, dysfunction of the temporomandibular joints, and toothaches are common in the DD population. These usually do not pose great diagnostic difficulties if the treating physician is mindful of them. Migraine, on the other hand, can be extremely difficult to diagnose in the more severely impaired DD patient. Symptoms of migraine can be very subjective and impossible to elicit in some cases. The presence of migraine equivalent symptoms helps with the correct diagnosis. Episodic confusion accompanied by vomiting, cyclic vomiting interspaced with normal health intervals and in the absence of other GI explanations for the symptoms, and episodes of transient lateralized weakness (hemiplegic migraine) accompanied by vomiting may be caused by migraine and usually respond to the appropriate treatment.

Apnea and Breath-Holding Spells

Of the two classic presentations of pediatric breath-holding spells, the pallid breath-holding attacks, although infrequent, can be seen in the adult institutionalized setting. These attacks follow minor trauma or startle and are accompanied by profound pallor. The individual may become hypotonic and may go into a convulsion as a result of the cerebral hypoperfusion. The diagnosis in these cases is made by the consistent association of the attacks with specific triggers.

With the increased survival of more fragile patients and aging of patients living in institutions, physicians caring for these patients are managing a growing number of DD patients with breathing disorders. Sleep apnea is common in patients with Down syndrome and those with skeletal deformities resulting in limited excursion of the chest. The usual symptoms of mental confusion and excessive daytime somnolence are seen in this population as well.

Of some concern is the association of sleep apnea with increased irritability and episodes of confused aggression. Aggressiveness and confused behavior can be episodic and unprovoked and may be mistaken for seizures. These are the DD patients that staff remember being more pleasant and lively, who became grouchier and irritable as they aged. Chronic sleep deprivation that accompanies sleep apnea may result in increased risk for seizures in some patients. Treatment for the sleep apnea should ameliorate all symptoms if the apnea is the primary cause of the problems.

Syncope

Syncope can mimic epileptic events in any age group. Presyncopal episodes can present as periods of agitation and confusion accompanied by autonomic symptoms that resemble complex partial seizures. Loss of consciousness can be gradual or abrupt, depending on posture and underlying etiology of the syncope. Syncopal episodes lasting longer than 10–12 seconds can be accompanied by salivation, tonic posturing, upward deviation of gaze, and, in some cases, multifocal clonic jerks (convulsive syncope). Syncope typically occurs in the upright or seating position, but this is not always the case. Cardiac arrhythmias and hypoglycemia of sudden onset can result in convulsive syncope in a recumbent patient. Convulsions that occur while eating are suggestive of glossopharyngeal neuralgia and typically occur in the absence of gagging symptoms. Carotid sinus hypersensitivity has also been reported in the DD population.

Spasticity and Clonus

The increased muscle tone and the jerking that accompany clonus can be confused with seizures. This is more often reported by staff involving in bathing, feeding, or suctioning the patient. The mechanism in these three situations is essentially the same: the distress produced by the unexpected contact of the body with water, the coughing and choking during feeding in dysphagic patients, and the coughing and discomfort produced by orotracheal suctioning.

The presence of clonus in DD patients with chronic, severe spasticity often results in contractures, and musculoskeletal deformities can be mistaken for seizures. A simple maneuver can clarify the diagnosis. If during the episode of clonus, the affected extremity is repositioned so that the agonists of the movement are unloaded (i.e., move the limb toward the direction of the movement), the clonus will improve or totally subside.

Reduction of sedatives such as barbiturates and benzodiazepines in patients with contractures can result in more noticeable hypertonia and clonus that may be confused with seizures by inexperienced staff. Hyper-excitability, tremors, irritability, and insomnia are usually but not always present and may persist for a few weeks after cessation of the drug.

Psychogenic Seizures

Simulation of seizures is more likely to occur in higher-functioning DD patients. It may occur "de novo" in patients with a previous diagnosis of epilepsy and also in patients without epilepsy who may "learn" the behavior, presumably attempting to change external circumstances. The episodes often have clinical features suggestive of malingering, with a voluntary production of symptoms and signs aiming at a secondary gain. Motivations are many, ranging from being excused from workshop and other chores all the way to trying to circumvent restrictions (i.e., smoking). Factors that help to differentiate epileptic and nonepileptic events when both coexist in the same patient include the following: (i) The epileptic seizures are the "older" seizures, usually going back several years, whereas the psychogenic events tend to be the more recent type of events; (ii) the clinical manifestations of the simulated episode are usually different from what is reported with the epileptic seizures; and finally, (iii) the presence of situational triggers also suggest a psychogenic etiology.

Anxiety and Affective Disorders

Anxiety and affective disorders are common in the DD patients. Diagnostic confusion with complex partial seizures may occur when anxiety presents as increased psychomotor agitation and tremulousness, which can be accompanied by autonomic symptoms. Recollection for these events may be sparse. Depression is another common confounder in the DD patient and may be iatrogenic, endogenous, or both. Endogenous depression is easy to miss and difficult to confirm, especially in the profoundly DD patient. Severe anhedonia and social withdrawal can be mistaken for subclinical seizures.

CONCLUSIONS

Some nonepileptic disorders that mimic seizures are more likely to occur in patients who have epilepsy, to be associated with epileptiform abnormalities in the EEG, or to be relieved by AEDs. This makes their differentiation from epilepsy even more difficult. However, many of these disorders are benign and do not carry the prognosis or stigmata attached to many of the epilepsies. They require no specific treatment and disappear spontaneously (8). The patient is ultimately the only person who knows what she or he experienced during the episodes in question and, whenever possible (i.e., higher-functioning patients), information should be obtained directly from him or her. In cases where history is not available, video-EEG recording of the events in question is the preferred method. It is important that someone who is familiar with the episodes be present during the recordings so that the specific behaviors and triggers can be identified.

References

1. Penfield W, Jasper H. Epilepsy and the functional anatomy of the brain. Boston: Little Brown, 1954.
2. Commission on Classification and Terminology of the ILAE. Proposal for revised classification of epilepsies and epileptic syndromes. *Epilepsia* 1989; 30:389–399.
3. DeToledo JC. Changing presentation of seizures with aging: clinical and etiological factors. *Gerontology* 1999; 45(6):329–335.
4. Devinsky O. What do you do when they grow up? Approaches to seizures in developmentally delayed adults. *Epilepsia* 2002; 43 Suppl 3:71–79.
5. Wolf P. Basic principles of the ILAE syndrome classification. *Epilepsy Res* 2006; 70 Suppl 1:S20–26.
6. DeToledo JC, Lowe MR, Haddad H. Behaviors mimicking seizures in institutionalized individuals with multiple disabilities and epilepsy: a video-EEG study. *Epilepsy Behav* 2002; 3(3):242–244.
7. Haddad H, Icovino J, DeToledo J. Chronic sleep deprivation and daytime naps confused with absence seizures in institutionalized patients. *Neurology* 1994; 44 Suppl 2:145.
8. Prensky A. An approach to the child with paroxysmal phenomenon with emphasis on nonepileptic disorders. In: Dodson E, Pellock J, eds. *Pediatric Epilepsy: Diagnosis and Therapy*. New York: Demos Publications, 1993:63–80.

IV

NEUROPSYCHOLOGIC FUNCTION

18 Memory Impairment and Its Cognitive Context in Epilepsy

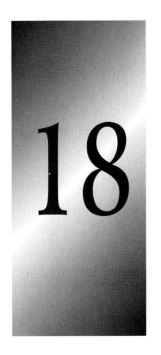

Bruce P. Hermann
Michael Seidenberg

A mong the cognitive problems that may be associated with epilepsy, its cause, and its treatment, memory is among the most serious. Surveys of persons with epilepsy consistently reveal elevated rates of complaints and concerns regarding cognitive function in general, and memory in particular (1–9). The degree to which those concerns reflect objective memory impairment has been the subject of investigation and will be discussed in this chapter, but complaints and concerns regarding mental status are prevalent. To better understand the problem of memory impairment in epilepsy, this chapter will briefly review the taxonomy of memory and the place of memory impairment in the context of cognitive impairment in epilepsy in general, followed by an empirical examination of declarative and procedural memory in persons with epilepsy in an attempt to understand and characterize patterns of cognitive morbidity in chronic epilepsy.

MODELS OF HUMAN MEMORY

Strictly defined, memory is the "the faculty by which the mind stores and remembers information" (10). It is now recognized that there are many types of memory and that they are dependent on varying neurobiological substrates.

Contemporary research has provided a taxonomy of human memory function (see Figure 18-1) and the pertinent underlying neural circutry (11). A fundamental distinction in human memory is the ability to consciously recollect facts and events, which has been termed declarative memory, in contrast to nonconscious learning ability (nondeclarative memory), which is expressed primarily through various types of performances. Declarative memory is especially pertinent to the discussion here, as some forms of epilepsy directly affect the neural regions involved in declarative memory processing.

Declarative memory for events (so called episodic memory) involves the recollection of events that occur in a temporal and spatial context, or what we would otherwise refer to as short-term memory. This form of memory is tested clinically by administration of either verbal (word lists, prose passages, word-pairs) or visual (geometric designs, faces, complex scenes) types of material, which assess the rate and degree of new learning and the ability to retain newly acquired information over delay intervals of varying lengths.

Another type of memory that will be presented for purposes of contrast is one form of nondeclarative memory: classical conditioning. Classical conditioning, a fundamental form of associative learning in humans and animals, is one type of nondeclarative memory, and conditioning of the eyeblink response is the most commonly

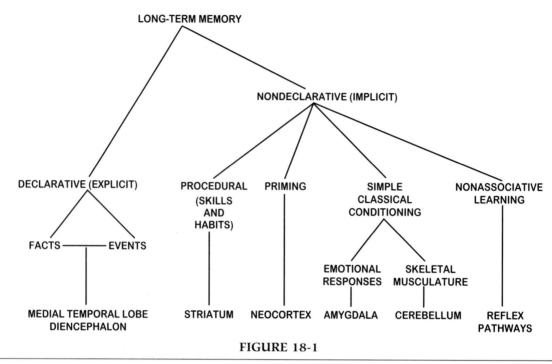

FIGURE 18-1

A contemporary taxonomy of memory.

investigated conditioning paradigm. The neural circuitry underlying this associative learning has been well characterized and shown to be dependent on the cerebellum (12). In that chronic epilepsy is known to increase the risk of cerebellar atrophy (13), it is possible that nondeclarative memory may be affected in epilepsy, and data to that effect will be presented.

In summary, there are actually many different types of memory, each with its own neural circuitry, procedures for assessment, and likelihood of impact by epilepsy and its treatment. We will turn first to the issue of declarative memory.

DECLARATIVE MEMORY AND TEMPORAL LOBE EPILEPSY

The issue of memory dysfunction in temporal lobe epilepsy has been of special interest. Temporal lobe epilepsy is a common syndrome, frequently with onset in childhood or adolescence, and often with a prolonged and intractable course (14, 15). Cognitive pathology is typically characterized by significant memory impairment (16); however, it is now appreciated that other neuropsychologic impairments may be observed as well (17, 18). In fact, comprehensive evaluation of patients with chronic temporal lobe epilepsy has revealed an average or mean pattern of relatively generalized cognitive dysfunction, with poorer performance compared to controls across all tested cognitive domains, including memory (19).

While informative, characterization of the *average* neuropsychologic profile of patients with chronic temporal lobe epilepsy does not provide insight into the possible distinct groupings or cognitive typologies that may exist within this common form of epilepsy. Further, the degree to which memory is impaired, in comparison to other cognitive abilities, remains to be characterized.

A yet untapped approach to understanding cognitive morbidity in epilepsy is taxonomic in nature. This involves addressing the question of whether empirically derived groupings of *persons* with similar profiles of cognitive function can be identified either within or across epilepsy syndromes. Taxonomies facilitate reliable clustering of individuals into meaningful groups, provide a common language and organizing influence in the field, and set the stage for further investigation of clinical and neurobiological correlates. To date, taxonomic approaches have rarely been used to advance understanding of the neurobehavioral complications of the epilepsies (20). That is, rather than grouping patients on the basis of *clinical seizure characteristics* (e.g., seizure frequency or seizure type) and examining the relationships of individual clinical seizure characteristics to cognition, one derives a grouping of *patients* based solely on their pattern of performance across several cognitive domains.

As an example of the potential utility of this approach, we recently applied cluster analysis to a large sample of patients with temporal lobe epilepsy and identified distinct cognitive subgroups or phenotypes. Patients were administered a comprehensive battery of neuro-psychologic tests, assessing the domains of intelligence, language, perception, memory, executive function, and cognitive and psychomotor processing speed. Adjusted (age, gender, education) z-scores were computed based on the performance of the controls, and domain scores were constructed for the epilepsy patients. The data for the epilepsy patients then were analyzed by cluster analysis, and several aspects of those findings are briefly presented here (21).

COGNITIVE PROFILES

First, from a neuropsychologic perspective, three distinct cognitive profiles were uncovered (Figure 18-2), suggesting that there are distinct groupings of patients with relatively characteristic cognitive profile types: (1) minimally impaired, (2) memory-impaired, and (3) memory-, executive-, and speed-impaired.

Cluster 1 (*minimally impaired*) consisted of approximately half (47%) the temporal lobe epilepsy subjects, who exhibited the most intact cognition of the three cluster groups. That said, their performance was significantly worse than controls across several cognitive domains including language, immediate and delayed memory, executive function, and psychomotor speed domains. While statistically significant, the pattern was one of mild but discernable cognitive dysfunction. Cluster 2 subjects (*predominantly memory-impaired*) consisted of 24% of the patient sample. They exhibited marked impairments in immediate and delayed memory, in the context of significantly poorer performance than controls across all other cognitive domains. Thus, memory was the most striking cognitive abnormality, but it occurred

in the context of a mild generalized depression of overall cognition compared to controls. Finally, Cluster 3 (*generally impaired*) consisted of 29% of the temporal lobe epilepsy subjects. They exhibited the poorest cognition across all domains compared to controls and also demonstrated significantly poorer performance across all cognitive domains compared to both Clusters 1 and 2. The most striking impairments in this group fell in the areas of executive function and cognitive/psychomotor speed. Thus, an underlying taxonomy characterized by the nature, pattern, and severity of evident cognitive complications can be identified. Memory impairment figures prominently in these groupings, but it occurs in the context of other cognitive pathology.

CLINICAL AND MORPHOMETRIC VALIDATION OF COGNITIVE PROFILES

Validation of these cognitive phenotypes was addressed by examination of the profiles of demographic features (age), clinical seizure features (duration of epilepsy, anti-epileptic drug [AED] polytherapy), and brain volumetrics (segmented whole-brain and lobar tissue volumes, cerebrospinal fluid [CSF], and hippocampus). In brief summary of the findings, the volumetric findings paralleled the cognitive findings (Figure 18-3). The most intact group (Cluster 1) showed significant abnormality in hippocampal volume with minimal change in other morphometric measurements. As the degree of cognitive impairment increased there was a pattern of corresponding volumetric abnormality, including greater hippocampal atrophy, and culminating in Cluster 3, where there was evidence of widespread volumetric abnormality.

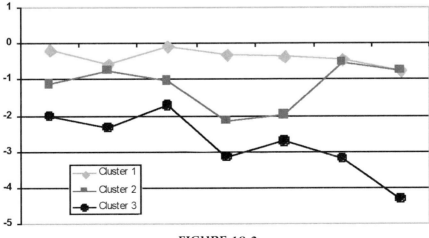

FIGURE 18-2

Cognitive profiles in temporal lobe epilepsy.

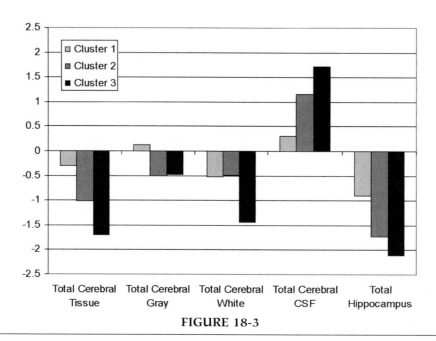

FIGURE 18-3

MRI volumetric findings in cognitive profile groups.

A closer examination of volumetric abnormality was undertaken. Looking specifically at the distribution of white-matter volume abnormality (Figure 18-4), Clusters 1 and 2 showed primary abnormality in the temporal lobe, with secondary and milder abnormality in the frontal and parietal lobes. Cluster 3, on the other hand, clearly exhibited diffuse white-matter abnormality that was evident across all lobar regions.

In addition, the most cognitively impaired group (Cluster 3) was older, had the longest duration of epilepsy, and took more medications than the other groups, especially Cluster 1. There were also meaningful but statistically nonsignificant trends in regard to other clinical seizure features. Cluster 3 had the highest proportions of patients with histories of >50 lifetime generalized tonic-clonic seizures, status epilepticus, and severe initial precipitating injuries. Thus, this appears to be a group that is most likely to have incurred both an earlier neurodevelopmental insult and a more protracted and severe course of epilepsy.

Thus, while mean profiles of cognition and volumetric abnormality are helpful and point to a relatively diffuse pattern of abnormality, discrete subgroups can be identified in terms of both cognition and volumetric abnormalities, with an interesting concordance between them.

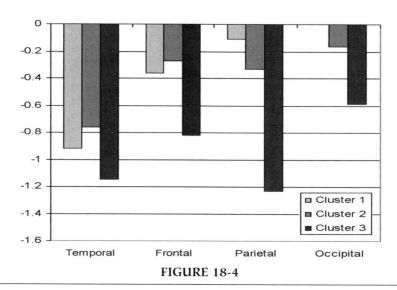

FIGURE 18-4

MRI white-matter volumetric abnormalities in cognitive profile groups.

PROSPECTIVE MEMORY CHANGE

Cross-sectional studies, as valuable as they may be, cannot provide insight into the prospective course of the disorder. Of considerable interest, but still controversial, is the degree to which abnormalities in mental status may progress over the duration of the disorder. The issue of cognitive progression in temporal lobe epilepsy is important, because curative surgical treatments exist but are frequently delayed (14, 22, 23). Patients with medication-resistant temporal lobe epilepsy often present with considerable cognitive and behavioral handicap when finally referred for surgical consideration, unfortunately sometimes after decades of unsuccessful medical management (24, 25).

Prospective cognitive studies of patients with epilepsy date back to the early part of the twentieth century (26), but these are often characterized by rather limited assessment of cognition (often IQ only), the inclusion of mixed seizure types, varying test-retest intervals, lack of control groups, and other methodological shortcomings. More common are cross-sectional studies (18, 27, 28), which, while informative, suffer from the obvious limitation of providing an indirect evaluation of neuropsychologic change over time, cohort effects, and other methodologic problems that prevent a clear and unequivocal characterization of the cognitive course of epilepsy (29). A recent review (26) concluded that progressive cognitive decline does occur in a proportion of patients and appears to be associated with markers of a difficult epilepsy course (e.g., number of lifetime generalized tonic-clonic seizures).

In this sample of patients, a subset of controls and epilepsy patients underwent cognitive reassessment four years later, and examination of their prospective memory and cognitive performance was undertaken. The statistical procedures used (regression-based norms for change) correct for sources of error in test-retest settings, such as regression to the mean, while comparing expected versus obtained performance based on the retest patterns of controls. Further, all test scores and cognitive domains are placed on the same metric, which allows comparison of relative performance across tests and cognitive domains.

We examined the implications of cluster membership for prospective cognitive course, including memory fucntion. Of the original sample, 45 epilepsy patients and 64 controls completed prospective cognitive reassessment 4 years following baseline assessment. Regression based z-scores (30–32) were calculated, and the three cluster groups were compared by MANOVA. Negative z-scores reflect lower-than-expected retest scores. All three cluster groups showed a poorer cognitive course compared to controls across the cognitive domains (Figure 18-5). However, Cluster 3 exhibited a significantly poorer course than Clusters 1 and 2 across all cognitive domains except intelligence, while Clusters 1 and 2 did not differ from each other on any of the cognitive domains. Thus, the cluster groupings have some predictive utility for cognitive prognosis.

We have examined only patients with temporal lobe epilepsy, and it is necessary to determine whether a similar phenotype classification can be detected in other epilepsy syndromes or whether there are different characteristic cognitive profiles. While a predominantly memory impaired group was observed in this sample of

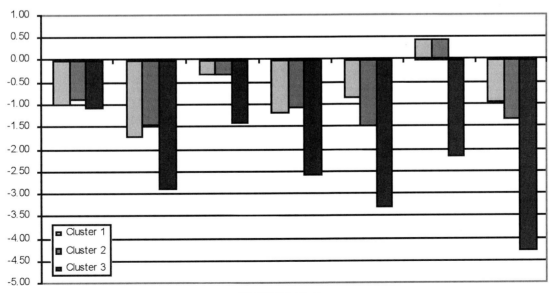

FIGURE 18-5

Prospective cognitive change in chronic temporal lobe epilepsy (regression-based norms for change).

subjects with temporal lobe epilepsy, it is conceivable that syndrome-specific typologies may be identified in other localization-related epilepsy syndromes (e.g., profiles of impaired executive function in frontal lobe epilepsy) and primary generalized epilepsies (29, 33, 34).

More generally, these results suggest that it is possible to derive meaningful neurobehavioral phenotypes of patients with temporal lobe epilepsy. Classification systems (i.e., seizure syndromes) have served the epilepsies well, and cognitive and neurobehavioral taxonomies might prove to be a useful addition for both clinical and research purposes.

Although cluster analysis is a powerful technique for simplifying a complex data set (35), the relatively small sample size examined here may limit the representativeness of patients with temporal lobe epilepsy. Additional phenotypes of patients with temporal lobe epilepsy may be obtained with larger and more representative samples. Further, the reproducibility of cognitive phenotypes across samples varying in patient characteristics, administered test batteries, data reduction procedures, and other methodological details will speak to the robustness of specific cognitive phenotypes across cohorts of epilepsy patients.

PROCEDURAL MEMORY AND CEREBELLAR ATROPHY

Cerebellar atrophy is a recognized complication of chronic epilepsy, including temporal lobe epilepsy (13). The traditional view of cerebellar function is that it contributes primarily to movement and motor control; however, converging animal and human studies indicate that the cerebellum contributes to a variety of higher cognitive abilities, including specific types of memory (36, 37), especially nondeclarative memory—a rarely studied form of memory in epilepsy.

To examine procedural memory in epilepsy patients, we used a task involving classical conditioning of the human eyeblink response—an often-used task in the procedural memory literature. Following established procedures (38), classical eyeblink conditioning consisted of pairing a conditioned stimulus (CS, a headphone-delivered 75-dB 1-kHz tone), with an unconditioned stimulus (US, a 5-psi air puff to the left eye) that elicited the unconditioned response (UR, an eyeblink). Special glasses contained an air puff delivery system and an infrared photobeam that recorded eyeblinks. Seventy acquisition trials were presented, and every tenth trial was a CS-alone trial to evaluate the *conditioned* eyeblink response (CR). The remaining trials were CS–US paired presentations. The tone CS was presented for 500 ms and co-terminated with the 100-msec US, producing a 400 msec interstimulus interval (ISI) (technically termed "delay conditioning"). The intertrial interval ranged from 8 to 16 sec ($M = 12$ sec)

with a background 65 dB white noise between trials. Following established procedures, a CR was defined as an eyeblink amplitude exceeding 10% of the subject's baseline UR amplitude (based on the mean UR amplitude for 10 US-alone trials presented prior to acquisition trials) occurring between 200 and 400 msec after CS onset. Eyeblinks occurring prior to 200 msec after CS onset (i.e., short-latency, tone-evoked nonassociative responses) were not counted as a CR. An experienced investigator made all decisions regarding CRs while blinded to group membership and MRI findings. Percentage of CRs exhibited during the acquisition phase was the primary dependent variable. Also assessed were CR latency and amplitude for CS-alone trials. Distributions of these variables were examined, and transformations performed when necessary.

Raw cerebellar volumes (cm^3) were 137.3 (12.6) for controls and 129.05 (13.95) for epilepsy subjects (6% reduction) ($p < 0.01$). Adjusted (for total ICV) cerebellar volumes were 135.7 for controls and 130.5 for epilepsy subjects (3.8% reduction, $p = 0.028$). Examination of relationships between classical eyeblink conditioning and brain volumetrics demonstrated a specific association between this form of learning and the cerebellum. Among healthy controls, conditioning performance was significantly associated only with cerebellar volume ($r = 0.49$, $p < 0.005$), with no significant association with other brain regions including total lobar tissue volumes (frontal, temporal, parietal, occipital) or total cerebral tissue or CSF volumes (Figure 18-6). In contrast, there was no association between classical conditioning performance and cerebellar volume in patients with chronic temporal lobe epilepsy. There was no relationship between any aspect of medication treatment (e.g., number, type) with conditioning performance or cerebellar volume.

Thus, other forms of memory may be affected by the neuropathology that may be associated with chronic epilepsy.

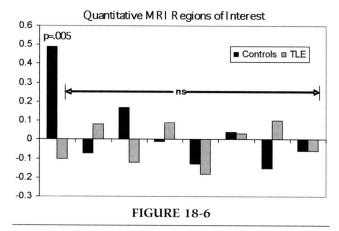

FIGURE 18-6

Correlation of classical conditioning with lobar volumetrics in chronic epilepsy and controls.

SUMMARY

Memory problems are a common neuropsychologic morbidity in epilepsy, but they appear in the context of other cognitive pathology. Reliable groupings of patients (clusters) with memory and other cognitive problems can be identified that have associations with underlying neuropathology and future cognitive course. Just as there are multiple memory systems in humans, it is also apparent that various forms of memory may be affected by the cause, course, or treatment of the disorder.

References

1. Thompson PJ, Corcoran R. Everyday memory failures in people with epilepsy. *Epilepsia* 1992; 33 Suppl 6:S18–20.
2. Au A, Leung P, Kwok A, Li P, et al. Subjective memory and mood of Hong Kong Chinese adults with epilepsy. *Epilepsy Behav* 2006; 9:68–72.
3. Giovagnoli AR, Mascheroni S, Avanzini G. Self-reporting of everyday memory in patients with epilepsy: relation to neuropsychological, clinical, pathological and treatment factors. *Epilepsy Res* 1997; 28:119–128.
4. Corcoran R, Thompson P. Epilepsy and poor memory: who complains and what do they mean? *Br J Clin Psychol* 1993; 32 (Pt 2):199–208.
5. Piazzini A, Canevini MP, Maggiori G, Canger R. The perception of memory failures in patients with epilepsy. *Eur J Neurol* 2001; 8:613–620.
6. Vermeulen J, Aldenkamp AP, Alpherts WC. Memory complaints in epilepsy: correlations with cognitive performance and neuroticism. *Epilepsy Res* 1993; 15:157–170.
7. Gleissner U, Helmstaedter C, Quiske A, Elger CE. The performance-complaint relationship in patients with epilepsy: a matter of daily demands? *Epilepsy Res* 1998; 32:401–409.
8. Lineweaver TT, Naugle RI, Cafaro AM, Bingaman W, et al. Patients' perceptions of memory functioning before and after surgical intervention to treat medically refractory epilepsy. *Epilepsia* 2004; 45:1604–1612.
9. Hendriks MP, Aldenkamp AP, van der Vlugt H, Alpherts WC, et al. Memory complaints in medically refractory epilepsy: relationship to epilepsy-related factors. *Epilepsy Behav* 2002; 3:165–172.
10. Soanes C, Stevenson A, eds. Concise Oxford English Dictionary. 11th ed. New York: Oxford University Press, 2004.
11. Squire LR, Zola SM. Structure and function of declarative and nondeclarative memory systems. *Proc Natl Acad Sci U S A* 1996; 93:13515–13522.
12. Wooduff-Pak D, Steinmetz J. Eyeblink classical conditioning: applications in humans. New York: Plenum Press, 2000.
13. Sandok EK, O'Brien TJ, Jack CR, So EL. Significance of cerebellar atrophy in intractable temporal lobe epilepsy: a quantitative MRI study. *Epilepsia* 2000; 41:1315–1320.
14. Engel J, Jr. Surgery for seizures. *N Engl J Med* 1996; 334:647–652.
15. Williamson PD, French JA, Thadani VM, Kim JH, et al. Characteristics of medial temporal lobe epilepsy: II. Interictal and ictal scalp electroencephalography, neuropsychological testing, neuroimaging, surgical results, and pathology. *Ann Neurol* 1993; 34:781–787.
16. Helmstaedter C. Effects of chronic epilepsy on declarative memory systems. *Prog Brain Res* 2002; 135:439–453.
17. Hermann BP, Seidenberg M, Schoenfeld J, Davies K. Neuropsychological characteristics of the syndrome of mesial temporal lobe epilepsy. *Arch Neurol* 1997; 54:369–376.
18. Oyegbile T, Hansen R, Magnotta V, O'Leary D, et al. Quantitative measurement of cortical surface features in localization-related temporal lobe epilepsy. *Neuropsychology* 2004; 18:729–737.
19. Oyegbile TO, Dow C, Jones J, Bell B, et al. The nature and course of neuropsychological morbidity in chronic temporal lobe epilepsy. *Neurology* 2004; 62:1736–1742.
20. Paradiso S, Hermann BP, Somes G. Patterns of academic competence in adults with epilepsy: a cluster analytic study. *Epilepsy Res* 1994; 19:253–261.
21. Hermann B, Seidenberg M, Lee EJ, Chan F, et al. Cognitive phenotypes in temporal lobe epilepsy. *J Int Neuropsychol Soc* 2007; 13:12–20.
22. Wiebe S, Blume WT, Girvin JP, Eliasziw M. A randomized, controlled trial of surgery for temporal-lobe epilepsy. *N Engl J Med* 2001; 345:311–318.
23. Engel J, Jr, Wiebe S, French J, Sperling M, et al. Practice parameter: temporal lobe and localized neocortical resections for epilepsy: report of the Quality Standards Subcommittee of the American Academy of Neurology, in association with the American Epilepsy Society and the American Association of Neurological Surgeons. *Neurology* 2003; 60:538–547.
24. Trevathan E, Gilliam F. Lost years: delayed referral for surgically treatable epilepsy. *Neurology* 2003; 61:432–433.
25. Burneo JG, McLachlan RS. When should surgery be considered for the treatment of epilepsy? *CMAJ* 2005; 172:1175–1177.
26. Dodrill CB. Neuropsychological effects of seizures. *Epilepsy Behav* 2004; 5 Suppl 1: S21–24.
27. Jokeit H, Ebner A. Long term effects of refractory temporal lobe epilepsy on cognitive abilities: a cross sectional study. *J Neurol Neurosurg Psychiatry* 1999; 67:44–50.
28. Helmstaedter C, Elger CE. The phantom of progressive dementia in epilepsy. *Lancet* 1999; 354:2133–2134.
29. Elger CE, Helmstaedter C, Kurthen M. Chronic epilepsy and cognition. *Lancet Neurol* 2004; 3:663–672.
30. Sawrie SM, Chelune GJ, Naugle RI, Luders HO. Empirical methods for assessing meaningful neuropsychological change following epilepsy surgery. *J Int Neuropsychol Soc* 1996; 2:556–564.
31. Hermann BP, Seidenberg M, Schoenfeld J, Peterson J, et al. Empirical techniques for determining the reliability, magnitude, and pattern of neuropsychological change after epilepsy surgery. *Epilepsia* 1996; 37:942–950.
32. Martin R, Sawrie S, Gilliam F, Mackey M, et al. Determining reliable cognitive change after epilepsy surgery: development of reliable change indices and standardized regression-based change norms for the WMS-III and WAIS-III. *Epilepsia* 2002; 43:1551–1558.
33. Lassonde M, Sauerwein HC, Jambaque I, Smith ML, et al. Neuropsychology of childhood epilepsy: pre- and postsurgical assessment. *Epileptic Disord* 2000; 2:3–13.
34. Nolan MA, Redoblado MA, Lah S, Sabaz M, et al. Intelligence in childhood epilepsy syndromes. *Epilepsy Res* 2003; 53:139–150.
35. Borgen FH, Barnett DC. Applying cluster analysis in counseling psychology research. *Journal of Counseling Psychology* 1987; 34:456.
36. Botez MI, Botez T, Elie R, Attig E. Role of the cerebellum in complex human behavior. *Ital J Neurol Sci* 1989; 10:291–300.
37. Schmahmann JD. The cerebellum and cognition. New York: Academic Press, 1997.
38. Sears LL, Andreasen NC, O'Leary DS. Cerebellar functional abnormalities in schizophrenia are suggested by classical eyeblink conditioning. *Biol Psychiatry* 2000; 48:204–209.

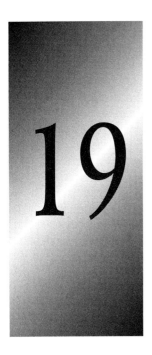

19 Cognition

Guy Vingerhoets

Numerous studies have documented cognitive dysfunctions in children and adults with epilepsy. The neuropsychologic deficits cover a wide range of brain-behavior domains, including attention, memory, mood, language, visuospatial and executive functions, intelligence, and social skills. Memory impairment, mental slowing, naming difficulties, and attentional deficits are the most frequently reported subjective complaints of cognitive dysfunction, but research has indicated that epilepsy patients tend to underestimate their cognitive impairments (1, 2). The exact cause of cognitive impairment in patients with epilepsy is difficult to establish given the vast number of factors that contribute to the resulting cognitive profile of an individual patient. The neuropathology underlying the epilepsy; the type, frequency, and duration of paroxysmal epileptic activity; and the adverse side effects of therapeutic interventions are considered the most relevant factors that give rise to the cognitive impairment. Because of the strong interrelations between these factors, it has proven very difficult to assess the relative contribution of each factor to the final neuropsychologic outcome. In humans, a number of methodological strategies have been used to disentangle the cognitive consequences of the different factors involved. Studies comparing the effects of different antiepileptic drug (AED) treatments or the pre- to ent antiepileptic drug (AED) treatments or the pre- to postsurgical changes on cognitive test performance aim to elucidate the impact of treatment variables. Cross-sectional and longitudinal neuropsychologic studies of strategically selected patient subgroups aim to differentiate the effects of lesion localization, epilepsy syndrome, and seizures. In general, these studies reveal that the AEDs' cognitive side effects predominantly affect attention and that the adverse effects are increased with rapid initiation, higher dosages, and polytherapy (3–5). Successful epilepsy surgery can arrest cognitive decline, but left temporal resections carry the risk of additional memory deficits (6). In addition, evidence has accumulated that idiopathic epilepsies show little if any clinically relevant cognitive impairments, whereas cryptogenic and symptomatic epilepsy disorders are accompanied by focal cognitive deficits that mirror the specific functions of the damaged brain areas. Early onset, long duration of the disease, and poor seizure control are associated with poor cognitive outcome (6).

This chapter focuses on the contribution of clinical neuropsychology to the assessment and description of cognitive deficits in the individual patient suffering from chronic epilepsy. Taking the different cognitive domains as a starting point, the major neuropsychologic observations for different types of epilepsy in children and adults are reviewed. The cognitive effects of therapeutic interventions, such as pharmacotherapy and epilepsy surgery, will not be discussed in detail here but can be found elsewhere in this volume.

INTELLIGENCE

Intelligence tests were initially designed to predict educational achievement in school-aged children. The success of this prediction popularized the concept of intelligence and broadened its use to adults, for whom it is widely regarded as a measure of general cognitive ability or problem-solving skills. An intelligence test is usually composed of different subtests that confront the individual with increasingly difficult problems within a specific skill, such as verbal reasoning, arithmetic, object assembly, and figure matching. Together, the performances on the entire test battery give rise to a single legendary measure: the full-scale intelligence quotient (IQ). Depending on the selected IQ test, several other subscales can be calculated, such as the verbal-scale IQ or the performance-scale IQ of the widely used Wechsler batteries measuring the performance for the verbal or performance subtests, respectively. Since IQ tests were not designed to investigate brain-behavior relationships, these measures may underestimate changes in a broader range of cognitive functions. It is also important to distinguish the intelligence batteries we described above from tests that offer an estimate of the IQ, such as the frequently used National Adult Reading Test. Tests of the latter category are typically short, unimodal, and psychometrically less grounded.

Adults

There exists very little information of whether cognition is already affected at the onset of epilepsy. A cross-sectional study compared 32 patients with temporal lobe epilepsy and their unaffected siblings, thereby minimizing genetic and environmental confounders (7). Significantly lower full-scale IQs of up to 1–2 standard deviations were found in the epileptic group, with greater differences in IQ with earlier onset of epilepsy, whereas no relation with disease duration was found. These results were taken as evidence that, at least in temporal lobe epilepsy, the functional impairment is not restricted to temporal functions but may reflect a more general disturbance in brain maturation that is already present at the time of epilepsy onset. These results are in line with age-at-onset studies and animal research (6).

Most prospective studies in adults with epilepsy reveal no, or only limited, intellectual decline over time (8–15). A significant association with seizure-related variables is rarely substantiated, and even status epilepticus appears to produce no subsequent intellectual decline (16). Other cognitive abilities seem to suffer more, again indicating the relative insensitivity of IQ for more specific

cognitive decline (17, 18). Cross-sectional studies showed that patients with longstanding refractory temporal lobe epilepsy and disease durations of more than 30 years have significantly lower full-scale IQs than do patients with a shorter disease course. The full-scale IQ of patients with higher educational attainment remained stable for a longer duration compared to less educated patients (19, 20). A recent study investigated the effect of seizure frequency on IQ in patients with secondary generalized seizures without any known etiology. Patients with a lifetime history of fewer than 10 seizures showed normal IQs, whereas a group with a history of more than 50 seizures performed below age-matched population norms (21).

Children

In comparison to normal controls, newly diagnosed children with idiopathic and cryptogenic epilepsies show no differences in intelligence, despite significantly worse scores across components of behavior and cognition (22, 23).

Most prospective studies in children revealed no significant adverse effects of (cumulative) seizures on full-scale IQ, although there appears to be a subgroup of about 10–25% of children that shows a clinically significant intellectual decline (14, 15, 23–29). Children with generalized symptomatic epilepsies, frequent seizures, high AED use, and early onset of epilepsy appear at risk for intellectual decline, although psychosocial factors may also play an important role (23, 30). Children with refractory epileptic seizures showed a significant decline of about 6 IQ points in full-scale and performance-scale IQ over a 3.5-year-period that was not observed in a similar adult patient group (28).

Cross-sectional studies reveal more robust findings of intellectual impairment (31–36). Children with generalized symptomatic epilepsies appear to be a high-risk group for intellectual and educational underachievement. Compared to normal children, even patients with benign forms of idiopathic epilepsy with centrotemporal or occipital localization and epileptic EEG discharges or short nonconvulsive seizures have been reported to have lower IQs (37–39). In children with centrotemporal spikes, deficits in IQ were associated with frequency of electroencephalographic (EEG) spikes, and a negative correlation was observed between the absolute delta and theta powers of quantitative EEG and performance IQ (37, 40). In line with the IQ test's ability to predict school achievement, children with idiopathic and cryptogenic epilepsies more often repeated a year at school and required significantly more special educational assistance than a healthy control group (22).

In severe childhood-onset epilepsies (West and Lennox-Gastaut syndromes), mental retardation is often an inherent part of the syndrome, and only few patients will achieve normal intelligence in adulthood. In rare childhood epilepsy syndromes with ongoing subclinical epileptiform discharges, the effect on IQ may be highly variable. In acquired epileptic aphasia (Landau-Kleffner syndrome), intellectual capacities often remain preserved, whereas in epilepsy with continuous spike-waves during sleep, global mental deficiency is common (41, 42).

ATTENTION

Clinically, several manifestations of attention can be evaluated. *Focused* attention is the ability to concentrate on a particular subset of the surrounding stimuli (focusing) and at the same time actively ignoring other stimuli (selecting). Increased distractibility or reduced concentration are typical complaints. The Stroop task, in which a person is asked to name the (incongruent) print color of color words, is a classical example of a focused attention task, because the reader must concentrate on the print color and suppress the overlearned tendency to read the color words. The ability to *divide* the attention between two (or more) simultaneously performed tasks is another manifestation of attention, and patients may report reduced proficiency when performing simultaneous tasks. Part B of the Trail Making Test, in which the individual has to alternate quickly between the numerical and alphabetical series to perform the task, is often used to evaluate divided attention. Finally, *sustained* attention is the ability to keep up the attentional effort over a period of time. This aspect of attention is frequently evaluated by investigating shifts in speed and accuracy during simple but lengthy cancellation tasks (43). Patients may complain about increased tiredness following a sustained mental effort or about the inability to read a book or watch a movie.

Adequate attention is a prerequisite for most cognitive tasks, and even subtle impairments may have an adverse effect on cognitive functions that are sensitive to this requirement, such as encoding and recall, naming, and the planning of behavior. Unlike other cognitive functions, attention has proven very difficult to localize in the brain, because many cortical and subcortical regions appear to contribute to this function, as can be derived from the impact of many different brain lesions on the attentional state.

Impaired attention is a frequent complaint in patients with epilepsy. It is often considered as an adverse side effect of AEDs. The complaints include impaired vigilance, difficulty focusing attention and maintaining this effort over time, and reduced mental and psychomotor speed.

Adults

On simple cancellation tasks (sustained attention) or on the Trail Making Test (divided attention), patients with frontal lobe epilepsy perform significantly worse than normal controls, but not always different from patients with temporal lobe epilepsy, although the frontal patients tend to be slower. Interestingly, patients with frontal lobe epilepsy reveal deficits in response inhibition on visual and verbal tasks of selective attention that are significantly worse than in patients with temporal lobe epilepsy (44–46). Attention deficits may be more prominent in patients whose epilepsy was caused by traumatic brain injury, and difficulties with divided attention and reduced information processing speed have been reported (47).

Children

Compared to normal controls, children with idiopathic occipital lobe epilepsy performed significantly worse on a battery of attention tests, including verbal span and visual search tasks (48). Heterogeneous samples of children with idiopathic generalized epilepsies display reduced processing time of semantic information in complex phonetic or semantic stimuli (but not in tonal or simple phonetic stimuli) and show impaired visual and auditory sustained attention (49, 50).

Among focal epilepsies, attentional dysfunctions are particularly prominent in children with frontal lobe epilepsies. Slowed visual search, poor response inhibition, and impaired sustained attention and performance speed differentiate children with frontal lobe epilepsy from children with other types of epilepsy. Successful surgery is reported to improve sustained attention in children with frontal and temporal lobe epilepsies (51–54).

Investigations on the cognitive effect of paroxysmal epileptic activity in children revealed that epileptiform EEG discharges have an independent but mild effect that is limited to transient mechanistic cognitive processes such as alertness and mental speed (55). Children with frequent epileptic EEG discharges displayed significant slowing of information processing speed, as demonstrated in simple and complex reaction-time tests, and visual searching speed. This effect can be distinguished from the effect of disease-related characteristics of epilepsy (such as type of epilepsy) on stable cognitive functions. However, it is argued that in certain cases, high seizure frequency or frequent epileptic EEG discharges have an accumulative effect that disrupts attention, leading to impaired acquisition and retention of new information and gradually worsening impairment of traitlike aspects of cognition, such as intelligence and educational achievement (55).

MEMORY

Memory encompasses the encoding, storage, and retrieval of information and has been particularly associated with frontal and temporal networks. Clinical assessment usually focuses on the evaluation of episodic (time- and context-dependent) memory by requiring the patient to learn lists of words or pictures, stories and complex figures, and by testing the consequent retention of these stimuli after a short or longer delay either through free recall or recognition or both. In testing patients with epilepsy, the evaluation of both verbal and nonverbal memory performance is essential, since material-specific memory impairment may indicate lateralization of the dysfunction with respect to the language-dominant hemisphere. Frequently used verbal episodic memory tests include the Auditory Verbal Learning Test and subtests of the Wechsler Memory Scale. The Complex Figure Test is often used to assess visual episodic memory. In addition, working memory can be evaluated using memory span tasks requiring the immediate repetition of increasingly longer lists of verbal or spatial stimuli or by using specific working memory paradigms such as the Sternberg task (43).

Adults

Memory impairments have been commonly associated with (medial) temporal lobe epilepsy due to structural lesions of the hippocampal formation (47). Lesion and functional neuroimaging studies have revealed stronger involvement of the medial temporal lobe structures of the language-dominant (usually the left) hemisphere in the encoding of verbal material and of the nondominant (usually the right) hemisphere during the retention of visuospatial material. Numerous investigators using a variety of approaches have documented a close association of both left-hemispheric temporal lobe epilepsy and left temporal lobectomy with verbal memory deficits, and a similar association of the right hemisphere with visuospatial memory deficits, although the latter association has been much more elusive (17, 56–58). In patients with right temporal lobe epilepsy, impairments on memory tasks using face stimuli have been most frequently reported (6). Left-sided temporal lobe epilepsy is commonly associated with impaired learning of stories or word lists, and also with reduced verbal working memory. Memory deficits have been reported in newly diagnosed and previously untreated adult patients with temporal lobe epilepsy suggesting that these dysfunctions cannot be attributed to the effects of AEDs or the chronic effects of recurrent seizures (59, 60). Poor performance on memory tests, including face recognition, word recognition, verbal recall, and complex figure recall, has also been reported in patients with idiopathic generalized epilepsy, suggesting that memory deficits in epilepsy may be due to neuronal dysfunction secondary to epileptic activity itself in the absence of any macroscopic brain abnormalities in the temporal lobes (61). The memory deficit is characterized by a reduced capacity to learn new

information (although the slope of the learning curve is similar to that of normal controls; initial retention is significantly reduced and never catches up on repeated trials) and impaired delayed recall (59, 60). Deficits in retrograde memory have also been reported in patients with temporal lobe epilepsy (62). Prospective studies on cognition in adults with temporal lobe epilepsy have documented a selective and gradual decline in visual and verbal memory performance over time (63). Associations with seizure-related variables are rarely substantiated, but in several cases persistent amnesia following status epilepticus has been described (8, 14). Follow-up studies after surgical treatment for temporal lobe epilepsy also reported progressive postsurgical memory decline, especially in patients with ongoing seizures or following anterior temporal lobectomy (64, 65).

Patients with frontal lobe epilepsy are also reported to show similar episodic memory deficits (impaired learning and delayed recall) as temporal lobe epilepsy patients. Compared to patients with temporal lobe epilepsy, patients with frontal lobe epilepsy also reveal significant problems with working memory, including significantly reduced verbal and visuospatial memory span. These deficits are in agreement with the involvement of frontal regions in human working memory (44–46). Significantly reduced activation in the dorsolateral prefrontal cortex and posterior parietal cortex during a Sternberg working memory paradigm has been described in patients with a high lifetime frequency (>50) of secondary generalized seizures. A similar group of patients with low frequency of seizures (<10) showed a brain activation pattern similar to that observed in healthy controls (21).

Impaired learning of new material and retrieval problems are more prominent in epilepsy patients with an etiology of traumatic brain injury and herpes simplex encephalitis. In the latter, and because of frequent medial temporal involvement, dense memory deficits have been reported, including anterograde and retrograde amnesia (47).

Children

Material-specific memory deficits have been described in both children and adults with unilateral temporal lobe epilepsy. An early age of disease onset (<5 years-of-age) appears associated with more severe verbal and nonverbal memory deficits, and successful surgery before puberty can limit the postsurgical memory deficits that are found in adults (66, 67).

Memory problems have been reported in children with benign idiopathic partial epilepsies. Children with epilepsy with centrotemporal spikes display problems with verbal learning and recall, and children with occipital lobe epilepsy show impaired memory for verbal and visual material (38, 48).

LANGUAGE

Tests of the execution of verbal commands (e.g., the Token Test); of the ability to retrieve the names of animals, objects, and actions (e.g., the Boston Naming Test); and of the ability to generate words fluently according to a set of prespecified rules (e.g., the Controlled Oral Word Association Test) constitute some of the tasks used to evaluate problems with speech comprehension, naming, and verbal fluency (43). Speech and language are lateralized cognitive functions, implying that one hemisphere (in right-handed individuals, usually the left hemisphere) is dominant for the processing of linguistic operations. Speech and language deficits have been frequently reported following frontal and temporal damage of the left hemisphere.

Adults

Despite the localization of important language areas in the epilepsy-prone frontal and temporal lobes, obvious language dysfunctions are rarely reported in adults with late-onset epilepsy. Patients with temporal lobe epilepsy in the language-dominant hemisphere frequently show naming deficits, supposedly as a result of spreading of the epileptic activity to lateral temporal areas (17). Functional neuroimaging has corroborated the findings of the intracarotid amobarbital procedure (Wada test) that atypical language dominance is more common in patients with early-onset epilepsies, in particular in those with left temporal lobe epilepsy. These findings suggest that the brain appears to be able to reorganize itself by relocating functions normally assigned to areas that were rendered dysfunctional by seizure activity to other, most often contralateral homologous, regions. Although there is evidence that the younger the brain, the more readily this relocation takes place, it remains to be determined whether relocation guarantees normal function and what criteria predict better outcome (68).

Left-sided hemispherectomies to achieve seizure control carry the risk of language dysfunction, particularly regarding expressive language and reading, even if surgery is performed before the age of 10 (69). The cognitive side-effects of AEDs are another treatment-related factor with a potential adverse effect on language. Higher doses of topiramate have been associated with deterioration of verbal IQ, word fluency, and verbal learning (3). Biochemical data and functional brain imaging suggest that treatment with topiramate disrupts frontal processing, leading to mental slowing and impairments of language production (21).

Children

The most dramatic language difficulties associated with epilepsy can be observed in children with the Landau-Kleffner syndrome (acquired epileptic aphasia). In this rare syndrome, 3- to 7-year-old children present with a gradual or sudden loss of the ability to understand and use spoken language, despite intact hearing and apparently normal previous development. All children with Landau-Kleffner syndrome show coincident abnormal electrical brain activity over both hemispheres, and the majority show seizures that usually occur at night. It remains unclear whether the paroxysmal EEG changes are causally related to the observed language dysfunction. Usually the seizures disappear and the EEG returns to normal by the age of 15. Language may improve, but receptive language problems usually continue into adulthood, and prognosis on language recovery is worse with an earlier disease onset (41, 42).

Minor language difficulties have been reported in children with idiopathic benign epilepsy with centrotemporal spikes (reduced verbal fluency) and idiopathic generalized epilepsy (increased processing time of semantic information) (38, 49, 70–72).

VISUOPERCEPTUAL AND SPATIAL SKILLS

Tasks that require the free drawing or copying of objects or figures, the comparison of figures or faces (e.g., the Facial Recognition Test), the construction of two- or three-dimensional assemblies (e.g., the Complex Figure Test or the Wechsler-subtest Block Design), and the orientation in space (e.g., the Money Road-Map Test, the Judgment of Line Orientation) often combine the use of visuoperceptual, motor, and spatial abilities. It is important to distinguish between the different functions underlying the impaired performance by comparing the performances of several visual-spatial tasks (43). The expression of visuospatial dysfunction is generally associated with damage to the right hemisphere, in particular with a more posterior localization.

Adults

Although visuoperceptual and spatial deficits can be expected in patients with occipital and parietal lobe epilepsies, there is little if any systematic information on the cognitive profile of these rare epilepsy types. Patients with frontal and temporal epilepsies may present with impairments on visual-spatial tests, but qualitative assessment should consider the possible contribution of mental and psychomotor slowing in the interpretation of these findings. On the other hand, structural brain imaging reveals widespread anatomic changes in patients with uncontrolled temporal lobe epilepsy including the parietal areas. In agreement with these findings, temporal lobe epilepsy patients perform significantly worse on visuoperceptual and spatial tasks compared to normal controls. Visuospatial performance correlates significantly with quantitative magnetic resonance imaging (MRI) volumetrics (17, 73, 74).

The ecological validity of neuropsychologic impairment is an important issue in the clinical management of the patient. In fact, many patients who have been diagnosed with epilepsy and respond favorably to drug treatment will not spontaneously report cognitive problems. Sensitive neuropsychologic measures may reveal subtle, yet significant discrepancies with normal performance that may be irrelevant for normal daily functioning. On the other hand, subtle deficits may manifest themselves in intellectually demanding professional or educational circumstances. Even in patients with well-controlled idiopathic epilepsy who maintain regular jobs, objective and subjective cognitive complaints can be demonstrated that have an impact on quality of life. Patients that are referred for neuropsychologic investigation often show a history of refractory or intractable symptomatic epilepsy. On this end of the spectrum, a much clearer relation between formal neuropsychologic assessment and ecologically valid mental limitations can be found. Frequently, these patients display obvious cognitive deficits that are reflected in daily life or educational achievement. Many factors, including intelligence, personality, and mood, will determine the final effect of cognitive impairment on daily behavior and perceived quality of life.

While the clinical relevance of cognitive impairment in epilepsy is increasingly recognized, there are no effective treatments available for epilepsy-related cognitive dysfunctions other than to avoid cognitive side effects in the treatment of seizures. Some experiments with behavioral or pharmacological interventions have addressed this question with moderate results (5). More exact delineation of the underlying cognitive deficits in the individual patient, coupled with new pharmacological agents or rehabilitative techniques that target specific cognitive functions, may pave the way towards more effective comprehensive treatment programs.

References

1. Thompson PJ, Corcoran R. Everyday memory failures in people with epilepsy. *Epilepsia* 1992; 33(suppl. 6):18–20.
2. Vermeulen J, Aldenkamp AP, Alpherts WC. Memory complaints in epilepsy: correlations with cognitive performance and neuroticism. *Epilepsy Res* 1993; 15:157–170.
3. Kwan P, Brodie MJ. Neuropsychological effects of epilepsy and antiepileptic drugs. *Lancet* 2001; 357(9251):216–222.
4. Meador K. Cognitive outcomes and predictive factors in epilepsy. *Neurology* 2002; 58(8): S21–S26.
5. Motamedi G, Meador K. Epilepsy and cognition. *Epilepsy Behav* 2003; 4:S25–S38.
6. Elger CE, Helmstaedter C, Kurthen M. Chronic epilepsy and cognition. *Lancet Neurology* 2004; 3(11):663–672.
7. Roeschl-Heils A, Bledowski C, Elger CE, Heils A, Helmstaedter C. Neuropsychological functioning among 32 patients with temporal lobe epilepsy and their discordant siblings. *Epilepsia*, 2002, 43 (suppl. 7):185.
8. Dodrill CB, Wilensky AJ. Intellectual impairment as an outcome of status epilepticus. *Neurology* 1990; 40(Suppl.2):23–27.
9. Selwa LM, Berent S, Giordani B, Henry TR, et al. Serial cognitive testing in temporal lobe epilepsy: longitudinal changes with medical and surgical therapies. *Epilepsia* 1994;35:743–749.
10. Holmes MD, Dodrill CB, Wilkus RJ, Ojemann LM, et al. Is partial epilepsy progressive? Ten-year follow-up of EEG and neuropsychological changes in adults with partial seizures. *Epilepsia* 1988; 39:1189–1193.
11. Dodrill CB. Progressive cognitive decline in adolescents and adults with epilepsy. In: Sutula T, Pitkänen A, eds. *Do Seizures Damage the Brain?* Progress in Brain Research 135. Amsterdam: Elsevier, 2002:399–407.
12. Helmstaedter C, Kurthen M, Lux S, Reuber M, et al. Chronic epilepsy and cognition: a longitudinal study in temporal lobe epilepsy. *Ann Neurol* 2003; 54:425–432.
13. Andersson-Roswall L, Engman E, Samuelsson H, Sjöberg-Larson D, et al. Verbal memory decline and adverse effects on cognition in adult patients with pharmacoresistant partial epilepsy: a longitudinal controlled study of 36 patients. *Epilepsy Behav* 2004; 5:677–686.
14. Dodrill CB. Neuropsychological effects of seizures. *Epilepsy Behav* 2004; 5:S21–24.
15. Vingerhoets G. Cognitive effects of seizures. *Seizure* 2006; 15(4):221–226.
16. Adachi N, Kanemoto K, Muramatsu R, Kato M, et al. Intellectual prognosis of status epilepticus in adult epilepsy patients: analysis with Wechsler Adult Intelligence Scale-Revised. *Epilepsia* 2005; 46(9):1502–1509.
17. Hermann BP, Seidenberg M, Schoenfeld J, Davies K. Neuropsychological characteristics of the syndrome of mesial temporal lobe epilepsy. *Arch Neurol* 1997; 54(4):369–376.
18. Thompson PJ, Duncan JS. Cognitive decline in severe intractable epilepsy. *Epilepsia* 2005; 46(11):1780–1787.
19. Jokeit H, Ebner A. Long term effects of refractory temporal lobe epilepsy on cognitive abilities: a cross sectional study. *J Neurol Neurosurg Psychiatry* 1999; 67:44–50.
20. Jokeit H, Ebner A. Effects of chronic epilepsy on intellectual functions. In: Sutula T, Pitkänen A, eds. *Do Seizures Damage the Brain?* Progress in Brain Research 135. Amsterdam: Elsevier, 2002:455–463.
21. Aldenkamp AR, Bodde N. Behaviour, cognition and epilepsy. *Acta Neurol Scand* 2005; 112:19–25.
22. Oostrom KJ, Smeets-Schouten A, Kruitwagen CLJJ, Peters ACB, Jennekens-Schinkel A. Not only a matter of epilepsy: early problems of cognition in children with "epilepsy only"—a prospective controlled study starting at diagnosis. *Pediatrics* 2003; 112:1338–1344.
23. Oostrom KJ, van Teeseling H, Smeets-Schouten A, Peters ACB, et al. Three to four years after diagnosis: cognition and behaviour in children with "epilepsy only": a prospective, controlled study. *Brain* 2005; 128:1546–1555.
24. Bourgeois BFD, Prensky AL, Palkes HS, Talent BK, et al. Intelligence in epilepsy: a prospective study in children. *Ann Neurol* 1983;14:438–444.
25. Ellenberg JH, Hirts DG, Nelson KB. Do seizures in children cause intellectual deterioration? *N Engl J Med* 1986; 314:1085–1088.
26. Aldenkamp AP, Alpherts WCJ, Bruine-Seeder DD, Dekker MJA. Test-retest variability in children with epilepsy: a comparison of WISC-R profiles. *Epilepsy Res* 1990; 7:165–172.
27. Neyens LG, Aldenkamp AP, Meinardi HM. Prospective follow-up of intellectual development in children with a recent onset of epilepsy. *Epilepsy Res* 1999; 34:85–90.
28. Bjornaes H, Stabell KE, Henriksen O, Loyning Y. The effects of refractory epilepsy on intellectual functioning in children and adults: a longitudinal study. *Seizure* 2001; 10:250–259.
29. Bjornaes H, Stabell KE, Henriksen O, Roste G, et al. Surgical versus medical treatment for severe epilepsy: consequences for intellectual functioning in children and adults. A follow-up study. *Seizure* 2002; 11:473–482.
30. Fastenau PS, Shen JZ, Dunn DW, Perkins SM, et al. Neuropsychological predictors of academic underachievement in pediatric epilepsy: moderating roles of demographic, seizure, and psychosocial variables. *Epilepsia* 2004; 45(10):1261–1272.
31. Schoenfeld J, Seidenberg M, Woodard A, Hecox K. Neuropsychological and behavioral status of children with complex partial seizures. *Dev Med Child Neurol* 1999; 37:159–167.
32. Nolan MA, Redoblado MA, Lah S, Sabaz M, et al. Intelligence in childhood epilepsy syndromes. *Epilepsy Res* 2003; 53(1–2):139–150.
33. Caplan R, Siddarth P, Gurbani S, Ott D, et al. Psychopathology and pediatric complex partial seizures: seizure-related, cognitive, and linguistic variables. *Epilepsia* 2004; 45(10):1273–1281.
34. Aldenkamp AP, Weber B, Overweg-Plandsoen WCG, Reijs R, et al. Educational underachievement in children with epilepsy: a model to predict the effects of epilepsy on educational achievement. *J Child Neurol* 2005; 20(3):175–180.
35. Hoie B, Mykletun A, Sommerfelt K, Bjornaes H, et al. Seizure-related factors and nonverbal intelligence in children with epilepsy. A population-based study from Western Norway. *Seizure* 2005; 14:223–231.
36. O'Leary SD, Burns TG, Borden KA. Performance of children with epilepsy and normal age-matched controls on the WISC-III. *Child Neuropsychol* 2006; 12:173–180.
37. Weglage J, Demsky A, Pietsch M, Kurlemann G. Neuropsychological, intellectual, and behavioral findings in patients with centrotemporal spikes wit hand without seizures. *Dev Med Child Neurol* 1997; 39:646–651.
38. Croona C, Kihlgren M, Lundberg S, et al. Neuropsychological findings in children with benign childhood epilepsy with centrotemporal spikes. *Dev Med Child Neurol* 1999; 41:813–818.
39. Aldenkamp A, Arends J. The relative influence of epileptic EEG discharges, short nonconvulsive seizures, and type of epilepsy on cognitive function. *Epilepsia* 2004; 45:54–63.
40. Tedrus GMAS, Fonseca LC, Tonelotto JMF, Costa RM, et al. Benign childhood epilepsy with centro-temporal spikes: Quantitative EEG and the Wechsler Intelligence Scale for children (WISC-III). *Clinical EEG and Neuroscience* 2006; 37(3):193–197.

41. Besag FMC. Cognitive and behavioral outcomes of epileptic syndromes: implications for education and clinical practice. *Epilepsia* 2006; 47(Suppl.2):119–125.

42. van Rijckevorsel K. Cognitive problems related to epilepsy syndromes, especially malignant epilepsies. *Seizure* 2006; 15(4):227–234.

43. Lezak MD, Howieson DB, Loring DW. Neuropsychological assessment, Fourth edition. Oxford/New York: Oxford University Press, 2004.

44. Helmstaedter C, Kemper B, Elger CE. Neuropsychological aspects of frontal lobe epilepsy. *Neuropsychologia* 1996; 34:399–406.

45. Upton D, Thompson PJ. General neuropsychological characteristics of frontal lobe epilepsy. *Epilepsy Res* 1996; 23:169–177.

46. Exner C, Boucsein K, Lange C, Winter H, et al. Neuropsychological performance in frontal lobe epilepsy. *Seizure* 2002; 11(1):20–32.

47. Jokeit H, Schachter M. Neuropsychological aspects of type of epilepsy and etiological factors in adults. *Epilepsy Behav* 2004; 5:S14–S20.

48. Gulgonen S, Demirbilek V, Korkmaz B, Dervent A, et al. Neuropsychological functions in idiopathic occipital lobe epilepsy. *Epilepsia* 2000; 41:405–411.

49. Henkin Y, Kishon-Rabin L, Pratt H, et al. Linguistic processing in idiopathic generalized epilepsy: an auditory event-related potential study. *Epilepsia* 2003; 44:1207–1217.

50. Henkin Y, Sadeh M, Kivity S, Shabtai E, et al. Cognitive function in idiopathic generalized epilepsy of childhood. *Dev Med Child Neurol* 2005; 47:126–132.

51. Lendt M, Gleissner U, Helmstaedter C, Sassen R, et al. Neuropsychological outcome in children after frontal lobe epilepsy surgery. *Epilepsy Behav* 2002; 3:51–59.

52. Riva D, Saletti V, Nichelli F, Bulgheroni S. Neuropsychological effects of frontal lobe epilepsy in children. *J Child Neurol* 2002; 17:661–667.

53. Hernandez MT, Sauerwein HC, Jambaque I, et al. Attention, memory, and behavioral adjustment in children with frontal lobe epilepsy. *Epilepsy Behav* 2003; 4:522–536.

54. Auclair L, Jambaqué I, Dulac O, Laberge D, et al. Deficit of preparatory attention in children with frontal lobe epilepsy. *Neuropsychologia* 2005; 43:1701–1712.

55. Aldenkamp AP, Arends J. Effects of epileptiform EEG discharges on cognitive function: Is the concept of "transient cognitive impairment" still valid? *Epilepsy Behav* 2004; 5:S25–34.

56. Moore PM, Baker GA. Validation of the Wechsler Memory Scale-Revised in a sample of people with intractable temporal lobe epilepsy. *Epilepsia* 1996; 37(12):1215–1220.

57. Giovagnoli AR, Avanzini G. Learning and memory impairment in patients with temporal lobe epilepsy: relation to the presence, type, and location of brain lesion. *Epilepsia* 1999; 40(7):904–911.

58. Hendriks MPH, Aldenkamp AP, Alpherts WCJ, Ellis J, et al. Relationship between epilepsy-related factors and memory impairment. *Acta Neurol Scand* 2004; 110:291–300.

59. Äikiä M, Kälviäinen R, Riekkinen PJ. Verbal learning and memory in newly diagnosed partial epilepsy. *Epilepsy Res* 1995; 22:157–164.

60. Aikia M, Salmenpera T, Partanen K, Kalviainen R. Verbal memory in newly diagnosed patients and patients with chronic left temporal lobe epilepsy. *Epilepsy Behav* 2001; 2:20–27.

61. Dickson JM, Wilkinson ID, Howell SJL, Griffiths PD, et al. Idiopathic generalised epilepsy: a pilot study of memory and neuronal dysfunction in the temporal lobes, assessed by magnetic resonance spectroscopy. *J Neurol Neurosurg Psychiatry* 2006; 77:834–840.

62. Lah S, Lee T, Grayson S, Miller L. Effects of temporal lobe epilepsy of retrograde memory. *Epilepsia* 2006; 47(3):615–625.

63. Hermann BP, Seidenberg M, Dow C, Jones J. et al. Cognitive prognosis in chronic temporal lobe epilepsy. *Annals of Neurology* 2006; 60:80–87.

64. Oxbury S, Oxbury J, Renowden S, et al. Severe amnesia: an unusual late complication after temporal lobectomy. *Neuropsychologia* 1997; 35:975–988.

65. Dietl T, Urbach H, Helmstaedter C, et al. Persistent severe amnesia due to seizure recurrence after unilateral temporal lobectomy. *Epilepsy Behav* 2004; 5:394–400.

66. Hermann BP, Seidenberg M, Haltiner A, Wyler AR. The relationship of age at onset, chronological age, and adequacy of preoperative performance to verbal memory change following anterior temporal lobectomy. *Epilepsia* 1995; 36:137–145.

67. Helmstaedter C, Lendt M. Neuropsychological outcome of temporal and extratemporal lobe resections in children. In: Jambaque I, Lassonde M, Dulac O, eds. *Neuropsychology of childhood epilepsies.* New York: Kluwer Academic, 2001:215–227.

68. Vingerhoets G, Deblaere K, Backes WH, Achter E, et al. Lessons for neuropsychology from functional MRI in patients with epilepsy. *Epilepsy Behav* 2004; 5:S81–S89.

69. Hertz-Pannier L, Chiron C, Jambaqué I, et al. Late plasticity for language in a child's non-dominant hemisphere: a pre- and postsurgery fMRI study. *Brain* 2002; 125:361–372.

70. Yung AWY, Park YD, Cohen MJ, Garrison TN. Cognitive and behavioral problems in children with centrotemporal spikes. *Pediatr Neurol* 2000; 23:391–395.

71. Northcott E, Connolly AM, Berroya A, Sabaz M, et al. The neuropsychological and language profile of children with benign rolandic epilepsy. *Epilepsia* 2005; 46(6):924–930.

72. Nicolai J, Aldenkamp AP, Arends J, Weber JW, et al. Cognitive and behavioral effects of nocturnal epileptiform discharges in children with benign childhood epilepsy with centrotemporal spikes. *Epilepsy Behav* 2006; 8:56–70.

73. Hermann BP, Seidenberg M, Bell B. The neurodevelopmental impact of childhood onset temporal lobe epilepsy on brain structure and function and the risk of progressive cognitive deficits. In: Sutula T, Pitkänen A, eds. *Do Seizures Damage the Brain?* Progress in Brain Research 135. Amsterdam: Elsevier, 2002:429–438

74. Hermann B, Seidenberg M, Bell B, Rutecki, et al. Extratemporal quantitative MR volumetrics and neuropsychological status in temporal lobe epilepsy. *J Int Neuropsychol Soc* 2003; 9:353–362.

75. Pulliainen V, Kuikka P, Jokelainen M. Motor and cognitive functions in newly diagnosed adult seizure patients before antiepileptic medications. *Acta Neurol Scand* 2000; 101:73–78.

76. Giordani B, Caveney AF, Laughrin D, Huffman JL, et al. Cognition and behavior in children with benign epilepsy with centrotemporal spikes (BECTS). *Epilepsy Res* 2006; 70:89–94.

77. Hernandez MT, Sauerwein HC, Jambaqué I, De Guise E, et al. Deficits in executive functions and motor coordination in children with frontal lobe epilepsy. *Neuropsychologia* 2002; 40:384–400.

78. Prevey ML, Delaney RC, Cramer JA, Mattson RH. Complex partial and secondarily generalized seizure patients: cognitive functioning prior to treatment with antiepileptic medication. *Epilepsy Res* 1998; 30:1–9.

79. Swartz BE, Simpkins F, Halgren E, et al. Visual working memory in primary generalized epilepsy: an [18]FDG-PET study. *Neurology* 1996; 47:1203–1212.

80. Devinsky O, Gershengorn J, Brown E, Perrine K, et al. Frontal functions in juvenile myoclonic epilepsy. *Neuropsychiatry Neuropsychol Behav Neurol* 1997; 10:243–246.

81. Jokeit H, Seitz RJ, Markowitsch HJ, Neumann N, et al. Prefrontal asymmetric interictal glucose hypometabolism and cognitive impairment in patients with temporal lobe epilepsy. *Brain* 1997; 120:2283–2294.

82. McDonald CR, Swartz BE, Halgren E, Patell A, et al. The relationship of regional frontal hypometabolism to executive function: A resting fluorodexoyglucose PET study of patients with epilepsy and healthy controls. *Epilepsy Behav* 2006; 9:58–67.

83. Savic I, Lekvall A, Greitz D, Helms G. MR spectroscopy shows reduced frontal lobe concentrations of N-acetyl-aspartate in patients with juvenile myoclonic epilepsy. *Epilepsia* 2000; 41:290–296.

84. Lassonde M, Sauerwein HC, Jambaque I, Smith ML, et al. Neuropsychology of childhood epilepsy: pre- and postsurgical assessment. *Epileptic Disorders* 2000; 2(1):3–13.

85. Culhane-Shelburne K, Chapieski L, Hiscock M, Glaze D. Executive functions in children with frontal and temporal lobe epilepsy. *J Int Neuropsychol Soc* 2002:8:623–632.

20 Atypical Language Organization in Epilepsy

Rachel Goldmann Gross
Alexandra J. Golby

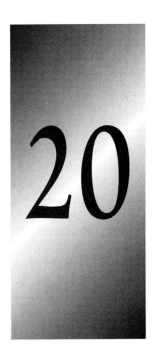

This chapter will explore the representation of language function in the brains of patients with epilepsy. In epilepsy, while abnormal electrical activity may disrupt brain function, there may be reorganization of functional units over time so that cognitive ability is preserved. Epilepsy therefore provides an interesting model in which to explore functional organization and neurologic response to injury. We investigate language function in particular because there is extensive knowledge of structural-functional relationships in this cognitive domain. Language function is made up of multiple linguistic subfunctions associated with particular brain regions, which, through interconnections, are thought to work together to generate language (1). Thus the study of language lends itself to a "neural networks" approach to brain reorganization.

There are various forms of epilepsy, with different seizure semiology, age of onset, severity, and underlying pathology. This chapter will focus on two types of epilepsy, both of which have been associated with language disturbance and functional reorganization: (1) hemispheric epilepsy of childhood requiring hemispherectomy, and (2) focal epilepsy, including mesial temporal lobe epilepsy (MTLE).

HEMISPHERIC EPILEPSY OF CHILDHOOD

Hemispheric epilepsy of childhood is characterized by a structural abnormality in one hemisphere, resulting in seizures arising from that hemisphere. Congenital etiologies include perinatal stroke, hemimegalencephaly, Sturge-Weber disease, and migrational disorders. Acquired causes include infection, Rasmussen encephalitis, head trauma, and vascular insults. Patients may have a combination of seizure types including tonic-clonic, atonic, focal motor, and complex partial seizures. Children with hemispheric epilepsy may be treated with hemispherectomy, in which one of the cerebral hemispheres is surgically removed or disconnected. Substantial improvement in seizure control is seen in 78–95% of patients after hemispherectomy (2).

It is striking that despite removal of the dominant hemisphere, language function is not devastated in most patients. Although children with a variety of unihemispheric abnormalities have baseline language impairment, function is often no worse after dominant-side hemispherectomy (2). Linguistic function may in fact improve postoperatively, in some cases from near-mutism to almost normal speech (2–5).

Indeed, if there is little to no linguistic consequence of hemispherectomy, it is assumed that the operated hemisphere is not necessary for language and that language is represented in the intact contralateral hemisphere. This notion has been supported by brain mapping techniques showing atypical language representation in patients with hemispheric epilepsy, including direct electrocortical stimulation (DCS) (6), intracarotid amobarbital testing (IAT, Wada test) (3), and functional magnetic resonance imaging (fMRI) (6).

Although many studies report impressive speech outcomes after hemispherectomy, some investigators have demonstrated impairment in particular linguistic domains. For instance, deficits have been observed during syntactic and morphological tasks in patients who have undergone left hemispherectomy (5, 7). In a study by Boatman et al. (7), language was assessed preoperatively and then followed after left hemispherectomy in six children with Rasmussen encephalitis. The authors noted that phoneme discrimination was intact in the immediate postoperative period, after which time the children showed single-word speech and improved comprehension. Naming continued to be impaired, and patients' speech remained largely telegraphic. These observations suggest that certain linguistic subfunctions may be inherent to or "hard wired" in a hemisphere and may be more or less readily reorganized to the contralateral hemisphere. Overall, there is likely some functional cost to transferring language to a formerly nondominant hemisphere.

There is significant discussion in the literature about the time course of language reorganization in patients with hemispheric epilepsy. When intact language function is observed immediately after hemispherectomy, the assumption is that language was already represented in the contralateral hemisphere or that language was transferred before surgery. In the latter case, language transfer could be induced either by seizure activity or by the presence of a structural lesion. On the other hand, when patients are significantly impaired postoperatively, and language function develops over time, the assumption is that language is gradually acquired by the nonoperated hemisphere after surgery. It is possible, however, that language was at least partially transferred preoperatively but was not immediately manifest after surgery because of "stunning" of the remaining hemisphere or time needed for reinforcement of connections that were not used while the dominant hemisphere was in place (7). Interestingly, in many patients there are significant preoperative linguistic deficits despite functional mapping techniques demonstrating preoperative language reorganization. Possible explanations include interference from seizure activity, transcallosal inhibition by the dominant hemisphere, expected functional level given overall cognitive development, medication effect, and insufficient preoperative language testing (4, 7).

Transfer of language may be influenced by patient age, both at seizure onset and at hemispherectomy. In general, the older the patient, the less likely language transfer is to occur (8). The literature reports older children and adolescents with good postsurgical linguistic outcomes, suggesting that in some cases sufficient plasticity is sustained into adolescence to enable effective language reorganization (3, 6, 7). In contrast, Loddenkemper et al. (8) report a 55-year-old man who underwent left hemispherectomy for intractable seizures due to trauma sustained at age five. This patient suffered significant postoperative aphasia despite a preoperative left IAT demonstrating intact language function. One explanation for this discrepancy is reduced neuronal plasticity in middle age, causing language to be less completely transferred to or less readily executed by the right hemisphere. However, other considerations are the subcortical location of the lesion (thought to induce less extensive functional reorganization and to be less completely inactivated by amobarbital relative to a cortical lesion) and intrahemispheric transfer of language to more posterior regions less reliably inactivated by IAT (8). Functional MRI may have provided more information than IAT in this case.

Curtiss et al. (9) emphasize etiology as predictive of language outcome after hemispherectomy. The authors show that postoperative language is superior in children with acquired lesions relative to those with developmental pathologies. Moreover, the various demographic factors thought to predict outcome (e.g., age at seizure onset or surgery, duration of epilepsy, side of seizure focus, preoperative cognitive function, and postoperative seizure control) have differential influence depending on etiology. They present etiology as an "all-inclusive variable" that can account for the effects of the other factors.

FOCAL EPILEPSY

Typically, focal epilepsy is secondary to a structural lesion in the brain such as tumor, stroke, vascular malformation, mesial temporal sclerosis, or focal dysplasia. However, focal epilepsy can be cryptogenic (i.e., no underlying lesion is identified) or associated with a specific epilepsy syndrome. Seizures may be focal or secondarily generalized, with clinical characteristics largely related to the location of the seizure focus and the propagation of ictal discharges. Mesial temporal lobe epilepsy (MTLE) is the most common type of focal epilepsy. MTLE can be difficult to control with anticonvulsant medications, but in selected patients it can respond well to surgical therapy.

In patients with focal epilepsy, various brain mapping techniques have been used to establish typical versus atypical language lateralization. Atypical language dominance (defined as right-sided or bilateral language representation) is more common in patients with epilepsy than in the general population, supporting the hypothesis that insult to the brain in epilepsy induces language reorganization.

IAT has long been the gold standard for language lateralization in patients with focal epilepsy being considered for surgical intervention (10). Indeed, IAT has shown higher rates of atypical language representation in patients with focal epilepsy than in the general population (11, 12). The major advantage of IAT is that by deactivating a large part of a hemisphere, the procedure simulates brain resection and provides an indication of potential postoperative deficits. Nevertheless, IAT cannot localize within a hemisphere and therefore has limitations in terms of detailed language mapping. Moreover, hemispheric inactivation is biased toward anterior territories, as amobarbital is typically injected into the anterior circulation via the carotid artery. Hence, there is the potential to inactivate only partially the more posterior areas involved in receptive language function, resulting in preserved linguistic capability and the false impression that the injected hemisphere is not critical for all language functions (10).

More recently, functional imaging techniques including fMRI, positron emission tomography (PET), and magnetoencephalography (MEG) have been used for mapping cognitive processes in the brain. Functional MRI studies have shown that atypical language lateralization is more prevalent in patients with focal epilepsy than in control populations (1, 13, 14). Moreover, Waites et al. (1) used fMRI to perform a resting-state functional connectivity analysis in 17 patients with left temporal lobe epilepsy and 30 healthy controls. Not only did fMRI show higher rates of atypical language lateralization in patients with epilepsy, but the authors demonstrated reduced connectivity among language areas in patients relative to control subjects. PET and MEG have also shown atypical language representation in patients with focal epilepsy (15, 16). Pataraia et al. (16) used MEG to map language function in 12 patients with temporal lobe epilepsy before and after anterior temporal lobectomy. Although the sample size was small, it was those patients with atypical (i.e., bilateral) language representation preoperatively who showed increased right-sided language function after surgery. This finding supports the notion of "readiness," either inherent or acquired, of the non-dominant hemisphere for language.

Newer imaging techniques such as fMRI, PET, and MEG differ from IAT in how language localization is inferred. IAT is a *deactivation* technique in that it creates a temporary brain lesion and tests for cognitive and behavioral changes. The other functional imaging methods, in contrast, demonstrate *activation* of brain regions associated with performance of particular tasks (10). The main strength of the newer techniques is their ability to localize function within a hemisphere, yielding detailed language maps. Furthermore, these methods are less invasive than IAT and can be repeated for serial assessment of language representation in the brain, which is essential for capturing the dynamic nature of brain reorganization in patients with epilepsy (10).

Nevertheless, there are several important limitations of the newer functional imaging techniques. Functional MRI and PET measure blood flow, from which (correctly or incorrectly) neural activity—and further, a cognitive process—is inferred. As MEG measures magnetic fields induced by electrical neuronal activity, it assesses brain activity more directly than fMRI or PET does. Moreover, these techniques highlight those areas that appear to *participate* in a given task, but not necessarily those *critical* for the execution of that task. They may therefore be sensitive, but less specific, as preoperative predictive tools (10). While there is good concordance with more established techniques such as IAT, where discrepancy exists, the newer techniques tend to show bilateral activation when IAT shows robust language lateralization (14, 17, 18).

In patients with focal epilepsy, language reorganization does not necessarily involve *en masse* language transfer to the contralateral hemisphere. This observation is based on cases of crossed dominance, in which an individual is right-dominant for some functions and left-dominant for others. The cases of crossed dominance observed with IAT primarily show dissociation between expressive and receptive function in patients with focal lesions involving anterior or posterior language areas (19). Functional imaging studies have also demonstrated crossed dominance in patients with focal epilepsy, showing dissociation between frontal and temporal activation (20). In general, patients with frontal seizure foci show reorganization of expressive functions, whereas those with temporal foci show transfer of receptive functions.

Observations of crossed dominance suggest that language function may selectively reorganize away from a diseased part of the brain but remain localized in a healthy region. The different reorganization patterns suggest that one could, in theory, find a wide variety of language networks (intra- and interhemispheric) in the brains of individuals or patient populations. Further studies using diffusion tractography and functional connectivity analysis may help to demonstrate how language areas work together within and across hemispheres to generate language.

Language reorganization in patients with focal epilepsy could be induced by seizure activity, the underlying structural or functional lesion, previous resection attempts, or some combination of these factors. Nevertheless, shift of language dominance is not seen in all patients with focal epilepsy, and patterns of reorganization seem to vary. These differences are likely due to a number of factors, including patient age at brain injury or seizure onset, duration of seizure activity, severity or frequency of seizures, patient or familial handedness, lesion size and location, and yet unknown (and likely idiosyncratic) characteristics of neural connectivity in individual patients' brains. The literature contains several discussions of the (often controversial) effects of these factors (12, 13, 21). Saltzman-Benaiah et al.

(21) identified predictors of atypical language representation in patients with focal epilepsy (e.g., left-sided seizure focus, seizure onset before age five, extratemporal seizure focus, and left-handedness) and showed that the likelihood of atypical language representation is related to the number of these factors present in a given case.

To the extent that language tasks engage particular brain regions, the choice of task can influence language localization by any mapping technique. It is therefore important to use multiple linguistic tasks that assess both receptive and expressive skills, which can be dissociated, in order to generate complete language maps (20). Failure to do so may cause brain areas involved in language function to be overlooked, with both neuroscientific and neurosurgical consequences. Rutten et al. (20) noted that many studies use only frontal activation to determine laterality because these areas are more uniformly activated by fMRI language tasks than temporal regions are. The cases of crossed dominance emphasize that this may be inadequate for language localization. This is particularly important for presurgical planning, as epilepsy surgery most often involves the temporal lobes. In addition, differences in the criteria used to establish language dominance may affect rates of atypical language representation reported by the various studies as well as the likelihood of identifying atypical representation in a particular patient (14).

CONCLUSION

Multiple lines of evidence demonstrate atypical language representation in patients with epilepsy, suggesting that

seizure activity can induce reorganization of language function. In patients with hemispheric epilepsy who undergo hemispherectomy, reorganization is inferred from the impressive preservation of language seen in many cases after removal of the dominant hemisphere. In patients with focal epilepsy, brain mapping techniques such as IAT, fMRI, PET, and MEG show that atypical language representation is more prevalent than in control populations. The literature also provides interesting cases of crossed dominance, in which certain linguistic functions are lateralized to one hemisphere while others are lateralized to the opposite hemisphere.

The study of language reorganization in epilepsy has implications for fundamental neuroscientific questions, including localization of function, hemispheric potential for particular cognitive tasks, and the ability of neural tissue to compensate for injury. A further goal for research in this area is more detailed language mapping, with assessment of injury-induced alterations in linguistic networks. To this end, it will be essential to develop and validate correlative imaging and fiber-tracking techniques that demonstrate anatomic and functional connectivity. Moreover, the nature, time course, and outcome of language reorganization in patients with epilepsy could be further elucidated by longitudinal studies that monitor for changes in language representation in the brain over time and with medical or surgical intervention. This kind of study is challenging, but possible, given the availability of noninvasive imaging methods such as fMRI. Greater understanding of these issues could assist in preoperative planning as well as guide the development of innovative therapeutic and rehabilitative interventions.

References

1. Waites AB, Briellmann RS, Saling MM, Abbott DF, et al. Functional connectivity networks are disrupted in left temporal lobe epilepsy. Ann Neurol 2006; 59(2):335–343.
2. Devlin AM, Cross JH, Harkness W, Chong WK, et al. Clinical outcomes of hemispherectomy for epilepsy in childhood and adolescence. Brain 2003; 126(Pt 3):556–566.
3. Loddenkemper T, Wyllie E, Lardizabal D, Stanford LD, et al. Late language transfer in patients with Rasmussen encephalitis. Epilepsia 2003; 44(6):870–871.
4. Vargha-Khadem F, Carr LJ, Isaacs E, Brett E, et al. Onset of speech after left hemispherectomy in a nine-year-old boy. Brain 1997; 120(Pt 1):159–182.
5. Vanlancker-Sidtis D. When only the right hemisphere is left: studies in language and communication. Brain Lang 2004; 91(2):199–211.
6. Spencer D, Poldrack R, Vaidya CJ, Temple E, et al. Functional brain organization following hemispherectomy using functional MRI. Epilepsia 1998; 39(Suppl. 6):254.
7. Boatman D, Freeman J, Vining E, Pulsifer M, et al. Language recovery after left hemispherectomy in children with late-onset seizures. Ann Neurol 1999; 46(4):579–586.
8. Loddenkemper T, Dinner DS, Kubu C, Prayson R, et al. Aphasia after hemispherectomy in an adult with early onset epilepsy and hemiplegia. J Neurol Neurosurg Psychiatry 2004; 75(1):149–151.
9. Curtiss S, de Bode S, Mathern GW. Spoken language outcomes after hemispherectomy: factoring in etiology. Brain Lang 2001; 79(3):379–396.
10. Golby A, McConnell K. Functional brain mapping options for minimally invasive surgery. In: Black P, Proctor M, eds. Minimally Invasive Neurosurgery. Totowa, NJ: Humana Press; 2005.
11. Janszky J, Jokeit H, Heinemann D, Schulz R, et al. Epileptic activity influences the speech organization in medial temporal lobe epilepsy. Brain 2003; 126(Pt 9):2043–2051.
12. Rasmussen T, Milner B. The role of early left-brain injury in determining lateralization of cerebral speech functions. Ann N Y Acad Sci 1977; 299:355–369.
13. Springer JA, Binder JR, Hammeke TA, Swanson SJ, et al. Language dominance in neurologically normal and epilepsy subjects: a functional MRI study. Brain 1999; 122 (Pt 11):2033–2046.
14. Adcock JE, Wise RG, Oxbury JM, Oxbury SM, et al. Quantitative fMRI assessment of the differences in lateralization of language-related brain activation in patients with temporal lobe epilepsy. Neuroimage 2003; 18(2):423–438.
15. Muller RA, Rothermel RD, Behen ME, Musik O, et al. Brain organization of language after early unilateral lesion: a PET study. Brain Lang 1998; 62(3):422–451.
16. Pataraia E, Billingsley-Marshall RL, Castillo EM, Breier JI, et al. Organization of receptive language-specific cortex before and after left temporal lobectomy. Neurology 2005; 64(3):481–487.
17. Tatlidil R, Xiong J, Luther S. Presurgical lateralization of seizure focus and language dominant hemisphere with O-15 water PET imaging. Acta Neurol Scand 2000; 102(2):73–80.
18. Papanicolaou AC, Simos PG, Castillo EM, Breier JI, et al. Magnetocephalography: a noninvasive alternative to the Wada procedure. J Neurosurg 2004; 100(5):867–876.
19. Kurthen M, Helmstaedter C, Linke DB, Solymosi L, et al. Interhemispheric dissociation of expressive and receptive language functions in patients with complex-partial seizures: an amobarbital study. Brain Lang 1992; 43(4):694–712.
20. Rutten GJ, Ramsey NF, van Rijen PC, Alpherts WC, et al. fMRI-determined language lateralization in patients with unilateral or mixed language dominance according to the Wada test. Neuroimage 2002; 17(1):447–460.
21. Saltzman-Benaiah J, Scott K, Smith ML. Factors associated with atypical speech representation in children with intractable epilepsy. Neuropsychologia 2003; 41(14):1967–1974.

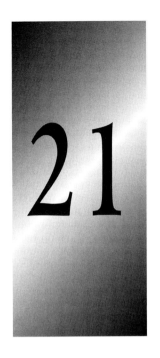

21 Interictal Perceptual Function

Arthur C. Grant

Disturbances of brain function induced by or associated with the epilepsies may be involved with an almost infinite variety of disorders of perception.

G.H. Glaser, 1970 (1)

INTRODUCTION

Only in the last decade has there been broad recognition that seizures are not the only, and for some patients not even the most distressing, epilepsy symptom. Interictal function of the epileptic brain may also be disrupted, resulting in corresponding cognitive disturbances. This chapter addresses the impact of epilepsy on human perception, outside of the peri-ictal interval. Although it may seem logical that olfactory dysfunction is associated with temporal lobe epilepsy (TLE) and visual disturbances with occipital lobe epilepsy (OLE), the underlying functional anatomy is not always straightforward. For instance, patients with medically uncontrolled TLE also have impaired tactile spatial acuity. The presence of specific perceptual disturbances in focal epilepsy syndromes is consistent with the view that epilepsy is a network disease, with the potential to affect neural circuits distant from the seizure focus. The cause of interictal perceptual dysfunction is unknown, but propagating epileptiform discharges may play a role. This chapter reviews the impact of epilepsy on each sensory modality. Concluding remarks highlight the potential for thoughtfully selected psychophysical perceptual tasks to provide additional insight into the cognitive impact of different epilepsy syndromes and of ablative epilepsy surgery.

OLFACTORY PERCEPTION

Most studies of olfaction in epilepsy have been in patients with TLE because of the close anatomical association of the olfactory system with limbic system structures often implicated in mesial temporal lobe epilepsy. In particular, the entorhinal cortex, prepiriform cortex, and amygdala are involved in olfactory perception (2, 3). West and Doty reviewed the literature on epilepsy and olfactory function in the mid-1990s and highlighted the remarkably inconsistent findings from one study to the next (2). They noted that studies differed with respect to odors used, testing methods, and subject selection.

A clearer picture has emerged from subsequent work, combined with a critical assessment of earlier studies. Epilepsy is *not* associated with increased olfactory thresholds (decreased sensitivity) to commonly used test odorants such as 1-butanol and phenyl ethyl alcohol (PEA) (2–5). In retrospect, this observation is hardly surprising in light of the findings in patient H. M. In this well-known and intensively studied patient, who underwent extensive bilateral temporal lobectomies for treatment of uncontrolled seizures, postoperative odor detection thresholds were normal (6). This case illustrates that the mesial temporal structures, indeed the majority of the temporal lobes bilaterally, are not necessary for normal odor detection in humans.

Epileptic subjects had *lower* olfactory thresholds (higher sensitivity) for pyridine, nitrobenzene, and thiophene than did controls in one relatively large study of taste and smell acuity in epilepsy (7). This effect was most pronounced in the patients with complex partial seizures (presumably of predominantly temporal lobe origin) without secondary generalization. There was no difference in odor detection thresholds between epileptic subjects who were taking antiepileptic drugs (AEDs) and those who were medication-free. Although all patients in this study had abnormal electroencephalograms (EEGs), specific EEG findings and other diagnostic criteria were not described.

In contrast to their normal or supranormal odor detection, epileptic subjects are usually impaired on tests of odor naming, discrimination, and recall. These deficits are often (3, 8), but not always (4, 9), found to be more pronounced in patients with right TLE than in those with left TLE or other epilepsy syndromes. Kohler and colleagues examined the monorhinic odor detection threshold to PEA and odor identification in 40 patients with schizophrenia, 14 patients with right TLE, 18 patients with left TLE, and 25 healthy controls matched for age, education, and smoking status (3). All TLE patients had uncontrolled seizures and were candidates for epilepsy surgery. As expected, there was no difference in PEA detection threshold between groups or nostrils. The right TLE and schizophrenic subject groups had impaired odor identification compared to controls. There were no within-group nostril differences.

Carroll et al. tested birhinic identification and recall of common odors in 30 patients with epilepsy (10 left TLE, 10 right TLE, 10 non-TLE) and 10 controls (8). All three epilepsy subject groups were substantially impaired in odor identification, but only the right TLE group had abnormally low retention of nameable odors in comparison to non-nameable odors. The authors hypothesized that right temporal lobe structures are crucially involved in short-term odor retention and that function of these olfactory memory-encoding circuits is disrupted in right TLE (8). The specificity of the retention deficit to nameable odors was speculated to result from lateralized involvement of the right temporal lobe in autobiographical memory, as nameable and distinct odors are "encoded primarily in terms of significant autobiographical episodes or events" (8).

One study found odor recognition and discrimination more impaired in left than in right TLE patients, with both groups performing worse than controls (9). All TLE patients had uncontrolled seizures and underwent the psychophysical olfactory testing while implanted with indwelling depth electrodes for definitive localization of the epileptogenic focus. In addition to the behavioral data, amygdalar chemosensory evoked potentials were recorded. Odors were presented monorhinally ipsilateral to the side of seizure origin. As with previous studies, impaired performance of the TLE group was attributed to abnormal olfactory encoding and short-term memory (9). Interestingly, the performance disparity between left and right TLE patients was tentatively attributed to group differences in psychosocial traits, as opposed to any difference in perceptual or memory processes. Specifically, the concept that right TLE patients "tended to exaggerate their desired qualities" while left TLE patients "tended to exaggerate their weaknesses" was proposed to explain corresponding differences in response bias and decision criteria employed in the psychophysical tests (9).

In summary, most research studies indicate that people with epilepsy have normal or supranormal olfactory thresholds and have impaired odor discrimination, identification, and recall. These olfactory deficits are probably more pronounced in right than in left TLE, consistent with the relatively frequent association of olfactory symptoms and disturbances to right TLE patients. Whether these psychophysically determined deficits result primarily from a disturbance of perception or of memory (or both) is not clear, as this distinction is particularly difficult to make in olfaction because of the central role of the limbic system in both processes.

TASTE PERCEPTION

Campanella et al. investigated taste acuity as well as odor detection thresholds (7). Epileptic subjects had substantially *increased* sensitivity (lower thresholds) to sucrose and urea compared to controls, while there were no group differences in sensitivity to sodium chloride or hydrochloric acid. The authors suggested that abnormal zinc metabolism may play a role in both epileptogenesis and alterations in taste and smell sensitivity.

Taste sensitivity to phenylthiocarbamide (PTC) was compared in 400 patients with epilepsy (200 idiopathic and 200 symptomatic) and 100 normal controls in northwestern India (10). PTC taste sensitivity is a genetic trait with autosomal dominant inheritance, and the "goitrogenic" thiocarbamides are found in edible plants of the *Brassica* genus, such as Brussels sprouts, cauliflower, and kale. Both epilepsy groups had a significantly higher fraction of nontasters (idiopathic 35.5%, symptomatic 32.5%) than did the control group (20.0%). Epilepsy diagnosis was based on clinical history, interictal EEG, and brain computed tomography. The authors hypothesized an elevated risk for epilepsy among PTC nontasters due to a complicated series of steps, beginning with increased intake of bitter-tasting goitrogenic substances and ending with disturbed brain development in utero or in early childhood (10). Although the hypothesis is clearly speculative, the data suggest that specific forms of dysgeusia may have an increased prevalence in people with epilepsy.

Recent functional neuroimaging studies may provide a functional anatomic basis for future studies of taste perception in TLE, especially mesial TLE. In a review of functional neuroimaging data from normal subjects, Small et al. conclude that major gustatory processing areas include the insula, parietal and frontal opercula, and orbitofrontal cortex (11). In addition, taste-processing regions were highly lateralized to the right hemisphere. A case report from the same group also illustrates the significance of mesial temporal structures to taste perception (12). A patient with intractable TLE and bilateral (right > left) mesial temporal atrophy had normal taste detection thresholds and intensity estimation but elevated taste recognition thresholds (12). Functional PET imaging revealed activation of the left amygdala associated with an aversive taste stimulus. After a left selective amygdalohippocampectomy the patient had a marked selective loss of taste recognition, while all other aspects of taste perception were unchanged. Taken together, these two studies demonstrate the significance of mesial temporal structures in taste recognition and identification and the potential for impaired taste function in patients with mesial TLE. No study has prospectively evaluated taste in a carefully selected TLE population, and this remains a potentially fruitful area of research.

SOMATIC PERCEPTION

Three studies have specifically investigated somatic sensation in epilepsy. Knecht et al. administered a tactile vibratory frequency discrimination task to nine patients with complex partial seizures (six of whom were not taking AEDs at the time of testing) and 11 normal controls (13). Subjects performed worse than controls on both hands, but performance on the side contralateral to the side of seizure onset was worse than on the ipsilateral side. The authors hypothesized that the impaired performance may be due to dysfunctional cortical plasticity induced by propagation of prior seizure activity. Since two-thirds of the epileptic subjects were AED-free, subnormal performance could not be attributed to nonspecific drug-induced cognitive slowing.

The author and colleagues used a tactile grating orientation (GOT) discrimination task associated with activation of parietooccipital cortex (14) to investigate tactile

perception in temporal lobe epilepsy (15). The task was administered at the index fingertip to 15 subjects with medically intractable TLE and 19 neurologically normal controls. TLE subjects were severely impaired bilaterally, with GOT discrimination nearly twice that of controls. In contrast to the previous study (13), we did not find a significant performance difference between hands in the TLE subjects. Mean within-group GOT discrimination thresholds did not differ in nine subjects tested on and off AEDs. These findings largely confirm and expand those of Knecht et al. (13) indicating impaired interictal somatosensory processing in TLE unrelated to AED effects.

Tactile extinction was measured with the Quality Extinction Test (QET) in 73 patients with epilepsy and 30 controls (16). In the QET the palms of both hands are brushed simultaneously with two different materials, and the blindfolded subject states which hands were touched. Subjects included 41 patients with focal epilepsy and 32 patients with primary generalized epilepsy. There was no difference between the latter group and controls. Patients with focal epilepsy had significantly more tactile extinctions on the palm contralateral to the side of seizure onset. The authors concluded that focal epilepsies are intrinsically more likely than generalized epilepsies to disrupt tactile perceptual networks and that this cerebral disturbance is more pronounced in the hemisphere ipsilateral to the seizure focus.

VISUAL PERCEPTION

Historically, visual evoked potentials (VEPs), and to a lesser extent event-related potentials (ERPs), have been the primary techniques used to study the effects of epilepsy on the visual system. Although quantitative, the VEP is behaviorally passive, and group differences in VEP waveform amplitude or latency do not correlate with performance on psychophysical visual tasks. Nonetheless, these studies represent the majority of available data on visual information processing in epilepsy.

Most VEP experiments included only subjects with photosensitive epilepsy (PSE) or childhood epilepsy with occipital paroxysms (CEOP), and focused on changes in cerebral physiology immediately prior to an induced photoparoxysmal response or seizure (17). An exception is an early study by Lucking and colleagues, who examined flash-evoked VEPs in 40 patients with epilepsy and 30 controls (18). The patients constituted a heterogeneous group with respect to epilepsy syndrome, seizure types, and EEG findings, but none had PSE. The VEP was recorded from occipital, central, and temporal head regions. Compared to controls, patient VEPs had much higher interindividual variability in all three head regions. Patients without interictal epileptiform discharges in their EEG had more uniform VEPs than those with such discharges, whether focal or generalized. There were no obvious morphological or latency distinctions between the VEPs of nine medication-free patients and 31 patients receiving AED treatment.

Faught and Lee used pattern reversal stimuli in 18 patients with PSE and 61 normal controls (19). All 18 patients had one or more types of generalized onset seizures and a photoparoxysmal response (PPR) to intermittent photic stimulation. Mean latency of the P2 wave was significantly *shorter* in patients (92.5 msec) than in controls (97.5 msec). Patients whose seizures were controlled had normal P2 latencies, while those with uncontrolled seizures had significantly shorter latencies. When retested after introduction of valproic acid, six patients with improved seizure control had a mean increase in P2 latency, while two patients without improvement did not. It is tempting to draw an analogy between the decreased P2 latency in PSE patients and the lowered olfactory thresholds observed in one study of TLE patients (7) and to suggest that the cortical hyperexcitability associated with epileptogenesis may heighten perceptual sensitivity in some circumstances.

More recent studies have capitalized on newly available methods to record brain responses to specific stimuli. Masuoka et al. used fMRI to measure occipital lobe blood flow changes in response to a pattern reversal visual stimulus in 10 patients with uncontrolled OLE and nine normal controls (20). Six of the OLE patients, but only one control subject, had asymmetric activation patterns, and all six correlated with the side of seizure onset. The other four patients failed to activate in both occipital lobes, while the remaining eight controls had symmetric bilateral activation. These results demonstrated the potential utility of this technique for seizure lateralization in OLE.

Magnetoencephalography (MEG) has also been used to measure photic-induced changes in neuronal activity (21). MEG was obtained during intermittent photic stimulation (IPS) in 10 patients with idiopathic PSE, three nonphotosensitive epilepsy patients, and five normal controls. The authors defined a phase clustering index (PCI) and compared phase synchrony in the gamma band (30–120Hz) in trials that did or did not evolve into a PPR. The PCI was much higher and spatially broader when IPS provoked a PPR than when it did not. The authors conclude that control of beta- and gamma-band oscillations is labile in PSE patients and that in the setting of IPS, "local resonances, excessive synchrony, and spatial spread of synchrony" can occur, leading to a PPR or a seizure (21).

Limbic ERPs during a visual object decision and naming task were recorded from bilateral hippocampal depth electrodes in patients with uncontrolled TLE being evaluated for epilepsy surgery (22). Visual stimuli consisted of either real or nonsense objects. Mean ERP amplitudes were significantly different between nonsense and real objects

in the nonepileptogenic hippocampus but were not significantly different in the epileptogenic hippocampus, even in the five patients with normal hippocampal pathology. These findings indicated that TLE can impair semantic processing of visual stimuli by the hippocampus.

AUDITORY PERCEPTION

Both ERPs and psychophysical perceptual tasks have been used to study auditory function in epilepsy. Despite fairly uniform auditory ERP methodology across research groups, results have been inconsistent (for instance, see 23, 24). Within-subject changes in auditory ERPs may be of greater clinical utility than between subject differences, as shown by Abubakr and Wambacq (24). Preictal, interictal, and postictal (≤6 hours after seizure) ERPs were obtained in 10 patients with uncontrolled TLE during inpatient video-EEG monitoring. Because the authors were interested in ERP variability in space and time, they performed a temporal principal-component analysis of the evoked waveform on 26 scalp electrodes. In 9 out of 10 patients, ERP amplitude was significantly reduced in postictal compared to preictal recordings in all electrodes ipsilateral to the epileptogenic focus (24).

Ehrlé et al. examined processing of rapid auditory information in 18 patients with intractable TLE and hippocampal atrophy, and six normal controls (25). Subjects performed a two-alternative, forced-choice, auditory anisochrony discrimination task. In each trial the subject had to decide whether the first or second series of five identical tones had one tone out of sequence—that is, a different interonset interval (IOI), with base IOIs of 80, 300, 500, 800, and 1,000 msec. There was no difference between controls, left TLE, and right TLE groups at 300 msec and longer IOIs, but subjects with left TLE were impaired with the shortest IOI of 80 msec. It was concluded that discrimination of rapid auditory sequences is impaired in patients with left hippocampal atrophy. The author and colleagues had similar results with a three-alternative, forced-choice, brief tone pitch discrimination task administered to 16 TLE patients (11 with uncontrolled seizures) and 15 controls (26). Patients had higher mean discrimination thresholds than controls with tone durations of both 10 and 100 msec, but a significant "group X tone duration" interaction indicated that patients were substantially more impaired with the shorter 10 msec tone. These two studies suggest that interictal auditory processing in TLE is comparable to that of healthy controls with stimuli of sufficient redundancy, but is relatively impaired with low-redundancy stimuli.

Dichotic listening paradigms provide an opportunity to explore relative hemispheric function in focal epilepsy, particularly TLE. In a large and well-designed study, 80 patients with medically uncontrolled TLE performed worse than 113 controls on a dichotic listening task with word stimuli (27). Both left and right TLE groups were impaired with both left and right ear stimuli. When the subject group was restricted to 51 right-handed, left language-dominant patients, there was no group difference in laterality index (a measure of relative ear preference), with both groups showing a strong right ear preference. Furthermore, the majority of both right and left TLE patients had a normal right ear advantage (REA), and differences at the group level were due largely to the influence of a small number of patients with large ear asymmetries.

Using consonant-vowel stimuli in a series of dichotic listening tasks, Hugdahl and colleagues concluded that left hemisphere cognitive dysfunction is an independent and stronger predictor of altered auditory perception than is side of seizure focus in TLE (28). Interestingly, the patient subgroup with left hemisphere dysfunction consistently performed significantly *better* than the subgroup with normal left hemisphere function in reporting stimuli to the left ear. This finding indicated that the left hemisphere dysfunction group lost the expected REA in a non-forced-attention condition—that is, when attention was not directed toward one ear or the other.

Though provocative, these results must be viewed in the context of the whole experiment. The authors assessed general, right hemisphere, and left hemisphere cognitive function using a composite score derived from several neuropsychologic measures, but primarily the Halstead-Reitan Battery (HRB). This battery was validated in patients with known structural brain damage, and its use in epilepsy populations has been limited. In fact, the authors found no significant difference between the left and right TLE subgroups on the composite left hemisphere neuropsychologic deficit scale (28). This result is clearly at odds with the well-described and clinically useful correlation between a temporal lobe seizure focus and ipsilateral hemisphere dysfunction, particularly (but not exclusively) in the areas of language and memory.

Mazzucchi et al. used both verbal and tonal stimuli in their study of 84 patients heterogeneous with respect to type and location of both lesions and seizure focus (29). In the 33 nonlesional patients, those with a left-sided seizure focus had a right ear preference for both verbal and tonal stimuli, while patients with a right-sided focus had a left ear preference for tonal stimuli and no significant laterality for verbal stimuli. Differences between these results and those of other groups are likely due to corresponding differences in inclusion criteria and methodology.

PATHOPHYSIOLOGY

The pathophysiology of interictal perceptual dysfunction in epilepsy is unknown. It is tempting to speculate that similar mechanisms underlie the well-known regional and sometimes bilateral lobar hypometabolism seen in unilateral mesial TLE (30). This hypothesis could be tested by correlating performance on psychophysical perceptual tasks with extent and severity of interictal hypometabolism in a group of patients with localization-related epilepsy. It would also be interesting to know whether performance on carefully selected perceptual tests correlated with postoperative metabolic normalization (31, 32). Interictal epileptiform discharges (IEDs) can disrupt cognition, and they may well play a causative role in disturbances of perception. If IEDs do disrupt sensory processing circuits, one might expect that the performance gap between patients and controls would widen as stimulus redundancy decreased, as was observed in two studies of low-level auditory perception (25, 26).

Nonspecific cognitive slowing induced by AEDs cannot account for altered perceptual function in epilepsy. First, most AEDs have little or no effect on cognition when used at recommended doses (33, 34). Second, no effect of AEDs on perceptual function was found in most studies that specifically addressed this issue (7, 13, 15, 18). Third, the correlation of specific perceptual disturbances with specific epilepsy syndromes cannot be explained as a consequence of nonspecific cognitive slowing induced by numerous AEDs.

FUTURE DIRECTIONS

We have learned a great deal about the relationship between perception and epilepsy since the prescient comment of Dr. Glaser quoted at the beginning of this chapter. We know that epilepsy can affect all five senses, resulting in both impaired and occasionally supranormal sensibility. The specificity of perceptual disturbances correlates, albeit somewhat loosely, with the underlying epilepsy syndrome. Both visual (20) and auditory (24) stimuli, combined with "recording" techniques of sufficient spatial resolution (e.g., fMRI, MEG, intracranial electrodes), may be valuable tools for lateralizing and localizing epileptogenic foci in appropriately selected patients. Furthermore, these techniques can provide new insight into the relationship between sensory stimuli and neuronal activity at a seizure focus and thus possibly shed light on the mechanisms of both reflex seizures and seizure disruption with sensory input. Perhaps most importantly, the body of evidence reviewed here largely supports the idea that focal epilepsies (and TLE in particular) are a network disease, involving brain regions distant from the seizure focus.

Acknowledgments

Supported in part by NINDS K23NS046347.

References

1. Glaser GH. Epilepsy and disorders of perception. *Res Publ Assoc Res Nerv Ment Dis* 1970; 48:318–333.
2. West SE, Doty RL. Influence of epilepsy and temporal lobe resection on olfactory function. *Epilepsia* 1995; 36(6):531–542.
3. Kohler CG, Moberg PJ, Gur RE, O'Connor MJ, et al. Olfactory dysfunction in schizophrenia and temporal lobe epilepsy. *Neuropsychiatry Neuropsychol Behav Neurol* 2001; 14(2):83–88.
4. Eskenazi B, Cain WS, Novelly RA, Mattson R. Odor perception in temporal lobe epilepsy patients with and without temporal lobectomy. *Neuropsychologia* 1986; 24(4):553–562.
5. Lehrner J, Baumgartner C, Serles W, Olbrich A, et al. Olfactory prodromal symptoms and unilateral olfactory dysfunction are associated in patients with right mesial temporal lobe epilepsy. *Epilepsia* 1997; 38(9):1042–1044.
6. Eichenbaum H, Morton TH, Potter H, Corkin S. Selective olfactory deficits in case H.M. *Brain* 1983; 106 (Pt 2):459–472.
7. Campanella G, Filla A, De Michele G. Smell and taste acuity in epileptic syndromes. *Eur Neurol* 1978; 17(3):136–141.
8. Carroll B, Richardson JT, Thompson P. Olfactory information processing and temporal lobe epilepsy. *Brain Cogn* 1993; 22(2):230–243.
9. Hudry J, Perrin F, Ryvlin P, Mauguiere F, et al. Olfactory short-term memory and related amygdala recordings in patients with temporal lobe epilepsy. *Brain* 2003; 126(Pt 8):1851–1863.
10. Pal SK, Sharma K, Pathak A, Sawhney IM, et al. Possible relationship between phenyl-thiocarbamide taste sensitivity and epilepsy. *Neurol India* 2004; 52(2):206–209.
11. Small DM, Zald DH, Jones-Gotman M, Zatorre RJ, et al. Human cortical gustatory areas: a review of functional neuroimaging data. *Neuroreport* 1999; 10(1):7–14.
12. Small DM, Bernasconi N, Bernasconi A, Sziklas V, et al. Gustatory agnosia. *Neurology* 2005; 64(2):311–317.
13. Knecht S, Henningsen H, Deppe M, Osinska L, et al. Persistent unihemispheric perceptual impairments in humans following focal seizures. *Neurosci Lett* 1996; 217(1):66–68.
14. Sathian K, Zangaladze A, Hoffman JM, Grafton ST. Feeling with the mind's eye. *Neuroreport* 1997; 8(18):3877–3881.
15. Grant A, Henry T, Fernandez R, Hill M, et al. Somatosensory processing is impaired in temporal lobe epilepsy. *Epilepsia* 2005; 46:534–539.
16. Scarone S, Gambini O, Pieri E, Canger R. Quality extinction test and lateralized EEG focality: preliminary observations in a group of epileptic patients. *Eur Neurol* 1985; 24(4):244–247.
17. Orren MM. Evoked potential studies in petit mal epilepsy. Visual information processing in relation to spike and wave discharges. *Electroencephalogr Clin Neurophysiol Suppl* 1978(34):251–257.
18. Lucking CH, Creutzfeldt OD, Heinemann U. Visual evoked potentials of patients with epilepsy and of a control group. *Electroencephalogr Clin Neurophysiol* 1970; 29(6):557–566.
19. Faught E, Lee SI. Pattern-reversal visual evoked potentials in photosensitive epilepsy. *Electroencephalogr Clin Neurophysiol* 1984; 59(2):125–133.
20. Masuoka LK, Anderson AW, Gore JC, McCarthy G, et al. Functional magnetic resonance imaging identifies abnormal visual cortical function in patients with occipital lobe epilepsy. *Epilepsia* 1999; 40(9):1248–1253.
21. Parra J, Kalitzin SN, Iriarte J, Blanes W, et al. Gamma-band phase clustering and photosensitivity: is there an underlying mechanism common to photosensitive epilepsy and visual perception? *Brain* 2003; 126(Pt 5):1164–1172.
22. Vannucci M, Dietl T, Pezer N, Viggiano MP, et al. Hippocampal function and visual object processing in temporal lobe epilepsy. *Neuroreport* 2003; 14(11):1489–1492.
23. Mervaala E, Nousiainen U, Kinnunen J, Vapalahti M, et al. Pre- and postoperative auditory event-related potentials in temporal lobe epilepsy. *Epilepsia* 1992; 33(6):1029–1035.
24. Abubakr A, Wambacq I. The localizing value of auditory event-related potentials (P300) in patients with medically intractable temporal lobe epilepsy. *Epilepsy Behav* 2003; 4(6):692–701.
25. Ehrlé N, Samson S, Baulac M. Processing of rapid auditory information in epileptic patients with left temporal lobe damage. *Neuropsychologia* 2001; 39(5):525–531.
26. Grant A, Fujikawa S, Zeng F, Nelson L, et al. Central auditory function in temporal lobe epilepsy. *Epilepsia* 2001; 42 (suppl 7):249.
27. Lee GP, Loring DW, Varney NR, Roberts RJ, et al. Do dichotic word listening asymmetries predict side of temporal lobe seizure onset? *Epilepsy Res* 1994; 19:153–160.
28. Gramstad A, Engelsen BA, Hugdahl K. Dichotic listening with forced attention in patients with temporal lobe epilepsy: significance of left hemisphere cognitive dysfunction. *Scand J Psychol* 2006; 47(3):163–170.
29. Mazzucchi A, Visintini D, Magnani G, Cattelani R, et al. Hemispheric prevalence changes in partial epileptic patients on perceptual and attentional tasks. *Epilepsia* 1985; 26(5):379–390.
30. Henry TR, Votaw JR. The role of positron emission tomography with [^{18}F]fluorodeoxyglucose in the evaluation of the epilepsies. *Neuroimaging Clin N Am* 2004; 14(3):517–535.
31. Spanaki MV, Kopylev L, DeCarli C, Gaillard WD, et al. Postoperative changes in cerebral metabolism in temporal lobe epilepsy. *Arch Neurol* 2000; 57(10):1447–1452.
32. Vermathen P, Ende G, Laxer KD, Walker JA, et al. Temporal lobectomy for epilepsy: recovery of the contralateral hippocampus measured by ^{1}H MRS. *Neurology* 2002; 59(4):633–636.
33. Asconape JJ. Some common issues in the use of antiepileptic drugs. *Semin Neurol* 2002; 22(1):27–39.
34. Vermeulen J, Aldenkamp AP. Cognitive side-effects of chronic antiepileptic drug treatment: a review of 25 years of research. *Epilepsy Res* 1995; 22(2):65–95.

22 Neuropsychologic Aspects of Frontal Lobe Epilepsy

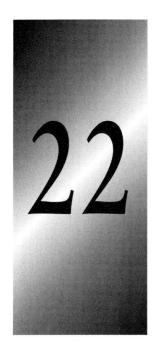

Helge Bjørnæs
Pål Gunnar Larsson

The frontal lobes occupy more than one-third of the total cerebral volume. The prefrontal parts are bidirectionally connected with all areas of association cortex in the brain, as well as with limbic structures and subcortical regions, including several of the thalamic nuclei and hypothalamus. Homotopic regions in the left and right parts are closely interconnected. This extensive system of connections makes it possible for the prefrontal cortex to receive information from practically all parts of the brain as well as to influence the information processing in those parts. The simultaneous processing of both somatosensory and limbic-sensory information seems to be a unique function of the prefrontal cortex.

Studies of children and adults with known affections of the frontal lobes, animal research, and recent imaging studies in healthy people and patient groups have accumulated much knowledge of the role played by these structures in human behavior. This knowledge has facilitated the selection of methods in assessing neuropsychologic effects of frontal lobe epilepsy, and it has pointed out the kinds of deficits to look for, assuming that epilepsy mimics other kinds of damage.

By and large, the assumed impairments have been sought within a class of abilities that may summarily be termed "executive functions." There are no strict definitions of the concept, and there is controversy about whether there is one central agency or several independent abilities, whether these functions are processed exclusively in the frontal lobes, and how to measure normal and impaired executive functions, among others. It is beyond the scope of the present chapter to discuss these topics. We adopt a pragmatic point of view in order to shed some light on the effects of frontal lobe epilepsy on cognition, mentioning research findings only sporadically, where they have relevance for the controversies within this field.

A loose description of the kinds of abilities that may be included in the concept is given by Shulman (1), who suggests: "Executive processes include (i) focusing attention on relevant information and inhibiting irrelevant information, (ii) switching focused attention between tasks, (iii) planning a sequence of subtasks to accomplish a goal, (iv) monitoring and updating the contents of working memory to determine the next step in a sequential task, and (v) coding representations in working memory for time and place of appearance." This description places weight mainly on the cognitive parts of the concept, in accordance with the scope of this chapter. The social and emotional aspects will be discussed in Chapter 23. We will focus mainly on cognition during the interictal period here.

It is believed that the prefrontal regions perform these important processes by means of their extensive network of connections to and from other parts of the brain. When parts of the frontal regions become epileptogenic, these interconnections seem to constitute part of the problem, as epileptic activity may easily propagate to contralateral parts of the frontal lobes and to remote regions throughout the brain, with the potential to disturb ongoing activity in these regions. In the same way, epileptiform activity in posterior parts of the brain may spread to the frontal lobes and disturb frontal activity.

IMPACT OF FRONTAL LOBE EPILEPSY ON COGNITION: STUDIES IN ADULTS

From a clinical point of view it is important to understand how frontal lobe epilepsy (FLE) affects the life of the patients, no matter whether the effects are "pure" frontal symptoms or not. To delineate these effects, one needs to compare patients with FLE to healthy controls on a wide range of relevant measures. This also applies to the study of neuropsychologic effects.

Unfortunately there is a scarcity of studies describing effects of frontal lobe epilepsy in general terms on standard neuropsychologic tests. The findings from these studies, however, reveal deficits in several neuropsychologic tests, including many of the subtests on the Wechsler Memory Scale, and tests demanding mental flexibility and rapid visuo-motor coordination. On the Wisconsin card sorting test—a test supposed to be particularly sensitive to frontal lobe dysfunction—the majority of FLE patients show impaired performance.

Findings indicating that FLE may affect cognition on a range of abilities are also supported when a series of tasks supposed to be particularly sensitive to frontal lobe lesions is administered. Patients with FLE, at least patients with a relatively severe and lasting seizure condition, reveal impaired performance on tests measuring different aspects of executive function, including tests of interference and response inhibition, of anticipation and planning, of verbal and nonverbal fluency, of concept formation, and of motor sequencing and motor coordination.

In contrast to deficits in executive functioning, the effect of FLE on intelligence is not clear. Most studies indicate that FLE is not strongly associated with reduced intellectual functioning, although mean IQ values substantially below average have been reported.

The Question of Localization-Related Cognitive Deficits

The frontal lobes may be divided in several different parts, according to their cytoarchitecture, with different cortical and subcortical connections. Studies of the effects of focal lesions in different parts have shown that the dorsolateral regions contribute to a range of cognitive functions, including working memory and regulatory abilities such as mental and motor flexibility, whereas the orbitofrontal parts seem to be involved in emotional and social cognition, appreciation of consequences of action, and inhibitive control of behavior. It is assumed that epileptic lesions will provoke the same kinds of deficits depending on location as focal structural lesions do, but this has not been easily proven in FLE.

Not even the specialization of the left and right hemispheres in predominantly verbal and nonverbal processing, respectively, has been easily demonstrated. In patients with lateralized frontal lobe damage, a "double dissociation" between verbal and figurative fluency tasks has been demonstrated; patients with left frontal lobe lesions were impaired on the verbal task, and vice versa (2). In patients with epilepsy there has been no clear support for the "double dissociation" in this respect. To the contrary, patients with left FLE seem to be impaired on both the verbal and the figurative fluency tasks, particularly if the tasks also require additional elements of set shifting. These findings suggest that the left frontal lobe (FL) may be particularly involved in set shifting.

The importance of the left FL in complex executive tasks has been shown in connection with the so called "20 Questions" task, in which patients with left frontal or bifrontal epileptic lesions were impaired in the selection of effective strategies, compared with patients with unilateral right frontal lobe epilepsy and patients with right or left temporal lobe lesions (3). In this task, patients with orbitofrontal epileptic lesions, irrespective of side, may generate more impulsive responses than patients with dorsolateral lesions.

The Question of Additional Effect of Seizure Related Factors

In studies of temporal lobe epilepsy (TLE), age at onset has emerged as an important factor for cognitive deficits. This has not been equally clear in FLE. Different studies have shown either no relation between test performance and seizure-related variables such as age at onset, duration of seizures, or seizure severity, or findings indicate an interaction between lateralization of lesion, age at onset, and type of task. For example, early right onset seems to be more related to perseverative errors than early left onset (4).

The Question of Pathognomonic Signs for FLE

Most studies have taken for granted that FLE may be associated with similar functional disturbances regardless of etiology. That this assumption probably is correct was shown in a study comparing FLE patients with patients who had frontal lobe tumors (FLT) (5): It was observed that FLE patients had impaired digit span forward compared with FLT patients, but no further differences occurred on any other measure of intelligence, memory, and attention. The findings agree with the results of a study of differential effects on neuropsychologic functioning of different kinds of etiology in FLE, including head injury, tumor, dysplasia, and vascular accidents (6). Lesions to the frontal lobes seem to disturb cognitive functions irrespective of etiology.

In summary, FLE may impair a wide range of cognitive functioning, including memory.

Differential Impact of FLE Compared to TLE

Even though findings of cognitive impairments in FLE do not constitute a firm pattern, evidence suggests that FLE may affect an array of abilities. Part of these deficits may stem from the impact of seizure activity on consciousness and attention, an impact that may be common to seizures originating in other parts of the brain as well. To scrutinize more closely the unique effects of FLE, comparisons have been performed between groups of patients with epileptogenic tissue in different cerebral locations. Most of these studies have focused on patients with frontal and temporal lobe epilepsy, many with a control group of healthy people in addition. These studies are of particular interest for differential diagnosis and for basal neuropsychologic knowledge.

The neuropsychologic effects of FLE do not seem to be very different from those of TLE when general neuropsychologic tests are used. On the great majority of test measures there are no significant differences between these two groups. However, both groups of patients seem to be impaired on most tests relative to the controls. The results demonstrate that both FLE and TLE can have devastating effects on cognition.

In order to differentiate neuropsychologically between patients with TLE and FLE, tests used for routine assessment may not be optimal, whereas highly specialized tests may be better suited for this purpose. For example, tests of emotional facial expressions have revealed TLE patients to be selectively impaired in remembering the emotional expressions, whereas patients with FLE may be impaired in the ability to remember faces in general.

Further qualitative differences between the two groups of patients may be obtained if a series of tasks supposed to measure different aspects of executive function is used. FLE patients tend to perform inferiorly to TLE patients on most such tasks, but statistical analyses may reveal different patterns of deficits among the patients. For example, TLE may be associated with impairment in speed and attention, whereas FLE may be associated with two distinct patterns: either with marked difficulties in learning, coordination, and alternating motor sequences or with problems in concept formation, planning, and response inhibition. Most patients with FLE could be classified according to one of these two patterns, but whether the patterns are characteristic for lesions in special locations within the frontal lobes is yet not established (7). In any case, the results speak against the presence of a unitary executive function.

Still other differences between TLE and FLE patients have been reported. The different findings obviously depend on what tests are chosen. Thus, patients with FLE may be impaired relative to patients with TLE on tests for motor sequencing, cost estimation, ability to resist interference, and mental flexibility. Moreover, greater impairment on these tasks was seen in patients with left frontal lobe epilepsy than in those with right frontal epilepsy.

Behavioral Disturbances

We will briefly mention the effects of FLE on behavior beyond cognition. As the frontal lobes are also involved in the initiation, planning, programming, and execution of motor activity, these parts of behavior may also be disturbed. Most salient are the ictal motor manifestations, which may range from subtle movements of one finger or a hand to the most violent, exaggerated movements, sometimes with vocalization. The violent movements, usually starting from sleep, may be mistaken as nightmares. Seizures may also manifest themselves as sudden changes in mood, agitated behavior, or sudden loss of spontaneity.

Interictally, patients with FLE, particularly children, may be hyperactive and impulsive. Conscientiousness, obsession, and addictive behavior have also been described in FLE.

Social Cognition

Patients with FLE may also have problems in certain aspects of what broadly might be called social cognition. Compared with healthy controls, they may be impaired in the perception of emotional expressions and in humor appreciation, but they may perform normally on tests of so called "theory of mind," in contrast to patients with autism (5, 8).

In summary, traditional neuropsychologic tests show impaired performance both in patients with FLE and TLE, with few clear differences between the groups. Experimental tasks may differentiate better between the two groups. Even though it is demonstrated that most patients with FLE may be characterized by certain cognitive patterns, these patterns to a large degree depend on the selected patients and the tests used.

FLE IN CHILDREN

The maturing processes of the frontal lobes are protracted. Myelination of the prefrontal lobes, for example, is not completed until young adulthood (9). The consequences of this long-lasting process for neuropsychologic functioning have been discussed. One question is whether focal lesions in the immature frontal lobes of children will give neuropsychologic deficits at all or whether these deficits, if present, will be different from those found in adults. As these discussions are beyond the scope of the present paper, we will mention only briefly findings with relevance for this topic in the following paragraphs.

Brain-imaging techniques combined with experimental neuropsychology have provided new options for studying the relationships between physiologic and psychologic maturing processes. There is converging evidence that the development of complex cognitive abilities partly reflects the development in executive functioning and the maturation of connections between association cortices in the posterior parts of the brain and the prefrontal lobes (10). Natural questions to be asked then from a clinical neuropsychologic point of view are about the consequences for children at different ages of epileptic lesions in the frontal lobes.

There are very few studies of the general impact of FLE on cognition in children. In children with no visible lesions on magnetic resonance imaging (MRI), only a few circumscribed deficits in verbal and figurative fluency tasks were revealed (e.g., the ability to rapidly generate words starting with specified letters [phonemic fluency] and abstract drawings [design fluency]), whereas measures of intelligence and verbal memory were normal (11). As seizure frequency did not seem to play a role for the deficits, the findings indicate that frontal epileptiform activity on its own may be sufficient to cause selective cognitive deficits.

Compared to patients with TLE, children with FLE seem to be more impaired on measures of performance speed. They are also more easily affected by distracting stimuli during learning and recall, as shown, for example, by making more intrusion errors (i.e., mixing up items from the learned task and the distracting task during recall) or by recalling fewer of the recently learned items after having been introduced to the distracter items. The increased distractibility may even affect attention, particularly when preparing for a quick response (12). They also have deficits in planning and impulse control relative to children with TLE and thus may be at greater risk for developing school problems (13, 14).

With respect to memory deficits, there are somewhat contradictory findings, but memory problems are probably not as pronounced in children with FLE as in those with TLE.

In summary, children with FLE may show cognitive impairment on a range of neuropsychologic tasks, similar to what is found in adults. Moreover, experimental tests may differentiate also between children with FLE and those with TLE. The most common deficits in FLE seem to be in executive functions including planning, impulse control, and resistance to distracters. As the age range of the children in the different studies here reviewed is between 5 and 16 years, executive deficits seem to be present despite incomplete maturation of the prefrontal lobes.

INHERITED FRONTAL LOBE EPILEPSY AND BEHAVIOR

Autosomal dominant nocturnal frontal lobe epilepsy (ADNFLE) is associated with behavior disturbances during sleep. The reported disturbances include a broad range of symptoms, from enuresis to violence, and are reported also in patients with well-controlled seizures on antiepileptic medication. The nocturnal symptoms present a diagnostic challenge, and these patients are often misdiagnosed as having benign parasomnias or psychiatric disorders.

METHODOLOGICAL CONSIDERATIONS

Studies with traditional neuropsychologic tests have shown impairment in a range of cognitive abilities in FLE as well as in TLE, with few clear differences between the two groups. This could mean that the functional contributions of the temporal and the frontal areas of the brain are not quite unique but to a certain degree overlap. This may apply even with respect to executive function. For example, not only children with FLE, but also children with TLE and generalized epilepsy, may perform below norms on measures of executive functions. Furthermore, when compared to healthy controls, even unselected groups of children with epilepsy or children with different kinds of epilepsy syndromes have been found to be impaired on a series of tasks supposed to measure executive functioning (15). Notably, a population-based study of a large group of children with epilepsy could find no significant differences in executive deficits in children with maximum involvement of electroencephalographic (EEG) pathology over the frontal lobes compared to those with more posterior pathology (16).

Even more specific findings suggesting that the hippocampus may contribute to card sorting, a test thought to be sensitive to frontal lobe dysfunction, have been reported. Thus, children with FLE as well as children with TLE and presence of hippocampal atrophy may be impaired on measures from this test relative to children with TLE without hippocampal atrophy and normal controls. Similar findings have been reported in adults.

One alternative explanation to the functional overlap hypothesis introduces the concept of "nociferous cortex": propagation of epileptic activity from a temporal lobe focus may disturb regions outside the temporal lobe, for example those involved in executive functions (17).

A third explanation focuses on the "purity" of the tests used to measure frontal and temporal processing: The tests may contain elements that tap both kinds of functions. To expand this view one can consider most, perhaps all, cognitive tasks to be complex and to require collaboration of several brain structures. This is in agreement with recent evidence that cognitive abilities are organized in functional networks, connecting different brain structures that contribute uniquely to the processes. For example, the ability to generate a series of words belonging to a certain semantic category (semantic word fluency) is thought to depend on the interaction of comprehensive neural networks, encompassing aspects of language functioning, executive processes, attention, and semantic memory. Damage to parts of such a network may result in deficits in the subserved cognitive abilities, but for different reasons: Temporal lobe damage may affect semantic memory (storage processes), whereas frontal lobe damage may impair executive processes (retrieval strategies).

Attempts to provide the patients with tools to compensate for their supposedly specific network deficits seem to be an interesting approach both to diagnostics and to treatment. Thus patients with seizures of frontal origin improved their performance significantly more than did those with seizures of temporal origin on semantic fluency tasks when provided with structured cuing aimed at compensating for deficits in retrieval strategies (18). The diagnostic value of providing patients with frontal lobe dysfunction with cues to compensate for executive deficits was noted already by Luria and Tsvetkova in 1964 (19).

Another approach to refining the differential neuropsychologic diagnostics between TLE and FLE is to increase the load on the assumed unique functions by making the tasks more demanding or by composing tasks in such a way that several subcategories of the functions in question are challenged at the same time (e.g., to present tasks requiring both fluency and the ability for set shifting in attempts to measure deficits in executive functioning).

Future studies in this field should ameliorate the limitations seen in most studies so far. The number of patients with FLE has been small in most studies—too small to allow further subdivision for statistical analyses. Moreover, when comparing patients with FLE and those with TLE, seizure-related variables should be reported, as such variables may make great differences in the functioning of TLE patients. Finally, the most important methodological improvements would be to control for remote functional disturbances, not only as measured with the EEG, but also by using positron emission tomography (PET) or functional MRI (fMRI) to evaluate changes beyond the focus.

Because of the scarcity of studies, conclusions about cognitive consequences in FLE must be drawn cautiously.

SUMMARY

FLE may disturb a wide range of neuropsychologic functions including memory and executive function. Apart from involvement of executive function there is no distinct pattern of deficits characterizing FLE, probably because of rapid propagation of epileptic activity. FLE usually does not strongly affect intelligence. There are similar deficits in adults and in studied children in the age range of 5–16 years. FLE may mimic effects of focal structural lesions but tends to give less circumscribed deficits. There are no clear effects of laterality on cognitive functioning in FLE. There are less clear effects of seizure history variables than in TLE.

Acknowledgment

Thanks to Dr. Svein I. Johannessen for kind advice during the preparation of the manuscript.

References

1. Shulman MB. The frontal lobes. *Epilepsy Behav* 2000; 1(6):384–395.
2. Jones-Gotman M, Milner B. Design fluency: the invention of nonsense drawings after focal cortical lesions. *Neuropsychologia* 1977; 15(4-5):653–674.
3. Upton D, Thompson PJ. Twenty questions task and frontal lobe dysfunction. *Arch Clin Neuropsychol* 1999; 14(2):203–216.
4. Upton D, Thompson PJ. Age at onset and neuropsychological function in frontal lobe epilepsy. *Epilepsia* 1997; 38(10):1103–1113.
5. Exner C, Boucsein K, Lange C, Winter H, et al. Neuropsychological performance in frontal lobe epilepsy. *Seizure* 2002; 11(1):20–32.
6. Upton D, Thompson PJ. Neuropsychological test performance in frontal-lobe epilepsy: the influence of aetiology, seizure type, seizure frequency and duration of disorder. *Seizure* 1997; 6(6):443–447.
7. Helmstaedter C, Kemper B, Elger CE. Neuropsychological aspects of frontal lobe epilepsy. *Neuropsychologia* 1996; 34(5):399–406.
8. Farrant A, Morris RG, Russell T, Elwes R, et al. Social cognition in frontal lobe epilepsy. *Epilepsy Behav* 2005; 7(3):506–516.
9. Yakovlev PI, Lecours AR. The myelogenetic cycles of regional maturation of the brain. In Minikiniwski A, ed. Regional Development of the Brain in Early Life. Oxford: Blackwell, 1967:3–10.
10. Menon V, Boyett-Anderson JM, Reiss AL. Maturation of medial temporal lobe response and connectivity during memory encoding. *Brain Res Cogn Brain Res* 2005; 25(1):379–385.
11. Riva D, Avanzini G, Franceschetti S, Nichelli F, Saletti V, et al. Unilateral frontal lobe epilepsy affects executive functions in children. *Neurol Sci* 2005; 26(4):263–270.

12. Auclair L, Jambaque I, Dulac O, LaBerge D, et al. Deficit of preparatory attention in children with frontal lobe epilepsy. *Neuropsychologia* 2005; 43(12):1701–1712.

13. Hernandez MT, Sauerwein HC, Jambaque I, De Guise E, et al. Deficits in executive functions and motor coordination in children with frontal lobe epilepsy. *Neuropsychologia* 2002; 40(4):384–400.

14. Hernandez MT, Sauerwein HC, Jambaque I, de Guise E, et al. Attention, memory, and behavioral adjustment in children with frontal lobe epilepsy. *Epilepsy Behav* 2003; 4(5):522–536.

15. Slick DJ, Lautzenhiser A, Sherman EM, Eyrl K. Frequency of scale elevations and factor structure of the Behavior Rating Inventory of Executive Function (BRIEF) in children and adolescents with intractable epilepsy. *Child Neuropsychol* 2006; 12(3):181–189.

16. Hoie B, Mykletun A, Waaler PE, Skeidsvoll H, et al. Executive functions and seizure-related factors in children with epilepsy in western Norway. *Dev Med Child Neurol* 2006; 48(6):519–525.

17. Hermann B, Seidenberg M. Executive system dysfunction in temporal lobe epilepsy: effects of nociferous cortex versus hippocampal pathology. *J Clin Exp Neuropsychol* 1995, 17(6):809–819.

18. Drane DL, Lee GP, Cech H, Huthwaite JS, et al. Structured cueing on a semantic fluency task differentiates patients with temporal versus frontal lobe seizure onset. *Epilepsy Behav.* 2006 Sep; 9(2):339–344.

19. Luria AR, Tsvetkova LD. The programming of constructive activity in local brain injuries. *Neuropsychologia* 1964, 2:95–108.

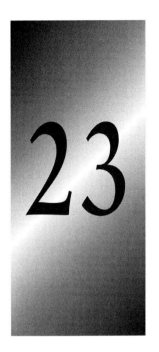

23 Social and Emotion Information Processing

Hazel J. Reynders

Neuropsychological function in epilepsy is a well researched field and has developed our general understanding of cognitive function in numerous ways. It is also well established that psychopathology and psychosocial problems are frequent among patients with epilepsy. It is also widely acknowledged that there are a number of different factors influencing social and emotional responses in epilepsy, including neurobiological factors such as age of onset, seizure control, and seizure type; psychosocial factors including perceived stigma, fear of seizures, and adjustment to epilepsy; and medication factors such as monotherapy versus polytherapy and the presence or absence of barbiturate medications. Adults with epilepsy have been found to have higher rates of social problems and social isolation difficulties than people in the general population.

Understanding the multi-etiological contributions to the social and emotional difficulties associated with epilepsy requires a move toward developing biopsychosocial frameworks for empirical investigation of the psychologic distress experienced by people with epilepsy. In this respect, neuropsychologic research acts as a bridging discipline between neurobiological explanations of emotional disturbance in epilepsy and the social and emotional disturbances often associated with the experience of epilepsy.

This chapter sets out to explore the evidence for social and emotional information processing deficits in epilepsy. The relationship between perception and experience of emotional responses in epilepsy is also examined, together with the consequences for future research and understanding of the multi-etiological contributions to social and emotional difficulties in epilepsy.

DEFINITIONS OF SOCIAL COGNITION

Over recent years, an evolving discipline of social cognition has emerged, which has increased understanding of the cognitive and neurobiological processes involved in social and emotion information processing within psychosocial environments.

Social cognition has been defined as encompassing those skills that are involved in the ability to recognize, understand, and respond appropriately to socially relevant information. The evidence in the literature suggests that social cognition is mediated by a number of component cognitive processes that are served centrally, at a neurologic level, via systems that link the amygdala with cortical regions including the ventromedial prefrontal cortex, the cingulate cortex, and the right somatosensory cortex (1, 2).

THE PREFRONTAL-AMYGDALAR SOCIAL COGNITION CIRCUITRY

The amygdala links cortical regions that process sensory information with the hypothalamus and brainstem effector systems. Via prefrontal and temporal connections, it integrates the emotional significance of sensory stimuli and guides complex behavior. Several findings are linked to the hypothesis that the human amygdala forms a crucial part of the neural circuitry involved in the appraisal of danger and the emotion of fear (3). Evidence from functional neuroimaging studies of healthy volunteers (4) and participants with socio-affective disorders (5) has converged with evidence from studies with patients with lesions in medial temporal lobe structures to identify temporo-limbic regions, especially the amygdala, as key components of the circuitry underlying emotion information processing in the human brain (6). Areas of research include perception of emotion expression, emotion and social experience and behavior, and emotional learning and memory.

The prefrontal–amygdalar pathways have also been linked to deficits in theory of mind (7, 8) and decision making (9), both of which are important aspects of social cognition. Damage to the ventromedial frontal cortex may result in profound disruption of social behavior and inability to observe social conventions, within the context of often well-preserved intellectual abilities. This region connects to the anterior cingulate and the amygdala and influences emotion perception, motivation, and the ability to make inferences about the mental state of others ("theory of mind").

EMOTIONAL PERCEPTION AND RECOGNITION

A number of investigations have shown the importance of the amygdala in the perception and processing of social information associated with negative affect (10). The consequences of human amygdala damage have been found to include problems in recognizing facial and vocal expressions of emotion, and a number of studies have shown specific impairments in the recognition of expressions of fear after amygdala damage (11–13) with sparing of other emotional expressions. Positron emission tomography (PET) and functional magnetic resonance imaging (fMRI) techniques have been used to demonstrate a selective response to facial expressions of fear in the normal amygdala (14), even when the faces are masked with neutral expressions to eliminate conscious perception of the fear stimuli (15).

The majority of the amygdala studies have focused on patients with bilateral amygdala damage. The evidence for impairments following unilateral damage is less clear.

Adolphs et al. (11) failed to find any significant deficits in six patients with unilateral amygdala damage included in their study. Nevertheless, a number of lesion studies have found some evidence for fear perception deficits to occur following unilateral amygdala damage. Again, there are some contradictory findings in the literature. Whilst most studies find a right side dominance for emotion perception, there is the case of D.R. (13), who showed fear perception deficits with relatively greater damage to the left side amygdala. Functional studies have also suggested a left side dominance for fear recognition (15). In contrast, Adolphs et al. (16) found significant impairments in emotion recognition among a subgroup of patients who had undergone right temporal lobotomies.

There is a growing body of recent research that shows emotion perception problems among patients with epilepsy. So far, however, the findings have been mixed. Meletti et al. (17) found impairments selectively among patients with right temporal lobe epilepsy. In contrast, other studies have found no evidence of laterality of impairments in temporal lobe epilepsy (18, 19). Nevertheless, there is growing evidence that some patients with epilepsy may be vulnerable to the emotion perception deficits usually associated with bilateral amygdala damage, even when the structural evidence suggests unilateral epilepsy-related lesions.

Although subgroups of temporal lobe epilepsy patients with a unilateral epilepsy focus show emotion recognition impairments, this may not be enough to suggest that unilateral damage is sufficient to produce fear recognition deficits. Seizures arising from mesial temporal lesions with clearly defined unilateral foci often spread to affect contralateral brain regions, and among patients with epilepsy there is often some compromise of both cerebral hemispheres. An alternative approach is to directly investigate the impact of the degree of amygdala damage in epilepsy on emotion perception abilities. Preliminary findings by Houghton et al. (20) indicated that emotion perception deficits, similar to those in amygdala damage, are related to reduced amygdala volume in temporal lobe epilepsy. However, a recent study by Fowler et al. (19) found inconsistent results. They assessed patients with mesial temporal lobe epilepsy and asymmetrical amygdala damage. Although no consistent impairments were found, seven of the 28 patients had significant difficulties recognizing emotional expressions.

Although the majority of the epilepsy studies have focused on assessing perception of facial expressions of emotion, Fowler et al. (19) extended their investigation of patients with temporal lobe epilepsy and amygdala damage to include other tasks known to be associated with amygdala function: sentences describing emotion-laden situations, nonverbal sounds, and prosody. In the subgroup they identified as having emotion recognition deficits, they found both auditory and visual emotion recognition impairments.

Types of Seizures

Few studies have examined the relationship between types of seizures and emotional recognition deficits. The amygdala is the mesial temporal structure most frequently associated with seizure related experiential phenomena, especially the sensation of fear-related experiences. Ictal fear is an involuntary emotional response experienced during seizure onset, and it is characterized by a profound sense of fear or foreboding (21). Further work links atrophy of the amygdala to symptoms of ictal fear in temporal lobe epilepsy (22). Two recent studies (18, 23) have sought to understand whether emotion perceptions are related to the clinical manifestation of fear occurring as part of a seizure.

Yamada et al. (23) carried out a single case study of a patient with left temporal lobe epilepsy and ictal fear before and after epilepsy surgery. They found that, although the patient correctly identified emotions before surgery, the patient attached enhanced emotions of fear, anger, and sadness to various expressions. After surgery, the patient no longer showed the abnormally high intensity ratings. The authors interpret their results as indicative of presurgery interictal hypersensitivity of the left mesial temporal circuit, including the amygdala, supported by the evidence of interictal epileptiform activity in the frontotemporal regions.

Reynders et al. (18) investigated social cognition based on clinical evidence of individuals with temporal lobe epilepsy and ictal fear compared with individuals with temporal lobe epilepsy but no ictal fear and individuals with idiopathic generalized epilepsy. They found that all three epilepsy groups had difficulty recognizing fear, with greater impairments among the patients with ictal fear. Consistent with a hypothesis of amygdala involvement, a significant number of patients with temporal lobe epilepsy and ictal fear made errors in fear recognition, often choosing surprise in place of fear as a response. Although the evidence suggests that mesial temporal regions are implicated in epilepsy as being more vulnerable to emotion perception deficits, the findings indicate that they may not be exclusively so. Reynders et al. (18) found evidence of emotion recognition difficulties among both temporal lobe epilepsy patents and those with idiopathic generalized epilepsy. A further study by Farrant et al. (24) found face emotion recognition deficits among patients with frontal seizures. In contrast, Meletti et al. (17) found normal emotion perception among patients with extratemporal seizure foci, including those in the frontal regions.

The variability found in the evidence of emotion recognition deficits among patients with epilepsy highlights the complex potential factors that might contribute to social cognition difficulties in a chronic condition such as epilepsy. In addition, the function of the amygdala may be compromised by epilepsy conditions, even when there is no established amygdalar atrophy. Seizures may originate simultaneously within both the amygdala and the hippocampus even when there is no structural evidence of an amygdalar lesion (25). Seizures characterized by fear auras are not produced exclusively by lesions or seizure foci within the amygdala, although the evidence suggests that these are usually associated with anterior hippocampal abnormalities or when sclerosis is found of both the hippocampus and the amygdala (26). Accordingly, it may be that even when there is no direct neuroanatomical evidence of amygdalar pathology, it would seem reasonable to suppose that there could be some compromise of the social cognition circuitry within which the amygdala plays a significant role.

Other Seizure Variables

Other seizure-related variables have also been examined. Meletti et al. (17) found that among all their subjects with right temporal lobe lesions, the degree of emotion recognition difficulties was related to earlier age of first seizure, either febrile or afebrile, and age of epilepsy onset. A significant relationship was also found by Reynders et al. (18) between anger recognition deficits and age of onset. The results suggest that there may be a vulnerability associated with early onset of seizures or epilepsy.

Duration of illness has also been found to increase vulnerability for fear recognition deficits among both temporal lobe epilepsy and patients with idiopathic generalized epilepsy. Such findings are consistent with those that show amygdalar atrophy in temporal lobe epilepsy to be associated with duration of the epilepsy disorder (27) and total number of seizures experienced (28) rather than with age of onset or etiology.

Even among patients with generalized seizures, the impact of seizures or duration of epilepsy may affect the amygdala's function via its interconnectedness with other brain regions such as the thalamus, the hypothalamus, and the brainstem. Generalized seizures are produced by an abnormal thalamocortical interaction (29) that involves pathways that link extensively with the amygdala. When seizures are frequent, longer duration of illness is likely to produce increasingly adverse effects as the total number of seizures accumulates. Evidence from research with other clinical conditions such as schizophrenia shows that emotion recognition deficits, particularly the recognition of fear in others, can occur without clear evidence of structural damage and that severity of illness is related to emotion recognition deficits (30). It is possible, therefore, to view a combination of duration and seizure frequency as a marker for the overall severity of epilepsy and as an important factor in producing a general vulnerability for emotion recognition deficits among patients with epilepsy. It would also account for the fact that not all patients with epilepsy, even those with clear evidence of amygdala involvement, have fear recognition deficits.

EMOTIONAL EXPERIENCE

It is well-established that damage to the amygdala and surrounding cortex in monkeys has been shown to have significant impact on social behavior and interaction with the environment. These changes are more likely to occur when the damage is early in life. In contrast to the animal studies, the research suggests that humans with acquired amygdala damage do not show impaired social behavior. They show a normal subjective sense of emotion in that they report their emotional states to be similar to those of control subjects and they are able to demonstrate appropriate facial expressions of emotion. There seems, therefore, to be a dissociation between their impaired abilities to correctly interpret negative emotions in others and their intact abilities to experience and express emotional and social information. One explanation is that the amygdalar damage in humans is sustained later in life, because early amygdalar damage is necessary for the development of adverse alterations in social behavior in adulthood. When amygdalar damage is acquired later, individuals may be able to cognitively compensate from learned experience, and the evidence suggests that there is a critical period for the development of amygdala-related social responses (31).

Although impairments in emotional recognition do not necessarily imply deficits in subjective experience or in the expression of emotions, a number of researchers have demonstrated an association between socioaffective disorders, such as autism (32) and schizophrenia (30), and abnormalities in the judgment of facial expressions of emotion. Evidence of the interconnectedness between emotional perception and affective responses comes from a different direction in a study by Birbaumer et al. (5), who found abnormal amygdala activation in subjects suffering from social phobia when they were shown a series of faces with neutral expressions.

In epilepsy, some individuals may acquire lesions or compromise to the amygdala early in life, and there is often reference to a specific personality presentation in temporal lobe epilepsy, often described anecdotally, as someone with a tendency to misinterpret social cues in others and to fail to respond appropriately in social situations. Although such a description is controversial, there has been some evidence of personality and social difficulties associated with temporal lobe epilepsy, particularly when seizures originate within the limbic regions. As part of their investigation of emotion perception

deficits in epilepsy, Reynders et al. (18) investigated the potential relationship between emotion perception and the experience of emotion, either directly in terms of the underlying neurobiology of temporal lobe epilepsy or more indirectly in relation to the impact of emotion and social cognitive impairments on psychosocial factors such as quality of life or psychologic distress. Three groups of patients (13 with temporal lobe epilepsy and ictal fear, 14 with temporal lobe epilepsy and nonfear auras, and 10 with idiopathic generalized epilepsy) completed tests of visual and face processing, face emotion recognition, and social judgment. In addition, the epilepsy groups also completed measures of mood (Hospital Anxiety and Depression Scale [HADS] and the SCL-90-R) and quality of life (QOLIE-31). Both the HADS and the SCL-90-R indicated high rates of affective disorder but did not indicate that patients with temporal lobe epilepsy are more vulnerable to psychologic disturbance than patients with other forms of epilepsy. The deficits in emotional perception, found in all groups of patients with epilepsy, did not correlate with measures of psychologic distress. Neither was interpretation of one's own emotional experience significantly related to emotion recognition.

These results provide evidence for dissociation between the experience and evaluation of one's own emotional experience and the ability to judge emotions in others. The results also suggest that, in relation to emotion recognition, a dissociation exists between a neurobiologically driven fear experience without psychologic context (i.e., a fear aura) and affective responses that, perhaps, reflect the multi-etiological nature of psychologic disorder in epilepsy (33). In a chronic neurologic condition such as epilepsy, psychologic effects and psychosocial impact interact with the direct effects of medication, lesion site, and seizure activity on emotional processing systems within the brain.

SOCIAL INTEGRATION SKILLS

Nevertheless, subtle deficits in social judgment have been identified among patients with amygdala damage and also in patients with epilepsy who show fear recognition deficits. Adolphs et al.'s (34) patients with bilateral damage to the amygdala judged unfamiliar individuals to be more approachable and more trustworthy than did control subjects from their perception of facial expressions. Reynders et al. (18) used the same assessment to measure social judgment among patients with epilepsy and found a significant negative correlation between the ability to recognize facial expressions of fear and the ability to make social judgments of trustworthiness of strangers from photographs of faces, regardless of type of epilepsy. An association was also found between perception of facial emotional expressions and subjective assessment of overall quality of life.

Most of the research in epilepsy has been carried out with patients with temporal lobe epilepsy. The social cognition neural circuitry is known to be influenced by the prefrontal pathways. The orbitofrontal region is particularly implicated in emotion perception and emotion-laden interpersonal behavior. The medial frontal area is associated with deficits in the regulation of emotional and motivation responses and in the ability to see another's perspective (theory of mind). Aspects of social cognition usually associated with the prefrontal pathways have not been extensively researched among patients with frontal lobe epilepsy. Deficits in emotion perception have been found, particularly in terms of the ability to rate relative emotional intensity. A recent study by Farrant et al. (24) used a range of social cognition tasks in addition to neuropsychologic tests to assess patients with frontal lobe epilepsy. The tasks included a theory of mind task, a faux pas task, an appreciation of humor in verbal descriptions task, an emotion perception task, and a task that demanded the inferring of mental states and emotion from gaze expression. They found no significant impairments on tests of theory of mind or faux pas. However, they did find that patients with frontal lobe epilepsy had significant impairments on tests of humor appreciation, recognition of facial emotions, and perception of eye-gaze expression.

COGNITIVE ABILITY VERSUS "EMOTIONAL INTELLIGENCE"

In the Farrant et al. (24) study, specific impairments of social cognition and executive function were found against a background of intact general intellectual ability and overall cognitive functions. A dissociation with general intellectual abilities has also been apparent in other studies of emotion and social information processing, with patients usually well-matched with controls on IQ tasks. Recent research has explicitly investigated the relationship between cognitive and emotional "intelligence." The concept of emotional intelligence has been developed to measure the multifactorial array of inter-related emotional, personal, and social competencies that influence the ability to actively and effectively cope with daily demands. One of the most widely used measures of emotional intelligence is the Emotional Quotient Inventory (35). Bar On et al. (36) used this measure of emotional intelligence on patients with lesions to the ventromedial cortex (six patients), amygdala (three patients), and right somatosensory cortex (three patients), structures hypothesised as being involved in social cognition and emotional aspects of decision making. All three experimental groups had significant impairments in the overall measure of

emotional intelligence in the context of intact cognitive intelligence. The authors interpret these results as being supportive of the hypothesis that emotional intelligence is separate and different from cognitive intelligence, and is also subserved by neural systems that overlap with other social cognition abilities.

A recent study by Walpole and colleagues (submitted for publication) aimed to establish the relationship between cognitive and emotional intelligence in people with temporal lobe epilepsy. Sixteen patients with temporal lobe epilepsy were matched with fourteen control subjects in terms of their overall intellectual ability. The results showed participants with temporal lobe epilepsy to have lower scores in total emotional intelligence, and on a number of domains of emotional intelligence, than control participants.

EMOTIONAL MEMORY

Studies of patients with amygdalar lesions have shown differential roles in the mesial temporal regions during learning and recall of emotionally laden memories, with a role for the amygdala in the consolidation and activation of emotional memories. Boucsein et al. (37) tested 22 patients after temporal lobe epilepsy surgery and found worse performance by patients with greater amygdala damage on tests of learning visual facial expressions. There was no effect of lateralization of surgery. Glogau et al. (38) found that patients with right temporal lobe epilepsy had significantly lower scores than healthy controls in face memory, whereas patients with left temporal lobe epilepsy demonstrated impairments both in face memory and in facial expression memory. The left temporal lobe epilepsy patients were also selectively impaired in their facial expression perception, and this significantly influenced their ability to learn facial emotional expressions. The investigators hypothesized that functional reorganization of verbal memory in left temporal lobe epilepsy may compromise visual memory. They also suggested that patients with right temporal lobe epilepsy may be able to verbalize visual material more successfully than those with left temporal lobe epilepsy.

CLINICAL IMPLICATIONS AND FUTURE RESEARCH

Future research questions might address the complex relationship between seizure variables and emotion recognition deficits. Are they related to duration of epilepsy, regardless of type or age of onset? Do newly diagnosed patients initially have intact emotion recognition skills that deteriorate relative to the duration of their disorder? Is the effect simply one of illness chronicity, or is the total number of seizures the major contributory factor? What role might medication play? What is the impact of using different tools and procedures for the assessment of emotion recognition deficits?

Patients are largely unaware of their emotion recognition impairments, and there is still little known about the impact of such impairments on quality of life and psychosocial well-being. The research indicates that assessing social cognition factors should become an integral part of the neuropsychologic examination of patients. As such, social cognition deficits need to be identified and addressed as part of routine neuropsychological examination and intervention.

It is widely accepted in the literature that, in a clinically complex condition such as epilepsy, there are a number of neurobiological, psychosocial, and psychologic factors that could produce psychosocial disturbance. This acknowledgment has often failed to influence the research models adopted, and the field remains, to a large extent, polarized between neurobiological and psychosocial explanations. Recent studies of emotion perception, together with other aspects of social cognition, including social judgment, emotional intelligence, and those tasks usually associated with compromise of the prefrontal pathways, are beginning to form the basis for a theoretical framework for the understanding of social cognition deficits in epilepsy and how these relate to emotional and social well-being.

Such work might have important implications for the theoretical understanding of affective abnormalities in epilepsy and might also add to our understanding of the mechanisms underlying the interrelationships between socio-neurocognitive variables and socio-affective disturbance.

Understanding the effects of emotion perception deficits and emotional learning difficulties may greatly enhance neuropsychologically informed approaches to developing meaningful coping strategies.

*R*eferences

1. Adolphs R. The neurobiology of social cognition. *Curr Opin Neurobiol* 2001; 11: 231–239.
2. Adolphs R. Cognitive neuroscience of human social behaviour. *Nat Rev Neurosci* 2003; 4:165–178.
3. LeDoux JE. Synaptic self. New York: Viking, 2002.
4. Ketter TA, Andreason PJ, George MS, et al. Anterior paralimbic mediation of procaine-induced emotional and psychosensory experiences. *Arch Gen Psychiatry* 1996; 53:59–69.
5. Birbaumer N, Grodd W, Diedrich O, Klose U, et al. fMRI reveals amygdala activation to human faces in social phobics. *Neuroreport* 1997; 9(6):1223–1226.
6. Davidson R J, Irwin W. The functional neuroanatomy of emotion and affective style. *Trends Cogn Sci* 1999; 3:11–21.
7. Shaw P, Lawrence EJ, Radbourne C, Bramham J, et al. The impact of early and late damage to the human amygdala on "theory of mind" reasoning. *Brain* 2004; 127:1535–1548.
8. Stone VE, Baron-Cohen S, Calder A, Keane J, et al. Acquired theory of mind impairments in individuals with bilateral amygdala lesions. *Neuropsychologia* 2003; 41(2):209–220.
9. Bechara A, Damasio H, Damasio AR, Lee GP. Different contributions of the human amygdala and ventromedial prefrontal cortex to decision-making. *J Neurosci* 1999; 19(13):5473–5481.
10. Adolphs R. Neural systems for recognising emotions. *Curr Opin Neurobiol* 2002; 12(2):169–177.
11. Adolphs R, Tranel D, Damasio H, Damasio AR. Impaired recognition of emotion in facial expressions following bilateral damage to the human amygdala. *Nature* 1994; 372: 669–672.
12. Broks P, Young AW, Maratos EJ, et al. Face processing impairments after encephalitis: amygdala damage and recognition of fear. *Neuropsychologia* 1998; 36(1):59–70.
13. Scott SK, Young AW, Calder AJ, Hellawell DJ, et al. Impaired auditory recognition of fear and anger following bilateral amygdala lesions. *Nature* 1997; 385:254–257.
14. Breiter HC, Etcoff NL, Whalen PJ, et al. Response and habituation of the human amygdala during visual processing of facial expression. *Neuron* 1996; 17:875–887.
15. Whalen PJ, Rauch SC, Etcoff NL, McInerney SC, et al. Masked presentations of emotional facial expressions modulate amygdala activity without explicit knowledge. *J Neurosci* 1998; 18(1):411–418.
16. Adolphs R, Tranel D, Damasio H. Emotion recognition from faces and prosody following temporal lobectomy. *Neuropsychology* 2001; 15:396–404.
17. Meletti S, Benuzzi F, Rubboli G, Cantalupo G, et al. Impaired facial emotion recognition in early-onset right mesial temporal lobe epilepsy. *Neurology* 2003; 60:426–431.
18. Reynders HJ, Broks P, Dickson JM, Lee CE, et al. Investigation of social and emotion information processing in temporal lobe epilepsy with ictal fear. *Epilepsy Behav* 2005; 7:419–429.
19. Fowler HL, Baker GA, Tipples J, et al. Recognition of emotion with temporal lobe epilepsy and asymmetrical amygdala damage. *Epilepsy Behav* 2006; 9:164–172.
20. Houghton JM, Broks P, Wing A, et al. Does temporal lobe epilepsy impair the ability to recognise cues to the emotional state of others? *Epilepsia* 2000; 41(suppl 7):249.
21. Gloor P, Olivier A, Quesney LF. The role of the limbic system in experiential phenomena of TLE. *Ann Neurol* 1982; 12:129–144.
22. Cendes F, Andermann F, Gloor P, et al. Relationship between atrophy of the amygdala and IF in TLE. *Brain* 1994; 117(Pt 4):739–746.
23. Yamada M, Toshiya M, Wataru S, Namiko C, et al. Emotion recognition from facial expressions in a temporal lobe epileptic patient with ictal fear. *Neuropsychologia* 2005; 43,434–441.
24. Farrant A, Morris RG, Russell T, et al. Social cognition in frontal lobe epilepsy. *Epilepsy Behav* 2005; 7:506–516.
25. Guerreiro C, Cendes F, Li LM, Jones-Gotman M, et al. Clinical patterns of patients with TLE and pure amygdalar atrophy. *Epilepsia* 1999; 40(4):453–461.
26. Feichtinger M, Pauli E, Schafer I, Eberhardt KW, et al. Ictal fear in temporal lobe epilepsy: surgical outcome and focal hippocampal changes revealed by proton magnetic resonanace spectroscopy imaging. *Arch Neurol* 2001; 58(5):771–777.
27. Miller LA, McLachlan RS, Bouwer MS, Hudson LP, et al. Amygdalar sclerosis: preoperative indicators and outcome after temporal lobectomy. *J Neurol Neurosurg Psychiatry* 1994; 57:1099–1105.
28. Kalviainen R, Salmenpera T, Partanen K, Vainio P Sr, et al. MRI volumetry and T2 relaxometry of the amygdala in newly diagnosed and chronic TLE. *Epilepsy Res* 1997; 28:39–50.
29. Smith DF, Appleton RE, MacKenzie JM, Chadwick DW. An atlas of epilepsy. New York, Carnforth UK: The Parthenon Publishing Group, 1997.
30. Evangeli M, Broks P. Face processing in schizophrenia: parallels with the effects of amygdala damage. *Cognit Neuropsychiatry* 1999; 4(2):1–24.
31. Phelps EA, LeDoux JE. Contributions of the amygdala to emotion processing: from animal models to human behaviour. *Neuron* 2005; 48:175–187.
32. Hobson RP. Emotion recognition in autism: co-ordinating faces and voice. *Psychol Med* 1988; 18:911–923.
33. Hermann BP, Whitman S, Anton M. A multietiological model of psychological and social dysfunction in epilepsy. In: Bennett TL, ed. *The Neuropsychology of Epilepsy*. New York: Plenum Press, 1992.
34. Adolphs R, Tranel D, Damasio AR. The human amygdala in social judgement. *Nature* 1998; 393(4):470–474.
35. Bar On R. The Emotional Quotient Inventory (EQ-i): a test of emotional intelligence. Toronto, Canada: Multi-Health Systems, 1997.
36. Bar On R, Tranel D, Denburg NL, Bechara A. Exploring the neurological substrate of emotional and social intelligence. *Brain* 2003; 126:1790–1800.
37. Boucsein K, Weniger G, Mursch K, Steinhoff BJ, et al. Amygdala lesion in temporal lobe epilepsy subjects impairs associative learning of emotional facial expressions. *Neuropsychologia* 2001; 39:231–236.
38. Glogau S, Ellgring H, Elger CE, Helmstaedter C. Face and facial expression memory in temporal lobe epilepsy patients: preliminary results. *Epilepsy Behav* 2004; 5: 106–112.

V

NEUROPSYCHIATRIC AND BEHAVIORAL DISORDERS IN PATIENTS WITH EPILEPSY

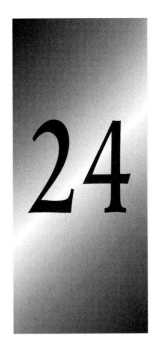

24 Classification of Neuropsychiatric Disorders in Epilepsy

Ennapadam S. Krishnamoorthy
Rema Reghu

The classification of psychiatric disorders in epilepsy has always been controversial. A well-established system of classification would ensure effective scientific communication among specialists around the world. This is especially true in a specialty, such as neuropsychiatry, with few well-defined parameters and diagnostic tests—a specialty that therefore relies on clear and concise clinical descriptions. Further, because epilepsy-specific neuropsychiatric disorders are well described empirically and have clear differences compared with generic psychiatric disorders, there is a felt need for a distinct classification (1).

The European psychiatrists of the nineteenth and early twentieth century were the first to suggest paradigms of classification for neuropsychiatric disorders in epilepsy. There was considerable disagreement among these "experts," which is documented in an elegant review by Schmitz and Trimble (2). The advent of electroencephalography (EEG) and its widespread use in epilepsy centers from the 1950s also had a major influence on classification at this interface. Clinician scientists such as Landolt (3, 4) at this time described classificatory systems that had EEG firmly at their helm. Subsequent to this, however, there have been few serious attempts to develop a classificatory system and, to our best knowledge, no organized consensus efforts backed by international academic bodies.

The scenario until recently was complicated by other factors as well. It is noteworthy that both the International League Against Epilepsy (ILAE) (5) and the World Health Organization (WHO) classifications of seizures and epilepsy (6) do not take psychopathology of epilepsy into account. Nor does the psychopathology of epilepsy find a place in the evolving ILAE classification proposal (7). Further, any modern attempt at classification of epilepsy-specific psychopathology may have the onerous task of having to consider the spectrum of psychiatric diagnoses as described in the current psychiatric classifications—ICD-10 (8) and DSM-IV (9)—and relate this to diagnoses at the seizures and epilepsy interface. The most recent attempt at developing such a classification came from the ILAE Commission on Psychobiology of Epilepsy, which had a dedicated subcommission on classification. The consensus paper of this commission, which was widely circulated among experts with an interest in epilepsy neuropsychiatry, is now in press (10). The approach of this commission is reviewed here and analyzed for the benefit of the reader.

THE ILAE CLASSIFICATION

The classificatory system of the ILAE has taken a clearly clinical approach based on semiology. In this the commission has differed from other, etiology-driven approaches, the basic premise being that clinical descriptions, at least at present, have greater cross-cultural validity than do etiological associations, whose scientific bases remain somewhat uncertain. The ILAE classification begins by differentiating comorbid disorders from epilepsy-specific neuropsychiatric disorders. The acknowledgment here is that people with epilepsy can, like their peers in the community, suffer from both minor and major psychiatric disorders that are putatively unrelated to the epilepsy process and mirror well-acknowledged descriptions in ICD-10 and DSM-IV. While somewhat unusual, this approach puts the focus of this classification firmly on neuropsychiatric disorders specific to epilepsy and ensures that it is in no way competing with established classificatory systems in psychiatry—a wheel that needs no reinvention. A parallel can be drawn between this approach and that taken by surgical epileptologists, who differentiate "epilepsy surgery" from surgical approaches that aim to tackle symptomatic seizures, the former being far more specific than the latter. The comorbid psychiatric disorders described in this classification include anxiety and phobic disorders, minor and major depression, obsessive compulsive disorder, bipolar affective disorders, and forms of schizophrenia not recognized as being typical of epilepsy (for example, disintegrative forms of the condition). It is recommended that conventional criteria as described in the psychiatric classificatory systems should be used to classify these comorbid mental disorders.

Another area about which the commission has chosen to include a mention in this classification is "cognitive dysfunction." Avoiding detailed review of various neuropsychologic constructs in epilepsy, the ILAE classification merely seeks to mention cognitive impairments, including difficulties with memory, language, executive functions, visuospatial ability, and sensorimotor/perceptual functions, which may be general or specific (11). Some specific neurocognitive deficits such as the Landau–Kleffner syndrome, which can be associated with specific EEG changes such as electrical status epilepticus of slow wave sleep (ESES) or continuous spike and wave in slow wave sleep (CSWS) to be included here (12), find mention here.

The logic in such limited coverage was the admittedly controversial differentiation between neuropsychiatric and neuropsychologic disorders in epilepsy, with the latter being considered outside the purview of the subcommission on classification. Further, apart from the observed links between cognitive disorders, behavioral dysfunction, and intractable epilepsy, with their neurobiological underpinnings, the firmest links to emerge between neuropsychology and neuropsychiatry in epilepsy have been in the learning disability/mental retardation literature (13), in the observation of both types of dysfunction with antiepileptic drug treatment (14), and more recently in the context of "memory complaints that

are associated with depression rather than actual cognitive impairment" (15).

Although there are different ways of classifying mental states, the clinical approach of observing patients over a prolonged period of time is by far the most important, and that approach is the basis of this proposal. Further, as mentioned earlier, while there is good empirical evidence to suggest that the psychiatric disorders of epilepsy are clinically distinct, they do not find a place in the current classificatory systems in psychiatry such as ICD-10 and DSM-IV. Besides, operational rules that exist ensure that they are subsumed within categories (organic mental disorder, for example), in a way that may be neither appropriate nor accurate. Because these disorders are phenomenologically distinct and may respond to specific therapeutic measures, as discussed, for example, by Blumer (16), that approach is clearly unsatisfactory. Modern efforts must be directed at developing a more comprehensive and acceptable system of classification for psychiatric disorders in epilepsy.

Thus, with regard to the well-defined ictal and interictal psychiatric disorders specific to epilepsy, the commission has chosen to be rather more prescriptive, as a wealth of empirical observation has accumulated over decades. Among psychiatric disorders, depression and psychoses predominate the epilepsy literature, followed by anxiety disorders and personality trait accentuation/disorder. The ILAE commission has also chosen to classify largely based on relationship to ictus: interictal (between seizures with no presumed specific relationship); preictal (preceding seizures, sometimes serving as an aura or warning); postictal (following seizures, sometimes after a lucid interval); and alternate (a paradoxical relationship where either seizures or behavioral dysfunction predominate at different times). The core elements of the new ILAE classification with regard to epilepsy-specific disorders are reproduced in this chapter for the benefit of the reader.

PSYCHOPATHOLOGY AS A PRESENTING FEATURE OF EPILEPTIC SEIZURES

Psychiatric symptoms are often a feature of the seizure itself. Auras of simple partial seizures include psychiatric symptoms such as anxiety and panic, hallucinations in various modalities, and even transient abnormal beliefs. Abnormal (sometimes bizarre) behavior can also characterize partial seizures arising from the frontal and temporal lobes that often do not generalize. Subclinical seizure activity (often nonconvulsive status) can also present with catatonic features and other neuropsychiatric manifestations such as apathy and aggression (17).

Well-defined ictal states are included as follows:

- Complex partial seizure status: presents with impaired awareness.

- Simple partial seizure status (aura continua): presents with intact awareness.
- Absence status (spike-wave stupor): presents with a stuporous state and at times with minor myoclonic manifestations.

PSYCHIATRIC DISORDERS WITH ICTAL ASSOCIATIONS THAT ARE SPECIFIC TO EPILEPSY

There are disorders that are seen specifically in patients with epilepsy and have specific ictal associations as well as distinct clinical descriptions that may respond to specific forms of treatment. These can be broadly divided into the following categories:

Psychoses of Epilepsy

Interictal Psychosis of Epilepsy. This is a paranoid psychosis with strong affective components but usually not affective flattening. Features may include command hallucinations, third-person auditory hallucinations, and other first-rank symptoms. There is a preoccupation with religious themes. Personality and affect tend to be well-preserved unlike in other forms of schizophrenic psychosis. Psychotic features are usually independent of seizures, although they may become manifest as seizure freedom lessens (17).

Include: Schizophrenia-like psychosis of epilepsy
Exclude: Cases fulfilling criteria for undifferentiated or hebephrenic schizophrenia

Alternative Psychosis. The patient alternates between periods of clinically manifest seizures and normal behavior, and other periods of seizure freedom accompanied by a behavioral disturbance. The behavioral disturbance is often accompanied by paradoxical normalization of the EEG (forced normalization) (3, 4). The behavioral disturbance is polymorphic, with paranoid and affective features. The diagnosis of Alternative Psychosis (18) should be made in the absence of the EEG. If EEG confirmation is available, the diagnosis should be qualified further as "with forced normalization of the EEG."

Include: Forced Normalization/Paradoxical Normalization (19). Include also cases with relative normalization as defined by Krishnamoorthy and Trimble (20).
Exclude: Continuing interictal psychosis or postictal psychosis (recent cluster of seizures); nonconvulsive status with psychiatric manifestations.

Postictal Psychosis. This follows clusters of seizures (rarely single seizures) usually after a 24–48 hour period of relative calm (the lucid interval). These episodes can last from a few days to several weeks but usually subside in 1–2 weeks. Confusion and amnesia may be present. The content of thought is paranoid, and visual and auditory hallucinations may be present. Manifestations are often polymorphic, with affective features and a strong religious theme (17).

Include: Cases with a clear history of a cluster of seizures or an isolated single seizure (in a patient who has been seizure-free). The first manifestation of abnormal behavior should occur within a 7-day period of the last seizure (21).
Exclude: Postictal confusion; nonconvulsive status with psychiatric manifestations.

Affective-Somatoform (Dysphoric) Disorders of Epilepsy

Intermittent affective-somatoform symptoms are frequently present in chronic epilepsy. They present in a pleomorphic pattern and include eight symptoms: irritability, depressive moods, anergia, insomnia, atypical pains, anxiety, and euphoric moods. They occur at various intervals and tend to last from hours to 2–3 days, although they might on occasion last longer. Some of the symptoms may be present continually at a baseline from which intermittent fluctuations occur. The presence of three symptoms or more generally coincides with significant disability (16). The same affective-somatoform symptoms occur during the prodromal and postictal phases and need to be coded as such if they are of clinical significance.

Interictal Dysphoric Disorder. Intermittent dysphoric symptoms (at least three of those just mentioned) are present, each to a troublesome degree. In women the disorder is manifest (or accentuated) in the premenstrual phase.

Prodromal Dysphoric Disorder. Irritability or other dysphoric symptoms may precede a seizure by hours or days and cause significant impairment.

Postictal Dysphoric Disorder. Symptoms of anergia or headaches as well as depressed mood, irritability, or anxiety may develop after a seizure and be prolonged or exceptionally severe.

Alternative Affective-Somatoform Syndromes. Depression, anxiety, depersonalization, derealization, and even nonepileptic seizures have been reported as presenting manifestations of forced normalization (19). These may be diagnosed in the absence of an EEG as described previously, and, in the face of EEG evidence, coded as "with forced normalization of EEG."

Include: Brief-lasting but disabling changes in affect.

Exclude: Patients fulfilling ICD-10 and DSM-IV criteria for major depression, dysthymia, and cyclothymia.

Personality Disorders

Patients with chronic epilepsy may show distinct personality changes that tend to be subtle. Three types are recognized:

1. A deepening of emotionality with serious, highly ethical, and spiritual demeanor (22)
2. A tendency to be particularly detailed, orderly, and persistent in speech and action, viz. viscosity (23)
3. A labile affect with suggestibility and immaturity (referred to as eternal adolescence) (24)

They may be coded as personality disorders only if present to a degree that interferes significantly with social adjustment.

- Hyperethical or hyperreligious groups
- Viscous group
- Labile group
- Mixed (two or more of the above)

Diagnosis should be coded in the category as follows:

- No personality trait accentuation or disorder
- Personality trait accentuation, but not disorder
- Personality disorder specific to epilepsy

Exclude: Patients fulfilling criteria for well-defined DSM-IV or ICD-10 personality disorders.

Specific Phobic Fears

Specific phobic fears such as fear of seizures (25), agoraphobia, and social phobia may occur as a result of recurrent seizures. They may occur either as part of the interictal dysphoric disorder, in which case that diagnosis is preferred, or alone, in which case they should be coded here. Unlike comorbid psychiatric disorder, the phobic fears revolve around epilepsy, and the fear of the situation and subsequent avoidance are linked to the fear of having a seizure in that situation and the possible consequences.

Other Relevant Information (to be Recorded in All Patients if Possible)

Relationship to EEG Change. Characteristic changes in EEG could accompany disorders with psychiatric presentations such as generalized absence status, simple and complex partial seizures, or encephalopathy (organic brain syndrome), or there may be an absence or reduction of EEG abnormalities compared to previous and subsequent EEGs, as in forced normalization. The EEG is thus an important investigative tool, and the findings at the time of psychiatric disturbance need to be coded separately as follows:

- EEG not available/not done
- EEG remains unchanged
- Nonspecific EEG change
- Specific EEG change (please specify)

Anticonvulsant-Induced Psychiatric Disorders. As drugs used in the treatment of epilepsy may contribute to the development of psychiatric disorders, it is important that this be specified as an additional category. As both anticonvulsant induction (14) and withdrawal (26) are known to precipitate behavioral change, this factor needs to be specified, as does the specific anticonvulsant probably responsible, if at all possible. This also has prognostic and therapeutic implications, because often the only course of action available to the treating professional is withdrawal of the offending agent.

- Details of AED therapy not known/not documented
- No change in AED treatment
- AED institution (in a 30-day period prior to psychiatric disorder)
- AED withdrawal (in a 7-day period prior to psychiatric disorder)
- Both AED institution and withdrawal during 30-day period
- Note: Specify AEDs

CONCLUSIONS

While this classificatory system is by no means the ideal to which researchers have aspired, its clinical basis, focus on epilepsy-specific psychopathology, and inherent simplicity are likely to make it applicable in many settings, both in the developing and in the developed world. This operational system needs to be piloted, suitably modified, and validated in several settings before it is widely acceptable. Nevertheless, it has provided a template that hitherto did not exist.

The emphasis on clinical semiology is a reminder and acknowledgment of the importance of clinical descriptions in classificatory systems across medical disciplines. It also reflects the prevailing view in epilepsy neuropsychiatry that the exponential growth in technological advances has yet to result in tangible breakthroughs in our understanding of this interface. Indeed, the paucity of knowledge about specific etiological factors that influence the development of neuropsychiatric disorders in epilepsy is in itself proof of the neglect that this interface suffers. In the absence of such specific knowledge and understanding, the ILAE commission has chosen to take the view that attempting an etiological classification may be fallacious. Yet the emphasis on EEG change as the predominant factor retains the biomedical emphasis in this classification.

Perhaps advances in our knowledge and understanding through imaging and molecular genetic studies will revolutionize our approach to this interface.

Until then, we must be content with adopting, and modifying through systematic operational research, this clinically based ILAE classification.

References

1. Krishnamoorthy ES. An approach to classifying neuropsychiatric disorders in epilepsy. *Epilepsy Behav* 2000; 1 373–377.
2. Schmitz B, Trimble MR. Epileptic equivalents in psychiatry: some 19th century views. *Acta Neurol Scand* 1992; 86(suppl. 140):122–126.
3. Landolt H. Some clinical electroencephalographical correlations in epileptic psychoses (twilight states). *Electroencephalogr Clin Neurophysiol* 1953; 5:121.
4. Landolt H. Serial electroencephalographic investigations during psychotic episodes in epileptic patients and during schizophrenic attacks. In: Lorentz de Haas AM, ed. *Lectures on Epilepsy*. Amsterdam: Elsevier, 1958:91–133.
5. Commission on Classification and Terminology of the ILAE. Proposal for revised classification of epilepsies and epileptic syndromes. *Epilepsia* 1989:30:389–399.
6. World Health Organization. Manual of the international statistical classification of diseases, injuries and causes of death. Based on the recommendations of the Eighth Conference, Geneva, 1965. Geneva: WHO, 1967.
7. Engel J Jr. Report of the ILAE Classification Core Group. *Epilepsia* 2006; 47(9):1558–1568.
8. World Health Organization. ICD-10 classification of mental and behavioral disorders. Geneva: WHO, 1992.
9. American Psychiatric Association. Diagnostic and statistical manual of mental disorders, DSM-IV. Washington, DC: American Psychiatric Association, 1994.
10. Krishnamoorthy ES, Trimble MR, Blumer D. The classification of neuropsychiatric disorders in epilepsy: a proposal by the ILAE Commission on Psychobiology of Epilepsy. *Epilepsy Behav* 2007; 10(3):349–353.
11. Perrine K, Kiolbasa T. Cognitive deficits in epilepsy and contribution to psychopathology. *Neurology* 1999; 53(Suppl. 2):S39–S48.
12. Besag FM. Treatment of state-dependent learning disability. *Epilepsia* 2001; 42 (Suppl. 1):52–54.
13. Steffenberg E, Steffenberg S. Epilepsy and other neuropsychiatric morbidity in mentally retarded children. In: Sillanpaa M, Gram L, Johannessen S, I, Tomson T, eds. *Epilepsy and Mental Retardation*. Petersfield, UK: Wrightson Biomedical, 1999:47–59.
14. Trimble MR. New antiepileptic drugs and psychopathology. *Neuropsychobiology* 1998; 38(3):149–151.
15. Piazzini A, Canevini MP, Maggiori G, Canger R. The perception of memory failures in patients with epilepsy. *Eur J Neurol* 2001; 8(6):613–620.
16. Blumer D. Dysphoric disorders and paroxysmal affects: recognition and treatment of epilepsy-related psychiatric disorders. *Harvard Rev Psychiatr* 2000; 8(1):8–17.
17. Trimble MR. The psychoses of epilepsy. New York: Raven Press, 1991.
18. Tellenbach H. Epilepsie als Anfallsleiden und als Psychose. Uber alternative Psychosen paranoider Pragung bei "forceiter Normalisierung" (Landolt) des Elektroencephallogramms Epileptischer. *Nervenarzt* 1961; 36:190–202.
19. Wolf P. Acute behavioral symptomatology at disappearance of epileptiform EEG abnormality: paradoxical or "forced" normalization. In: Smith DB, Treiman DM, Trimble MR, eds. *Neurobehavioral Problems in Epilepsy*. Advances in Neurology 55. New York: Raven Press, 1991:127–142.
20. Krishnamoorthy ES, Trimble MR. Forced normalization: clinical and therapeutic relevance. *Epilepsia* 1999:40(suppl. 10); S57–S64.
21. Logsdail SJ, Toone BK. Post-ictal psychoses: a clinical and phenomenological description. *Br J Psychiatry* 1988:152; 246–252.
22. Geschwind N. Behavioral change in temporal lobe epilepsy. *Arch Neurol* 1977; 34:453.
23. Blumer D. Personality disorders in epilepsy. In: Ratey JJ. *Neuropsychiatry of Personality Disorders*. Boston: Blackwell Science, 1995:230–263.
24. Trimble M. Cognitive and personality profiles in patients with juvenile myoclonic epilepsy. In. Schmitz B, Sander T. *Juvenile Myoclonic Epilepsy: The Janz Syndrome*. Petersfield, UK: Wrightson Biomedical, 2000:101–111.
25. Newsom-Davis I, Goldstein LH, Fitzpatrick D. Fear of seizures: an investigation and treatment. *Seizure* 1998:7; 101–106.
26. Ketter TA, Malow BA, Flamini R, White SR, et al. Anticonvulsant withdrawal-emergent psychopathology. *Neurology* 1994; 44(1):55–61.

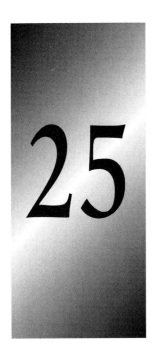

Mood Disorders in Epilepsy: Two Different Disorders with Common Pathogenic Mechanisms?

Andres M. Kanner

Multiple studies have documented the high comorbidity between mood disorders (MD) and epilepsy. Such comorbidity is not limited to studies carried out in tertiary centers but can be identified in population-based studies. For example, Ettinger et al. investigated the presence of symptoms of depression among 775 people with epilepsy (PWE), 395 people with asthma, and 362 healthy controls identified from a cohort of 85,358 adults aged 18 years and older using the Centers of Epidemiologic Studies-Depression (CES-D) Instrument (1). One-third of PWE (36.5%) had a CES-D score high enough to suggest the presence of severe or moderately severe depressive episode. The prevalence rate of such depressive episode was higher than that identified in people with asthma (27.8%) and healthy controls (11.8%). The same group of investigators compared the lifetime prevalence rates of bipolar symptoms and past diagnoses of bipolar I and II disorder with the Mood Disorder Questionnaire (MDQ) among subjects who identified themselves as having epilepsy and those with migraine, asthma, diabetes mellitus, or a healthy comparison group (2). Bipolar symptoms, evident in 12.2% of epilepsy patients, were 1.6 to 2.2 times more common in subjects with epilepsy than with migraine, asthma, or diabetes mellitus, and 6.6 times more likely to occur than in the healthy comparison

group. A total of 49.7% of patients with epilepsy who screened positive for bipolar symptoms were diagnosed with bipolar disorder by a physician, nearly twice the rate seen in other disorders. However, 26.3% of MDQ-positive epilepsy subjects carried a diagnosis of unipolar depression, and 25.8% had neither a uni- or bipolar depression diagnosis.

Investigators have attributed the high prevalence of MD to a variety of factors including reactive processes, iatrogenic causes, genetic predisposition, and seizure-related endogenous changes impacting neurochemical and neurophysiologic processes. These have been reviewed extensively in other review articles by this and other authors and will not be repeated here (3–5).

For a long time, investigators, clinicians, and patients have assumed a unidirectional relationship between epilepsy and MD, whereby the presence of the former is a risk factor for the latter. In fact, several population-based studies have demonstrated the existence of a bidirectional relationship between epilepsy and MD. In a population-based, case-control study carried out in Sweden, Forsgren and Nystrom found that newly diagnosed adult-onset epilepsy was seven times more frequent among patients with a history of depression *preceding the onset of epilepsy* than among age- and sex-matched controls (6). Similarly, in a population-based, case-control study of the incidence of new-onset epilepsy among adults aged 55 and older,

Hesdorffer et al. found that patients were 3.7 more likely to have a history of depression preceding their initial seizure than controls were (7). In this study, the authors also controlled for medical therapies for depression. These investigators provided further compelling evidence of a bidirectional relationship between MD and epilepsy in a population-based study carried out in Iceland (8). In this study, the investigators identified any psychiatric symptom and disorder that preceded the occurrence of the seizure disorder in all children and adults with epilepsy and in a group of age-matched controls free of any epilepsy. They found that a history of major depression (OR: 1.7, 95% CI: 1.1–2.7) and a history of attempted suicide (OR: 5.1, 95% CI: 2.2–11.5) *independently* increase the risk of experiencing unprovoked seizures and epilepsy. It should be noted, however, that the credit for the initial recognition of a bidirectional relationship between MD and epilepsy should go to Hippocrates, when he wrote 26 centuries ago that "melancholics ordinarily become epileptics, and epileptics melancholics: what determines the preference is the direction the malady takes; if it bears upon the body, epilepsy, if upon the intelligence, melancholy" (9).

The bidirectional relationship between MD and epilepsy should not be interpreted to suggest the existence of a causal relationship between the two. Rather, it suggests that both disorders share pathogenic mechanisms that, in turn, may explain their high comorbidity. This chapter reviews these common pathogenic mechanisms and their therapeutic implications for treatment of seizure disorders and of MD in PWE.

NEUROBIOLOGIC BASES OF MOOD DISORDERS

Neuroanatomy of Primary Mood Disorders

In a review of the literature, Sheline described morphologic and volumetric changes in neuroanatomical structures that form a "limbic-cortical-striatal-pallidal-thalamic circuit in patients with major depressive disorders (MDD)" (10). She proposed a limbic-thalamic-cortical branch as one of its arms, which includes the amygdala, hippocampus, medial-dorsal nucleus of the thalamus, and medial and ventrolateral prefrontal cortex. She also suggested the existence of a second arm running in parallel and linking the caudate, putamen, and globus pallidus with limbic and cortical regions. Depression in PWE has been associated more frequently with seizure disorders of temporal and frontal lobe origin, with prevalence rates ranging from 19% to 65% in various patient series (11–15). It is not surprising to find structural and functional changes of frontal and temporal lobe structures in patients with primary MD.

Structural changes identified on MRI

Temporal lobe structures. The temporal structures affected in patients with primary MDD and bipolar disorders (BPD) include the hippocampal formation, amygdala, entorhinal cortex, and parahippocampal gyrus (10). In 1996, Sheline et al. reported on the presence of smaller hippocampal volumes, bilaterally, of ten patients with a history of MDD in remission when compared to hippocampal volumes of 10 age-, sex-, and height-matched normal controls (16). They also identified large hippocampal low-signal foci ($\geq$4.5mm in diameter), and their number correlated with the total number of days depressed. A significant inverse correlation between the duration of depression and left hippocampal volume was also demonstrated, suggesting that patients with more chronic and active disease were more likely to have hippocampal atrophy. These authors replicated these findings in a larger study of 24 patients and 24 matched controls for age, sex, and height, in which they also found that core amygdala nuclei volumes correlated with hippocampal volumes. Hecimovic et al. carried out a review of all the published studies to date on the volumetric changes of various neuroanatomical structures (17). These are summarized in Table 25-1. As shown in the table, Sheline's findings were replicated by various investigators but not all. A reduction of the hippocampal formation was associated with an early age of onset of the MDD, a greater number of previous episodes, or longer duration of untreated depression (17). As shown in Table 25-1, findings of hippocampal volume change in bipolar disorder have not been uniform, as some studies found an increase, but others a decrease or no change in the hippocampal volume. The discrepancy in the data may stem from differences in the technique to measure the neuroanatomical structures, the number of MDD, the use of antidepressant medication, and duration of untreated illness (see subsequent discussions). None of the studies showed any significant differences in the total intracranial volume between patients with depression and healthy subjects. Nevertheless, most authors use relative measurements for comparison of regions of interest or with a total intracranial volume as a covariate in the statistical analysis.

Some authors have associated the severity of depression with the development of hippocampal atrophy. For example, Shah and colleagues compared hippocampal volumes of 20 patients with treatment-resistant MDD to 20 patients who responded to therapy and 20 healthy controls (23). Patients with treatment-resistant MDD were more likely to have hippocampal atrophy.

Lower verbal memory scores are a functional consequence of hippocampal damage, as demonstrated in a study by MacQueen and colleagues, who compared hippocampal volumes and hippocampal-dependent memory tests between 20 patients with first episode that was never

TABLE 25-1
Volumetric Changes in Primary Mood Disorders

NEUROANATOMIC STRUCTURE	N TYPE OF MD	FINDINGS OF VOLUME CHANGES	AUTHOR
Hippocampus-amygdala complex	48 MDD	No significant between-group difference	Coffey et al., 1993 (18)
Hippocampus-amygdala complex	40 MDD	No significant between-group difference	Ashtari et al., 1999 (19)
Hippocampus	20 MDD	Reduction in the volume	Krishnan et al. 1991 (20)
Hippocampus	19 MDD	No significant between-group difference	Axelson et al., 1993 (21)
Hippocampus	19 MDD	No significant between-group difference	Pantel et al., 1997 (22)
Hippocampus	20 MDD	Reduction in the left hippocampal volume	Shah et al., 1998 (23)
Hippocampus	24 MDD (women)	Reduction in the volume	Sheline et al., 1999 (4)
Hippocampus	34 MDD	Reduction in the left hippocampal volume	Mervaala et al., 2000 (24)
Hippocampus	38 MDD	No significant between-group difference	Vakili et al., 2000 (25)
Hippocampus	14 MDD	No significant between-group difference	Von Gunten et al., 2000 (26)
Hippocampus	66 MDD	Reduction in the right hippocampal volume	Steffens et al., 2000 (27)
Hippocampus	25 MDD	No significant between-group difference	Rusch et al., 2001 (28)
Hippocampus	30 MDD	Reduction in the right hippocampal volume	Bell-McGinty et al., 2002 (29)
Hippocampus	30 MDD	Reduction in the volume with a first episode	Frodl et al., 2002 (30)
Hippocampus	38 MDD	Reduction in the volume	Sheline et al., 2003 (31)
Hippocampus	20 MDD	Reduction in the volume	MacQueen et al., 2003 (32)
Hippocampus	31 MDD	Reduction in the volume	Caetano et al., 2004 (33)
Hippocampus	38 MDD	No significant between-group difference	Vythilingam et al., 2004 (34)
Hippocampus	30 MDD	No significant between-group difference after 1 year follow-up	Frodl et al., 2004 (35)
Hippocampus	40 MDD	Reduction in the volume if allele L/L of the 5-HTTLPR	Frodl et al., 2004 (36)
Hippocampus	31 MDD	Reduction in the total and posterior hippocampal volume	Neumeister et al., 2005 (37)
Amygdala	19 MDD	No significant between-group difference	Pantel et al., 1997 (22)
Amygdala	27 MDD	Reduction in the left amygdala volume	Pearlson et al., 1997 (38)
Amygdala	20 MDD	Bilaterally reduced core nuclei volumes	Sheline et al., 1998 (39)
Amygdala	34 MDD	Asymmetry (left smaller than right)	Mervaala et al., 2000 (24)
Amygdala	14 MDD	Reduction in the left amygdala volume	Von Gunten et al., 2000 (26)
Amygdala	30 MDD	Increase in the volume with a first episode	Frodl et al., 2002 (40)
Amygdala	30 MDD	No significant between-group difference after 1 year follow-up	Frodl et al., 2004 (35)
Temporal lobe	17 MDD	Reduction in the volume on the left and right	Hauser et al., 1989 (41)
Temporal lobe	48 MDD	No significant between-group difference	Coffey et al., 1993 (18)
Temporal lobe	30 MDD	Reduction in the left medial temporal volume	Greenwald et al., 1997 (46)

*All studies listed are in comparison with healthy controls. MDD: major depressive disorder; BD: bipolar disorder.

treated and normal age-matched controls (32). The same comparisons were carried out between a second patient group that included 17 patients with recurrent depressive episodes and matched controls and the patients with a single depressive episode. While patients with a single and multiple episodes had verbal memory deficits, only patients with multiple episodes had hippocampal atrophy. As in Sheline's studies, there was a significant correlation between the duration of the depressive illness and the degree of hippocampal atrophy.

Atrophy has also been identified in other mesial temporal structures. Bell-McGinty and colleagues found an inverse relationship between the volumes of hippocampus and entorhinal cortex and the time since the first lifetime depressive episode in a study of 30 patients with MDD and 47 matched controls (29).

In a recent study, Posener and colleagues suggested the need to study the shape of the hippocampus in addition to the measurement of its volume, because the former can identify structural changes even in the absence of volumetric decrements (43). Using the method of high-dimensional brain mapping, these authors generated 10 variables, or components of the hippocampal shape, in a study that compared high-dimensional mapping of 27 patients with MDD and 42 healthy controls. In depressed patients, these authors identified hippocampal deformation suggestive of specific involvement of the subiculum, while finding no differences in hippocampal volumes between the two groups.

As previously mentioned, exposure to treatment with antidepressant drugs may have an impact on the development of hippocampal atrophy. Indeed, Sheline and colleagues demonstrated that pharmacotherapy with antidepressants may protect patients with MDD from developing hippocampal atrophy (31). In a study of 38 female patients, they found a significant correlation between reduction in hippocampal volume and the duration of depression that went untreated. On the other hand, there was no correlation between hippocampal volume loss and time depressed while taking antidepressant medication or with lifetime exposure to antidepressants. Vakili and colleagues supported the same findings (25). In a study of 38 patients with MDD they found no difference in hippocampal volumes between patients and controls, yet they identified a possible relationship between hippocampal volumes and disease severity (left hippocampal volumes correlated with Hamilton Depression Rating Scale at baseline), as well as with treatment response (female responders to fluoxetine therapy had significantly larger right hippocampal volumes).

Changes in amygdala. As shown in Table 25-1, volumetric changes of the amygdalae of patients with MDD are less consistent than those in the hippocampal formation. This is not surprising, because measurement of the volume of the amygdala and its nuclei is technically much more difficult than that of hippocampal structures. Sheline and colleagues found the core volume of amygdala nuclei, but not its total volume, to be decreased bilaterally among 20 patients with a history of MDD, free of any neurologic disorder, compared to those of 20 matched controls (39). Conversely, Frodl and colleagues found increased amygdala volumes in 30 inpatients with a first episode of MDD, compared to matched controls. The authors attributed these changes to enhanced blood flow (40).

Structural changes of temporal lobe structures in PWE are well known and include atrophy of hippocampus, amygdala, entorhinal cortex, and parahippocampal gyrus in patients with mesial temporal sclerosis (MTS), the most frequent type of temporal lobe epilepsy (TLE). In one study of patients with TLE, higher scores of depression were associated with the presence of MTS (43). In a recent study, Gilliam et al. investigated the association of an indicator of hippocampal function measured with magnetic resonance spectroscopy (MRSI) with severity of depression symptoms in 31 patients with pharmaco-resistant TLE (44). They found that the extent of hippocampal ^{1}H-MRSI abnormalities correlated with severity of depression but other clinical factors did not.

MRI structural changes in frontal lobes. Structural changes have been investigated in various structures of the frontal lobes of patients with primary MD, including the prefrontal cortex and cingulate gyrus as well as in their white matter, revealing a decrease in volume of these structures. These data were also reviewed by Hecimovic et al. (17), and a summary appears in Table 25-2. For example, Bremner and colleagues found that orbitofrontal cortical volumes of 15 patients with MDD in remission were significantly smaller than the volume of orbitofrontal cortex and other frontal cortical regions of 20 controls (45). Coffey and colleagues also found smaller frontal lobe volumes in 48 inpatients with severe depression who had been referred for electroshock therapy, compared to 76 controls (46). Lai and colleagues found smaller bilateral orbital frontal cortex volumes in 20 elderly patients with MDD compared to 20 matched controls (47). Taylor and colleagues also found smaller orbitofrontal cortex volumes in 41 elderly patients with MDD than in 40 controls (48). Furthermore, these authors found that smaller volumes were independently associated with cognitive impairment. Kumar and colleagues found that the magnitude of prefrontal volume changes was related to the severity of the depression, as elderly patients with minor depression had lesser changes than those with MDD (49).

The presence of white matter hyperintensities in frontal lobes has also been associated with depression in the elderly. Kumar and colleagues found that decreased frontal lobe volumes and the number of white matter hyperintensities on MRI represent relatively independent pathways to late-life MDD (50). Tupler and colleagues on their part compared the number and volumes of white matter hyperintensities on MRI between 69 patients with late-onset depression, 49 with early onset depression, and 37 controls (51). Patients with late-onset depression had more severe hyperintensity ratings in deep white matter than controls or patients with early onset, while both groups of depressed patients had worse ratings than controls. Of note, left-sided white matter lesions were significantly associated with an older age at the onset of depression.

Functional Changes

Temporal lobes. The use of positron emission tomography (PET) and single-photon emission tomography (SPECT) studies have yielded significant data suggestive of abnormal serotonergic activity in primary MD and in epilepsy, and in particular as it pertains to the serotonin

TABLE 25-2
Structural Changes in Frontal Lobe Structures in Patients with Primary MDs

BRAIN STRUCTURE	SAMPLE	FINDINGS	AUTHORS
Prefrontal cortex	23 MDD	Reduction in the subgenual prefrontal cortex volume	Drevets et al., 1997 (52)
Prefrontal cortex	30 MDD (young women)	Reduction in the left anterior cingulate volume	Botteron et al., 2002 (53)
Prefrontal cortex	15 MDD	Reduction in the gyrus rectus volume	Bremner et al., 2002 (45)
Prefrontal cortex	18 MDD	No significant change in the pregenual area	Brambilla et al., 2002 (54)
Prefrontal cortex	30 MDD	Reduction in the volume	Steffens et al., 2003 (55)
Prefrontal cortex	24 MDD (elderly)	Reduction in the anterior cingulate, the gyrus rectus and the orbitofrontal cortex volume	Ballmaier et al., 2004 (56)
Prefrontal cortex	10 MDD (with psychotic features)	Reduction in the left subgenual prefrontal cortex volume	Coryell et al., 2005 (57)
Prefrontal cortex	31 MDD	Reduction in the anterior cingulate volume	Caetano et al., 2006 (58)
Posterior cingulate	31 MDD	Reduction in the volume	Caetano et al., 2006 (58)
Frontal lobe	48 MDD	Reduction in the volume	Coffey et al., 1993 (18)
Prefrontal cortex	30 BD	Reduction in the midsagittal areas	Coffman et al., 1990 (59)
Prefrontal cortex	17 BD	Reduction in the volume	Sax et al., 1999 (60)
Prefrontal cortex	27 BD	No significant between-group difference in the pregenual cortex	Brambilla et al., 2002 (54)
Prefrontal cortex	17 BD	Reduction in the left and right prefrontal cortex volumes	Lopez-Larson et al., 2002 (61)
Prefrontal cortex	27 BD	Reduction in the left anterior cingulate volume	Sassi et al., 2004 (62)
Prefrontal cortex	32 BD	Increase in the anterior cingulate volume	Adler et al., 2005 (63)
Prefrontal cortex	32 BD	Increase in the volume	Adler et al., 2005 (63)
Prefrontal cortex	36 BD	Reduction in the volume	Nugent et al., 2005 (64)
Prefrontal cortex	16 BD (children)	Reduction in the left anterior cingulate volume	Kaur et al., 2005 (65)
Prefrontal cortex	15 BD	No significant between-group difference in the subgenual cortex	Sanches et al., 2005 (66)
Fusiform gyrus	32 BD	Increase in the volume	Adler et al., 2005 (63)
Posterior cingulate	16 BD (children)	Reduction in the volume	Kaur et al., 2005 (65)
Posterior cingulate	36 BD	Reduction in the volume	Nugent et al., 2005 (64)
White matter	36 BD	Increase in the white matter hyperintensities	Dupont et al, 1995 (67)
White matter	70 BD	Increase in the hyperintense lesions volume in the subependymal region, subcortical gray nuclei, and the deep white matter	McDonald et al., 1999 (68)
White matter	48 MDD	Increase in the periventricular white matter hyperintensities	Coffey et al., 1993 (18)
White matter	48 MDD	Increase in the periventricular white matter hyperintensities	Coffey et al., 1993 (18)
White matter	30 MDD	No significant between-group difference	Dupont et al., 1995 (67)
White matter	35 MDD	Increase in the left frontal and left putaminal deep white matter hyperintesities	Greenwald et al., 1998 (68)
White matter	24 MDD (women)	No significant between-group difference	Lenze et al, 1999 (70)
White matter	41 MDD (elderly)	Increase in the deep white matter hyperintensities	Kramer-Ginsberg et al., 1999 (71)
White matter	115 MDD	Increase in the white matter hyperintensities	Tupler et al., 2002 (51)
White matter	133 MDD (elderly)	Increase in the white matter hyperintensities	Taylor et al., 2003 (48)
White matter	253 MDD (elderly)	Increase in the white matter hyperintensities	Taylor et al., 2003 (48)

*All studies listed are in comparison with healthy controls. MDD: major depressive disorder; BD: bipolar disorder.

(5-hydroxytryptamine, 5HT) receptor most frequently involved in MD and epilepsy: the $5HT_{1A}$ receptor. Deficits in 5HT transmission in human MD are thought to be partially related to a paucity of serotonergic innervation of terminal areas, suggested by a scarcity of 5HT levels in brain tissue, plasma, and platelets (72–76) and with a deficit in serotonin transporter binding sites in postmortem human brain (77–79). Serotonin stores and transporter protein are important components of serotonin terminals, so a combined deficit is a plausible indicator of reduced axonal branching and synapse formation.

With respect to abnormal serotonergic activity in functional neuroimaging studies of patients with primary MDD, Sargent et al. demonstrated reduced $5HT_{1A}$ receptor binding potential values in frontal, temporal, and limbic cortex with PET studies using [^{11}C]WAY-100635 in both unmedicated and medicated depressed patients compared with healthy volunteers (80). Of note, binding potential values in medicated patients were similar to those in unmedicated patients. Drevets et al., using the same radioligand, reported a decreased binding potential of $5HT_{1A}$ receptors in mesial-temporal cortex and in the raphe in 12 patients with familial recurrent major depressive episodes, compared to controls (81). A deficit in the density or affinity of postsynaptic $5HT_{1A}$ receptors was identified in the hippocampus and amygdala of untreated depressed patients who committed suicide (82). In addition, impaired serotonergic transmission has been associated with defects in the dorsal raphe nuclei of suicide victims with MDD, consisting of an excessive density of serotonergic somatodendritic impulse–suppressing $5HT_{1A}$ autoreceptors (83).

Similar abnormalities have been reported in PWE. In a PET study of patients with TLE using the $5HT_{1A}$ receptor antagonist [^{18}F] *trans*-4-fluoro-N-2-[4-(2-methoxyphenyl)piperazin-1-yl]ethyl-N-(2-pyridyl) cyclohexanecarboxamide, reduced $5HT_{1A}$ binding was found in mesial temporal structures ipsilateral to the seizure focus in patients with and without hippocampal atrophy. Reduced serotonergic activity was independent of the presence or absence of hippocampal atrophy on MRI, and reduced volume of distribution and binding remained significant after partial volume correction (84). In addition, a 20% binding reduction was found in the raphe and a 34% lower binding in the thalamic region ipsilateral to the seizure focus. In a separate PET study aimed at quantifying $5HT_{1A}$ receptor binding in 14 patients with TLE, a decreased binding was identified in the epileptogenic hippocampus, amygdala, anterior cingulate, and lateral temporal neocortex ipsilateral to the seizure focus, as well as in the contralateral hippocampi, but to a lesser degree, and in the raphe nuclei (85). Other investigators using the $5HT_{1A}$ tracer 4,2-(methoxyphenyl)-1-[2-(N-2-pyridinyl)-*p*-fluorobenzamido]ethylpiperazine ([^{18}F]MPPF) found that the decrease in binding of $5HT_{1A}$

was significantly greater in the areas of seizure onset and propagation identified with intracranial electrode recordings. As in the other studies, reduction in $5HT_{1A}$ binding was present even when quantitative and qualitative MRI were normal (86).

In a recent study of 46 patients with TLE, Theodore et al. demonstrated an inverse correlation between increased severity of symptoms of depression identified on the Beck Depression Inventory and $5HT_{1A}$ receptor binding at the hippocampus ipsilateral to the seizure focus and, to a lesser degree, at the contralateral hippocampus and midbrain raphe (87).

Reduction in $5HT_{1A}$ receptor binding is not restricted to patients with TLE. PET studies with the $5HT_{1A}$ receptor antagonist carbonyl carbon-11 WAY-100635 ([^{11}C]WAY-100635) found a decreased binding potential in the dorsolateral prefrontal cortex, raphe nuclei, and hippocampus of 11 patients with juvenile myoclonic epilepsy, compared to 11 controls (88).

Frontal lobes. Involvement of frontal lobes in primary MD has also been demonstrated with functional neuroimaging using PET, SPECT, and neuropsychologic studies (89–91). PET studies of major depression have revealed resting-state abnormalities in the prefrontal and cingulate cortices. In one of the leading studies, Liotti et al. investigated common and differential changes in regional blood flow among three groups: euthymic unipolar patients in remission, acutely depressed patients, and never-depressed volunteers (92). Subjects were studied before and after transient sad mood challenge with [^{15}O]H$_2$O PET after provocation of sadness with autobiographical memory scripts. Mood provocation in both depressed groups resulted in regional cerebral blood flow (rCBF) decreases in medial orbitofrontal cortex Brodmann's area 10/11, which were absent in the healthy group. In the remitted group, mood provocation produced a unique rCBF decrease in pregenual anterior cingulate 24a. The main effects in healthy subjects, an rCBF increase in subgenual cingulate Brodmann's area 25 and a decrease in right prefrontal cortex Brodmann's area 9, were not present in the depressed groups.

Executive abnormalities are consistently found among studies of patients with MDD and are more apparent in more severe depressive disorders. These neuropsychologic disturbances correlated with reduced blood flow in mesial prefrontal cortex (93). Furthermore, in tests demanding executive function, cingulate cortex and striatum could not be activated in patients with major depressive disorders (94, 95).

Functional disturbance of frontal lobe structures has been recognized in TLE as well (96) and particularly among patients with TLE and comorbid depression, as they have been found to have bilateral reduction in inferofrontal metabolism (14, 96). Likewise, neuropsychologic testing with the Wisconsin Card Sorting Test, which is highly sensitive to executive dysfunction, has revealed poor performance in patients with TLE and comorbid depression (97–102). Of note, inferior frontal cortex is the main target of the meso-limbic dopaminergic neurons and provides input to the serotonergic neurons of the dorsal raphe nucleus.

Neumeister et al., using the selective $5HT_{1A}$ radioligand [^{18}F]-FCWAY, found reduced $5HT_{1A}$ receptor binding in the anterior and posterior cingulate in patients with panic disorder with and without comorbid depression (103). These findings probably account for the high comorbidity of symptoms of anxiety and panic in primary MD (discussed subsequently) both in patients with and in patients without epilepsy.

Finally, a relationship between abnormal 5HT activity and suicidal behavior associated with several psychiatric diagnoses has been suggested in multiple studies, including quantitative autoradiography studies of brain tissues obtained from suicide victims, in studies of serotonin transporter sites, and in studies of $5HT_{1A}$ receptor binding, to name a few (89). These studies suggest abnormal serotonergic function, primarily at the ventral prefrontal cortex. As discussed below, these abnormalities may account for the higher suicidality encountered in PWE.

Mechanisms of Hippocampal Atrophy

Hippocampal atrophy in primary major depressive disorders has been attributed to two potential pathogenic mechanisms: (1) a high glucocorticoid exposure, and (2) an alteration in neurotrophic factors resulting from the mood disorder (104).

High Glucocorticoid Exposure

This mechanism mediating hippocampal atrophy is based on the excessive activation of the hypothalamic-pituitary-adrenal (HPA) axis, identified in almost half of individuals with depression, resulting in impaired dexamethasone suppression of adrenocorticotropin (ACTH) and cortisol. This effect is partially reversed by antidepressant treatment (105).

The high glucocorticoid exposure can be traced back to the increased activity of neurons in the paraventricular nucleus of the hypothalamus that secrete corticotropin-releasing factor (CRF); this neuropeptide stimulates the synthesis and release of ACTH from the anterior part of the pituitary gland. CRF is a major mediator of stress responses in the central nervous system (CNS) and its levels have been found to be increased in the cerebrospinal fluid in suicide victims and in persons with depression. Hypersecretion of CRF in some depressed patients was also reversed with antidepressant treatment (106, 107). CRF receptors CRF_1 and CRF_2 are abundant in the brain, and they are thought to be involved in response to stress (108, 109). Central administration of the CRF_1 antisense oligodeoxynucleotides has resulted in anxiolytic effects against both high CRF secretion and psychologic stressors. There were also observations (110) that there is a down-regulation in the CRF receptor number in the frontal cortex of depressed patients compared to controls. Further, chronic administration of CRF to normal volunteers resulted in HPA axis alterations indistinguishable from those of patients with major depression (106).

Several brain structures control the activity of the HPA axis, including the hippocampus (with an inhibitory effect on hypothalamic neurons), and the amygdala (with a direct excitatory influence) (104). Glucocorticoids from the circulation exert powerful feedback on the HPA axis and, under physiologic conditions, appear to enhance hippocampal inhibition of the HPA activity and probably hippocampal function in general (111). In experimental studies with rats and monkeys, prolonged increased concentrations of glucocorticoids have been found to damage hippocampal neurons, particularly CA3 pyramidal neurons, possibly by reduction of dendritic branching and loss of dendritic spines that are included in glutamatergic synaptic inputs (112). Hypercortisolemia has also been found to interfere with the development of new granule cell neurons in the adult hippocampal dentate gyrus (113). Deleterious effects of chronic glucocorticoid exposure may lead initially to a transient and reversible atrophy of the CA3 dendritic tree, then to an increased vulnerability to a variety of insults, and finally to cell death under extreme and prolonged conditions (114).

Of note, a proconvulsant effect of CRF has been suggested by several authors in animal models of epilepsy and in human studies. For example, Wang et al. demonstrated that the expression of CRH, CRH-binding protein, and CRH-R1 (a CRH membrane receptor) were significantly elevated in cortical tissue obtained from six children with generalized epilepsy (mean age 8.2 ± 1.5 years) relative to age-matched controls (mean age 7.8 ± 1.4 years) (114). Baram et al. demonstrated that CRF induces limbic seizures in the immature rat that are abolished by selective blocking of the CRF1 receptor. CRF1 messenger RNA levels were maximal in sites of seizure origin and propagation during the age when CRF is most potent as a convulsant (115).

BDNF Theory

Acute and chronic stress decreases levels of brain-derived neurotrophic factor (BDNF) in the dentate gyrus and the pyramidal cell layer of hippocampus, amygdala, and neocortex, which may contribute to structural hippocampal changes (116). These changes are mediated by glucocorticoids and can be overturned with antidepressant therapy, as chronic administration of antidepressant drugs increases BDNF expression and also prevents a stress-induced decrease in BDNF levels (117). There is also evidence that antidepressant drugs can increase hippocampal BDNF levels in humans (118). These data indicate that antidepressant-induced up-regulation of BDNF can hypothetically repair damage to hippocampal neurons and protect vulnerable neurons from additional damage.

Neuropathologic Data

There have been very few neuropathologic studies of the human hippocampal formation in patients with primary major depressive disorder. Lucassen et al. carried out a neuropathologic study of 15 hippocampi of patients with a history of major depressive disorder and compared them to those of 16 matched controls and nine steroid-treated patients (119). In 11 of 15 depressed patients, rare but convincing apoptosis was identified in entorhinal cortex, subiculum, dentate gyrus, CA1, and CA4. Apoptosis was also found in three steroid-treated patients and one control. However, no apoptosis of pyramidal cells in CA3 was identified. In a neuropathologic study of amygdala and entorhinal cortex, Bowley and colleagues carried out a neuronal and glial cell count in brains from seven patients with MDD, 10 with BPD, and 12 control cases (120). The specimens of MDD patients and those of patients with BPD not treated with lithium and valproic acid had a significant reduction of glial cells and of the glial/neuron ratio in left amygdala and to a lesser degree in left entorhinal cortex.

In patients with TLE, the magnitude of hippocampal atrophy is significantly greater than that in major depressive disorder, while the neuropathologic findings are different. In MTS, neuropathologic findings consist of neuronal cell loss and astrocytosis in the hippocampal formation (including areas CA1, CA2, CA3, and CA4, dentate gyrus, and subiculum), amygdala, entorhinal cortex, and parahippocampal gyrus (121).

Neuropathological studies have also documented structural cortical changes in frontal lobes of depressed patients. Rajkowska and colleagues found decreases in cortical thickness, neuronal sizes, and neuronal densities in layers II, III, and IV of the rostral orbitofrontal region in the brains of depressed patients (122). In the caudal orbitofrontal cortex there were significant reductions in glial densities in cortical layers V and VI that were also associated with decreases in neuronal sizes. Finally, in the dorsolateral prefrontal cortex there was a decrease in neuronal and glial density and size in all cortical layers.

Neurotransmitter Abnormalities in Epilepsy and Depression

Neurotransmitter abnormalities are the other major group of pathogenic mechanisms that are shared by epilepsy and MD. The changes in $5HT_{1A}$ receptor binding in patients with TLE and major depressive disorders are a clear example. In fact, there is ample evidence that serotonin, norepinephrine (NE), dopamine (DA), gamma-aminobutyric acid (GABA), and glutamate are operant in the pathogenesis of both disorders.

Animal models of epilepsy with two strains of genetic epilepsy-prone rats (GEPR), GEPR-3 and GEPR-9, provide experimental data on the pathogenic role played by 5HT and NE in seizure predisposition. Indeed, these rats are characterized by predisposition to sound-induced generalized tonic-clonic seizures (123–125) and, particularly in GEPR-9s, a marked acceleration of kindling (126). Both strains of rats have innate serotonergic and noradrenergic pre- and postsynaptic transmission deficits. Noradrenergic deficiencies in GEPRs appear to result from deficient arborization of neurons arising from the locus coeruleus (127, 128), coupled with excessive presynaptic suppression of NE release in the terminal fields and lack of postsynaptic compensatory up-regulation (126, 129). GEPR-9 rats have a more pronounced NE transmission deficit and, in turn, exhibit more severe seizures than GEPR-3 rats do (130). There also is evidence of deficits in serotonergic arborization in the GEPR's brain as well as deficient postsynaptic serotonin$_{1A}$-receptor density in the hippocampus (131). Of note, patients with MDD display endocrine abnormalities similar to those identified in GEPRs, including increased corticosterone serum levels, deficient secretion of growth hormone, and hypothyroidism (132).

Increments of either NE or 5-HT transmission can prevent seizure occurrence, while reduction will have the opposite effect (126, 133). For example, drugs that interfere with the release or synthesis of NE or 5-HT exacerbate seizures in the GEPRs, including the NE storage vesicle inactivators reserpine or tetrabenazine; the NE false transmitter alpha-methyl-*m*-tyrosine; the NE synthesis inhibitor alpha-methyl-*p*-tyrosine; and the 5-HT synthesis inhibitor *p*-chlorophenylalanine. Conversely, drugs that enhance serotonergic transmission, such as the selective serotonin reuptake inhibitor (SSRI) sertraline, resulted in a dose-dependent seizure frequency reduction in the GEPR that correlates with the extracellular thalamic serotonergic concentration (134). The 5-HT precursor 5-hydroxy-L-tryptophan (5-HTP) has anticonvulsant effects in GEPRs when combined with the SSRI, fluoxetine (135). SSRIs and monoamine oxidase inhibitors (MAOIs) can exert anticonvulsant effects in experimental animals, such as mice and baboons, that are genetically prone to epilepsy (133, 136) as well as non-genetically-prone cats (137), rabbits (138), and rhesus monkeys (139). In addition, an antiepileptic effect of 5-HT1A receptors has been correlated to a membrane-hyperpolarizing response, which is associated with increased potassium conductance in hippocampally kindled seizures in cats and in intrahippocampal kainic-acid–induced seizures in freely moving rats (140, 141).

Antiepileptic drugs (AEDs) with established psychotropic effects (carbamazepine, valproic acid, and lamotrigine) can cause an increase in 5HT (142–147). In GEPRs, the anticonvulsant protection of carbamazepine can be blocked with 5HT-depleting drugs (142). In addition, the anticonvulsant effect of the vagal nerve stimulator (VNS) in the rat may be mediated by activation of the locus coeruleus (148). Deletion of noradrenergic and serotonergic neurons in the rat prevents or significantly reduces the anticonvulsant effect of VNS against electroshock or pentylenetetrazol-induced seizures (149). Furthermore, the effect of VNS on the locus coeruleus may be responsible for its antidepressant effects identified in humans.

The role of DA, GABA, and glutamate in primary mood disorders has been recognized in recent studies but is yet poorly understood. Changes in glutamate neurotransmission seem to be involved in the etiology of the major psychiatric disorders including schizophrenia, major depression, and bipolar disorders. Studies employing in vivo magnetic resonance spectroscopy have revealed altered cortical glutamate levels in depressed subjects. Consistent with a model of excessive glutamate-induced excitation in mood disorders, several antiglutamatergic agents, such as riluzole and lamotrigine, have demonstrated potential antidepressant efficacy. Glial cell abnormalities commonly associated with mood disorders may at least partly account for the impairment in glutamate action, because glial cells play a primary role in synaptic glutamate removal (150). Given the significant pathogenic role played by glutamate in epilepsy, it is worth reviewing the available data on primary MD. Indeed, a study by Sanacora et al. recently suggested that antagonists of glutamate neurotransmission may show antidepressant activity (151). Ten patients with treatment-resistant depression had the glutamate antagonist riluzole added to their ongoing medication regimen for 6 weeks, followed by an optional 6-week continuation phase. Depression and anxiety severity were assessed using the Hamilton Depression Rating Scale (HDRS) and the Hamilton Anxiety Rating Scale (HARS). Subjects' HDRS and HARS scores declined significantly following the initiation of riluzole augmentation therapy. This effect was significant at the end of the first week of treatment and persisted for the 12-week duration of the study.

Human Studies

In contrast to animal studies, the impact of pharmacologic augmentation or reduction in 5HT and NE transmission on seizures in humans has been rather sparse and mostly based on uncontrolled data. For example, depletion of monoamines with reserpine has been associated with an increase in frequency and severity of seizures in PWE (152, 153), while the use of reserpine at doses of 2 to 10 mg/day was found to lower the electroshock seizure

threshold and the severity of the resulting seizures in patients with schizophrenia (154–156). The tricyclic antidepressant imipramine, with reuptake inhibitory effects of NE and 5HT, was reported to suppress absence and myoclonic seizures in double-blind placebo-controlled studies (157–159). Open trials with the SSRIs fluoxetine and citalopram yielded an improvement in seizure frequency, but no controlled studies with this class of antidepressants have been performed as of yet (160–162).

Yet the data of the previously cited animal studies appear to be applicable as well to humans. Indeed, Alper et al. reviewed data from Food and Drug Administration Phase II and III clinical trials as Summary Basis of Approval (SBA) reports that noted seizure incidence in trials of several SSRIs and the SNRI venlafaxine and the alpha-2 antagonist mirtazapine (163). They compared seizure incidence among active drug and placebo groups in psychopharmacological clinical trials and the published rates of unprovoked seizures in the general population. The incidence of seizures was significantly lower among patients assigned to antidepressants than in those assigned to placebo (standardized incidence ratio = 0.48; 95% CI, 0.36–0.61). In patients assigned to placebo, seizure incidence was greater than the published incidence of unprovoked seizures in community nonpatient samples.

CLINICAL IMPLICATIONS

The data presented in the foregoing sections can have clinical implications with respect to the clinical manifestations of MD in epilepsy, the safety of antidepressant medications in PWE, and the response of PWE to antiepileptic therapies.

Implications with Respect to the Clinical Manifestations of MD in PWE

The data just reviewed clearly suggest an abnormal secretion pattern of 5HT in PWE, particularly those with TLE, that is more accentuated in the presence of MDD. A consequence of a deficient 5HT secretion can result in (i) the high prevalence of dysphoric disorders in PWE, particularly those with TLE; (ii) the high comorbidity of mood disorders with anxiety symptoms or disorders; (iii) a high suicidal risk of PWE.

Dysphoric Disorders in Epilepsy

The presence of dysphoric disorders in epilepsy has been recognized since the beginning of the twentieth century. Kraepelin (164) and then Bleuler (165) were the first authors to describe a pleomorphic pattern of symptoms that included affective symptoms consisting of prominent irritability intermixed with euphoric mood, fear, and symptoms of anxiety, as well as anergia, pain, and insomnia. Gastaut (166) confirmed Kraepelin and Bleuler's observations, leading Blumer to coin the term "interictal dysphoric disorder" to refer to this type of depression in epilepsy (4). Blumer described the chronic course of the disorder as having recurrent symptom-free periods and as responding well to low doses of antidepressant medication (4). Other investigators have been impressed as well by the pleomorphic presentation of depressive disorders in epilepsy, which were rich in dysphoric symptoms. For example, among 97 consecutive patients with refractory epilepsy and depressive episodes severe enough to merit pharmacotherapy, Kanner et al. found that 28 (29%) met DSM-IV criteria for MDD (167). The remaining 69 patients (71%) failed to meet criteria for any of the DSM-IV categories and presented with a clinical picture consisting of anhedonia (with or without hopelessness), fatigue, anxiety, marked irritability, poor frustration tolerance, and mood lability with bouts of crying. Some patients also reported changes in appetite and sleep patterns and problems with concentration. Most symptoms presented with a waxing and waning course, with repeated, interspersed symptom-free periods of one to several days' duration. The semiology most resembled a dysthymic disorder, but the intermittent recurrence of symptom-free periods precluded DSM criteria for this condition. Kanner and colleagues referred to this form of depression as "dysthymic-like disorder of epilepsy."

In a separate study of 199 consecutive patients with epilepsy, 132 (64%) failed to meet any DSM-IV-TR axis I diagnosis with two structured psychiatric interviews (i.e., the Structural Clinical Interview for DSM-IV Axis I [SCID] and the MINI-International Neuropsychiatric Interview [MINI]); yet, using the self-rating instruments Beck Depression Inventory and the Center of Epidemiologic Studies—Depression, 36 patients (18%) were identified with symptoms of depression of mild to moderate severity (168). Furthermore, of the 36 patients, symptoms of anxiety were identified in 35, irritability in 36, physical symptoms in 24, and increased energy in 18 patients. The patients' ratings of quality of life revealed a significant negative impact on their quality of life compared with asymptomatic patients. The depressive episode identified in these 36 patients reflect a "subsyndromic" type of dysphoric mood disorders, which psychiatrists are also recognizing in nonepilepsy patients as a cause of poor quality of life.

Comorbid Anxiety Symptoms in Depression

As just stated, a frequent comorbidity of mood and anxiety disorders has been identified in patients with and without epilepsy, with rates ranging between 50% and 80% in patients with primary mood disorders. Similar observations have been made in patients with epilepsy and depression. In a study of 174 patients with epilepsy from five epilepsy centers, 73% of patients with a history of depression also met DSM-IV criteria for an anxiety disorder (169). Recognition of comorbid symptoms of anxiety is of the essence, as they may worsen the quality of life of depressed patients and significantly increase their risk of suicide (170). Thus, evaluation of mood disorders must include investigation of comorbid symptoms of anxiety and vice versa.

Increased Suicidality Risk

Depression in patients with epilepsy is associated with a significantly higher suicide rate than in the general population. In a review of 11 studies, Harris and Barraclough (171) found the overall suicide rate in people with epilepsy to be five times higher than in the general population and 25 times greater for patients with complex partial seizures of temporal lobe origin. In a review of the literature, Jones et al. (172) identified a lifetime average suicide rate of 12% in people with epilepsy, compared to 1.1% to 1.2% in the general population. Similarly, Kanner et al. identified a 13% prevalence of habitual postictal suicidal ideation among 100 patients with refractory epilepsy (173).

Implications for the Treatment of Mood Disorders in Patients with Epilepsy

As previously shown, the use of SSRIs and SNRIs in the general population is safe. The higher incidence of seizures among patients with depression randomized to placebo identified in the study by Alper et al. (163) supports the bidirectional relationship between MD and epilepsy. Indeed, it is likely that the higher incidence of seizures among patients randomized to placebo reflects the increased risk that patients with MD have of suffering from epilepsy. These data also support the protective effect of serotonergic and noradrenergic agents demonstrated in the animal models of epilepsy reviewed in this chapter. Furthermore, in a recent critical review of the literature, Jobe concluded not only that the use of SSRIs is safe but that the proconvulsant effects of antidepressants cannot be accounted for by their serotonergic or noradrenergic effects (126). In a study from our center, sertraline was found to *definitely* worsen seizures in only one out of 100 patients (167). In another five patients, a transient increase in seizure frequency was attributed to this antidepressant with a probable, but not definite, causality. Four of these five patients were maintained on sertraline therapy. Following adjustment of the dose of their AED, none of these patients experienced further seizure exacerbation. Blumer has also reported using tricyclic antidepressants alone and in combination with SSRIs in epileptic patients without seizure exacerbation (4). No data have been published on the safety of SNRIs in PWE. We have used the SNRI venlafaxine in more than 100 patients with epilepsy, a significant proportion of whom suffered from intractable epilepsy, without observing any worsening in seizure frequency or severity (Kanner, unpublished data). Finally, monoamine oxidase-A inhibitors (MAOI) are not known to cause seizures in nonepileptic patients (173, 174). Bupropion, maprotiline, and amoxapine are the antidepressant drugs with the strongest proconvulsant properties and should be avoided in epileptic patients (173, 174). Furthermore, the occurrence of seizures in nonepileptic patients has been identified following an overdose or in slow metabolizers who are found to have high serum concentrations of the antidepressant drug (175).

Implications for Seizure Control in Patients with Comorbid Mood Disorder

Can any of the pathogenic mechanisms operant in MD worsen the course of a comorbid seizure disorder? There are data that support this hypothesis. In a study of 890 patients with new onset epilepsy, Mohanraj and Brodie found that individuals with a history of psychiatric disorders were more than three times *less likely* to be seizure-free with antiepileptic drugs (median follow-up period was 79 months) than patients without a history of psychiatric disorders (176). Similarly, among 121 patients who underwent a temporal lobectomy, Anhoury et al. reported a worse postsurgical seizure outcome for patients with a psychiatric history compared with those without a psychiatric history (177).

Given that depression (along with anxiety) is one of the most frequent psychiatric comorbidities in epilepsy, can depression predict a worse postsurgical outcome for patients who undergo a temporal lobectomy? In a study of 100 patients who had a temporal lobectomy and were followed for a mean period of 8.1 ± 3.3 years, Kanner et al. investigated the role of a lifetime history of depression as a predictor of postsurgical seizure outcome (178). Using a multivariate logistic regression model, the investigators evaluated the covariates of a lifetime history of depression, cause of temporal lobe epilepsy (i.e., mesial temporal sclerosis, lesional, or idiopathic), duration of seizure disorder, occurrence of generalized tonic-clonic seizures, and extent of resection of mesial temporal structures. They found that a lifetime history of depression and, to a smaller extent, resection of mesial structures predicted persistent auras in the absence of disabling seizures, whereas the cause of the temporal lobe epilepsy, extent of resection of mesial structures, having GTC seizures, and a lifetime history of depression and other psychiatric disorders predicted a failure to achieve freedom from disabling seizures. The data in these three studies raise the question of whether a history of depression may be a marker of a more severe form of epilepsy.

CONCLUSION

The data reviewed in this chapter provide a different perspective on the relation between depression and epilepsy. They explain the high comorbidity of these disorders and offer an alternative hypothesis on the association between mood disorders and refractory epilepsy. These data clearly demonstrate the safety of using antidepressant drugs in the general population and in PWE.

References

1. Ettinger A. Reed M, Cramer J, Epilepsy Impact Group. Depression comorbidity in community-based patients with epilepsy or asthma. *Neurology* 2004; 63: 1008–1014.
2. Ettinger AB, Reed ML, Goldberg JF, Hirschfeld RM. Prevalence of bipolar symptoms in epilepsy vs other chronic health disorders. *Neurology* 2005; 65:535–540.
3. Kanner AM, Balabanov A. Depression in epilepsy: how closely related are these two disorders? *Neurology* 2002; 58(Suppl 5):S27–39.
4. Hermann B, Whitman S. Psychosocial predictors of interictal depression. *J Epilepsy* 1989; 2:231–237.
5. Blumer D, Altshuler LL. Affective disorders. In: Engel J, Pedley TA, eds. *Epilepsy: a Comprehensive Textbook*, Vol. II. Philadelphia: Lippincott-Raven, 1998:2083–2099.
6. Forsgren L, Nystrom L. An incident case referent study of epileptic seizures in adults. *Epilepsy Res* 1990; 6:66–81.
7. Hesdorffer DC, Hauser WA, Annegers JF, et al. Major depression is a risk factor for seizures in older adults. *Ann Neurol* 2000; 47:246–249.
8. Hesdorffer DC, Hauser WA, Olafsson E, Ludvigsson P, et al. Depression and suicidal attempt as risk factor for incidental unprovoked seizures. *Ann Neurol* 2006; 59(1): 35–41.
9. Lewis A. Melancholia: a historical review. *J Mental Sci* 1934; 80:1–42.
10. Sheline YI. Neuroimaging studies of mood disorder effects on the brain. *Biol Psychiatry* 2003; 54(3):338–352.
11. Septien L, Giroud M, Didi-Roy R. Depression and partial epilepsy: relevance of laterality of the epileptic focus. *Neurol Res* 1993; 15:136–138.
12. Altshuler LL, Devinsky O, Post RM, Theodore W. Depression, anxiety, and temporal lobe epilepsy. *Arch Neurol* 1990; 47:284–288.
13. Stevens J. Interictal clinical manifestation of complex partial seizures. In: Penry J, Daly D, eds. *Complex Partial Seizures and Their Treatment*. Advances in Neurology 11. New York: Raven Press, 1975:85–88.
14. Bromfield EB, Altshuler L, Leiderman DB, Balish M, Ketter TA, Devinsky O, Post RM, Theodore WH. Cerebral metabolism and depression in patients with complex partial seizures. *Arch Neurol.* 1992 June; 49(6):617–23. Erratum in: *Arch Neurol* 1992 Sep; 49(9):976.
15. Hermann BP, Seidenberg M, Bell B. Psychiatric comorbidity in chronic epilepsy: identification, consequences, and treatment of major depression. *Epilepsia* 2000; 41(Suppl 2):S31–41.
16. Sheline YI, Wang PW, Gado MH, et al. Hippocampal atrophy in recurrent major depression. *Proc Natl Acad Sci U S A* 1996.93(9):3908–3913.
17. Hecimovic H, Santos J, Gilliam F, Kanner AM. Neuroanatomical and neurobiological bases of psychiatric disorders. In: Ettinger AB, Kanner AM, eds. *Psychiatric Issues in Epilepsy: A Practical Guide to Diagnosis and Treatment*, 2nd ed. Philadelphia: Lippincott Williams and Wilkins, 2007:93–118.
18. Coffey CE, Wilkinson WE, Weiner RD, Parashos IA, et al. Quantitative cerebral anatomy in depression: a controlled magnetic resonance imaging study. *Arch Gen Psychiatry* 1993; 50(1):7–16.
19. Ashtari M, Greenwald BS, Kramer-Ginsberg E, Hu J, et al. Hippocampal/amygdala volumes in geriatric depression. *Psychol Med* 1999; 29(3):629–638.
20. Krishnan KR, Doraiswamy PM, Figiel GS, Husain MM, et al. Hippocampal abnormalities in depression. *J Neuropsychiatry Clin Neurosci* 1991; 3(4):387–391.
21. Axelson DA, Doraiswamy PM, McDonald WM, Boyko OB, et al. Hypercortisolemia and hippocampal changes in depression. *Psychiatry Res* 1993; 47(2):163–173.
22. Pantel J, Schroder J, Essig M, Popp D, et al. Quantitative magnetic resonance imaging in geriatric depression and primary degenerative dementia. *J Affect Disord* 1997; 42(1): 69–83.
23. Shah PJ, Ebmeier KP, Glabus MF, Goodwin GM. Cortical grey matter reductions associated with treatment-resistant chronic unipolar depression: controlled magnetic resonance imaging study. *Br J Psychiatry* 1998; 172:527–532.

24. Mervaala E, Fohr J, Kononen M, Valkonen-Korhonen M, et al. Quantitative MRI of the hippocampus and amygdala in severe depression. *Psychol Med* 2000; 30(1):117–125.
25. Vakili K, Pillay SS, Lafer B, Fava M, et al. Hippocampal volume in primary unipolar major depression: a magnetic resonance imaging study. *Biol Psychiatry* 2000; 47(12): 1087–1090.
26. von Gunten A, Fox NC, Cipolotti L, Ron MA. A volumetric study of hippocampus and amygdala in depressed patients with subjective memory problems. *J Neuropsychiatry Clin Neurosci* 2000; 12(4):493–498.
27. Steffens DC, Byrum CE, McQuoid DR, Greenberg DL, et al. Hippocampal volume in geriatric depression. *Biol Psychiatry* 2000; 48(4):301–309.
28. Rusch BD, Abercrombie HC, Oakes TR, Schaefer SM, et al. Hippocampal morphometry in depressed patients and control subjects: relations to anxiety symptoms. *Biol Psychiatry* 2001; 50(12):960–964.
29. Bell-McGinty S, Butters MA, Meltzer CC, Greer PJ, et al. Brain morphometric abnormalities in geriatric depression: long-term neurobiological effects of illness duration. *Am J Psychiatry* 2002; 159(8):1424–1427.
30. Frodl T, Meisenzahl EM, Zetzsche T, Born C, et al. Hippocampal changes in patients with a first episode of major depression. *Am J Psychiatry* 2002; 159(7):1112–1118.
31. Sheline YI, Gado MH, Kraemer HC. Untreated depression and hippocampal volume loss. *Am J Psychiatry* 2003; 160(8):1516–1518.
32. MacQueen GM, Campbell S, McEwen BS, Macdonald K, et al. Course of illness, hippocampal function, and hippocampal volume in major depression. *Proc Natl Acad Sci U S A* 2003; 100(3):1387–1392.
33. Caetano SC, Hatch JP, Brambilla P, Sassi RB, et al. Anatomical MRI study of hippocampus and amygdala in patients with current and remitted major depression. *Psychiatry Res* 2004; 132(2):141–147.
34. Vythilingam M, Vermetten E, Anderson GM, Luckenbaugh D, et al. Hippocampal volume, memory, and cortisol status in major depressive disorder: effects of treatment. *Biol Psychiatry* 2004; 56(2):101–112.
35. Frodl T, Meisenzahl EM, Zetzsche T, Hohne T, et al. Hippocampal and amygdala changes in patients with major depressive disorder and healthy controls during a 1-year follow-up. *J Clin Psychiatry* 2004; 65(4):492–499.
36. Frodl T, Meisenzahl EM, Zill P, Baghai T, et al. Reduced hippocampal volumes associated with the long variant of the serotonin transporter polymorphism in major depression. *Arch Gen Psychiatry* 2004; 61(2):177–183.
37. Neumeister A, Wood S, Bonne O, Nugent AC, et al. Reduced hippocampal volume in unmedicated, remitted patients with major depression versus control subjects. *Biol Psychiatry* 2005; 57(8):935–937.
38. Pearlson GD, Barta PE, Powers RE, Menon RR, et al. Ziskind-Somerfeld Research Award 1996. Medial and superior temporal gyral volumes and cerebral asymmetry in schizophrenia versus bipolar disorder. *Biol Psychiatry* 1997; 41(1):1–14.
39. Sheline YI, Gado MH, Price JL. Amygdala core nuclei volumes are decreased in recurrent major depression. *Neuroreport* 1998; 9(9):2023–2028.
40. Frodl T, Meisenzahl E, Zetzsche T, Bottlender R, et al. Enlargement of the amygdala in patients with a first episode of major depression. *Biol Psychiatry* 2002; 51(9): 708–714.
41. Hauser P, Altshuler LL, Berrettini W, Dauphinais ID, et al. Temporal lobe measurement in primary affective disorder by magnetic resonance imaging. *J Neuropsychiatry Clin Neurosci* 1989; 1(2):128–134.
42. Greenwald BS, Kramer-Ginsberg E, Bogerts B, Ashtari M, et al. Qualitative magnetic resonance imaging findings in geriatric depression: possible link between later-onset depression and Alzheimer's disease? *Psychol Med* 1997; 27(2):421–431.
43. Posener JA, Wang L, Price JL, Gado HM, et al. High-dimensional mapping of the hippocampus in depression. *Am J Psychiatry* 2003; 160:83–89.
44. Gilliam FG, Maton BM, Martin RC, Sawrie SM, et al. Hippocampal 1H-MRSI correlates with severity of depression symptoms in temporal lobe epilepsy. *Neurology* 2007; 68(5):364–368.
45. Bremner JD, Vithilingham M, Vermetten E, Nazeer A, et al. Reduced volume of orbitofrontal cortex in major depression. *Biol Psychiatry* 2002; 51:273–279.
46. Coffey CE, Wilkinson WE, Weiner RD, et al. Quantitative cerebral anatomy in depression: a controlled magnetic resonance imaging study. *Arch Gen Psychiatry* 1993; 50:7–16.
47. Lai T, Payne ME, Byrum CE, Steffens DC, et al. Reduction of orbital frontal cortex volume in geriatric depression. *Biol Psychiatry* 2000; 48(10): 971–975.
48. Taylor WD, Steffens DC, McQuoid DR, Payne ME, et al. Smaller orbital frontal cortex volumes associated with functional disability in depressed elders. *Biol Psychiatry* 2003; 53(2):144–149.
49. Kumar A, Zhisong J, Warren B, Jayaram U, et al. Late-onset minor and major depression: early evidence for common neuroanatomical substrates detected by using MRI. *Proc Natl Acad Sci U S A* 1998; 95(13):7654–7658.
50. Kumar A, Bilker W, Jin Z, Udupa J. Atrophy and high intensity lesions: complementary neurobiological mechanisms in late-life major depression. *Neuropsychopharmacology* 2000; 22(3):264–274.
51. Tupler LA, Krishnan KR, McDonald WM, Dombeck CB, et al. Anatomic location and laterality of MRI signal hyperintensities in late-life depression. *J Psychosom Res* 2002; 53(2):665–676.
52. Drevets WC, Price JL, Simpson JR, Jr., Todd RD, et al. Subgenual prefrontal cortex abnormalities in mood disorders. *Nature* 1997; 386(6627):824–827.
53. Botteron KN, Raichle ME, Drevets WC, Heath AC, et al. Volumetric reduction in left subgenual prefrontal cortex in early onset depression. *Biol Psychiatry* 2002; 51(4): 342–344.
54. Brambilla P, Nicoletti MA, Harenski K, Sassi RB, et al. Anatomical MRI study of subgenual prefrontal cortex in bipolar and unipolar subjects. *Neuropsychopharmacology* 2002; 27(5):792–799.
55. Steffens DC, McQuoid DR, Welsh-Bohmer KA, Krishnan KR. Left orbital frontal cortex volume and performance on the Benton visual retention test in older depressives and controls. *Neuropsychopharmacology* 2003; 28(12):2179–2183.
56. Ballmaier M, Toga AW, Blanton RE, Sowell ER, et al. Anterior cingulate, gyrus rectus, and orbitofrontal abnormalities in elderly depressed patients: an MRI-based parcellation of the prefrontal cortex. *Am J Psychiatry* 2004; 161(1):99–108.
57. Coryell W, Nopoulos P, Drevets W, Wilson T, et al. Subgenual prefrontal cortex volumes in major depressive disorder and schizophrenia: diagnostic specificity and prognostic implications. *Am J Psychiatry* 2005; 162(9):1706–1712.
58. Caetano SC, Kaur S, Brambilla P, Nicoletti M, et al. Smaller cingulate volumes in unipolar depressed patients. *Biol Psychiatry* 2006; 59:702–706.
59. Coffman JA, Bornstein RA, Olson SC, Schwarzkopf SB, et al. Cognitive impairment and cerebral structure by MRI in bipolar disorder. *Biol Psychiatry* 1990; 27(11):1188–1196.
60. Sax KW, Strakowski SM, Zimmerman ME, DelBello MP, et al. Frontosubcortical neuroanatomy and the continuous performance test in mania. *Am J Psychiatry* 1999; 156(1):139–141.
61. Lopez-Larson MP, DelBello MP, Zimmerman ME, Schwiers ML, et al. Regional prefrontal gray and white matter abnormalities in bipolar disorder. *Biol Psychiatry* 2002; 52(2):93–100.
62. Sassi RB, Brambilla P, Hatch JP, Nicoletti MA, et al. Reduced left anterior cingulate volumes in untreated bipolar patients. *Biol Psychiatry* 2004; 56(7):467–475.
63. Adler CM, Levine AD, DelBello MP, Strakowski SM. Changes in gray matter volume in patients with bipolar disorder. *Biol Psychiatry* 2005; 58(2):151–157.
64. Nugent AC, Milham MP, Bain EE, Mah L, et al. Cortical abnormalities in bipolar disorder investigated with MRI and voxel-based morphometry. *Neuroimage* 2006; 30:485–497.
65. Kaur S, Sassi RB, Axelson D, Nicoletti M, et al. Cingulate cortex anatomical abnormalities in children and adolescents with bipolar disorder. *Am J Psychiatry* 2005; 162(9): 1637–1643.
66. Sanches M, Sassi RB, Axelson D, Nicoletti M, et al. Subgenual prefrontal cortex of child and adolescent bipolar patients: a morphometric magnetic resonance imaging study. *Psychiatry Res* 2005; 138(1):43–49.
67. Dupont RM, Jernigan TL, Heindel W, Butters N, et al. Magnetic resonance imaging and mood disorders. Localization of white matter and other subcortical abnormalities. *Arch Gen Psychiatry* 1995; 52(9):747–755.
68. McDonald WM, Tupler LA, Marsteller FA, Figiel GS, et al. Hyperintense lesions on magnetic resonance images in bipolar disorder. *Biol Psychiatry* 1999; 45(8):965–971.
69. Greenwald BS, Kramer-Ginsberg E, Krishnan KR, Ashtari M, et al. Neuroanatomic localization of magnetic resonance imaging signal hyperintensities in geriatric depression. *Stroke* 1998; 29(3):613–617.
70. Lenze E, Cross D, McKeel D, Neuman RJ, et al. White matter hyperintensities and gray matter lesions in physically healthy depressed subjects. *Am J Psychiatry* 1999; 156(10):1602–1607.
71. Kramer-Ginsberg E, Greenwald BS, Krishnan KR, Christiansen B, et al. Neuropsychological functioning and MRI signal hyperintensities in geriatric depression. *Am J Psychiatry* 1999; 156(3):438–444.
72. Brown GL, Ebert MH, Goyer PF, et al. Aggression, suicide, and serotonin: relationships to CSF amine metabolites. *Am J Psychiatry* 1982; 139:741–746.
73. Brown GL, Linnoila MI. CSF serotonin metabolite (5-HIAA) studies in depression, impulsivity, and violence. *J Clin Psychiatry* 1990; 51 Suppl:31–41.
74. Roy A, De Jong J, Linnoila M. Cerebrospinal fluid monoamine metabolites and suicidal behavior in depressed patients: a 5-year follow-up study. *Arch Gen Psychiatry* 1989; 46:609–612.
75. Langer SZ, Galzin AM. Studies on the serotonin transporter in platelets. *Experientia* 1988; 44:127–130.
76. Nemeroff CB, Knight DL, Krishnan RR, et al. Marked reduction in the number of platelet–tritiated imipramine binding sites in geriatric depression. *Arch Gen Psychiatry* 1988; 45:919–923.
77. Malison RT, Price LH, Berman R, et al. Reduced brain serotonin transporter availability in major depression as measured by [123I]-2 beta-carbomethoxy-3 beta-(4-iodophenyl)tropane and single photon emission computed tomography. *Biol Psychiatry* 1998; 44:1090–1098.
78. Ogilvie AD, Harmar AJ. Association between the serotonin transporter gene and affective disorder: the evidence so far. *Mol Med* 1997; 3:90–93.
79. Ogilvie AD, Battersby S, Bubb VJ, et al. Polymorphism in serotonin transporter gene associated with susceptibility to major depression. *Lancet* 1996; 347:731–733.
80. Sargent PA, Kjaer KH, Bench CJ, Rabiner EA, et al. Brain serotonin$_{1A}$ receptor binding measured by positron emission tomography with [11C]WAY-100635: effects of depression and antidepressant treatment. *Arch Gen Psychiatry* 2000; 57:174–180.
81. Drevets WC, Frank E, Price JC, Kupfer DJ, et al. PET imaging of serotonin 1A receptor binding in depression. *Biol Psychiatry* 1999; 46:1375–1387.
82. Oguendo MA, Placidi GP, Malone KM, et al. Positron emission tomography of regional brain metabolic responses to a serotonergic challenge and lethality of suicide attempts in major depression. *Arch Gen Psychiatry* 2003; 60:14–22.
83. Leake A, Fairbairn AF, McKeith IG, Ferrier IN. Studies on the serotonin uptake binding site in major depressive disorder and control post-mortem brain: neurochemical and clinical correlates. *Psychiatry Res* 1991; 39:155–165.
84. Toczek MT, Carson RE, Lang L, Ma Y, et al. PET imaging of 5-HT$_{1A}$ receptor binding in patients with temporal lobe epilepsy. *Neurology* 2003; 60:749–756.
85. Savic I, Lindstrom P, Gulyas B, Halldin C, et al. Limbic reductions of 5-HT$_{1A}$ receptor binding in human temporal lobe epilepsy. *Neurology* 2004; 62:1343–1351.

86. Merlet I, Ostrowsky K, Costes N, Ryvlin P, et al. 5-HT$_{1A}$ receptor binding and intracerebral activity in temporal lobe epilepsy: an [^{18}F]MPPF-PET study. *Brain* 2004; 127:900–913.

87. Theodore WH, Hasler G, Giovacchini G, Kelley K, Reeves-Tyer P, Herscovitch P, Drevets W. Reduced Hyppocampal 5HT1A PET Receptor Binding and Depression in Temporal Lobe Epilepsy. *Epilepsia*, 2007, in press.

88. Meschaks A, Lindstrom P, Halldin C, Farde L, et al. Regional reductions in serotonin 1A receptor binding in juvenile myoclonic epilepsy. *Arch Neurol* 2005; 62:946–960.

89. Baxter LR, Schwartz JM, Phelps ME, Mazziotta JC, et al. Reduction of the prefrontal cortex glucose metabolism common to three types of depression. *Arch Gen Psychiatry* 1989; 46:243–250.

90. Starkstein SE, Robinson RG. Depression and frontal lobe disorders. In: Miller BL, Cummings JL, eds. *The Human Frontal Lobes, Functions and Disorders*. New York: The Gilford Press, 1998:3–26:537–546.

91. Bench CJ, Friston KJ. Regional cerebral blood flow in depression measured by positron emission tomography: the relationship with clinical dimensions. *Psychol Med* 1993; 23:579–590.

92. Liotti M, Mayberg H, McGinnis S, Brennan SL, et al. Unmasking disease specific cerebral blood flow abnormalities: mood challenge in patients with remitted unipolar depression. *Am J Psychiatry* 2002; 159:1830–1840.

93. Bench CJ, Friston KJ. Regional cerebral blood flow in depression measured by positron emission tomography: the relationship with clinical dimensions. *Psychol Med* 1993; 23:579–590.

94. Dolan RJ, Bench CJ. Neuropsychological dysfunction in depression: the relationship to cerebral blood flow. *Psychol Med* 1994; 24:849–857.

95. Elliott R, Baker SC. Prefrontal dysfunction in depressed patients performing a complex planning task: a study using positron emission tomography. *Psychol Med* 1997; 27:931–942.

96. Jokeit H, Seitz RJ, Markowitsch HJ, Neumann N, et al. Prefrontal asymmetric interictal glucose hypometabolism and cognitive impairment in patients with temporal lobe epilepsy. *Brain* 1997; 120:2283–2294.

97. Hempel A, Risse GL, Mercer K, Gates J. Neuropsychological evidence of frontal lobe dysfunction in patients with temporal lobe epilepsy. *Epilepsia* 1996; 37|suppl5|:119.

98. Hermann BP, Wyler AR, Richey ET. Wisconsin card sorting test performance in patients with complex partial seizures of temporal-lobe origin. *J Clin Exp Neuropsychol* 1988; 10:467–476.

99. Horner MD, Flashman LA, Freides D, Epstein CM, et al. Temporal lobe epilepsy and performance on the Wisconsin Card Sorting Test. *J Clin Exp Neuropsychol* 1996; 18:310–313.

100. Hermann B, Seidenberg M. Executive system dysfunction in temporal lobe epilepsy: effects of nociferous cortex versus hippocampal pathology. *J Clin Exp Neuropsychol* 1995; 17:809–819.

101. Hermann BP, Seidenberg M, Schoenfeld J, Davies K. Neuropsychological characteristics of the syndrome of mesial temporal lobe epilepsy. *Arch Neurol* 1997; 54:369–376.

102. Corcoran R, Upton D. A role for the hippocampus in card sorting? *Cortex* 1993; 29:293–304.

103. Neumeister A, Bain E, Nugent AC, Carson RE, et al. Reduced serotonin type 1A receptor binding in panic disorder. *J Neurosci* 2004; 24:589–591.

104. Nestler EJ, Barrot M, DiLeone RJ, Eisch AJ, et al. Neurobiology of depression. *Neuron* 2002; 34(1):13–25.

105. Holsboer F. Stress, hypercortisolism and corticosteroid receptors in depression: implications for therapy. *J Affect Disord* 2001; 62(1-2):77–91.

106. Holsboer F. Corticotropin-releasing hormone modulators and depression. *Curr Opin Investig Drugs* 2003; 4:46–50.

107. Reul JM, Holsboer F. Corticotropin-releasing factor receptors 1 and 2 in anxiety and depression. *Curr Opin Pharmacol* 2002; 2(1):23–33.

108. Brunson KL, Eghbal-Ahmadi M, Bender R, Chen Y, et al. Long-term, progressive hippocampal cell loss and dysfunction induced by early-life administration of corticotropin-releasing hormone reproduce the effects of early-life stress. *Proc Natl Acad Sci U S A* 2001; 98(15):8856–8861.

109. Brunson KL, Khan N, Eghbal-Ahmadi M, Baram TZ. Corticotropin (ACTH) acts directly on amygdala neurons to down-regulate corticotropin-releasing hormone gene expression. *Ann Neurol* 2001; 49(3):304–312.

110. Nemeroff CB, Owens MJ. Treatment of mood disorders. *Nat Neurosci* 2002; 5 Suppl:1068–1070.

111. Nestler EJ, Gould E, Manji H, Buncan M, et al. Preclinical models: status of basic research in depression. *Biol Psychiatry* 2002; 52(6):503–528.

112. Sapolsky RM. Glucocorticoids and hippocampal atrophy in neuropsychiatric disorders. *Arch Gen Psychiatry* 2000; 57:925–935.

113. Fuchs E, Gould E. Mini-review: in vivo neurogenesis in the adult brain: regulation and functional implications. *Eur J Neurosci* 2000; 12:2211–2214.

114. Wang W, Dow KE, Fraser DD. Elevated corticotropin releasing hormone/corticotropin releasing hormone-R1 expression in postmortem brain obtained from children with generalized epilepsy. *Ann Neurol* 2001; 50:404–409.

115. Baram TZ, Chalmers DT, Chen C, Koutsoukos Y, et al. The CRF1 receptor mediates the excitatory actions of corticotropin releasing factor (CRF) in the developing rat brain: in vivo evidence using a novel, selective, non-peptide CRF receptor antagonist. *Brain Res* 1997; 770(1-2):89–95.

116. Smith MA, Makino S, Kvetnansky R, Post RM. Effects of stress on neurotrophic factor expression in the rat brain. *Ann N Y Acad Sci* 1995; 771:234–239.

117. Nibuya M, Morinobu S, Duman RS. Regulation of BDNF and trkB mRNA in rat brain by chronic electroconvulsive seizure and antidepressant drug treatments. *J Neurosci* 1995; 15:7539–7547.

118. Chen B, Dowlatshahi D, MacQueen GM, Wang JF, et al. Increased hippocampal BDNF immunoreactivity in subjects treated with antidepressant medication. *Biol Psychiatry* 2001; 50:260–265.

119. Lucassen PJ, Muller MB, Holsboer F, Bauer J, et al. Hippocampal apoptosis in major depression is a minor event and absent from subareas at risk for glucocorticoid overexposure. *Am J Pathol* 2001; 158:453–468.

120. Bowley MP, Drevets WC, Ongur D, Price JL. Low glial numbers in the amygdala in major depressive disorder. *Biol Psychiatry* 2002; 52(5):404–412.

121. Mathern GW, Babb TL, Armstrong DL. Hippocampal sclerosis. In: Engel J, Pedley TA, eds. *Epilepsy: A Comprehensive Textbook*. Philadelphia and New York: Lippincott-Raven, 1997:133–155.

122. Rajkowska G, Miguel-Hidalgo JJ, Wei J, Dilley G, et al. Morphometric evidence for neuronal and glial prefrontal cell pathology in major depression. *Biol Psychiatry* 1999; 45(9):1085–1098.

123. Jobe PC, Dailey JW. Genetically epilepsy-prone rats (GEPRs) in drug research. *CNS Drug Rev* 2000; 6:241–260.

124. Coffey LL, Reith MEA, Chen NH, Jobe PC, et al. Amygdala kindling of forebrain seizures and the occurrence of brainstem seizures in genetically epilepsy-prone rats. *Epilepsia* 1996; 37:188–197.

125. Jobe PC, Mishra PK, Dailey JW, Ko KH, et al. Genetic predisposition to partial (focal) seizures and to generalized tonic/clonic seizures: Interactions between seizure circuitry of the forebrain and brainstem. In: Berkovic SF, Genton P, Hirsch E, Picard F, eds. *Genetics of Focal Epilepsies*. Avignon, France: John Libbey & Company, Ltd., 1999:251.

126. Jobe PC, Dailey JW, Wernicke JF. A noradrenergic and serotonergic hypothesis of the linkage between epilepsy and affective disorders. *Crit Rev Neurobiol* 1999; 13:317–356.

127. Clough RW, Peterson BR, Steenbergen JL, et al. Neurite extension of developing noradrenergic neurons is impaired in genetically epilepsy-prone rats (GEPR-3s): an in vitro study on locus coeruleus. *Epilepsy Res* 1998; 29:135–146.

128. Ryu JR, Jobe PC, Milbrandt JC, et al. Morphological deficits in noradrenergic neurons in GEPR-9s stem from abnormalities in both the locus coeruleus and its target tissues. *Exp Neurol* 1999; 156:84–91.

129. Yan QS, Jobe PC, Dailey JW. Thalamic deficiency in norepinephrine release detected via intracerebral microdialysis: a synaptic determinant of seizure predisposition in the genetically epilepsy-prone rat. *Epilepsy Res* 1993; 14:229–236.

130. Jobe PC, Mishra PK, Adams-Curtis LE, et al. The genetically epilepsy-prone rat (GEPR). *Ital J Neurol Sci* 1995; 16:91–99.

131. Dailey JW, Mishra PK, Ko KH, Penny JE, et al. Serotonergic abnormalities in the central nervous system of seizure-naive genetically epilepsy-prone rats. *Life Sci* 1992; 50:319–326.

132. Jobe PC and Weber RJ. Co-morbidity of neurologic and affective disorders: the model of the epilepsy-prone rat. In Gilliam F, Kanner AM, Sheline Y, eds. *Depression and Brain Dysfunction*, Taylor & Francis, London, 2006, pp. 121–157.

133. Meldrum BS, Anlezark GM, Adam HK, and Greenwood DT. Anticonvulsant and proconvulsant properties of viloxazine hydrochloride: pharmacological and pharmacokinetic studies in rodents and epileptic baboon. *Psychopharmacology (Berl)* 1982; 76:212–217.

134. Yan QS, Jobe PC, Dailey JW. Further evidence of anticonvulsant role for 5-hydroxytryptamine in genetically epilepsy prone rats. *Br J Pharmacol* 1995; 115:1314–1318.

135. Yan QS, Jobe PC, Dailey JW. Evidence that a serotonergic mechanism is involved in the anticonvulsant effect of fluoxetine in genetically epilepsy-prone rats. *Eur J Pharmacol* 1993; 252(1):105–112.

136. Lehmann A. Audiogenic seizures data in mice supporting new theories of biogenic amines mechanisms in the central nervous system. *Life Sci* 1967; 6:1423–1431.

137. Polc P, Schneeberger J, and Haefely, W. Effects of several centrally active drugs on the sleep wakefulness cycle of cats. *Neuropharmacology* 1979; 18:259–267.

138. Piette Y, Delaunois AL, De Shaepdryver AF, and Heymans C. Imipramine and electroshock threshold. *Arch Int Pharmacodyn Ther* 1963; 144:293–297.

139. Yanagita T, Wakasa Y, and Kiyohara H. Drug-dependence potential of viloxazine hydrochloride tested in rhesus monkeys. *Pharmacol Biochem Behav* 1980; 12:155–161.

140. Beck SG, Choi KC. 5-Hydroxytryptamine hyperpolarizes CA3 hippocampal pyramidal cells through an increase in potassium conductance. *Neurosci Lett* 1991; 133:93–96.

141. Okuhara DY, Beck SG. 5-HT$_{1A}$ receptor linked to inward-rectifying potassium current in in hippocampal CA3 pyramidal cells. *J Neurophysiol* 1994; 71:2161–2167.

142. Yan QS, Mishra PK, Burger RL, Bettendorf AF, et al. Evidence that carbamazepine and antiepilepsirine may produce a component of their anticonvulsant effects by activating serotonergic neurons in genetically epilepsy-prone rats. *J Pharmacol Exp Ther* 1992; 261:652–659.

143. Dailey JW, Reith MEA, Yan QS, Li MY, et al. Anticonvulsant doses of carbamazepine increase hippocampal extracellular serotonin in genetically epilepsy-prone rats: dose response relationships. *Neurosci Lett* 1997; 227(1):13–16.

144. Dailey JW, Reith ME, Steidley KR, Milbrandt JC, et al. Carbamazepine-induced release of serotonin from rat hippocampus in vitro. *Epilepsia* 1998; 39(10):1054–1063.

145. Dailey JW, Reith ME, Yan QS, Li MY, et al. Carbamazepine increases extracellular serotonin concentration: lack of antagonism by tetrodotoxin or zero Ca^{2+}. *Eur J Pharmacol* 1997; 328(2–3):153–162.

146. Southam E, Kirkby D, Higgins GA, Hagan RM. Lamotrigine inhibits monoamine uptake in vitro and modulates 5-hydroxytryptamine uptake in rats. *Eur J Pharmacol* 1998; 358(1):19–24.

147. Whitton PS, Fowler LJ. The effect of valproic acid on 5-hydroxytryptamine and 5-hydroxyindoleacetic acid concentration in hippocampal dialysates in vivo. *Eur J Pharmacol* 1991; 200:167–169.

148. Naritokku DK, Terry WJ, and Helfert RH. Regional induction of *fos* immunoreactivity in the brain by anticonvulsant stimulation of the vagus nerve. *Epilepsy Res* 1995; 22:53–62.

149. Browning RA, Clark KB, Naritoku, DK, Smith DC, et al. Loss of anticonvulsant effect of vagus nerve stimulation in the pentylenetetrazol seizure model following treatment with 6-hydroxydopamine or 5,7-dihydroxytryptamine. *Soc Neurosci* 1997; 23:2424 (Abstract).

150. Kugaya A, Sanacora G. Beyond monoamines: glutamatergic function in mood disorders. *CNS Spectr* 2005; 10(10):808–819.

151. Sanacora G, Kendell SF, Levin Y, Simen AA, et al. Preliminary evidence of riluzole efficacy in antidepressant-treated patients with residual depressive symptoms. *Biol Psychiatry* 2007; 61:822–825.

152. Lewis JJ. Rauwolfia derivates. In: Root WS, Hofmann FG, eds. *Physiological Pharmacology*. New York: Academic Press, 1974:79.

153. Maynert EW, Marczynski TJ, Browning RA. The role of the neurotransmitters in the epilepsies. In: Friedlander WJ, ed. *Advances in Neurology*. New York: Raven Press, 1975:79.

154. Naidoo D. The effects of reserpine (serpasil) on the chronic disturbed schizophrenic: a comparative study of rauwolfia alkaloids and electroconvulsive therapy. *J Nerv Ment Dis* 1956; 123:1–13.

155. Noce RH, Williams DB, Rapaport W. Reserpine (serpasil) in management of the mentally ill. *JAMA* 1955; 158:11–15.

156. Tasher DC, Chermak MW. The use of reserpine in shock-reversible patients and shock-resistent patients. *Ann N Y Acad Sci* 1955; 61:108–116.

157. Fromm GH, Rosen JA, Amores CY. Clinical and experimental investigation of the effect of imipramine on epilepsy. *Epilepsia* 1971; 12:282.

158. Fromm GH, Wessel HB, Glass JD, Alvin JD, et al. Imipramine in absence and myoclonic-astatic seizures. *Neurology* 1978; 28:953–957.

159. Fromm GH, Amores CY, Thies W. Imipramine in epilepsy. *Arch Neurol* 1972; 27:198–204.

160. Favale E, Rubino V, Mainardi P, Lunardi G, et al. The anticonvulsant effect of fluoxetine in humans. *Neurology* 1995; 45:1926–1927.

161. Specchio LM, Iudice A, Specchio N, et al. Citalopram as treatment of depression in patients with epilepsy. *Clin Neuropharmacol* 2004; 27:133–136.

162. Hovorka J, Herman E, Nemcova I. Treatment of interictal depression with citalopram in patients with epilepsy. *Epilepsy Behav* 2000; 1:444–447.

163. Alper K, Schwartz KA, Kolts RL, Khan A. Seizure incidence in psychopharmacological clinical trials: an analysis of Food and Drug Administration (FDA) Summary Basis of Approval reports. *Biol Psychiatry* 2007; [Epub ahead of print]

164. Kraepelin E. *Psychiatrie*, Vol 3. Leipzig: Johann Ambrosius Barth, 1923.

165. Bleuler E. *Lehrbuch der Psychiatrie*. 8th ed. Berlin: Springer, 1949.

166. Gastaut H, Roger J, Lesèvre N. Différenciation psychologique des épileptiques en fonction des formes électrocliniques de leur maladie. *Rev Psychol Appl* 1953; 3:237–49.

167. Kanner AM, Kozak AM, Frey M. The use of sertraline in patients with epilepsy: is it safe? *Epilepsy Behav* 2000; 1(2):100–105.

168. Kanner AM, Wuu J, Barry J, Hermann B, et al. Atypical depressive episodes in epilepsy: A study of their clinical characteristics and impact on quality of life. *Neurology* 2004; 62:(Suppl 5):A249.

169. Jones JE, Herman BP, Barry JJ, Gilliam F, et al. Clinical assessment of Axis I psychiatric morbidity in chronic epilepsy: a multicenter investigation. *J Neuropsychiatry Clin Neurosci* 2005; 17(2):172–179.

170. Sareen J, Cox BJ, Afifi TO, deGraaf R, et al. Anxiety disorders and risk for suicidal ideation and suicide attempts: a population-based longitudinal study of adults. *Arch Gen Psychiatry* 2005; 62:1249–1257.

171. Harris EC, Barraclough B. Suicide as an outcome for mental disorders: a meta-analysis. *Br J Psychiatry* 1997; 170:205–228.

172. Jones JE, Hermann BP, Barry JJ, Gilliam FG, et al. Rates and risk factors for suicide, suicidal ideation, and suicide attempts in chronic epilepsy. *Epilepsy Behav* 2003; 4 Suppl 3:S31–8.

173. Kanner AM, Soto A, Gross-Kanner H. Prevalence and clinical characteristics of postictal psychiatric symptoms in partial epilepsy. *Neurology* 2004; 62:708–713.

174. Curran S, DePauw K. Selecting an antidepressant for use in a patient with epilepsy: safety considerations. *Drug Safety* 1998; 18:125–133.

175. Swinkels J, Jonghe F. Safety of antidepressants. *Int Clin Psychopharmacol* 1995; 9 (supp 4):19–25.

176. Mohanraj R, Brodie MJ. Predicting outcomes in newly diagnosed epilepsy. *Epilepsia* 2003; 44(Suppl 9):15 (abstract).

177. Anhoury S, Brown RJ, Krishnamoorthy ES, Trimble MR. Psychiatric outcome after temporal lobectomy: a predictive study. *Epilepsia* 2000; 41:1608–1615.

178. Kanner AM, Byrne R, Chicharro AV, Frey M, et al. A lifetime history of depression is the sole predictor of post-surgical auras in seizure-free patients that underwent an antero-temporal lobectomy. *Epilepsia* 2006; 44:(Suppl 4):198 (abstract).

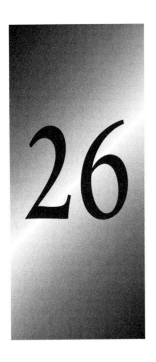

26 Interictal Dysphoric Disorder

Dietrich Peter Blumer

Unique for an illness classified as a neurologic disease, epilepsy is a disorder with an abundance of mental and behavioral changes. In fact, until about half a century ago, epilepsy was widely considered one of the major psychiatric disorders, with etiology and symptomatology distinct from manic-depressive, schizophrenic, or sexual disorders. Following World War II, psychiatry entered a phase of disinterest both in genetics and disorders that could be ascribed to brain dysfunction, and consequently the field of epilepsy, together with the electroencephalography (EEG) laboratories, was turned over to the discipline of neurology. This change resulted in the remarkable modern progress of understanding the neurologic aspects of epilepsy and of achieving seizure control, while the psychiatric aspects were neglected if not ignored. As was fashionable at the time, neurologists considered the psychiatric aspects of epilepsy a mere psychosocial problem and deemed vigorous efforts to free their patients from the stigma of having a psychiatric disorder to be most helpful for them.

Fortunately, such a one-sided view of epilepsy is now being remedied. In the ongoing debate about the presence of mood changes, anxiety, irritability ("aggression"), suicidality, and psychosis among patients with epilepsy, it is of importance to consider the early findings of Kraepelin, the pioneer of modern psychiatric classification, who first pointed out the presence of the interictal dysphoric disorder *(Verstimmungszustand)* as a core finding among the patients with epilepsy.

PREMODERN VIEW OF THE AFFECTIVE DISORDERS OF EPILEPSY

Kraepelin's observations are recognized as the basis for our modern psychiatric diagnostic classification. They were based on the daily, long-term observations of his patients with psychiatric disorders at a university hospital. In his psychiatric textbook of 1923, Kraepelin precisely described the affective changes of patients with epilepsy as they presented before the modern era of anticonvulsant therapy as the interictal dysphoric disorder (1). Periodic dysphorias, he stated, represent the most common of the psychiatric disorders of epilepsy. The dysphoric episodes are characterized particularly by irritability, with or without outbursts of fury. Depressive moods and anxiety, as well as headaches and insomnia, are also present, while euphoric moods are seen less often. These pleomorphic dysphoric episodes occur intermittently without external triggers and without clouding of consciousness. They begin and end rapidly and recur fairly regularly in a uniform manner, occurring every few days to every few months and lasting from a few hours up to 2 days. The dysphoric symptoms can be observed in both the prodromal and postictal phases of an attack, but they most commonly appear as phenomena independent of the overt seizures. A patient just awakens with the dysphoria, or it develops insidiously through the course of a day. While the intermittent dysphoric state with its disturbing irritable moods was marked in many patients, it must be emphasized that Kraepelin noted very positive personality traits in the majority of patients with epilepsy, describing them as "quiet, modest, devoted, amicable, helpful, industrious, thrifty, honest, and deeply religious." One must add here that the general prevalence of these traits explains the remorse that characteristically follows an episode of irritability.

Kraepelin described interictal hallucinatory or delusional episodes of epilepsy that occurred without clouding of consciousness, usually lasting a few days but at times persisting for weeks or even months; he viewed these psychotic episodes as mere expansions of the dysphoric moods. Chronic interictal psychoses were rarely observed, and suicide among patients with epilepsy was reported as a rare event in the era preceding modern antiepileptic treatment with its "forced normalization."

In the German-language literature, the dysphoric disorder was recognized as the principal psychiatric disorder of epilepsy as long as epilepsy was considered an important part of psychiatry. Thus, Bleuler, in his 1949 textbook of psychiatry (2), described the pleomorphic and intermittent dysphoric moods of epilepsy according to Kraepelin's concept. Bleuler did not label the psychoses of epilepsy as "schizophrenia-like" but clearly differentiated them from those of schizophrenia by the fact that the former present with only the accessory (nowadays labeled "positive") symptoms in the absence of the fundamental ("negative") symptoms of schizophrenia.

Upon the acceptance of epilepsy as a neurologic disorder, the large number of patients with chronic epilepsy and psychiatric complications, while representing a majority of those presenting with refractory seizures at epilepsy centers, received only limited attention. Though the occurrence of psychoses in epilepsy could not be overlooked and the frequency of suicide among patients with chronic epilepsy was repeatedly noted, these serious complications have tended to be viewed by neurologists as belonging to the psychiatric field and were not properly dealt with. Even today, there exists no general agreement about the most common affective disorder identified among patients with epilepsy long ago: the interictal dysphoric disorder, which precedes both interictal psychoses and suicides. The modern classification of psychiatric disorders includes no reference at all to epilepsy-related psychopathology, and there has been a trend to view the affective changes among patients with epilepsy as symptoms of a depressive or other psychiatric disorder defined by the merely descriptive criteria of the conventional DSM classification, instead of a unique disorder based on specific etiology and requiring specific treatment.

Concomitant with ignorance of the importance of epilepsy, modern psychiatry does not include an understanding of the general importance of what is termed "irritability," the unique trait of the interictal dysphoric disorder. The affective change of irritability refers to the paroxysmal trend of penting up the affective symptoms of anger, hate, rage, and fury to an explosive degree (as opposed to being good-natured). Aggression, in contrast, may not be associated with these affective symptoms and merely consists of the tendency to attack (as opposed to being passive).

MODERN CONFIRMATION OF THE INTERICTAL DYSPHORIC DISORDER

The histories systematically obtained from patients with epilepsy at the Epi-Care Center (Memphis, Tennessee) have confirmed the premodern observations by showing that irritability, depressive moods, anergia, insomnia, atypical pains, anxiety, fears, and euphoric moods are all frequently present; they are viewed as the eight key symptoms of interictal dysphoric disorder (3). Longitudinal assessment of these eight symptoms with an appropriate instrument (the Seizure Questionnaire) (4) documented that they indeed occur in the same intermittent and pleomorphic pattern noted by premodern psychiatrists. Patients with interictal psychiatric features had a mean of five of these symptoms; the presence of at least three symptoms generally coincided with significant impairment requiring treatment, and this number became to be considered the minimum for establishing the diagnosis of the interictal dysphoric disorder.

Presumably as an undesirable result of the modern antiepileptic drugs, the dysphoric symptoms now appear to be somewhat more protracted compared with the premodern psychiatric description of the dysphoric disorder, and the depressive symptoms may at times be more pronounced than the irritability. For the same reason, chronic interictal psychoses are now more frequent, and suicidality has become a significant problem (5).

The important items from the questionnaire for identifying the dysphoric disorder are listed in Figure 26-1. The questions are completed by the patient and next of kin as part of the Seizure Questionnaire. The examiner then reviews the questionnaire for completeness and accuracy with both the patient and next of kin. The answers concerning the eight symptoms of the dysphoric disorder are clarified by asking for characteristic examples of their manifestations, and their

Depressive Mood
1   Do you have frequent depressive moods?
        Since about when?
        Are they present all the time or off and on?
        How long do they last (hours, days, or weeks)?
        How often do they occur?

Anergia
2   Do you often lack energy?
        Since about when?
        Do you lack energy all the time or episodically?
        If episodically, indicate how often and how
        long they last (hours, days, weeks)

Pain
3   Do you have many aches and pains (please
    describe pain and location)?
        Since about when?
        How often and for how long?

Insomnia (hypersomnia)
4   Do you have trouble with your sleep?
        Since about when?
        How often and what kind of trouble?

Irritable explosive affect
5   Are you often very irritable?
        Do you have outbursts of temper?
        Since about when?
        How often do you become irritable?
        How do you react when you become very
        irritable?

Euphoric Mood
6   Do you have sudden moods of great happiness?
        Since about when?
        How often and for how long?

Fear
7   Do you have fears of certain situations?
        Since about when?
        What fears do you have (being in crowds, being
        alone, or other)?

Anxiety
8   Do you have frequent worries (anxieties)?
        Since about when?
        How often do you feel very worried?

FIGURE 26-1

Inquiry for the symptoms of the interictal dysphoric disorder. The listed set of questions from the Seizure Questionnaire (4) aims to establish presence or absence of the eight key symptoms of the interictal dysphoric disorder. They are answered jointly by patient and next of kin. The answers are then reviewed by the examiner for completeness and accuracy. A symptom is rated as positive if it can be judged troublesome in the life of the patient, and the particular number is circled. Each troublesome symptom becomes a target for treatment.

severity is assessed. If an individual symptom represents a problem in the life of the patient, it is rated as positive. During the treatment of the dysphoric disorder (the goal being complete remission), progress is assessed by checking every symptom for clearly troublesome presence, mild presence, or absence.

The dysphoric disorder, commonly present among patients with known epilepsy, can also be identified in other populations. Noteworthy are the observations of Himmelhoch, who identified a significant number of the patients from his center for affective disorders as suffering from epilepsy-related affective disorders (6). He referred to Kraepelin and the German psychiatric literature on epilepsy of the first half of the twentieth century when he noted the considerable number of affectively ill patients who had epilepsy-related mood disorders, often in the absence of manifest seizures. In an epidemiologic survey of patients from his clinic for affective disorders, he found that 10% of 748 patients had a final diagnosis of interictal or *subictal* affective illness. He arrived at the diagnosis of "*dysthymic*" interictal or subictal mood disorder for this subgroup of affectively ill patients. Himmelhoch used the term *dysthymic* in quotation marks for the disorder he described in the early 1980s as identical to Kraepelin's dysphoric disorder *(Verstimmungszustand)* among patients with epilepsy. Indeed, *dysthymia* refers to a chronic state of moderate ("neurotic") depression; to be *verstimmt* means being "out of tune or in a bad mood" and is more accurately translated as being *dysphoric*, a term that serves to imply episodicity rather than chronicity of the mental state.

Himmelhoch based his description of the syndrome on his experience with over 3,000 affectively ill patients. He recognized that the disorder did not belong to the spectrum of manic-depressive disorders but rather to epilepsy. He made the important point that there are in fact patients with the characteristic psychiatric changes associated with epilepsy who do not present with overt seizures but experience a subictal disorder and do belong to the spectrum of epilepsy-related disorders. Furthermore, he recognized early the marked premenstrual exacerbation of the disorder in women. The authors of the current psychiatric classification appropriately chose the term *dysphoric disorder* for the labile and pleomorphic mood state of the premenstrual phase with its notable irritability, a state that is identical by symptomatology and etiology to the interictal or subictal mood disorder (7).

For a global appreciation of the psychiatric aspects of temporal lobe epilepsy in modern times, the contributions of two outstanding neurologists with interest in the psychiatric aspects of epilepsy need to be cited. Norman Geschwind recognized a characteristic interictal syndrome of behavioral change in temporal lobe epilepsy, including an increased concern with ethical or religious issues, a contrasting irritability of varying degree, hyposexuality, and a trend toward hypergraphia. He considered the presence of a spike focus in temporal limbic structures as the primary pathogenetic mechanism of the interictal change with its characteristic deepening of the emotional life of these patients (8). Henri Gastaut noted the striking relationship of behavior after bilateral temporal lobectomy (Klüver-Bucy syndrome) and behavior upon the presence of a mesial temporal epileptogenic focus (9). The three major behavioral changes of Klüver-Bucy syndrome are placidity, inability to stay focused (hypermetamorphosis of attention), and hypersexuality. Supported by a series of his own studies, Gastaut noted that patients with chronic mesial temporal lobe epilepsy tend to show changes opposite to those seen in Klüver-Bucy syndrome: intensified emotionality, heightened attention to details, and hyposexuality. He pointed out that this finding was not surprising, considering that, due to the effect of the irritative lesion, patients with temporal lobe epilepsy present with an interictal state of increased (excitatory and inhibitory) activity of the temporal-limbic system as opposed to the state of globally decreased activity following the ablation experiment.

The most important symptoms of the heightened emotional intensity among patients with chronic mesial temporal lobe epilepsy are irritability, intensified moods, and anxiety—all key symptoms of interictal dysphoric disorder. These intermittent changes tend to be associated with more subtle, yet specific, personality changes. As noted by observers since premodern times, and again emphasized by Norman Geschwind, these changes consist of a general deepening or intensification of emotionality and a serious, highly ethical, and spiritual demeanor that contrasts with the episodic irritability. A second distinct personality change has frequently been debated. As opposed to the fleeting attention span seen in Klüver-Bucy syndrome, patients with epilepsy tend to be particularly detailed, persistent, and orderly in speech and behavior. These traits have been referred to by several different names, including "viscosity" or "stickiness," and in premodern times were often considered to be a leading aspect of the personality changes associated with epilepsy. A third change among patients with chronic temporal lobe epilepsy, opposite to what is observed in Klüver-Bucy syndrome, is a global hyposexuality, including decreased libidinous and genital arousal, as first described by Gastaut and Collomb (10). The common hyposexuality tends to be a specific handicap, but the sexual changes tend to reach obvious clinical significance only in the uncommon event of a reversal of the hyposexuality to a marked hypersexuality after complete surgical elimination of the epileptogenic zone (11). The distinct personality changes of chronic temporal lobe epilepsy include very positive traits, as noted by early psychiatric observers, that obviously do not require any

treatment. The interictal dysphoric changes, on the other hand, commonly require therapeutic intervention.

Epilepsy is an intermittent paroxysmal disorder. Its psychiatric features tend to be manifest in an intermittent pattern and present in a far more rapid pattern than those of bipolar disorder. The dysphoric disorder of epilepsy was first clearly identified by Kraepelin, based on the daily observations of long-term inpatients with epilepsy at university hospitals. The modern psychologic assessments routinely carried out by cross-sectional inquiry are clearly inadequate for recognizing the characteristically intermittent dysphoric disorder.

Refractory epilepsy tends to be of mesial temporal origin. As expected in a disorder that disrupts the regular activity of limbic centers, mesial temporal epilepsy is associated with psychiatric symptoms, not only intermittent but also pleomorphic in nature. Among patients with refractory epilepsy with psychiatric features, the interictal dysphoric disorder tends to be ubiquitous.

Recognizing the affective changes associated with epilepsy as the pleomorphic interictal dysphoric disorder with its intermittent symptomatology is of major importance, since the disorder with all its diverse symptoms is well treatable by adding the appropriate psychotropic medication to the antiepileptic medication. Furthermore, effective treatment of the dysphoric disorder can prevent its serious complications of interictal psychoses and suicide. The prevalence of psychosis of any type in epilepsy has been reported to be between 4% in a neurologic outpatient seizure clinic and 60% among epileptic inpatients of a psychiatric hospital. Suicide in populations from epilepsy centers has been reported as high as 20% of the causes of death—a prevalence similar to that among patients with bipolar disorder. The effective prevention of suicide in epilepsy—by properly treating the interictal dysphoric disorder—has been well documented by our experience with a large number of patients at the Epi-Care Center (5). Treatment must proceed with an understanding of the pathogenesis of the interictal psychiatric changes.

PATHOGENESIS

In 1951, Gibbs observed that the epileptic and psychiatric components of psychomotor epilepsy appeared to be physiologically antithetical (12). A few years later, Landolt (13) observed a patient whose epileptiform EEG had normalized each time he was dysphoric, ascribed the findings to a "supernormal braking action," and developed the concept of "forced normalization." Related studies focused particularly on the alternating pattern of interictal psychoses and seizures, and the term "forced normalization" came into current use. Trimble, in particular, has emphasized the importance of forced normalization in many studies and a recent monograph (14). Engel (15) postulated that the psychiatric disorder of epilepsy may result from the inhibitory activity that develops in reaction to the excessive excitatory activity of the chronic seizure disorder. The following findings are in accordance with this postulate (3):

1. The development of the interictal dysphoric and psychotic disorders is delayed (by about 2 years and 12 years, respectively) following onset of the epilepsy as inhibitory mechanisms become increasingly established. This finding accords with the particular linkage of the psychiatric disorders of epilepsy with its common refractory form, mesial temporal lobe epilepsy.

2. Upon decrease of seizures, and particularly upon full control, dysphoric or psychotic symptoms tend to be exacerbated or to emerge *de novo* ("forced normalization" or "alternating psychosis").

3. Psychiatric changes emerge at times when severe exacerbation of the seizure activity engages an enhanced inhibitory response. Thus, the prodromal phase of seizures may be associated with dysphoric symptoms (such as elated mood or heightened irritability), and the postictal phase is commonly associated with dysphoric symptoms (such as anergia, pain, depression, and, in rare cases, even suicidality) and at times (usually after a flurry of seizures) with psychosis. Dysphoric symptoms frequently intensify with the increased seizure activity of the premenstrual phase (7).

4. There is a delayed phasing-out of the psychiatric changes over 6 to 18 months after complete surgical elimination of the epileptogenic zone, presumably upon the gradual fading of inhibitory mechanisms that have then become unnecessary.

As noted by Himmelhoch, paroxysmal excessive neuronal activity with its major psychiatric manifestation of a dysphoric disorder, characteristic for the interictal phase of chronic mesial temporal epilepsy, may occur likewise in the absence of overt seizures among individuals with various cerebral disorders involving limbic areas and may be identified as subictal dysphoric disorder (3, 6). Of particular interest is the finding that the common premenstrual dysphoric disorder presents with a pleomorphic and labile symptomatology identical to that of interictal dysphoric disorder (7). More than two-thirds of women with epilepsy experience their seizures predominantly or exclusively in a catamenial pattern, and many experience severe premenstrual dysphoria (16). This finding has been related to a shift in the estradiol/progesterone ratio in favor of the proconvulsant estradiol over the anticonvulsant progesterone. It has been suggested that premenstrual dysphoric

disorder—as a subictal disorder—may be best treated, like interictal dysphoric disorder, with the combination of an antidepressant and an anticonvulsant.

TREATMENT

Our experience in treating the psychiatric disorders of epilepsy dates back some 25 years, with an initial publication in 1988 (17). Subsequent reports of series of patients with epilepsy treated for their dysphoric disorder (18) and for interictal psychosis (19) documented key findings from our experience at the Epi-Care Center in Memphis from 1987 to 1999. Of the 10,739 patients with epilepsy seen at the Center during that period, a majority underwent psychiatric evaluation.

According to the foregoing hypothesis of the pathogenesis of the psychiatric disorders of epilepsy, their pharmacological treatment has to be directed primarily against the inhibitory mechanisms. The proconvulsant tricyclic antidepressant drugs, at modest doses, appear to serve as effective antagonists to excessive inhibition and may be indispensable for successfully treating the interictal dysphoric and psychotic disorders. Gastaut and colleagues (20) pointed out that, as measured by their response to metrazol, patients with temporal lobe epilepsy (in contrast to those with primary generalized epilepsy) show, surprisingly, a higher interictal seizure threshold than do persons without epilepsy. The bias against the use of antidepressants for the psychiatric disorders of epilepsy, on the grounds that they may lower the seizure threshold, is erroneous on both empirical and theoretical grounds. Modest amounts of tricyclic antidepressant medication do not increase seizure frequency in patients with chronic epilepsy whose dysphoric disorder indicates the presence of marked inhibition, and the selective serotonin reuptake inhibitors (SSRIs), which we commonly use as adjuncts to the tricyclic antidepressants, are not known to lower the seizure threshold. The combination appears more effective than the use of a tricyclic or of an SSRI alone. Tricyclic antidepressants tend to lower the seizure threshold more than other psychotropic drugs do, and their proconvulsant effect may serve to mitigate and eliminate the psychotoxic effects of excessive inhibition; effectiveness of the SSRI suggests different mechanisms of action. Patients with primary generalized epilepsy (who occasionally experience dysphoric symptoms, presumably due to secondary involvement of mesial temporal structures), as noted by Gastaut, have a lower interictal seizure threshold than those with mesial temporal lobe epilepsy (and of course a lower seizure threshold than do individuals without epilepsy); they need a more cautious dose of antidepressant medication. Such patients appear to respond well to particularly low doses of these medications.

Based on the experience with seizure patients suffering from a dysphoric disorder, at least three of the eight key symptoms of the dysphoric disorder are usually present when treatment with antidepressant medication is indicated (18). We add 100 to 150 mg of imipramine or 75 to 125 mg of nortriptyline at bedtime to the antiepileptic medication, making sure that the insomnia (i.e., difficulty initiating and maintaining sleep) common among these patients is corrected; the more sedative nortriptyline is preferred over imipramine for that purpose, and amitriptyline, doxepin, or trimipramine may have to be substituted at 100 to 150 mg at bedtime. If anergia is troublesome, we tend to choose a more activating tricyclic drug, such as desipramine (at 50 mg twice daily to 50 mg three times daily) or protriptyline (at 5 to 20 mg daily). In a commonly necessary second step, if the patient does not respond sufficiently, we promptly proceed to double antidepressant treatment by adding an SSRI to the tricyclic, which is then usually kept at 100 mg. As opposed to the choice of the tricyclic drug, the choice of the SSRI is not guided by any clinical findings, and another SSRI is substituted readily if response to the initial drug is not satisfactory. Paroxetine had been our preferred SSRI at 20 mg once or twice daily; however, a different SSRI often may be more effective, such as sertraline (at 50 to 100 mg in the morning) or fluoxetine or citalopram (at 20 to 40 mg daily). If sleep is not disturbed, one may also proceed in the reverse order by starting with the SSRI and then adding a tricyclic drug if necessary. The modest dose of tricyclic medication required avoids the many side effects of this type of antidepressant and allows for a safe combination with an SSRI. We have rarely used the selective serotonin-norepinephrine reuptake inhibitor venlafaxine with its relatively broad-spectrum effect, which may be helpful in treating the dysphoric disorder, in order to address the sleep disorder and anergia of the disorder more flexibly with the combination of a tricyclic drug and an SSRI. In a third step, the action of the antidepressants may have to be enhanced by adding a small dose of neuroleptic, such as 1 to 2 mg of risperidone at bedtime. Importantly, if lethargy remains troublesome, a stimulant medication (e.g., methylphenidate) may need to be added.

At each therapeutic intervention, the status of each of the eight symptoms of the dysphoric disorder is assessed (Figure 26-2). Response to the treatment usually can be achieved for all the symptoms of the dysphoric disorder—irritability, depressive and elated moods, insomnia, anergia, anxiety, fears, and pains—and can be expected *as soon as the therapeutic dose is reached,* allowing a rapid modification of the dose as needed. The mechanism of action of the antidepressant drugs in the interictal dysphoric disorder clearly is different than in traditional depressive disorders: the drugs are effective rapidly, at lower doses, and have a broad-spectrum effect

INTAKE	+	−
Depressive mood	(+)	
Anergia		−
Atypical pain		−
Insomnia/hypersomnia	+	
Irritable/explosive affect	+	
Euphoric mood	+	
Fear	+	
Anxiety	+	
AFTER 1 MONTH	+	−
Depressive mood		−
Anergia		−
Atypical pain		−
Insomnia/hypersomnia		−
Irritable/explosive affect	(+)	
Euphoric mood		−
Fear		−
Anxiety	(+)	
AFTER 2 MONTHS	+	−
Depressive mood		−
Anergia		−
Atypical pain		−
Insomnia/hypersomnia		−
Irritable/explosive affect		−
Euphoric mood		−
Fear		−
Anxiety		−

FIGURE 26-2

Scoring of symptoms during treatment of an illustrative case. Case 1 required a brief treatment period of 2 months. At each of the three visits, presence or absence of the eight key symptoms was checked. A symptom checked positive but within parentheses indicates that it is now significantly less troublesome but requires further treatment.

for the entire range of symptoms, not just for depressive moods, anergia, and insomnia.

It must be noted that the described treatment of the interictal (and subictal) dysphoric disorder also needs to be used for treating interictal psychoses. As noted early by Kraepelin, the interictal psychotic symptoms of epilepsy (hallucinations, delusions, paranoid ideas) may develop among patients with dysphoric disorders and could be termed "dysphoric disorders with psychotic symptomatology." These patients require double antidepressant treatment enhanced by the addition of antipsychotic medication (risperidone or olanzapine) and, in general, are well treatable (19).

Case studies of particularly severe or atypical dysphoric disorders requiring prolonged or unusual therapeutic interventions have been reported elsewhere (3).

We include here an illustrative case of typical prompt recovery.

ILLUSTRATIVE CASE

This 17-year-old female had experienced generalized seizures from age 3 to 4 and had taken anticonvulsants until age 10. At age 16, she had four generalized seizures over a 3-day period, was treated with topiramate 200 mg twice a day, and had no further seizures.

Since about age 13, following menarche, she experienced frequent hour-long elated moods with rapid speech, as well as daily spells of anxiety and outbursts of temper. She also began to have fears of suffering a seizure and death. During the premenstrual phase, her irritability would increase and she had crying spells. After the brief episode of recurrent seizures and the successful treatment with topiramate, she began to suffer more severe and more frequent anxiety attacks (3–10 daily) and an increased lability of moods with daily verbal outbursts of anger. She began missing school, made poor grades, and had to start home schooling. Two months prior to being seen by us, she started citalopram 60 mg daily, but 6 weeks later she had a serious argument with her father and put a gun to her chest. She was admitted for a few days to a psychiatric hospital, where valproic acid 500 mg was added to her medication. After discharge, she had less anxiety but slept 12 to 16 hours daily, and her neurologist referred her to us. We stopped both the valproic acid and the citalopram and added the combination of sertraline 50 mg in the morning and imipramine 50 mg twice per day to her topiramate. At follow-up 1 month later, her only symptoms were minor irritability (three times per week) and two very brief anxiety attacks. Her sertraline was increased to 100 mg in the morning, and over the follow-up period of 3 years her dysphoric symptoms have remained in complete remission (Figure 26-2).

Comment: A longstanding but mild seizure disorder had become associated after menarche with irritability, anxiety, fears, and elated moods; depressive moods occurred only during the premenstrual phase. We replaced an ineffective SSRI with sertraline and chose imipramine as a tricyclic with little sedative and good antianxiety effect, achieving remission of all dysphoric symptoms.

DIAGNOSTIC VALIDITY OF INTERICTAL DYSPHORIC DISORDER AND THE GENERAL SIGNIFICANCE OF THE PAROXYSMAL AFFECTS

The effectiveness of antidepressant medication to treat interictal moods has contributed to an assumption that the disorder could be described as depressive in nature ("dysthymic-like"). But it must be noted that the very prompt effect of antidepressant drugs at a low dose in epilepsy on the irritable, anxious, depressive, and elated moods, as well as on sleep and anergia, is quite different from their delayed effect at higher doses in depressive states. The pleomorphic and intermittent phenomenology of the dysphoric disorder, with its key symptom of irritability, is obviously dissimilar to what could be termed a "dysthymic-like" state. The term "schizophrenia-like" used in the past for the psychoses associated with epilepsy, is likewise inappropriate. Geschwind has pointed out that the use of terms borrowed from the standard psychiatric nomenclature may serve only to obscure the characteristic features of the psychiatric changes in temporal lobe epilepsy (8).

Interictal dysphoric disorder may become associated with suicidal episodes, is present prior to and concomitant with interictal psychoses, and can be recognized as the major psychiatric disorder that is specifically related to epilepsy. The disorder can be identified by the practical method described in this chapter and requires specific treatment. An optimal treatment of the dysphoric disorder is eminently feasible but requires a careful observation of the persistence or remission of every key symptom of the disorder.

Robins and Guze (21) outlined four criteria for a valid diagnosis of psychiatric disorders: clinical phenomenology, genetics (i.e., etiology), course, and treatment response. Our current psychiatric classification is based merely on clinical phenomenology and course of the disorders and is recognized as tentative; in particular, it does not include genetic considerations. The interictal dysphoric disorder meets all four criteria and represents the most important among the subictal and premenstrual dysphoric disorders in the spectrum of epilepsy-related dysphoric disorders. Every major psychiatric disorder with independent inheritance has not only a distinct etiology, phenomenology, course, and treatment response, but also distinct personality and psychodynamic features. Patients with epilepsy and psychiatric symptomatology likewise tend to reveal distinct personality and psychodynamic features (3, 8, 20).

The current practice of psychiatrists viewing epilepsy as an ordinary neurologic disorder must be remedied, not only to provide appropriate diagnosis and treatment for the many patients with epilepsy-related psychiatric disorders but also for a more complete understanding of human nature. The key symptom of the dysphoric disorder, referred to simply as "irritability," represents not aggression but an accentuation of the general human tendency to build up and explosively discharge the paroxysmal affects of anger, hate, rage, envy, and jealousy (3, 22). These paroxysmal affects are associated in the same patients with epilepsy, characteristically, with enhanced opposite tendencies to be exceptionally good-natured, helpful to others, and devoutly religious. With its link to passionate religiosity, epilepsy had earned the historical label of the "Sacred Disease" (23), and the significance of the conflict associated with the disorder is well understood—since the early history of Cain and Abel—by religious thinkers who are concerned with the profound conflict of good and evil in human nature. The unfortunate fact that religious fervor may become associated with intolerance and hatred of the "infidels" has been evident all too often through the history of humankind.

Among psychiatrists, Szondi assigned epilepsy a central role for the understanding of human nature (22). His work was ignored earlier, when psychiatry disregarded its biologic basis, because it was based on genetic considerations, but also because epilepsy had come to be considered an ordinary neurologic disorder. He assumed the existence of specific drive genes, present in every individual and, in a minority, to a pathogenetic degree; the dynamic nature of every drive factor is based on the polarity of two opposite drive tendencies. In the drive factor associated with epilepsy, the tendency to accumulate and discharge angry affects is paired with the tendency to make good; this drive factor determines ethical behavior—to be good or evil (conscientious or unscrupulous, tolerant or intolerant, good-natured or malicious, healing or wounding, pious or blasphemous). This drive factor is of a paroxysmal nature, manifesting itself in three principal phases: "First, the energies of the crude affects are accumulated; anger or rage, hate or vengeance, envy or jealousy are incited . . . then follows the explosive discharge in some form of paroxysm . . . then the phase of trying to make good, the hyperethical and often hyperreligous phase."

In our patients with epilepsy, the dysphoric affects are intertwined with the highly positive personality traits noted early by Kraepelin, as outbursts of anger are commonly followed by remorse, the need to atone, and depressive mood to the extreme of feeling suicidal.

Beyond specific personality changes, the psychiatric manifestations of epilepsy consist of the common dysphoric disorder and the less common psychoses. Their pathogenesis appears related to the inhibitory response to chronic paroxysmal neuronal hyperactivity of the mesial temporal limbic system. Treatment aimed at mitigating this process tends to be highly successful for the interictal dysphoric disorder and similarly for interictal psychoses. Renewed recognition, after a half century, of the importance of epilepsy for psychiatry is overdue. More than in any established psychiatric disorder, the relationship of psychopathology to cerebral changes is evident in epilepsy. Neurologists who choose to deal with the intricate complexities of the neural substrate of epilepsy exclusively must have psychiatrists available who can assist them in dealing with the psychiatric aspects of the disorder.

SUMMARY

The unawareness of psychiatrists of the nature of the disorders related to epilepsy dates back half a century, when epilepsy came to be considered an ordinary neurologic disorder. Epileptic seizures, however, can be provoked in every human being. Epilepsy is an extraordinary disorder that, beyond its well-known neurologic complexities, tends to become complicated with a wide range of specific psychiatric changes; they occur upon the establishment of a temporal-limbic focus of intermittent excessive neuronal excitatory activity that produces increasingly inhibitory responses. These changes are distinct from those related to the two major psychiatric spheres for which a genetic basis is established (i.e., the manic-depressive and schizophrenic disorders) and represent a genetic sphere of their own.

Apart from more subtle personality changes and the serious late complications of interictal psychoses and suicidal episodes, the key affective syndrome associated with epilepsy consists of the interictal dysphoric disorder with its characteristic intermittent and pleomorphic symptomatology. This disorder was clearly identified about a century ago by Kraepelin, when he established a comprehensive basis for the modern classification of the psychiatric disorders, at a time when epilepsy represented an area of major interest to psychiatrists. A practical method of recognizing the dysphoric disorder is reported. The disorder tends to be very treatable by combining psychotropic (chiefly antidepressant) with the antiepileptic medication.

Psychiatrists must become familiar with the psychiatric aspects of epilepsy to be able to assist the neurologists who focus on the neural complexities of the illness. They also must become able to recognize, among their own patients, the presence of a subictal dysphoric disorder that requires the same treatment as the interictal dysphoric disorder; combined treatment with antidepressant and antiepileptic medication is likewise indicated for the premenstrual dysphoric disorder, a condition that appears to belong to the spectrum of epilepsy-related psychiatric disorders. Furthermore, they must learn how an ignored population in their care—the epilepsy patients confined to state hospitals—can be properly treated. Of particular importance is the need for psychiatrists to become familiar with the role of the paroxysmal affects in the general human condition, with their basic conflict to be intermittently angry and irascible yet otherwise good-natured, helpful, and religious—a conflict that tends to be particularly accentuated among patients with the "Sacred Disease."

References

1. Kraepelin E. Psychiatrie. 8th ed. Leipzig: Barth, 1923.

2. Bleuler E. Lehrbuch der Psychiatrie. 8th ed. Berlin: Springer, 1949.

3. Blumer D, Montouris G, Davies K. The interictal dysphoric disorder: recognition, pathogenesis, and treatment of the major psychiatric disorder of epilepsy. *Epilepsy Behav* 2004; 5:826–840.

4. Blumer D, Davies K. Psychiatric issues in epilepsy surgery. In: Ettinger AB, Kanner AM, eds. *Psychiatric Issues in Epilepsy: A Practical Guide to Diagnosis and Treatment.* Philadelphia: Lippincott Williams & Wilkins, 2001:231–249.

5. Blumer D, Montouris G, Davies K, Wyler A, et al. Suicide in epilepsy: psychopathology, pathogenesis, and prevention. *Epilepsy Behav* 2002; 3:232–241.

6. Himmelhoch JM. Major mood disorders related to epileptic changes. In: Blumer D, ed. *Psychiatric Aspects of Epilepsy.* Washington, DC: American Psychiatric Press; 1984:271–294.

7. Blumer D, Herzog AG, Himmelhoch J, Salgueiro CA, et al. To what extent do premenstrual and interictal dysphoric disorders overlap? Significance for therapy. *J Affect Disord* 1998; 48:215–225.

8. Geschwind N. Behavioural changes in temporal lobe epilepsy. *Psychol Med* 1979; 9:217–219.

9. Gastaut H. Interpretation of the symptoms of psychomotor epilepsy in relation to physiological data on rhinencephalic function. *Epilepsia* 1954; 3:84–88.

10. Gastaut H, Collomb H. Étude du comportement sexuel chez les épileptiques psychomoteurs. *Ann Med Psychol (Paris)* 1954; 112:657–696.

11. Blumer D. Hypersexual episodes in temporal lobe epilepsy. *Am J Psychiatry* 1970; 126:1099–1106.

12. Gibbs FA. Ictal and non-ictal psychiatric disorders in temporal lobe epilepsy. *J Nerv Ment Disease* 1951; 113:522–528.

13. Landolt H. Über Verstimmungen, Dämmerzustände und schizophrene Zustandsbilder bei Epilepsie: Ergebnisse klinischer und elektroenzephalographischer Untersuchungen. *Schweiz Arch Neurol Psychiatrie* 1955; 76:313–321.

14. Trimble MR, Schmitz B, eds. Forced normalization and alternative psychoses of epilepsy. Petersfield, UK and Bristol, PA, USA: Wrightson Biomedical, 1998.

15. Engel J. Seizures and epilepsy. Philadelphia: Davis, 1989.

16. Herzog AG, Klein P, Ransil BJ. Three patterns of catamenial epilepsy. *Epilepsia* 1997; 38:1082–1088.

17. Blumer D, Zielinski J. Pharmacologic treatment of psychiatric disorders associated with epilepsy. *J Epilepsy* 1988; 1:135–150.

18. Blumer D. Antidepressant and double antidepressant treatment for the affective disorder of epilepsy. *J Clin Psychiatry* 1997; 58:3–11.

19. Blumer D, Wakhlu S, Montouris G, Wyler A. Treatment of the interictal psychoses. *J Clin Psychiatry* 2000; 61:110–122.

20. Gastaut H, Morin G, Lesèvre N. Étude du comportement des épileptiques psychomoteurs dans l'intervalle de leurs crises: les troubles de l'activité globale et de la sociabilité. *Ann Med Psychol (Paris)* 1955; 113:1–27.

21. Robins E, Guze SB. Establishment of diagnostic validity in psychiatric illness: its application to schizophrenia. Am J Psychiatry 1970; 126:938–947.

22. Szondi L. Schicksalsanalytische Therapie: ein Lehrbuch der passiven und aktiven analytischen Psychotherapie. Bern: Huber, 1963.

23. Temkin O. The falling sickness: a history of epilepsy from the Greeks to the beginnings of modern neurology. Baltimore: Johns Hopkins Press, 1971.

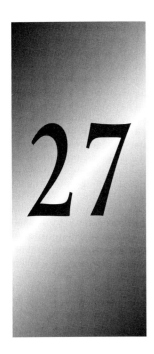

Epilepsy and Anxiety

Martin Schöndienst
Markus Reuber

nxiety disorders are twice as common in people with epilepsy as in the general population, and several large studies have shown that mood disorders are more common in epilepsy than in other chronic medical conditions such as diabetes or asthma. Although most attention has focused on depression or dysphoric states, anxiety may actually be more common (1). For instance, one recent study looking for psychopathology using a standardized diagnostic interview in inpatients with epilepsy found that the one-year prevalence of anxiety disorders was 25% and of mood disorders 19% (2). However, in some secondary care and specialist settings the prevalence of disabling anxiety symptoms may exceed 50% (1).

In fact, if "fear" is defined as the perception of a *specific* danger and "anxiety" as the experience of a *nonspecific* threat, it would be hard to think of a medical disorder that should predispose more to fear or anxiety than epilepsy. Having epilepsy is associated with a large number of threats, including the unpredictability of seizures, the feeling of loss of control, the risk of ictal injury (or even death), and negative social effects. This array of factors with anxiogenic potential actually makes it more difficult to answer the question why anxiety symptoms do not feature more prominently in our patients than to answer the question why epilepsy is often associated with

disabling anxiety. Unfortunately, the former question has received little attention to date.

The *Diagnostic and Statistical Manual of Mental Disorders IV* (DSM-IV) and the *International Classification of Mental and Behavioral Disorders*—10th edition (ICD-10) distinguish over 11 (DSM-IV) or 16 (ICD-10) different categories of anxiety disorders. However, most are excluded when a significant explanatory medical condition (such as epilepsy) is present. The International League Against Epilepsy (ILAE) has proposed its own classification of neuropsychiatric disorders associated with epilepsy. This classification (see Chapter 24) aims to be more specific and describes a number of additional mental disorders thought to be etiologically linked to epilepsy. It emphasizes the importance of a multifactorial organic approach (including the relationship of neuropsychiatric symptoms to EEG abnormalities or anticonvulsant drug treatment), but it contains very little detail about anxiety symptoms associated with epilepsy.

What is more, neither the DSM-IV, the ICD-10, nor the ILAE approach to classification take full account of personality or interactional features that may not be extreme or disabling enough to amount to a "personality disorder" but are nevertheless highly relevant for resilience toward disabling anxiety symptoms and for the way they clinically present. In fact, almost all anxiety disorders, including those associated with epilepsy, develop in patients with particular vulnerabilities, and treatment of more refractory anxiety disorders is unlikely to be successful without an understanding of the patient's personality or ego-structural background. Although epileptologists often deal with patients with character traits that psychoanalysts would call "ego-structural deficits," their neurologic training has often not equipped them to recognize or respond to such traits. It may seem an irritating overextension of their clinical focus to expect neurologists to observe such details as patients' introspective abilities, their ability to understand internal processes in others, maladaptive patterns in interpersonal relationships, patterns of attachment, and their preferred defense mechanisms (e.g., projection, isolation, splitting, denial) (3). However, neurologists may recognize that these features guide their clinical intuition already, and it may be a relatively small step for them to register these psychodynamic and interactional features more explicitly.

In this chapter we will approach the complex relationship between anxiety and epilepsy by focusing on a number of important clinical scenarios. Some will be illustrated with excerpts of (translated) transcripts of initial outpatient visits to the Bethel Epilepsy Centre, Germany, and (original) transcripts of clinical encounters at the Sheffield Teaching Hospitals in the UK. We will then discuss aspects of the pathophysiology, personality-related, psychologic, and psychodynamic features of each typical presentation of anxiety. The final part of this chapter will present a multidimensional therapeutic approach to anxiety in patients with epilepsy.

COMMON CLINICAL SCENARIOS

Epilepsy-Related Fear in Everyday Life

Fear and anxiety are phylogenetically ancient, naturally occurring affective states that are essential to learning and survival. The mental and somatic manifestations of these states are generated by a cascade of physical and chemical changes in a dispersed network of neuronal systems involving attention, stimulus perception and recognition, and memory retrieval and association as well as motor and autonomic control. One important conceptualization has described the psychophysiology of anxiety as a carefully counterbalanced system involving a "behavioral activation system" (BAS) and a "behavioral inhibition system" (BIS), the latter mediating passive avoidance and approach-avoidance conflict (4). Both systems are continuously involved in the monitoring of perceptions and cognition and cannot be "switched off" at will. On this basis, challenging thoughts or adverse experiences related to epilepsy may cause fear or trigger anxiety symptoms that

would not be considered as evidence of psychopathology or mental illness because they were adequately explained by the patient's medical disorder. For instance, a small study in which we examined patients with panic disorder ($n = 7$) and patients with epileptic anxiety-auras ($n = 5$) using the Structured Clinical Interview for the DSM-IV (SCID) and a range of anxiety scales showed that patients with epilepsy experienced more anxiety symptoms and exhibited more avoidance behavior than panic patients, although several patients with epilepsy did not fulfill the DSM-IV criteria for a mental disorder (5). The term "seizure phobia," which has been applied to 20–30% of patients with epilepsy (6), reframes some of these epilepsy-related anxiety symptoms in terms of a mental disorder but is not included in the current diagnostic manuals.

Example 1. In the following transcripts, capital letters signify emphasis (This is more emphatic than this, and THIS is even more emphatic); all other prosodic details have been omitted to enhance readability. The incomplete and broken sentences are not a consequence of a language deficit or poor translation but reflect the nature of verbal communication.

A patient with focal motor seizures affecting the right arm associated with speech arrest reports that the frequency of her seizures has increased.

Patient: an'uh I worry that I might Have them at work. . . . Tuesday NIGHT . . . Late at night you see . . .

Physician: why do you worry aBOUT . . . work, . . . or HAving them at work, what what's the, . . .

Patient: because uh' . . . you know there's LOTS of CUStomers, . . . around n' they're strangers and I don't want to . . .

Physician: you'd be embarrassed . . .

Patient: well a LIttle bit yeah . . . I mean the PEOple that I work wi' . . . I wouldn't be embarrassed in front of THEM, but . . . eh in front of strangers yeah I would . . . I mean.. usually I get a . . . COUple of seconds WARning an' . . . I'll eh go in t'back or . . . I KNOW . . . I mean I have HAD . . . one or two at work and I've gone in Ladies.

Physician: I see . . .

Patient: Been on t' shop floor an' I thought . . . uhm QUICK run in the ladies n' I've . . . managed to get OUTa way or I've run in CASH office . . . Managed to get OUT of way . . . I'd SOOner Nobody KNOW . . . at work.

Anxiety arising from the seizures themselves or from the actual or anticipated response of others can be difficult to process and communicate. The resulting affect is often isolated. As in this example, it is implied in a particular narrative, but not described explicitly. Alternatively, it can be projected completely onto other people. An attentive physician can identify this distressing affect and help patients to work through it. The first step in this process would be to support the patient in being more explicit about the things she is afraid of.

Preictal Anxiety

Whereas the phenomenologic and pathophysiologic delineation of ictal anxiety, including anxiety auras, is relatively straightforward, preictal anxiety is harder to distinguish and describe. Recent neurophysiologic studies looking at electroencephalographic (EEG) changes for the purpose of seizure prediction suggest that states with a high seizure risk exist and last for several hours. However, these studies provide very little information about the subjective experience of patients in such preictal states. This means that there is no clear relationship between particular segments of EEG-recordings categorized as "preictal" by nonlinear mathematical coherence measures and symptoms that patients or their relatives interpret as indicating that a seizure is imminent (7).

Example 2. A patient with idiopathic generalized epilepsy (IGE) gives this description of mornings when the patient is going to have a seizure. On such a morning:

Patient: it is eh— my PERsonal feeling, a completely different, then I feel eh . . . much more insecure, then I almost feel ANxious, you could compare it to, and eh . . . you notice, you come out in a SWEAT, eh . . . sweat on your hands and feet, so probably very CLASSical FEATures, eh . . . put PLAINly in one sentence, these are the kind of things, which try to get you DOWN, as if following the motto (fall in tone) stay calm, you KNOW, you are somehow not completely aWAKE, and it will take a while now, a little while, sit yourself down, eh . . . this doesn't have to and then you tell yourself, this DOESn't have to turn things topsy turvy, what is happening around you and eh . . . you don't have to get upset about your parents eh . . . staring at you or somehow CRIticising you.

As this example demonstrates, patients' spontaneous descriptions of preictal states often hint at physical, perceptive, and affective (predominantly anxiety-related) symptoms that are tightly interlaced with psychosocial or biographical facts. It may be difficult to pick up prodromal anxiety symptoms in such a highly condensed account, which combines apparently conflicting descriptions of prodromal symptoms, the specific fear of a seizure, the reactive denial of this fear, its projection onto caregivers or seizure witnesses, the report of behavior precipitating seizures, and maneuvers intended to control the developing seizure. From a psychodynamic point of view these difficulties can be explained by an ego-structural conflict between autonomy-oriented versus dependent traits that are reactivated and played out by the patient during the description of the preictal state.

Ictal Anxiety

By comparison, ictal anxiety is a relatively well understood clinical phenomenon. Ictal anxiety is typically related to epileptic activity affecting the amygdala, especially on the right side. However, ictal fear not only is a feature of temporal lobe seizures but also is associated with seizures arising in the anterior cingulate, orbitofrontal cortex, or other limbic structures (1). To date, differences in the anxiety-related symptomatology associated with epileptic activity in these different temporal or frontal lobe structures have not been formally examined. However, it seems that no affect can be elicited more readily by electrical stimulation of brain structures than anxiety. This does not mean that the diagnosis of ictal anxiety is always easy. Anxiety symptoms may not be readily volunteered. If they are described, it may be difficult to distinguish between ictal anxiety and panic attacks.

Example 3. The following patient, a student with left hippocampal sclerosis, does not mention anxiety symptoms spontaneously, although the physician has indicated that he is giving the patient time to talk about his own concerns. Eventually the physician asks specifically about seizure warnings. The patient replies:

Patient: well, I have to say, I rarely have any eh . . . warnings, which tell me that a seizure may be coming ON, well other patients who I've MET often say, they really NOtice, I'll have a seizure in a minute and can DO something, I practically NEver have that, I mean that I can guarantee to preDICT that, well that

Physician: But instead?

Patient: sometimes I have a kinda sickness beFOREhand, so that I MIGHT have a kinda suspicion, well, may have, something might happen, what I notice, when I am PANicking, when I'm Anxious, insecurity, whether before a SEIzure or just WELL, can I MASter my life, well for real, whether for instance the oral examination in my high school finals, whether it is about an exercise or something, well then I DO feel at risk of a seizure, for instance I had an ABsence there, the other worry is just, I want to be elsewhere, so really almost the wish, perhaps also SUicide, eh, exaggerated, so really the wish DEAD, perhaps this is also a reason, why you sometimes go into such an absence.

Following his initial denial of any seizure warning, this patient eventually responds to the physician's prompt by describing a complex, multimodal symptomatology involving panic and anxiety. His account begins with an apparently physical sensation. The existential challenge posed by the (pre) ictal symptomatology becomes clear only after both interlocutors have invested considerable communication effort in the reconstruction of the subsequent seizure experience.

The hesitant disclosure of affective (pre) ictal symptoms evident in this example was the most important distinguishing feature in a comparative Conversation Analytic study of the communication behavior of eight patients with panic attacks and seven patients with epileptic anxiety auras (5) (for other distinguishing clinical, interactional features and investigations, see Table 27-1). Patients with epilepsy typically failed to provide a more detailed description of the terrifying nature of their symptoms unless they were prompted and the description was facilitated by the physician. Their interictal processing of anxiety symptoms was characterized by omission, suggesting that they had a tendency to displace or forget ictal affective symptoms, regardless of the distress they cause during a seizure. This was in marked contrast to the interactive behavior of patients with panic attacks, who readily volunteered their anxiety symptoms. If physicians treating patients with epilepsy are not aware of the fluctuating recall or recognition of affective symptoms that their patients exhibit, ictal anxiety can easily remain undiagnosed. Conversely, careful prompting may allow patients to share aspects of their ictal experience that they had previously suppressed or avoided.

Postictal Anxiety

Postictal anxiety is not thought to be caused directly by epileptic discharges. Postictal dysphoric states can last from minutes to days. In one study, anxiety was the commonest postictal symptom (affecting 45 of 100 patients), although it rarely occurred in isolation and was often associated with depressive and neurovegetative symptoms (8). The

subgroup of patients with depression and anxiety was characterized by postictal feelings of guilt. This is reminiscent of the established psychoanalytical theory, discussed by Janz, that some seizures are related to conflict-generating and guilt provoking aggressive impulses (9).

Panic Disorder in Patients with Epilepsy

We have already mentioned the sometimes difficult differentiation of ictal anxiety and panic disorder. Unfortunately, the situation is complicated by the fact that there is also an increased incidence of panic disorder in patients with epilepsy (i.e., of patients having both ictal anxiety and panic disorder). Example 4 (later in this chapter) illustrates how complex the relationship between panic and anxiety can be.

From a psychodynamic point of view, panic patients often exhibit a striking self-conflict, oscillating between complete helplessness and a marked urge to dominate. The cognitive-behavioral understanding of panic attack has changed significantly over the last decade. Whereas

---

TABLE 27-1
Differential Diagnosis of Panic Attack versus Ictal Anxiety Caused by a Focal Epileptic Seizure

	PRIMARY PANIC ATTACK	FOCAL EPILEPTIC SEIZURE
Clinical features		
Consciousness	Alert	May progress to impairment
Duration	5–10 minutes	0.5–2 minutes
Automatisms	Very rare	Common with progression to CPS
Nocturnal attacks	Occur from state of wakefulness	May wake patient up
Subjective symptoms		
Déjà vu, hallucinations	Very rare	>5%
Depressive symptoms	Common, severity associated	Not uncommon, severity not associated
Anticipatory anxiety	Very common	Can occur but not common
Relation to "normal" anxiety	No clear subjective difference between "normal" fear and panic states	Clear difference between "normal" and ictal fear
Investigations		
Interictal EEG	Usually normal	Often abnormal
Ictal EEG	Usually normal	Usually abnormal (may be normal in SPS)
MRI of temporal structures	Usually normal	Often abnormal*
Linguistic and interactional features in the history		
Anxiety symptoms as a topic	Usually volunteered	Not volunteered without prompting
Anxiety symptoms	Discussed extensively	Discussed sparingly
	Volunteered quickly	Hesitant disclosure
	Self-initiated as a topic	Often not discussed without prompting
	Frequent use of formulaic expressions	Apparently difficult to describe, descriptions characterized by high formulation effort.
	Are described as focused on particular objects	Ictal fear is described as nonspecific, untargeted anxiety

CPS = complex-partial seizure, SPS = simple partial seizure, * = explicit search for hippocampal sclerosis or other discrete amygdala lesion with appropriate magnetic resonance imaging

the "false-suffocation alarm" model, particularly supported by Klein (10), predominated during the late 1990s, the currently favored model hypothesizes that there is an extensive anxiety network that can develop *selective* hypersensitivity toward *specific physical* sensations related to threshold changes mediated by the amygdalar-hippocampal complex. As a consequence, relatively minor internal or external stimuli can trigger a cascade that gives rise to anxiety symptoms. The effects of the amygdala on the prefrontal cortex appear to play a crucial role in the development of anticipatory anxiety, catastrophizing cognition, and phobic avoidance. Conversely, prefrontal effects on the amygdala can extinguish anxiety or panic reactions (11). Secondary avoidance behavior means that a distressing panic experience is never counterbalanced by the experience of toleration of a particular trigger and thus the perception of danger associated with the trigger is perpetuated. This means that the observation of situational triggers for many panic attacks is now usually attributed to context learning.

Generalized Anxiety Disorder in Patients with Epilepsy

One might expect a large number of patients with epilepsy to fulfill the DSM-IV criteria for generalized anxiety disorder (GAD). Contemplating the risks associated with their seizure disorder, many could experience "excessive anxiety and worry (apprehensive expectation), occurring more days than not for at least six months, about a number of events or activities." For this reason it was surprising that only 12% of 77 patients with medically refractory epilepsy we examined using the Structured Diagnostic Interview for the DSM-IV (SCID) were formally diagnosed with GAD (Trentowska M, Brandt C, Schöndienst M, in preparation). This suggests that there are factors that protect people who are persistently exposed to particular dangers from developing chronic anxiety.

Unfortunately, little research has focused on the causation, phenomenology, or processing of interictal anxiety in patients with epilepsy, and the neurobiologic or psychodynamic evidence base is slim. Hence, the following comments are based on the psychologic understanding of patients with GAD but no epilepsy.

One of the most striking neuropsychologic findings in GAD is that patients have a positive attentional bias to threatening stimuli or information (12). Patients also have a tendency to interpret neutral (but unclear or low-threshold) stimuli as threatening. This means that GAD patients face a constant barrage of anxiety-provoking perceptions and cognitions. These are processed in a specific, abstract, and incomplete way. Borkovec et al. showed that in their mental processing of fear, GAD patients mentally stop short of or shy away from imagining the

thing or issue that they are particularly fearful of (13). Instead, they have a tendency to launch into constantly renewed sequences of more abstract worry. From a psychodynamic point of view this characteristic combination of expectation-fear and tension represents cognitive avoidance. The resulting constant worry paradoxically perpetuates the patient's distressing anxiety. Supposing that GAD phenomenology in patients with epilepsy has an equivalent etiology, the provision of nonspecific reassurance or emotional support (or even constraints placed on activities) would be ineffective. Conversely, a detailed exploration and open verbalization of particular fears (such as fear of unpredictable falls, of loss of control in public, or of sudden death) could aid the cognitive processing of the specific issue and thereby reduce the issue's anxiogenic potential.

It should be noted that psychodynamic models and a cognitive-behavioral understanding of GAD are not mutually exclusive. The two approaches are complementary. Crits-Christoph et al. pointed out that patients with GAD often have a history of unstable personal relationships or traumatic experiences (14). On this background, patients develop central conflicts relating to reliability and avoidance. When these conflicts become acute, patients displace threatening cognitions to less anxiogenic domains of cognition and leave a residue of the damaging, fear-evoking thought content behind.

Obsessive-Compulsive Disorder in Patients with Epilepsy

Obsessive-compulsive disorder (OCD) is characterized by recurrent intrusive and unpleasant thoughts that may be combined with compulsive actions. It has been related to dysfunction in a number of brain areas including the limbic system, basal ganglia, and orbitofrontal region. OCD usually manifests as an inter- or postictal symptom; however, obsessive thoughts can occasionally be part of a temporal lobe aura as "forced thinking." The most comprehensive study of OCD in patients with epilepsy found no increased prevalence in IGE but identified clinical levels of obsessionality and compulsivity in 9 of 62 (14.5%) patients with temporal lobe epilepsy (versus 1.2% of 82 healthy controls) (15). The OCD risk was not related to epilepsy variables such as focus lateralization, choice of antiepileptic drug (AED), duration of epilepsy, or seizure frequency, but OCD was more common in patients with a previous history of depression.

The psychodynamic properties of obsessionality and compulsivity in patients with epilepsy have not been studied in detail. Interestingly, the study mentioned in the previous paragraph, and a number of other studies, have also indicated that patients with epilepsy have elevated scores on trait-measures of obsessionality. Janz formulated the marked difference he perceived in this respect between his patients with IGE and seizures on awakening and patients with focal epilepsy with sleep-related seizures in psychoanalytical terms: Patients with IGE were characterized by "denial of irrepressible aggressive tendencies"; that is, they "used the infantile defence mechanism of denial for the purpose of daily conflict management." In contrast, patients with focal seizures from sleep predominantly used "defence mechanisms of the so-called anankastic [obsessive compulsive] group," so that their "enechetic [orderly, particular, viscous] character should be understood as a control strategy for hate and aggressive tendencies" (9).

MULTIDIMENSIONAL THERAPEUTIC APPROACH

The preceding presentations of anxiety in patients with epilepsy show that the successful therapy of anxiety symptoms usually requires a multidimensional, and sometimes a multidisciplinary, approach.

Example 4. A 51-year-old woman had an episode of meningitis when she was 14. She had three generalized tonic-clonic seizures on awakening while aged 15 to 17, but she then achieved complete seizure control on phenytoin. When she was 40, she developed anxiety symptoms in supermarkets, which were diagnosed as panic attacks. Aged 50, she had two generalized tonic-clonic seizures in supermarkets that were preceded by "panic attacks." These seizures triggered an episode of major depression with anxiety symptoms:

Patient: since then I feel as if someone had extinguished my LIFE, this PHYsical exhaustion was immense. I had forgotten an awful lot and what do you call it eh . . . these word-finding difficulties and such like. and that is the problem, which I have now, yeah, to go out and feel safe, I'm afraid, of simply not managing the distance, but also afraid, of having a seizure, which causes problems, with going into shops, these lights.

Unexpectedly, an EEG did not support the clinical working diagnosis of postmeningitic symptomatic epilepsy but showed generalized 3-Hz spike-waves with photosensitivity. An ambulatory EEG recording demonstrated that neon lighting in supermarkets could trigger spike-wave paroxysms that were accompanied by panic symptoms. The spontaneous spike-wave activity and photosensitivity subsided after the AED treatment had been changed. During a repeat visit to the supermarket no ictal discharges were seen in an ambulatory EEG recording, but the patient continued to experience agoraphobic symptoms. These symptoms improved more gradually with repeat exposure ("in vivo exposition") on the one hand and psychodynamic psychotherapy on the other. The psychotherapy focused on this patient's low self-esteem, which had been reinforced since puberty by her family's persistent devaluation.

Understanding this patient's symptomatology required epileptological and psychodynamic expertise. It is unclear whether the development of "panic attacks" at the age of 40 was initially triggered by epileptic discharges (perhaps the problem had not manifested earlier in her life because of changes in lighting technology or shopping habits), or whether the epileptic discharges were triggered by panic symptoms (perhaps mediated by hyperventilation). It is evident that at the time of presentation the triggers, panic symptoms, and epileptic discharges were closely linked. The appropriate adjustment of antiepileptic therapy was not sufficient to control the panic attacks. Anxiety symptoms also failed to settle fully with exposure treatment. A satisfactory outcome was achieved only by additional treatment that aimed to increase the patient's resilience to anxiogenic stimuli or cognitions. In other words, the clinical approach to this patient's anxiety symptoms involved a number of distinct but interlinked components.

Optimizing Treatment for Epilepsy

Although the control of epileptic seizures may conversely increase fear and avoidance in some patients with seizure phobia, optimal seizure control represents a better basis for more specific treatments addressing pathological anxiety than ongoing seizures. This is most clearly evident after successful epilepsy surgery, which has been shown to be associated with a gradual decline in anxiety scores (16). Epilepsy surgery has also been reported to be helpful for obsessive-compulsive phenomena (1).

In fact, the benefits of optimized seizure control by the most appropriate treatment may well be more significant than any direct anxiolytic effects that have been reported in anxiety patients without epilepsy with a range of AEDs including gabapentin, pregabalin, tiagabine, vigabatrin, valproate, benzodiazepines, or barbiturates (1). What is more, any potential anxiolytic benefits related to AEDs may be outweighed by anxiety symptoms caused by toxicity. Side effects are particularly likely to cause anxiety if patients were not warned about them in advance. For instance, patients may become anxious when they develop paraesthesias with topiramate, zonisamide, acetazolamide, or sultiam. Lamotrigine, ethosuximide, or zonisamide can cause anxiety, sometimes in the context of insomnia and psychosis-like symptoms. Cognitive and memory deficits associated with most AEDs may give rise to concerns about a dementing process, although some patients with marked cognitive problems (such as those that may be seen with phenobarbitone or topiramate) can appear surprisingly unconcerned about their mnestic deficits.

Despite these provisos (and the absence of controlled studies proving the anxiolytic effects of AEDs in people with epilepsy), there may be circumstances in which one could choose an AED with anxiolytic potential in a patient with epilepsy who also has symptoms of an anxiety disorder. Although, as Example 4 demonstrates, it is rarely possible to alleviate anxiety symptoms satisfactorily with an adjustment of medication alone, GABAergic drugs in particular can reduce anxiety in animal experiments and clinical practice, and it seems reasonable to try and harness this "side effect" if the AED in question is also suitable for the patient's seizure disorder.

Psychologic Treatment

The psychologic treatment of anxiety in patients with epilepsy is not only the task of psychotherapists; it begins in the neurologic outpatient setting. Appropriate communication can help patients to process epilepsy-related fears and may alleviate anxiety. Anxiety can significantly reduce the effectiveness of verbal communication in the clinic setting. It may be helpful to back up information given at clinic visits with a letter, leaflets, or advice on sources of additional information. The support of epilepsy nurses can be invaluable. The psychologic models of panic disorder and generalized anxiety discussed in preceding sections both suggest that specific information, or the explicit discussion of the patient's particular fears, is more effective than general reassurance.

For patients who need more than basic information, support, and reassurance, more advanced psychologic interventions are useful (17). In fact, psychologic treatment may not only reduce psychologic symptoms and improve quality of life but also reduce the number of epileptic seizures. Psychotherapeutic strategies can be combined with pharmacological treatments, but successful treatment may require a close collaboration between epileptologist and psychotherapist.

Neurologists may find it difficult to engage some of their patients in a psychotherapeutic process. In our experience, patients with epilepsy find it more difficult to disclose avoidance or phobic cognitions than do patients with simple agora- or social phobias. A behavioral entry into a therapeutic relationship (for instance, the development of an anxiety hierarchy and exposition plan) is often a useful first step. But the exposition itself can reveal the complex background of ego-structural deficits or conflicts, which would be most appropriately targeted with focal psychodynamically oriented or even psychoanalytic therapy. These approaches would aim to reduce anxiety symptoms by increasing self-understanding, self-control, and reflexivity (i.e., the ability to reflect on one's own ways of thinking and be prepared to change them) (18).

Treatment with Medication

Although there are no studies of anxiolytic drug treatments in patients with epilepsy, there is a large body of evidence that has examined the effectiveness of pharmacological treatments in panic, obsessive–compulsive, and phobic anxiety disorders. The most important substances for the medical therapy of anxiety disorders are antidepressants, including selective serotonin reuptake inhibitors (SSRIs), serotonin and noradrenaline reuptake inhibitors, tricyclic antidepressants, reversible monoamine oxidase (MAO) inhibitors, benzodiazepines, and buspirone. The evidence for the use of these substances is not easy to summarize, but on the whole, treatment effect sizes of pharmacological treatment are similar to those of psychologic interventions, although pharmacological treatment is associated with a risk of drug dependence or symptom relapse on discontinuation of treatment (17). In addition, in patients with epilepsy, psychotropic medication is associated with a small risk of seizure exacerbation. This risk can be specified to some extent (see Table 27-2).

In practical terms, SSRIs are often chosen because of their advantageous side-effect profile, their relatively small effect on neuronal excitability, and their favorable pharmacokinetic properties with low potential for drug-drug interactions. The beneficial effects of SSRIs or tricyclic antidepressants is thought to be mediated by the effects of these medications on raphe nuclei and the locus coeruleus, which are involved in some of the downstream effects of the anxiety cascade. Benzodiazepines (e.g., clonazepam, alprazolam) are also very effective in anxiety disorders and clearly anticonvulsant,

TABLE 27-2
Risk of Seizures Associated with Drugs Prescribed for Anxiety Disorders (1).

Drug	Approximate Risk (%)
High risk (5% or higher risk of seizure)	
Chlorpromazine (high dose)	9
Medium risk (0.5–5% risk of seizure)	
Olanzapine	1
Quetiapine	1
Clomipramine (high dose)	1
Bupropion	0.5
Imipramine	0.5
Low risk (less than 0.5% risk of seizure)	
Risperidone	0.3
Venlafaxine	0.3
SSRIs	0.1
Mirtazepine	0.05

but they carry a risk of dependence. Buspirone, a partial agonist at the serotonin-1A-receptor, lowers the seizure threshold in animal experiments but (like the beta blocker propranolol) is considered as relatively safe in patients with epilepsy (1). Although almost all antidepressant drugs interact with different cytochrome P450 enzymes and therefore have the potential to interact with enzyme-inducing and enzyme-inhibiting AEDs, such interactions are rarely relevant in clinical practice.

CONCLUSIONS

In this chapter we have used our current physiologic, psychologic, and psychodynamic understanding to explore the topic of anxiety in people with epilepsy. This approach has not only challenged our ability to integrate some usually unconnected scientific views but has also demonstrated very clearly how deficient our understanding of anxiety remains in this context. However, these deficits should not serve as an excuse for clinicians and researchers to ignore this important area of epileptology.

We have demonstrated that anxiety symptoms are particularly hard to recognize in patients with epilepsy. The detection of anxiety symptoms is complicated by the coping strategies they elicit. Some of these strategies involve the collaboration of physicians—for instance, when the unpleasant affect is isolated by an over-rational approach to the patient's symptoms. What is more, patients and physicians find it difficult to distinguish between epilepsy- or treatment-related symptoms and psychopathology. Nevertheless, neuropsychiatrically oriented epileptologists should be able to appreciate the intensity of their patients' experience of threat, fear, or anxiety; to assess the potential contribution of ictal, organic, and pharmacological factors; and to recognize the intrapsychic filtering and defense processes that patients employ. The recognition and correct understanding of anxiety symptoms and the formulation of a therapeutic approach are likely to be facilitated if physicians look beyond the symptom level (avoidance behavior, phobic traits, somatic anxiety symptoms, catastrophizing cognitions, etc.) and take account of the influence of their patients' personality on symptoms and coping strategies.

Several studies have shown that anxiety is one of the most significant predictors of reduced health-related quality of life (HRQoL) in patients with epilepsy, explaining more of the variance in self-report measures than depression, seizure-related, clinical, or demographic variables. This means that addressing and alleviating anxiety symptoms could produce marked improvements in patients' quality of life. While our examples show why neurologists may have to be very attentive to identify patients' anxiety symptoms, they also demonstrate that patients' signals can be picked up by those who are willing to listen.

References

1. Beyenburg S, Mitchell A, Schmidt D, Elger CE, et al. Anxiety in patients with epilepsy: systematic review and suggestions for clinical management. *Epilepsy Behav* 2005; 7:161–171.
2. Swinkels WAM, Kuyk J, De Graaf EE, van Dyck R, et al. Prevalence of psychopathology in Dutch epilepsy inpatients: a comparative study. *Epilepsy Behav* 2001; 2:441–447.
3. OPD Task Force. Operationalized psychodynamic diagnostics: foundation and manual. Seattle, Toronto, Göttingen, Bern: Hogrefe & Huber, 2001.
4. Gray JA. The psychology of fear and stress. Cambridge, UK: Cambridge University Press, 1987.
5. Guelich E, Woermann FG, Rullkoetter N, Gerhards S, et al. Ictal fear versus panic attacks: first results from conversation analysis of clinical interviews. *Epilepsia* 2005; 46 (Suppl 6):343.
6. Newsom-Davis I, Goldstein LH, Fitzpatrick D. Fear of seizures: an investigation and treatment. *Seizure* 1998; 7:101–106.
7. Lehnertz K, Litt B. The first international collaborative workshop on seizure prediction. *Clin Neurophysiol* 2005; 116(3):489–588.
8. Kanner AM, Soto A, Gross-Kanner H. Prevalence and clinical characteristics of postictal psychiatric symptoms in partial epilepsy. *Neurology* 2004; 62:708–713.
9. Janz D. Die Epilepsien: spezielle Pathologie und Therapie. Stuttgart: Thieme, 1969.
10. Klein DF. False suffocation alarms, spontaneous panics, and related conditions: an integrative hypothesis. *Arch Gen Psychiatry* 1993; 50:306–317.
11. Goldmann-Rakic PS. The prefrontal landscape: implications for functional architecture for understanding human mentation and the central executive. *Philos Trans R Soc Lond B Biol Sci* 1996; 351:1445–1453.
12. Matthews A. Why worry? The cognitive function of anxiety. *Behav Res Ther* 1990; 28: 455–468.
13. Borkovec TD, Costello E. Efficacy of applied relaxation and cognitive-behavioral therapy in the treatment of generalized anxiety disorder. *J Consult Clin Psychol* 1993; 61:611–619.
14. Crits-Cristoph P, Connolly MB, Azarian K, Crits-Cristoph K, et al. An open trial of brief supportive-expressive psychotherapy in the treatment of generalized anxiety disorder. *Psychotherapy* 1996; 33:418–430.
15. Monaco F, Cavanna A, Magli E, Barbagli D, et al. Obsessionality, obsessive-compulsive disorder, and temporal lobe epilepsy. *Epilepsy Behav* 2005; 7:491–496.
16. Reuber M, Andersen B, Elger CE, Helmstaedter C. Depression and anxiety before and after temporal lobe epilepsy surgery. *Seizure* 2004; 13:129–135.
17. Roth A, Fonagy P. What works for whom? A critical review of psychotherapy research. New York: Guilford, 2005.
18. Schöndienst M. The role of psychotherapy in the treatment of epilepsies. In: Trimble M, Schmitz B, eds. *The Neuropsychiatry of Epilepsy*. New York: Raven Press, 2002: 313–322.

28 Biting Behavior as a Model of Aggression Associated with Seizures

Michelangelo Stanzani Maserati
Stefano Meletti
Gaetano Cantalupo
Federica Pinardi
Guido Rubboli
Antonio V. Delgado-Escueta
Carlo Alberto Tassinari

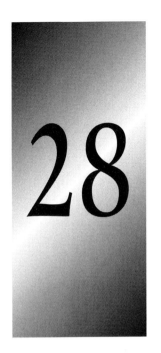

The relation between aggressive behaviors and epilepsy has been widely debated since the very first observations (1–3). The prevalence and incidence of this phenomenon in patients with epilepsy is still unknown (4), but it is more often related to frontal or temporal lobe brain pathology: 23% of patients show aggressiveness during a postictal psychosis after a temporal lobe seizure, while 5% display aggressive behaviors in interictal periods (5, 6). Patients with temporal lobe epilepsy (TLE) and episodes of interictal affective aggression ("intermittent explosive disorder") have been studied, revealing a reduction of frontal neocortical grey matter (7) or severe amygdala atrophy (5). These data suggest the presence of a distributed brain dysfunction in subjects displaying interictal episodes of aggressive behavior (5).

Three different types of aggressive behaviors have been distinguished on the basis of their relation to the seizure event: interictal, ictal, and postictal aggression (5, 8, 9). All three types are considered to be defensive, in that they are episodes of "reactive" aggression: they occur in the context of high emotional arousal, anger, or fear. For the ictal or postictal types of aggression, very few articles have provided clear and detailed descriptions of the nature and types of aggressive display shown by patients (1, 8, 10–14). In particular, ictal and postictal episodes of aggression have been rarely documented by means of direct video-electroencephalographic (EEG) recording (8). Ictal and postictal aggression has usually been reported when the patient is exhibiting undirected automatisms in a confused postictal state (9). In this setting, it has been observed that aggressive behaviors often occur in response to a minimally unpleasant stimulation and particularly in response to attempts to restrain the patient (13, 15). In fact, according to novel laboratory models, this type of aggression is presumed to be linked to a dramatic disruption of brain function associated with a strong emotional and autonomic hyperarousal (16).

Experimentally, the act of threatening or biting a prey, or a conspecific, has been extensively studied in animal behavioral research. W. R. Hess (17) first established that species-specific patterns of attack and defense, such as biting, could be brought out by direct stimulation of specific brain areas, specifically the diencephalic structures. Indeed, biting constitutes the prototypical display of cat and rat aggressive behavior and can be observed after direct stimulation of the hypothalamus (18, 19). Moreover, the act of biting is strongly affected by activity of temporolimbic structures acting on the hypothalamus. The hippocampus, the amygdala, and the frontal cortex can act in a complex manner on biting behavior (BB), facilitating or inhibiting it, depending on the stimulation site (20–23). In animals, biting has been observed in relation to spontaneous seizures, especially when the epileptic discharges involved the limbic system (24–28).

This chapter complements the previously quoted papers on violence and aggressive behaviors overall, confirming the results of Delgado-Escueta et al. (8). We will focus on seizure-related biting as a model for aggressive behavior, interpreting this behavior as particularly relevant in the context of our ethologic approach, which considers biting in relation to epileptic seizures in man as the emergence of innate behavior, not previously described.

The data are based on our paper (29) dealing with BB observed in eleven patients and on personal observations (four additional cases). The analysis of biting acts was performed on video-polygraphic recordings of seizures (over 60 hours) in patients with drug-resistant focal epilepsy undergoing presurgical evaluation. The data can be summarized as in the following paragraphs.

Incidence and Frequency

Spontaneous report of BB by the patient or the patient's relatives is rare. The spontaneous observation of biting by patients or relatives occurred in only three of our cases; actual effective biting with objective evidence (usually light skin snaps or painful ecchymosis) in their relatives occurred in two instances: in a wife and in a 7-year-old daughter (Tassinari, unpublished personal data).

Patients and relatives, when confronted with video evidence of the biting, recognized such behavior with some reluctance. One family admitted being aware of the biting but withdrew, at the last moment, permission to publish photos or part of the video showing BB. In one instance, BB was also directed to bedsheets, confirming the anamnestic data. In a second instance, the biting of a member of the family, previously unreported, was reluctantly admitted by the parents after video documentation.

Taking this into account, spontaneous report of BB underestimates the frequency of this behavior.

Ictal and Postictal Occurrence

BB occurred similarly during and after the seizure, with variable delay from seizure onset. Recall of BB was not investigated properly, nor was the subjective feeling of explanation for such behavior. In the majority of our cases we can say that the patients were amnesic for the

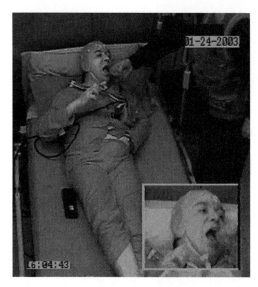

FIGURE 28-1

Postictal BB evoked by the intrusion of the examiner's hand in the patient's face and peripersonal space without touching the skin; patient 3 (29): 49-year-old male; MRI: right hippocampal sclerosis plus temporobasal focal cortical dysplasia. The intrusion was performed while the patient was presenting left-hand automatisms (genital grooming). Note the simultaneous reaching-grasping of the right arm/hand during the mouth opening.

episode when investigated. This should deserve further investigation, trying eventually to correlate the objective and subjective semiology and recall in seizures with and without BB in the same subject.

Triggering of the BB

Considering only the BB as observed by video documentation, we admit that the material is s-canty. It can allow, however, useful information for future research in the field.

1. BB occurred mostly as a reflex act when the examiner touched the patient's mouth-face region or by the intrusion of the examiner (usually the hands) in the space around the face/peripersonal space of the patient, without touching the skin (Figure 28-1).
2. Much less frequently, biting was directed toward the patient's hand or fingers or to the bedsheet, the handkerchief, or most inappropriately, to a thermometer (Figure 28-2).
3. While grasping to reach a moving target in the peripersonal space for biting it, the patient shows correct overall coordination between mouth opening, lip retraction, and hand grasping, with well-directed gaze and concomitant head and shoulder coordination.

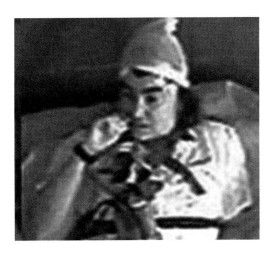

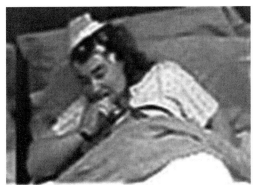

FIGURE 28-2

Ictal BB: (upper) The patient spontaneously bites the thermometer she was holding in the right hand before the beginning of a focal seizure arising from right temporal lobe structures; (lower) the same patient moves the right hand close to her mouth and bites her own fingers at the onset of another seizure. Patient 4 (29): 42-year-old female; MRI: right hippocampal sclerosis plus hypoplastic temporal lobe.

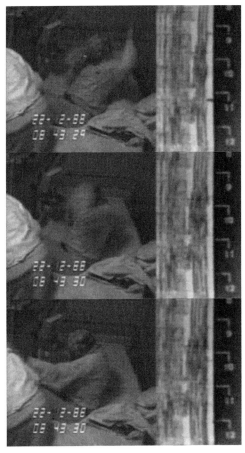

FIGURE 28-3

Ictal hitting and grabbing (sequence): The patient, while screaming, strikes and snatches the examiner who is trying to restrain his motor behavior. Patient 1 (29): 44-year-old male; MRI: right frontomesial focal cortical dysplasia.

AGGRESSIVE GESTURES AND FACIAL EXPRESSION CONCOMITANT TO BB

Clear violent behavior was documented during a seizure in a patient with diurnal and nocturnal hypermotor seizures (30, 31), likely related to a right frontomesial cortical dysplasia (Figure 28-3). Patient E. C. (44 years old at our observation) had a history of childhood seizures, misdiagnosed as psychiatric aggressive behavior either during school or later in life. For this reason he could not complete his education, and later he was repeatedly fired from places of employment for aggressive behaviors. On two occasions during a hospitalization, seizures were witnessed, and violent behavior involved two doctors. In one instance the female neurologist was grabbed in the corridor, falling with the patient;

in a second instance, during polygraphic recording, the patient started to grab the male doctor, holding him with repetitive grasping of the right arm, while with the left arm the patient repeatedly hit his head and shoulder. In both instances no serious harm was done; the patient did not remember the hitting behavior, and when confronted with the evidence he felt extremely embarrassed and displeased.

It is noteworthy that BB, in more than half of the instances, could be evoked or occurred when the patient had masticatory, lip smacking and chewing automatisms. This is suggestive of some contextual facilitation of the oromasticatory system (32), "prepared" or "ready" to respond actively (see discussion). Other than this single event described in the preceding paragraph, we did not observe any organized violent behavior in any recorded seizures, either with or without the presence of BBs.

Gestures and facial expressions with emotional valence were frequently observed ictally and postictally in

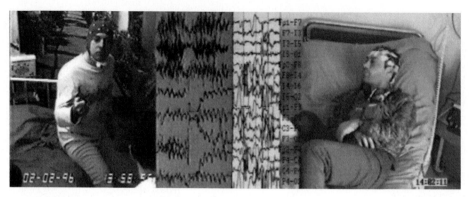

FIGURE 28-4

Postictal aggressive behaviors. (Left) The patient threatens the examiner with the fist while displaying an angry facial expression. Patient 8 (29): 34-year-old male; MRI: left temporopolar dysplasia. (Right) The patient abruptly kicks the examiner with his right leg, apparently lacking corresponding aggressive facial expression. 35-year-old male; MRI: left hippocampal sclerosis.

all patients. We found that (a) facial expression of anger, and especially aggressive arms/hands behaviors (i.e., to hit or threaten someone), were present in most patients and were displayed frequently; however, these gestures were never organized to result in a physical assault, but were rather fragmentary (Figure 28-4); (b) aggressive displays were frequently intermixed in the same patient and even in the same seizure event with other facial expressions such as fear or even happiness (33); (c) the relation between the expression of such facial and bodily gestures and the actions of the examiner could not be precisely quantified as done for biting acts. However, many of the facial expressions and hand behaviors displayed by the patient were clearly "evoked" by the action performed by the examiner on the patient.

In the majority of cases, we observed a particular attitude of the patient toward the persons in the environment. The patients did not appear to be angry; rather, they showed disappointment and frustration.

APPEARANCE, DURATION, AND DISAPPEARANCE OF THE BB

BB was not systematically looked for, and consequently in the majority of reflex BB we cannot precisely determine whether it already was present before our testing. In some instances of reflex BB we documented that it disappeared up to 10 to 20 seconds after the first evoked biting act.

In spontaneous BB the duration could be very short—so short as to be, in some instances, barely visible on real-time video inspection, becoming evident only with frame-by-frame video analysis, allowing recognition of the BB *a posteriori*. Similar features can be observed in spontaneous biting behavior as the expression of focal seizures in dogs (34; Figure 28-5).

ENDING OF THE SEIZURES WITH AGGRESSIVE BEHAVIORS OR BB

Schematically, based on video inspection and on the behavior of the patient interacting with the surroundings (examiner, surrounding people), we could describe two kinds of behaviors:

Sudden End. The patient quickly readapts to his surroundings, adjusting to his primitive normal position and looking as if almost nothing happened. Asked what he did or why he did it (eventually the BB), the patient answers without any apparent concern, almost as if what had just happened did not interest or concern him, or as if he "didn't do it." This behavior greatly puzzles the patient, even if the patient could recall and was conscious during the BB; the patient is surprisingly "cool"; he just performed it because "he had to do it" (see also discussion).

Only minutes later, or on being told about this behavior, the patient will say he is sorry, and displeased, apologizing for the "involuntary and yet conscious behavior!" (see discussion; 35).

Prolonged End. The second type can be quite different. The recovery is lengthy, with a waxing and waning of contact, with alternating degrees of memory impairment and embarrassment, interrupted at times by brief reappearances of oral and hand automatisms. The emotional expression switches from anxiety and avoidance toward a search of inappropriate, excessive positive emotional contact, with caresses or kisses; followed by an inappropriate jocular attitude intermixed with expression of embarrassment before recovery of full contact with the environment occurs. Memory for the episode is lost.

These two different modes of recovery usually distinguish two groups of seizure types: the first typically occurs with hypermotor seizures (31); the second occurs with

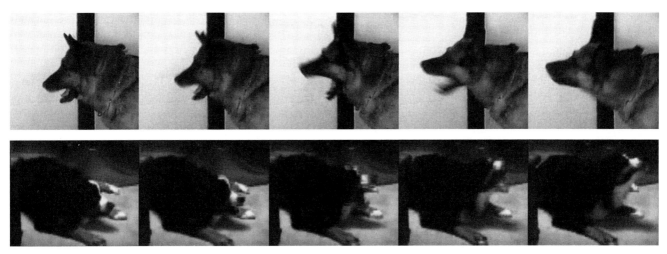

FIGURE 28-5

Epileptic ictal "fly-biting" behavior: the term is used by veterinary neurologists since the dog appears to be snapping at imaginary flies. Fly-biting is a recognized epileptic phenomenon (34). The upper filmstrip shows the sequence of a fly-snapping act in an epileptic dog treated with carbamazepine at the Department of Clinical Veterinary Medicine, University of Bologna (courtesy of Prof. G. Gandini and S. Cinotti). Note that the biting act is completed within 4 consecutive frames at 25 fps, so its duration is about 160 milliseconds. The lower filmstrip includes five consecutive frames from a video downloaded from http://www.canine-epilepsy.net within the "Fly-Biting" section by Dennis O'Brien, University of Missouri, College of Veterinary Medicine.

seizures originating in temporomesial structures, with diffuse-bilateral involvement of limbic structures (36).

GENDER DIFFERENCES IN THE EXPRESSION OF AGGRESSIVE GESTURES

We observed aggressive behaviors in eight male and three female subjects, and these data are consistent with those of the literature. Indeed, considering the patients described by Delgado-Escueta (8), eleven of 13 subjects were male, and a male predominance is also present in other publications on ictal/postictal aggression (2, 11, 13, 14). In patients with interictal affective aggression (TLE patients), intermittent explosive disorder, and other psychiatric conditions, a similar male sex preponderance for such behaviors has been reported (5, 7, 37, 38). Besides the different etiologies and contexts, aggressive behaviors observed during or after seizures and in the other mentioned conditions are considered *reactive* or *affective*: no planning occurs, behaviors occur during high emotional arousal, and afterward patients are remorseful and embarrassed.

AGGRESSIVE GESTURES AND FACIAL EXPRESSIONS

We frequently observed gestures and facial expressions with emotional valence during or after the seizures in all patients. We found that (1) facial expression of anger

and especially aggressive arms/hands behaviors (i.e., to hit or threaten someone) were present in most patients and were displayed frequently but without an organized assault; (2) expressions of fear or even happiness were frequently intermixed with aggressive displays in the same seizure event. Many of these facial expressions and hand behaviors displayed by the patient were clearly evoked by the action performed by the examiner on the patient.

ANATOMOELECTROCLINICAL CONSIDERATIONS

Our patients had heterogeneous etiologies and lesion locations. Only one of the patients had mesial TLE with evidence of isolated hippocampal sclerosis. Six of 11 subjects had evidence of lesions involving both the frontal and the temporal lobes, and three had MRI evidence of double pathology involving the temporal lobe (e.g., hippocampal sclerosis plus focal cortical dysplasia). Moreover, BB and related aggressive gestures were constantly observed when the ictal discharges involved the frontal and temporal regions.

Based on our observations, BB has no precise localizing or lateralizing value with respect to the site and side of seizure origin, but the appearance of this motor behavior is related to widespread and mainly bilateral dysfunction involving both the temporal and frontal regions. This is evident in the Stereo-EEG findings in one patient, who bit and grasped the examiner only during seizures in which the ictal discharge propagated to the ventromedial prefrontal cortex and the amygdala/hippocampal region of the right hemisphere. The same temporolimbic and prefrontal regions of the right hemisphere were reported to be involved in a patient described by Bartolomei et al. (39). These two patients showed a compulsive urge to bite something in association with high emotional arousal, fear, and agitation when ictal discharges involved the ventral prefrontal region. It is conceivable that dysfunction involving at least the mesial temporal and the prefrontal cortex is necessary for the expression of aggressive behaviors during or after seizures. These data support the hypothesis that the amygdalar-hippocampal region and the ventromedial prefrontal cortex are the critical regions whose involvement could be necessary and sufficient to lead to the overt expression of biting and of the other reported behaviors. This is consistent with current hypotheses about functional neuroanatomy of anger and aggression (40). In fact, these behaviors are hypothesized to be associated with dysfunction/hypofunction of the ventral prefrontal cortex, both in normal subjects and in different pathologic conditions (7, 38, 41, 42). Amygdalar pathology is thought to result in dysfunctional states of hyperarousal triggered by minor life events (5, 43). In cases of simultaneous frontal lobe pathology, impulsive aggressive behavior may result.

GENERAL CONCLUSION

The Nature of Biting and Role of the Patient's Peripersonal Space

Two conditions are necessary to observe BB in our subjects during a seizure: (1) An ictal discharge has to develop, disrupting frontotemporal limbic networks; (2) someone has to enter into the space near the patient and especially has to touch or simply carry out some activity in the space around the patient's face. This explains why these behaviors can be observed during as well as after the seizure, depending on when someone enters into close contact with the patient.

To evoke a reflex behavior, the patient's brain has (a) to detect that something, in many instances the hand of the examiner, is approaching him and especially his face; (b) to detect the exact space coordinates of the examiner's hand; and (c) to transform this sensory information into output, in this case, a brief (~600 ms) motor sequence constituting BB.

Occasionally, we observed a clear association of mouth and hand movements, suggesting the co-occurrence of a sort of grasping with the hand and mouth (Figure 28-1).

The neural correlates of these behaviors can be represented by structures that, both in other animals and in humans, have been demonstrated to encode the face and hand peripersonal space (44) and to select the appropriate motor response in accordance with the stimulus valence. Animal and human data demonstrate that the processing of space is not unitary but distributed among several brain areas. In monkeys, data showed that the premotor cortex (area 6), the putamen, and the ventral intraparietal area (VIP) are especially involved in the processing of the space near the body. In the monkey's premotor cortex many cells are bimodal; that is, they respond also to visual stimuli located in the space near their tactile receptive fields (45). Therefore in animals, multisensory neurons can control movements on the basis of both tactile and visual information coding the position of a stimulus relative to the hand, head, or both. This information can be used to perform simple actions such as avoiding a stimulus or reaching to grasp an object or bringing food to the mouth. Interestingly, and more relevant to the seizure-related behaviors observed in this study, several lines of evidence support the following: first, monkeys' premotor cortex can encode head movements, mouth grasping, and coordinated mouth/hand actions (46); and second, the neural structures involved in the evaluation of the peripersonal space and in the successive sensorimotor integration are outside the control of top-down influences, but rather are bottom-up processes (47). Indeed, it has been proposed that relatively automatic, fast, and encapsulated multisensory processing of nearby space might serve important primitive preservative functions and could represent an evolutionary advantage (47). Recent evidence supports the idea that multisensory-motor interfaces might encode defensive movements (48–50).

Seizures and Violence

Only one of our patients whom we analyzed (Figure 28-3) displayed violent behavior against another person, and the rarity of this phenomenon is in accordance with previous papers about aggression during or after seizures (3, 8, 11, 51). In the multicentric study performed by Delgado-Escueta to ascertain the relation and incidence of seizure-related aggression, only 13 subjects were identified out of 5,400 patients with epilepsy (8). Conversely, our behavioral analysis clearly showed that patients' behaviors are closely related to the actions of other subjects acting in the environment; therefore, the occurrence of some behavioral phenomena, such as the act of biting, could be underestimated. Attempts to restrain the patient's behavior are the most critical factor that promotes the progression of undirected aggressive displays to more organized violent behaviors (11).

Our results support the following inferences:

1. Aggressive behaviors resulting in physical violence toward persons (striking, stabbing people) are exceptional events.

2. Violence occurs exceptionally during epileptic seizures; second, postictal *confusion* "per se" cannot be generically related to violence.

3. Before one assumes that violent behavior is the manifestation of an epileptic seizure, direct recording of the presumed seizure-related violent act is required.

4. A clear distinction should be made between aggression during postictal psychosis and seizure-related behaviors.

NEUROETHOLOGICAL CONSIDERATIONS

Biting in man is viewed as an act of "aggression" resulting from a loss of self-control; in an epileptic seizure this same behavior is due to a transient dysfunction mainly of frontolimbic networks.

The BB, however, is expressed as a physiologic sequence of visual-hand-mouth coordination, as an "innate instinctive" behavior in defense of the peripersonal space, in most cases. BB can also be viewed as the expression of an "urge," a "need" directed not only to an intruder but also to inappropriate or dangerous objects (a glass thermometer, a bedsheet) or eventually to himself.

The patient sees what he is doing and cannot restrain from doing it. He is able to "pursue" the intruder's hand and grab it. The patient can see the objects without recognizing them. This can evoke the "psychic blindness" as described by Klüver and Bucy in animals with bilateral temporal lobectomy (52), which were apparently unable to recognize the meaning of objects by visual inspection.

A significant urge to bite and emotional hyperactivity characterize our patients as well as patients affected by Klüver-Bucy syndrome in the context of hyperorality (32, 53). The patient is in a condition, described by Caldecott-Hazard and Engel, in which "mental clouding could be viewed as a loss of cognitive and emotional responses that are normally attached to the perception of sensory stimuli," considering his postictal "ability to respond to stimuli without experiencing consciousness" (35). Biting, as we previously suggested for other motor sequences occurring in a variety of instances (29, 33, 36, 54–57), can result from "a loss of control" of higher centers on lower centers (namely the Central Pattern Generators networks) in a Jacksonian meaning and in agreement with the Jasper and Penfield view on epileptic automatisms as "paretic" phenomenon; that is, the expression of "loss of control" (58). This is also in accord with the theories of Tinbergen (59) and Lorentz (60), in which instinctive behavioral actions are triggered by sequences leading up to the final "consummatory act" (see also 61, 62). Biting, like other so-called "aggressive behaviors" related to an epileptic event, is not part of a plan originating from an intention to "go against another" to take advantage nor to first attack in order to prevent.

BB is above all a restricted, limited, involuntary and yet "necessary" self-defense behavior, sometimes self-directed. *Stricto sensu*, in this context, biting is not "aggression," which stems from Latin *aggredi*, compound of *ad* (toward) and *gradi* (to walk). We perfectly agree with the concept of Lorentz (63) and Eibl-Eibesfeldt (64), who propose that "aggressivity" in animals, as in man, is not synonymous with violence.

References

1. Schachter SC. Aggression in epilepsy. In: Kanner AM and Ettinger A, eds. *Psychiatric Issues in Epilepsy: A Practical Guide to Diagnosis and Treatment*. Second Edition. Baltimore: Wolters Kluwer/Lippincott Williams & Wilkins, 2007; 306–320.

2. Marsh L, Krauss GL. Aggression and violence in patients with epilepsy. *Epilepsy Behav* 2000; 1:160–168.

3. Rodin EA. Aggression and epilepsy. In: Riley TL, Roy A, ed. *Pseudoseizures*. Baltimore: Williams & Wilkins, 1982:185–212.

4. Alper KR, Barry JJ, Balabanov AJ. Treatment of psychosis, aggression and irritability in patients with epilepsy. *Epilepsy Behav* 2002; 3:S13–S18.

5. van Elst LT, Woermann FG, Lemieux L, et al. Affective aggression in patients with temporal lobe epilepsy: a quantitative MRI study of the amygdala. *Brain* 2000; 123:234–243.

6. Kanemoto K, Kawasaki J, Mori E. Violence and epilepsy: a close relation between violence and postictal psychosis. *Epilepsia* 1999; 40:107–109.

7. Woermann FG, van Elst LT, Koepp MJ, et al. Reduction of frontal neocortical grey matter associated with affective aggression in patients with temporal lobe epilepsy: an objective voxel by voxel analysis of automatically segmented MRI. *J Neurol Neurosurg Psychiatry* 2000; 68:162–169.

8. Delgado-Escueta AV, Mattson RH, King L, et al. Special report: the nature of aggression during epileptic seizures. *N Engl J Med* 1981; 305:711–716.

9. Treiman DM. Psychobiology of ictal aggression. *Adv Neurol* 1991; 55:341–356.

10. Ashford JW, Schulz C, Walsh GO. Violent automatism in a partial complex seizure: report of a case. *Arch Neurol* 1980; 37:120–122.

11. Rodin EA. Psychomotor epilepsy and aggressive behaviour. *Arch Gen Psychiatry* 1973; 28:210–213.

12. Saint-Hilaire JM, Gilbert M, Bouvier G, et al. [Epilepsy with aggressive behaviour: two cases with depth electrode recordings] (in French). *Rev Neurol (Paris)* 1981; 137:161–179.

13. Gerard ME, Spitz MC, Towbin JA, et al. Subacute postictal aggression. *Neurology* 1998; 50:384–388.

14. Janszky J, Rasonyia G, Szues A, et al. Subacute postictal aggressions. *Neurology* 1999; 52:221.

15. Borum R, Appelbaum KL. Epilepsy, aggression and criminal responsibility. *Psychiatr Serv* 1996; 47:762–763.

16. Haller J, Kruk MR. Normal and abnormal aggression: human disorders and novel laboratory models. *Neurosci Biobehav Rev* 2006; 30(3):292–303.

17. Hess WR. *The functional organization of the diencephalons*. New York: Grune & Stratton, 1957.

18. Wasman M, Flynn JP. Directed attack elicited from hypothalamus. *Arch Neurol* 1962; 6:220–227.

19. Flynn JP. Patterning mechanisms, patterned reflexes, and attack behavior in cats. *Nebr Symp Motiv* 1972; 20:125–153.

20. Block CH, Siegel A, Edinger H. Effects of amygdaloid stimulation upon trigeminal sensory fields of the lip that are established during hypothalamically elicited quiet biting attack in the cat. *Brain Res* 1980; 197:39–55.

21. Dalsass M, Siegel A. The bed nucleus of the stria terminalis: electrophysiological properties and responses to amygdaloid and hypothalamic stimulation. *Brain Res* 1987; 425: 346–350.

22. Edinger HM, Siegel A, Troiano R. Effect of stimulation of prefrontal cortex and amygdala on diencephalic neurons. *Brain Res* 1975; 97:17–31.

23. Siegel A, Edinger HM. Role of the limbic system in hypothalamically elicited attack behaviour. *Neurosci Biobehav Rev* 1983; 7:395–407.

24. Watson RE Jr, Edinger HM, Siegel A. An analysis of the mechanisms underlying hippocampal control of hypothalamically elicited aggression in the cat. *Brain Res* 1983; 269:327–375.

25. Wasman M, Flynn JP. Directed attack behavior during hippocampal seizures. *Arch Neurol* 1966; 14:408–414.

26. Pinel JP, Treit D, Rovner LI. Temporal lobe aggression in rats. *Science* 1977; 197:1088–1089.

27. Siegel A, Brutus M, Shaikh MB, et al. Effects of temporal lobe epileptiform activity upon aggressive behavior in the cat. *Int J Neurol* 1985; 19–20:59–73.

28. Griffith N, Engel J Jr, Bandler R. Ictal and enduring interictal disturbances in emotional behaviour in an animal model of temporal lobe epilepsy. *Brain Res* 1987; 400:360–364.

29. Tassinari CA, Tassi L, Calandra-Buonaura G, et al. Biting behavior, aggression, and seizures. *Epilepsia* 2005; 46:654–663.

30. Lüders HO, Acharya J, Baumgartner C, et al. Semiological seizure classification. *Epilepsia* 1998; 39:1006–1013.

31. Holthausen H, Hoppe M. Hypermotor seizures. In: Lüders HO, Noachtar S, eds. *Epileptic Seizures: Pathophysiology and Clinical Semiology*. New York: Churchill-Livingstone, 2000.

32. Janszky J, Fogarasi A, Magalova V, Tuxhorn I, et al. Hyperorality in epileptic seizures: periictal incomplete Klüver–Bucy syndrome. *Epilepsia* 2005; 46(8):1235–1240.

33. Tassinari CA, Gardella E, Rubboli G, et al. Facial expression of emotion in human frontal and temporal lobe epileptic seizures. *Ann N Y Acad Sci* 2003; 1000:393–394.

34. Heynold Y, Faissler D, Steffen F, Jaggy A. Clinical, epidemiological and treatment results of idiopathic epilepsy in 54 Labrador retrievers: a long-term study. *J Small Anim Pract* 1997; 38(1):7–14.

35. Caldecott-Hazard S, Engel J Jr. Limbic postictal events: anatomical substrates and opioid receptor involvement. *Prog Neuropsychopharmacol Biol Psychiatry* 1987; 11(4):389–418.

36. Tassinari CA, Gardella E, Meletti S, et al. The neuroethological interpretation of motor behaviours in "nocturnal-hyperkinetic-frontal seizures": emergence of "innate" motor behaviours and role of central pattern generators. In: Beaumanoir A, Andermann F, Chauvel P, Mira L, et al., eds. *Frontal Seizures and Epilepsies in Children*. London: John Libbey Eurotext, 2003:43–48.

37. Herzberg JL, Fenwick PB. The aetiology of aggression in temporal-lobe epilepsy. *Br J Psychiatry* 1988; 153:50–55.

38. Best M, Williams JM, Coccaro EF. Evidence for a dysfunctional prefrontal circuit in patients with an impulsive aggressive disorder. *Proc Natl Acad Sci U S A* 2002; 99: 8448–8453.

39. Bartolomei F, Guye M, Wendling F, et al. Fear, anger and compulsive behavior during seizure: involvement of large scale fronto-temporal neural networks. *Epileptic Disord* 2002; 4:235–241.

40. Davidson RJ, Putnam KM, Larson CL. Dysfunction in the neural circuitry of emotion regulation: a possible prelude to violence. *Science* 2000; 289:591–594.

41. Raine A, Lencz T, Bihrle S, et al. Reduced prefrontal gray matter volume and reduced autonomic activity in antisocial personality disorder. *Arch Gen Psychiatry* 2000; 57: 119–127.

42. Pietrini P, Guazzelli M, Basso G, et al. Neural correlates of imaginal aggressive behavior assessed by positron emission tomography in healthy subjects. *Am J Psychiatry* 2000; 157:1772–1781.

43. van Elst LT, Trimble MR, Ebert D. Dual brain pathology in patients with affective aggressive episodes. *Arch Gen Psychiatry* 2001; 58:1187–1188.

44. Ladavas E, Zeloni G, Farne A. Visual peripersonal space centered on the face in humans. *Brain* 1998; 121:2317–2326.

45. Rizzolatti G, Scandolara C, Matelli M, et al. Afferent properties of periarcuate neurons in macaque monkeys, II: visual responses. *Behav Brain Res* 1981; 2:147–163.

46. Rizzolatti G, Luppino G, Matelli M. The organization of the cortical motor system: new concepts. *Electroencephalogr Clin Neurophysiol* 1998; 106:283–296.

47. Farne A, Dematte ML, Ladavas E. Beyond the window: multisensory representation of peripersonal space across a transparent barrier. *Int J Psychophysiol* 2003; 50:51–61.

48. Cooke DF, Graziano MS. Sensorimotor integration in the precentral gyrus: polysensory neurons and defensive movements. *J Neurophysiol* 2004; 91:1648–1660.

49. Graziano MS, Taylor CS, Moore T. Complex movements evoked by microstimulation of precentral cortex. *Neuron* 2002; 34:841–851.

50. Graziano MS, Taylor CS, Moore T, et al. The cortical control of movement revisited. *Neuron* 2002; 36:349–362.

51. Ramani V, Gumnit RJ. Intensive monitoring of epileptic patients with a history of episodic aggression. *Arch Neurol* 1981; 38:570–571.

52. Kluver H, Bucy PC. Psychic blindness and other symptoms following bilateral temporal lobectomy in rhesus monkeys. *Am J Physiol* 1937; 119:352–353.

53. Karli P. *L'homme aggressif*. Paris: Odile Jacob eds, 1970.

54. Meletti S, Cantalupo G, Stanzani-Maserati M, et al. The expression of interictal, preictal, and postictal facial-wiping behavior in temporal lobe epilepsy: a neuro-ethological analysis and interpretation. *Epilepsy Behav* 2003; 4:635–643.

55. Meletti S, Cantalupo G, Volpi L, et al. Rhythmic teeth grinding induced by temporal lobe seizures. *Neurology* 2004; 62:2306–2309.

56. Tassinari CA, Meletti S, Gardella E, et al. Emergence de comportements moteurs innes communs aux crises frontales nocturnes et au parasomnies. In: Amann JP, Chiron C, Dulac O, Fagot-Largeault A, eds. *Épilepsie Connaissance du Cerveau et Société*. Laval, France: Les Presses, 2006:81–91.

57. Tassinari CA, Rubboli G, Gardella E, et al. Central pattern generators for a common semiology in fronto-limbic seizures and in parasomnias: a neuroethologic approach. *Neurol Sci* 2005; 26:s225–s232.

58. Jasper HH. Some physiological mechanisms involved in epileptic automatisms. *Epilepsia* 1964; 23:1–20.

59. Tinbergen N. *The study of instinct*. London: Oxford University Press; 1969.

60. Lorentz K. *Vergleichende Verhaltensforschung: Grundlagen der Ethologie*. Vienna: Springer, 1978.

61. Eibl-Eibesfeldt I. *Grundriß der vergleichenden Verhaltensforschung*. München: R. Piper & Co., 1987.

62. Eibl-Eibesfeldt I. *Krieg und Frieden aus der Sicht der Verhaltensforschung*. München: Piper & Co., 1983.

63. Lorentz K. *Das sogenannte Böse: zur Naturgeschichte der Aggression*. Vienna: Borotha Schöler, 1963.

64. Eibl-Eibesfeldt I. *Liebe und Hass*. München: Piper, 1970.

29 Psychoses and Forced Normalization

Bettina Schmitz
Michael Trimble

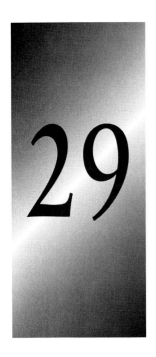

ompared to affective disorders, psychoses are rare complications in epilepsy, affecting about 4–6% of patients in clinical case series. Among the various types of psychoses, those occurring in a direct relationship to seizures are most common. The most common type of psychosis in epilepsy is postictal psychosis. Psychoses without a clear relationship to seizures—so-called interictal psychoses—may develop after several years of active epilepsy, most often of the temporal lobe type. Despite some psychopathological peculiarities, these psychoses resemble a chronic schizophrenia-like illness, and recent findings suggest subtle underlying limbic pathology, analogous to similar observations in "endogenous" schizophrenia. Psychoses can also be triggered by antiepileptic drugs (AEDs). Drugs that have strong anticonvulsive properties, especially, may trigger psychotic reactions. Some of these psychoses may be considered toxic, because they are often dose related. Psychoses that are associated with seizure freedom and electroencephalographic (EEG) normalization are covered by the terms "forced normalization" and "alternative psychosis." Although seizure control is often associated with milder behavioral problems, emotional instability, or insomnia, psychotic reactions are relatively rare. A precise etiological classification of psychoses, considering the biographical or genetic predisposition for

psychiatric problems, recent treatment changes, seizure frequency, and EEG activity as well as psychosocial stressors, is clinically very important, because therapeutic strategies are very different depending on the individual situation.

EPIDEMIOLOGY

Stefansson (1), in a case control study, compared the prevalence of nonorganic psychiatric disorders in patients with epilepsy to the prevalence among those with other somatic diseases, the groups being taken from a disability register in Iceland. Although the difference in psychiatric diagnoses overall was not significant, there was a higher rate of psychoses, particularly schizophrenia and paranoid states, among males with epilepsy.

Qin et al. (2), in a study from Denmark, confirmed the increased risk of schizophrenia and schizophrenia-like psychoses in epilepsy, and in this study a family history of psychoses and a family history of epilepsy were significant risk factors for psychosis. Bredkjaer et al. (3), in a record linkage study, looked for associations between epilepsy from the national patient register of Denmark and the equivalent psychiatric register. The incidence of nonorganic, nonaffective psychoses, which included schizophrenia and schizophrenia-spectrum disorders, was significantly increased in epilepsy even when patients with learning disability or substance abuse were excluded.

Higher prevalence rates for psychoses were found in studies of much more selected populations, such as hospital case series. Thus, Gureje (4), in patients attending a neurologic clinic, quoted that 37% of patients were psychiatric cases and that 29% of these were psychotic. Mendez et al. (5), in a retrospective investigation, reported that interictal psychotic disorders were found in over 9% of a large cohort of patients with epilepsy, in contrast to just over 1% in patients with migraine. Studies from Japan examining new referrals for epilepsy quote a 6% prevalence of psychoses in those with normal intelligence (in contrast to 24% in those with learning disability) (6).

CLASSIFICATION

There is no internationally accepted syndromic classification of psychoses in epilepsy. For pragmatic reasons, it remains convenient to group psychoses in epilepsy according to their temporal relationship to seizures.

Syndromes of Psychoses in Relation to Seizure Activity

The various syndromes are described in Table 29-1. The ictal psychoses are more likely to be linked to simple or complex partial seizure status than to absence status, but have never been examined in any detail. In clinical practice they are most frequently seen with seizures of temporal lobe origin, but some are secondary to frontal lobe seizures. Simple focal status or aura continua may cause complex hallucinations, thought disorders, and affective symptoms. The continuous epileptic activity is restricted and may escape scalp EEG recordings. Insight usually is maintained, and true psychoses emerging from such a state have not been described. Nonconvulsive status epilepticus requires immediate treatment with intravenous AEDs.

Postictal Psychoses

Most postictal psychoses are precipitated by a series or status of secondary generalized tonic-clonic seizures. More rarely, psychoses occur after single "grand mal" seizures or following a cluster of complex partial seizures (7). In the elderly a postictal psychosis may be the first presentation of a new-onset epilepsy disorder.

Postictal psychoses account for approximately 25% of psychoses in epilepsy. The relationship to the type of epilepsy is not clear. Dongier (8, 9) described a preponderance of generalized epilepsies, and Logsdail and Toone (10) noted a higher frequency of postictal psychosis in patients with focal epilepsies and complex focal seizures. One of the more comprehensive studies has been that of Kanemoto (11), and his distinctions between postictal and interictal psychoses are shown in Table 29- 2. Essentially, the postictal psychoses occur with later age of onset of epilepsy and at a later age than the interictal psychoses do. They are significantly associated with temporal lobe epilepsy, complex partial seizures, and temporal plus extratemporal structural lesions on magnetic resonance imaging (MRI). Patients are less likely to have learning disability and are less likely to have generalized

---

TABLE 29-1
Clinical Characteristics of Psychoses in Relation to Seizure Activity

	INTERICTAL	ICTAL	POSTICTAL	PARICTAL	ALTERNATIVE
Relative frequency	~20%	~10%	~50%	~10%	~10%
Consciousness	Normal	Impaired	Impaired or normal	Impaired	Normal
Typical features	Schizophrenia-like psychopathology	Mild motor symptoms	Lucid interval	Occurs often during presurgical evaluation	Initial symptom insomnia
Duration	Months	Hours to days	Days to weeks	Days to weeks	Weeks
EEG	Unchanged	Status epilepticus	Increased slowing, increased epileptic	Increased slowing, increased epileptic	Normalized
Primary treatment	Antipsychotics	AEDs intravenous	Benzodiazepines, seizure control	Benzodiazepines, seizure control	Sleep regulation, reduction of AEDs

TABLE 29-2
Significant Differences between Postictal (PIP) and Interictal Psychoses (IIP)

	PIP (*n* = 45)	IIP (*n* = 126)
Reduced intelligence (<70 IQ)	4	39
Complex partial seizures	37	84
Déjà vu aura*	10/43	10/103
Temporal MRI lesion	16	25
Temporal lobe epilepsy	39	74
Generalized spike waves	1	21
Age at epilepsy onset (years)	16	11
Age at psychosis onset (years)	35	25
Interval between onset of epilepsy and psychosis (years)	18	13

* Calculated for the subgroup of patients with focal epilepsies.

spike wave abnormalities on the EEG. Kanemoto also noted an association with déjà vu auras (11). Others have suggested an association between ictal fear and postictal psychosis (12).

A characteristic lucid interval is described in most patients, during which time the mental state appears to be normal. This interval can last from 1 to 6 days between the epileptic seizures and onset of psychosis (13). Failure to appreciate the presence of this lucid interval can lead to a misdiagnosis of this condition.

The psychopathology of postictal psychosis is polymorphic, but most patients present with abnormal mood and paranoid delusions (10). Some patients are confused throughout the episode; others present with fluctuating impairment of consciousness and orientation; and sometimes there is no confusion at all. Dominant are delusions of grandiosity and religiosity, often associated with an elevated mood when compared with interictal psychoses. Patients may also be anxious, and a typical symptom is fear of impending death. Because patients often have a clear sensorium and may receive command hallucinations if the latter relate to violence or suicide, it is during such states that violent attacks on the self or others may occur (14).

The EEG during postictal psychosis is usually deteriorated, with increased epileptiform as well as slow-wave activity; but there are few reliable studies, since people with acute psychoses are difficult to examine.

The psychotic symptoms spontaneously remit within days or weeks, often without need for psychotropic drug treatment. However, in some cases, chronic psychoses develop from recurrent and even a single postictal psychosis (10, 15). This is estimated to occur in about 25% of cases.

The pathophysiology is not known. Savard et al. (12) noted the clinical analogy of psychoses following complex partial seizures to other postictal phenomena such as Todd's paresis or postictal memory loss. Logsdail and

Toone (10) hypothesized that postictal psychosis results from increased postsynaptic dopamine sensitivity. Ring et al. (16) tested this hypothesis using single-photon emission computed tomography (SPECT) and the D2 ligand [^{123}I]iodobenzamide ([^{123}I]IBZM). They noted that patients with epilepsy and psychoses had decreased binding to the ligand, suggesting that there was increased release of endogenous dopamine in the psychotic state. Kanemoto (11) suggested that a restricted limbic status epilepticus was involved, but limited functional imaging studies produced contradictory results (17).

Parictal Psychosis

Most authors do not distinguish parictal and postictal psychoses. In parictal psychosis, psychotic symptoms develop gradually and parallel to increases in seizure frequency. The relationship to seizures is easily overlooked if seizure frequency is not carefully documented over prolonged periods. More rapid development of parictal psychoses can be seen, especially during the presurgical assessment of patients with intractable epilepsy, when a series of epileptic seizures may be provoked by withdrawal of AEDs. Impairment of consciousness is more frequent than in classical postictal psychosis.

Interictal Psychoses

Interictal psychoses occur between seizures (or, better, independently of seizures) and cannot directly be linked to the ictus. They are less frequent than peri-ictal psychoses (including preictal, ictal, parictal, and postictal psychoses) and account for 10–30% of diagnoses in unselected case series (9). Interictal psychoses are, however, clinically more significant in terms of severity and duration than are peri-ictal psychoses, which usually are brief and self-limiting.

In the early studies by Slater et al. it was stated that, in the absence of epilepsy, the psychoses in their study group would have been diagnosed as schizophrenia. The frequent presence of Schneiderian first-rank symptoms was noted (18). However, there have been persistent arguments as to the exact relationship between the two disorders and the phenomenology of the interictal epileptic psychoses. Slater maintained there was a distinct difference between schizophrenia and the schizophrenia-like psychoses associated with epilepsy, and he highlighted the preservation of affect, a high frequency of delusions and religious mystical experiences, and few motor symptoms.

Other authors have stressed the rarity of negative symptoms and the absence of formal thought disorders and catatonic states (19). McKenna et al. (20) pointed out that visual hallucinations were more prominent than auditory hallucinations. Tellenbach (21) stated that delusions were less well organized, and Sherwin (22) remarked that neuroleptic treatment was less frequently necessary. There have been other authors, however, who denied any clear psychopathologic differences between epileptic psychosis and schizophrenia.

Using the Present State Examination and the CATEGO computer program, which is a semi-standardized and validated method for quantifying psychopathology, it has been possible to compare the presentation of psychosis in epilepsy with process schizophrenia. Very few significant differences emerged from such studies (23), which suggests that, assuming that the patients are representative, a significant number will have a schizophrenia-like presentation, virtually indistinguishable from schizophrenia in the absence of epilepsy.

Phenomenology apart, Slater argued that long-term prognosis of psychosis in epilepsy was better than that in process schizophrenia. In a follow-up study on his patients, he found that chronic psychotic symptoms tended to remit, and personality deterioration was rare (24). Other authors have also described the outcome to be more favorable and long-term institutionalization to be less frequent than in schizophrenia (22). Unfortunately, there have been no longitudinal studies comparing the long-term outcome of psychosis in epilepsy and process schizophrenia.

Risk Factors

The pathogenesis of psychotic episodes in epilepsy is likely to be heterogeneous. In most patients, a multitude of chronic and acute factors can be identified that are potentially responsible for the development of a psychiatric disorder. These factors are difficult to investigate in retrospect, and the interpretation of them as either causally related or simply intercorrelated is arguable.

The literature on risk factors is highly controversial; studies are difficult to compare because of varying definitions of the epilepsy, the psychiatric disorder, and the investigated risk factors. Most studies are restricted to interictal psychoses.

Genetic Predisposition. With few exceptions (2), most authors did not find any evidence for an increased rate of psychiatric disorders in relatives of epilepsy patients with psychoses (25). This was one reason why Slater suggested that these psychoses were truly symptomatic, a representative phenotype of the genotype.

Sex Distribution. There has been a bias toward female sex in several case series, but this has not been confirmed in controlled studies (26, 27).

Duration of Epilepsy. The interval between age at onset of epilepsy and age at first manifestation of psychosis has been remarkably homogeneous, in the region of 11 to 15 years, in many series (28). This interval has been used to postulate the etiologic significance of the seizure disorder and a kindling-like mechanism. However, some authors (29) have argued that the supposedly specific interval represents an artifact. They have drawn attention to the wide range, with a significantly shorter interval in patients with later onset of epilepsy. They also have pointed out that patients whose psychoses did not succeed their epilepsy were excluded in most series, and that there is a tendency in the general population for the age of onset of epilepsy to have an earlier peak than that of schizophrenia.

Type of Epilepsy. There is a clear excess of temporal lobe epilepsy (TLE) in almost all case series of patients with epilepsy and psychosis. Among the pooled data of ten studies, 217 (76%) of 287 patients suffered from TLE (28).

The nature of a possible link of psychoses to TLE is, however, not entirely clear, partly because of ambiguities in the definition of TLE in the literature, based on either seizure symptomatology (e.g., psychomotor epilepsy), involvement of specific functional systems (e.g., limbic epilepsy), or anatomic localization as detected by depth EEG or neuroimaging (e.g., amygdalohippocampal epilepsy). Unfortunately, most authors have not sufficiently differentiated frontal and temporal lobe epilepsy.

The temporal lobe hypothesis has further been criticized for being based on uncontrolled case series, such as in the studies by Gibbs (30) and Slater and Beard (31). It was argued that TLE is the most frequent type of epilepsy in the general population and that there is an overrepresentation of this type of epilepsy in patients attending specialized centers.

Comparing psychosis rates in TLE and in idiopathic generalized epilepsy, some studies (32) note significant differences in the frequency of psychoses in temporal lobe epilepsy, but several do not (29). However, many patients with generalized epilepsy show pathology of temporal structures, making classification difficult, and, again, many reports lack the sophisticated brain imaging that is now required for such hypotheses to be tested.

There are several studies showing that psychoses in generalized epilepsies differ from psychoses in TLE (28). The former are more likely to be of short duration and confusional. Alternative psychoses, which are relatively common in generalized epilepsy, are usually mild and often remit before any development of paranoid-hallucinatory symptoms. Schneiderian first-rank symptoms and chronicity are more frequent in patients with TLE. This has considerable significance for psychiatrists attempting to unravel the underlying "neurology" of schizophrenia, and the findings from epilepsy were instrumental in altering the view of schizophrenia away from a psychosocial to a biological model.

There is a general consensus that psychoses are less common in patients with neocortical extratemporal epilepsies (33). Adachi (26) suggested that psychoses in patients with frontal lobe epilepsy may be overlooked because of a differing psychopathology, hebephrenic symptoms in particular dominating the presentation.

Type of Seizures. There is evidence from several studies that focal seizure symptoms that indicate ictal mesial temporal or limbic involvement are overrepresented in patients with psychosis. Hermann and Chabria (34) noted a relationship between ictal fear and high scores on paranoia and schizophrenia scales of the Minnesota Multiphasic Personality Inventory (MMPI). Kristensen and Sindrup (27) found an excess of dysmnesic and epigastric auras in their psychotic group. They also reported a higher rate of ictal amnesia. In another controlled study, ictal impairment of consciousness was related to psychosis, but simple seizure symptoms indicating limbic involvement were not (35).

No seizure type is specifically related to psychosis in generalized epilepsies. Most patients with psychosis and generalized epilepsies have absence seizures (9).

Severity of Epilepsy. The strongest risk factors for psychosis in epilepsy are those that indicate severity of epilepsy (28). These are long duration of active epilepsy, multiple seizure types, history of status epilepticus, and poor response to drug treatment. Seizure frequency, however, is reported by most authors to be lower in psychotic epilepsy patients than in nonpsychotic patients (36). It has not been clarified whether seizure frequency was low before or during the psychotic episode. This may represent a variant of forced normalization (see subsequent discussion).

Laterality. Left lateralization of temporal lobe dysfunction or temporal lobe pathology as a risk factor for

schizophreniform psychosis was originally suggested by Flor-Henry (25). Studies supporting the laterality hypothesis have been made using surface EEG, depth electrode recordings, computed tomography, neuropathology, neuropsychology, and positron emission tomography (PET), and more recently with MRI. The earlier literature has been summarized by Trimble (28). In a synopsis of 14 studies with 341 patients, 43% had left, 23% right, and 34% bilateral abnormalities. This is a striking bias toward left lateralization. However, lateralization of epileptogenic foci was not confirmed in all controlled studies (32). Again, it may be that certain symptoms rather than any syndrome are associated with a specific side of focus. Trimble pointed out that a specific group of hallucinations and delusions, defined by Schneider and referred to as first-rank symptoms, which usually (but by no means exclusively) signifies schizophrenia (28), may be relevant. He suggested that these may be signifiers of temporal lobe dysfunction, representing as they do disturbances of language and symbolic representation. In this sense he equated then to a Babinski sign for a neurologist; that is, as pointing to a location and lateralization of an abnormality in the central nervous system.

These laterality findings have received support from brain imaging studies, especially SPECT and MRI. Mellers et al. (37), using a verbal fluency activation paradigm and [^{99m}Tc]hexamethylpropylene amine oxime ([^{99m}Tc]HMPAO) SPECT, compared patients with schizophrenia-like psychoses of epilepsy ($n = 12$), with schizophrenia ($n = 11$), and with epilepsy and no psychoses ($n = 16$). The psychotic epilepsy patients showed lower blood flow in the superior temporal gyrus during activation than the other two groups. Using MR spectroscopy, Maier et al. (38) were able to compare hippocampal-amygdalar volumes and hippocampal N-acetyl aspartate (NAA) levels in patients with TLE and schizophrenia-like psychoses of epilepsy ($n = 12$), TLE and no psychoses ($n = 12$), schizophrenia and no epilepsy ($n = 26$), and matched normal controls ($n = 38$). The psychotic patients showed significant left-sided reduction of NAA, and this was more pronounced in the psychotic epilepsy group. Regional volume reductions were noted bilaterally in this group, and in the left hippocampus-amygdala in the schizophrenic group.

Flugel et al. (39) have recently examined 20 psychotic and 20 nonpsychotic cases with temporal lobe epilepsy using magnetization transfer imaging. They reported significant reductions of the magnetization transfer ratio (an index of signal loss) in the left superior and middle temporal gyri in the psychotic patients; this was unrelated to volume changes and best revealed in a subgroup with no focal MRI lesions.

Structural Lesions. The literature on brain damage and epileptic psychosis is very controversial. Some authors have suggested a higher rate of pathologic neurologic examinations, diffuse slowing on the EEG, and mental retardation (27, 40), but others could not find an association with psychosis (41). Neuropathologic studies of resected temporal lobes from patients with TLE have suggested a link between psychosis and the presence of cerebral malformations, such as hamartomas and gangliogliomas, as compared with mesial temporal sclerosis (42). These findings have been seen as consistent with findings of structural abnormalities, arising during fetal development, in the brains of schizophrenic patients without epilepsy.

Bruton (43) noted enlarged ventricles, periventricular gliosis, and an excess of acquired focal damage in brains of institutionalized psychotic epileptic patients compared with nonpsychotic controls. That study also reported that schizophrenia-like psychoses were distinguished by an excess of perivascular white matter softenings.

In a study specifically looking at hippocampal and amygdala volumes, Tebartz van Elst and colleagues (44) examined 26 patients with epileptic psychoses, 24 with temporal lobe epilepsy and no psychosis, and 20 healthy controls. The psychotic patients had significantly increased amygdala sizes in comparison with the other two groups, which was bilateral, not related to the laterality of the focus, or length of epilepsy history. No hippocampal differences were noted in this study. In a complementary study on the same groups, Rüsch et al. (45) were unable to find any neocortical volumetric differences.

Although the underlying pathology may be different, the absence of gliosis in the hippocampus and related structures characterizing schizophrenia, the site of the pathology, the timing of the lesions, and the consequent functional changes in the brain may all be crucial to the later development of any behavior changes in both epilepsy and schizophrenia. Thus, the behavior changes should be viewed as an integral part of the process of epilepsy that are manifest in some patients. However, the recent evidence, especially from brain imaging studies, suggests that Slater's original hypothesis was part right but part wrong. Thus, the interictal psychoses seem different from schizophrenia, especially with regards to the admixture with affective symptoms and the long-term prognosis. While hippocampal changes may relate to both disorders, the increased amygdala size (bilateral and around 17–20%) and the lesser volumetric changes in the hippocampus suggest that the two psychopathological states are biologically quite different. While the laterality findings with regards to the functioning of the left hemisphere seem to hold up, the data point away from fundamentally cortical abnormalities in these psychoses and bring the amygdala and related structures to the center of interest in pathogenesis.

FORCED NORMALIZATION

At the beginning of the twentieth century, reports appeared that suggested there was some kind of antagonism between epilepsy and psychosis. This was one of the reasons that led von Meduna to introduce convulsive therapy for the treatment of schizophrenia. In the 1950s, Landolt (46) published a series of papers on patients with epilepsy who became psychotic when their seizures were under control. He defined *forced normalization* thus: "Forced normalisation is the phenomenon characterised by the fact that, with the recurrence of psychotic states, the EEG becomes more normal, or entirely normal, as compared with previous and subsequent EEG findings." Forced normalization was thus essentially an EEG phenomenon. The clinical counterpart of patients becoming psychotic when their seizures came under control, and their psychosis resolving with return of seizures, was referred to as *alternative psychosis* by Tellenbach (21).

These phenomena have now been well documented clinically. The following are important to note, however. First, the EEG does not need to become "normal," but the interictal epileptiform disturbances decrease and in some cases disappear. Second, the clinical presentation need not necessarily be a psychosis. In childhood or in the mentally handicapped, aggression and agitation are common. Other manifestations include psychogenic nonepileptic seizures or other conversion symptoms, depression, mania, and anxiety states. Some patients experience some irritability and insomnia, which may either spontaneously resolve or develop into a psychotic state. Third, the disturbed behavior may last days or weeks. It is often terminated by a seizure, and the EEG abnormalities then return. Fourth, Landolt originally associated this phenomenon with focal epilepsies, but with the introduction of the succinimide drugs, he noted an association with the generalized epilepsies. Certainly, forced normalization may be provoked by the administration of anticonvulsants and has been reported with almost all AEDs. Drugs that have a higher propensity to control seizures even in pharmacoresistant patients, such as vigabatrin, topiramate, and levetiracetam of the newer AED generation, are associated with an increased risk to induce forced normalization (47, 48, 49).

Fifth, it is unlikely that forced normalization occurs at the beginning of an epileptic disorder. Most patients develop psychotic reactions only when seizures are switched off following many years of active epilepsy. It was therefore hypothesized that molecular effects of long-term epilepsy, such as dopaminergic hypersensitization, play a role (50).

The literature on antagonism between epilepsy and psychosis has been held to be incompatible with the suggestion, outlined in preceding sections, that there is an increased association between epilepsy and psychosis. This has been resolved by more careful understanding of the original literature. Thus, within the association or link between psychosis and epilepsy, there may be an antagonism of symptoms between seizures and the symptoms of psychosis. It is the longitudinal course of the disorders that has to be followed, and forced normalization, as opposed to alternative psychosis, requires serial EEG recordings before the diagnosis can be made.

It is often denied that forced normalization occurs, probably with good reason. Thus, it is certainly rarer than made out by Landolt, and studies are few and far between. It is difficult to document cases precisely, EEG recordings being difficult to obtain at the right times. However, studies that systematically analyze the etiology in consecutive case series identify forced normalization or alternative psychoses accounting for about 10% of cases (9), suggesting that this condition may often be overlooked in clinical settings.

Other reasons to ignore forced normalization relate to the fact that the concept brings psychiatry uncomfortably close to neurology, revealing a close biological link between seizures and psychosis. It also affects treatment. Thus, if, in some patients, suppression of seizures provokes psychopathology, it reinforces the fact, often ignored or misunderstood, that seizures and epilepsy are not synonymous and that an understanding of the epileptic process and its treatment goes far beyond the control of seizures. In clinical practice, to ignore the fact that some patients manifest these problems as their seizures come under control can lead to the continuation of severe behavior disturbances, with all of the social disruption that then emerges, and a failure to manage the epilepsy appropriately.

PSYCHOSIS FOLLOWING SURGERY

Temporal lobectomy is an established treatment for patients with intractable epilepsy. Ever since the early series, the possibility that surgery itself may be associated with the development of psychiatric disturbance, in particular psychosis, has been discussed. Some of the best evidence comes from the Maudsley series, initially described by Taylor (51) and more recently by Bruton (43). Most centers have stopped operating on floridly psychotic patients, based on the observation that psychoses generally do not improve with the operation. A few centers, however, regularly include psychiatric screening as part of their preoperative assessment, but postoperative psychiatric follow-up is often nonexistent. Assessment of psychosocial adjustment is rarely performed, in contrast to the often scrupulous recording of neuropsychologic deficits.

The Maudsley series shows that some patients develop new psychosis postoperatively, and there is an increased reporting of depression. Bruton (43) has suggested that the development of postoperative psychoses may be more common with certain pathologies (gangliogliomas). Patients

with right-sided temporal lobectomies may be more prone to these psychiatric disturbances (28). In some cases, the sudden relief of seizures that occurs following surgery may suggest a mechanism similar to forced normalization, although no persistent clear relationship emerges between success of the operation and the development of psychotic postoperative states. In recent times, there have been several small series reported of patients with psychoses who have been successfully operated on, without worsening of their psychosis but with marked improvement in seizure control (52).

DIAGNOSIS

The principles of diagnosis of psychiatric problems in epilepsy are essentially the same as when a patient does not have epilepsy. However, it is not possible to apply the strict DSM-IV classifications (53), and in many patients there are subtle aspects to the clinical picture that may suggest the underlying neurologic flavor of the phenomenology. In the schizophrenia-like psychoses, these include the retention of affective responses, lack of personality deterioration, and the development of some of the personality features noted in the interictal personality syndrome. An inclination to mysticism with developing religiosity is one of the most common.

Close attention to the relationship of the development of the psychoses to the seizure pattern is essential if the parictal disorders are to be distinguished from the interictal, although in many patients this is not always clear, and the pattern may change with time. In particular, there are reports of ictally driven psychoses evolving to a chronic interictal syndrome, subtle at first but then more enduring. In other cases, the acute psychoses may erupt in the absence of an obvious cluster of seizures, even though on previous occasions the relationship has been obvious. The EEG in some cases is very important in clarifying the diagnoses, especially for nonconvulsive status and states of forced normalization.

Because many patients with psychoses of epilepsy display prominent affective symptoms, it is important to identify those patients with an affective disorder, as opposed to a schizophrenia-like state or a paranoid illness, that may respond initially to effective antidepressant therapy.

TREATMENT

Most patients with psychoses should be treated with antipsychotic medications, although these, like most antidepressants, can lower the seizure threshold.

Ictal psychoses may only occasionally need neuroleptic drugs; they usually settle rapidly with intravenous AED treatment.

Postictal psychoses often do not require psychotropic medication, resolving over a few hours. However, it is important to stress how dangerous these cases can be, and it is essential to take note of any command hallucinations or delusions of harm to the self or others and protect accordingly. In the first instance, treatment with a benzodiazepine is helpful, since there is a risk, especially with some of the antipsychotics, of precipitating further seizures and exacerbating the psychosis. Regular benzodiazepines for perhaps 48 hours is often sufficient. In longer-term management, it is important to realize that postictal psychoses have a tendency to recur. It is therefore important to warn about this and to try, with effective AED therapy, to prevent clusters of seizures. It is sometimes possible to prevent such a cluster and hence the later psychosis by telling patients to take a benzodiazepine following a first seizure and continue then for about 48 hours. Sometimes all these measures fail, and so intermittent or even continuous antipsychotic treatment becomes important.

Interictally, the paranoid or schizophrenia-like states need to be evaluated in terms of their relationship to seizure frequency. Thus, in patients who stop having seizures in association with the onset of psychosis, a first therapeutic procedure might be lowering AEDs in order to allow seizures to reoccur. When neuroleptic drugs are used, a drug should be chosen that decreases the seizure threshold; even clozapine may be a logical prescription in this situation.

Where patients with epilepsy have no alteration of the seizure frequency, or the psychosis is occurring in the setting of increased seizure frequency, a neuroleptic less likely to precipitate seizures, such as a modern atypical antipsychotic, is recommended. Olanzapine and risperidone have been used most frequently in epilepsy; both drugs have relatively low risks of inducing seizures, risperidone possibly even lesser than olanzapine (54).

It should be recalled that patients taking anticonvulsants that increase hepatic metabolism will show lower serum levels of neuroleptics and may therefore require somewhat higher doses than patients not on these medications to achieve a similar clinical effect. For long-term treatment, side effects should be considered, particularly in patients taking AEDs with similar side effect profiles. Olanzapine is more sedating than risperidone; there is also a risk for a reduced glucose tolerance, relevant for elderly patients, but extrapyramidal side effects are less common compared to risperidone. Weight gain should also be considered when prescribing olanzapine, particularly in combination with an AED that also induces weight gain, such as valproate or pregabalin. Potential cardiotoxic effects of antipsychotics (QT prolongation with, for example, pimozide and ziprosidone) should be considered in elderly patients, particularly when they take carbamazepine or phenytoin. Clozapine is only exceptionally prescribed in epilepsy because of the well-known

epileptogenic risks. Clozapine causes weight gain and salivation. Because of its hematotoxicity, a combination with carbamazepine should be avoided.

As with all psychiatric problems, psychopharmacologic management alone is not sufficient. Although the role of psychotherapy in the management of psychotic conditions has not proved to be of any substantial value, it is important to acknowledge that epileptic patients with psychosis bear the burden of epilepsy in addition to their psychosis. Patients with intermittent psychotic states are often perplexed and embarrassed about what has happened to them while psychotic and fear further continuing bouts with a descent into insanity. Patients with continuous psychosis require the skills of paramedical intervention, and the full resources of community care may be needed to help them rehabilitate and to assist their families in coping with their difficulties. In many patients with chronic psychoses of epilepsy, the preservation of affect and lack of personality disintegration over years sustains them well in their communities and may enable them to live with their families or even marry. Maintaining them and bringing such support to them is important, so that they may be sustained in the community and less likely to need recurrent admission to the hospital. Further, in a good family environment with adequate medical facilities and follow-up care, patient compliance will tend to be good. Deterioration of an otherwise delicate situation, induced by poor compliance, leading to more seizures and exacerbation of psychopathology, with loss of control by the family and the physician, may thereby be avoided.

SUMMARY AND CONCLUSIONS

There is evidence that psychoses are overrepresented in patients with epilepsy, and few physicians who manage epilepsy have not seen patients with either an ictal, postictal, or interictal psychosis. The link to temporal lobe epilepsy is strong, both clinically and theoretically, because there is an acknowledged link between the limbic system and the modulation of emotional and social behaviors (55). It has to be of profound interest that epilepsy, which is so often associated with lesions in medial temporal structures that tend to be present from an early phase in life, is linked to psychoses, which often resemble paranoid and schizophreniform states found in the absence of epilepsy. Thus, the latter can also be shown to have pathology in the same areas of the brain (55), and schizophrenia is now viewed as a developmental disorder associated with anomalous CNS development in the fetal or perinatal era of life.

Finally it has to be repeated that epilepsy is not synonymous with seizures, and the latter are but one manifestation of the disordered cerebral function of patients with epilepsy.

References

1. Stefansson SB, Olafsson E, Hauser WA. Psychiatric morbidity in epilepsy: a case controlled study of adults receiving disability benefits. *J Neurol Neurosurg Psychiatry* 1998; 64(2):238–241.

2. Qin P, Xu H, Laursen TM, Vestergaard M, et al. Risk for schizophrenia and schizophrenia-like psychosis among patients with epilepsy: population based cohort study. *BMJ* 2005; 331(7507):23.

3. Bredkjaer SR, Mortensen PB, Parnas J. Epilepsy and non-organic non-affective psychosis: national epidemiologic study. *Br J Psychiatry* 1998; 172:235–238.

4. Gureje O. Interictal psychopathology in epilepsy: prevalence and pattern in a Nigerian clinic. *Br J Psychiatry* 1991; 158:700–705.

5. Mendez MF, Grau R, Doss RC, Taylor JL. Schizophrenia in epilepsy: seizure and psychosis variables. *Neurology* 1993; 43(6):1073–1077.

6. Matsuura M, Adachi N, Muramatsu R, Kato M, et al. Intellectual disability and psychotic disorders of adult epilepsy. *Epilepsia* 2005; 46 Suppl 1:11–14.

7. Slater E, Beard AW. The schizophrenia-like psychoses of epilepsy. V. Discussion and conclusions. *Br J Psychiatry* 1963; 109:143–150.

8. Dongier S. Statistical study of clinical and electroencephalographic manifestations of 536 psychotic episodes occurring in 516 epileptics between clinical seizures. *Epilepsia* 1959–1960; 1:117–142.

9. Schmitz B, Robertson M, Trimble MR. Depression and schizophrenia in epilepsy: social and biological risk factors. *Epilepsy Res* 1999; 35:59–68.

10. Logsdail SJ, Toone BK. Postictal psychoses: a clinical and phenomenological description. *Br J Psychiatry* 1988; 152:246–252.

11. Kanemoto K. Postictal psychosis revisited. In: Trimble MR, Schmitz B, eds. *The Neuropsychiatry of Epilepsy*. Cambridge, UK: Cambridge University Press, 2002:117–134.

12. Savard G, Andermann F, Olivier A, Remillard GM. Postictal psychosis after partial complex seizures: a multiple case study. *Epilepsia* 1991; 32:225–231.

13. Sommer W. Postepileptisches Irresein. *Arch Psychiatr Nervenkr* 1881; 11:549–612.

14. Kanemoto K, Kawasaki J, Mori E. Violence and epilepsy: a close relation between violence and postictal psychosis. *Epilepsia* 1999, 40(1):107–109.

15. Wolf P. Psychosen bei Epilepsie. Ihre Bedingungen und Wechselbeziehungen zu Anfaellen. Habilitationsschrift, Freie Universitaet Berlin 1976.

16. Ring HA, Trimble MR, Costa DC, Moriarty J, et al. Striatal dopamine receptor binding in epileptic psychoses. *Biol Psychiatry* 1994; 35:375–380.

17. Leutmezer F, Podreka I, Asenbaum S, Pietrzyk U, et al. Postictal psychosis in temporal lobe epilepsy. *Epilepsia* 2003; 44(4):582–590.

18. Slater E, Beard AW, Glithero E. The schizophrenia-like psychoses of epilepsy. *Br J Psychiatry* 1963; 109:95–150.

19. Köhler GK. Epileptische Psychosen: Klassifikationsversuche und EEG-Verlaufsbeobachtungen. *Fortschr Neurol Psychiatr* 1975; 43:99–153.

20. McKenna PJ, Kane JM, Parrish K. Psychotic symptoms in epilepsy. *Am J Psychiatry* 1985; 142:895–904.

21. Tellenbach H. Epilepsie als Anfallsleiden und als Psychose. Üeber alternative Psychosen paranoider Prägung bei "forcierter Normalisierung" (Landolt) des Elektroencephalogramms Epileptischer. *Nervenarzt* 1965; 36:190–202.

22. Sherwin I. Differential psychiatric features in epilepsy; relationship to lesion laterality. *Acta Psychiatr Scand* [Suppl] 1984; 313:92–103.

23. Perez MM, Trimble MR. Epileptic psychosis: diagnostic comparison with process schizophrenia. *Br J Psychiatry* 1980; 137:245–249.

24. Glithero E, Slater E. The schizophrenia-like psychoses of epilepsy. IV: Follow-up record and outcome. *Br J Psychiatry* 1963; 109:134–142.

25. Flor-Henry P. Psychosis and temporal lobe epilepsy: a controlled investigation. *Epilepsia* 1969; 10:363–395.

26. Adachi N, Onuma T, Nishiwaki S, Murauchi S, et al. Inter-ictal and post-ictal psychoses in frontal lobe epilepsy: a retrospective comparison with psychoses in temporal lobe epilepsy. *Seizure* 2000; 9(5):328–335.

27. Kristensen O, Sindrup HH. Psychomotor epilepsy and psychosis. I. Physical aspects. *Acta Neurol Scand* 1978; 57:361–369.

28. Trimble M. *The psychoses of epilepsy*. New York: Raven Press, 1991.

29. Stevens JR. Psychiatric implications of psychomotor epilepsy. *Arch Gen Psychiatry* 1966; 14:461–471.

30. Gibbs FA. Ictal and non-ictal psychiatric disorders in temporal lobe epilepsy. *J Nerv Ment Dis* 1951; 113:522–528.

31. Slater E, Beard AW, Glithero E. The schizophrenia-like psychoses of epilepsy. *Br J Psychiatry* 1963; 109:95–150.

32. Shukla GD, Srivastava ON, Katiyar BC, et al. Psychiatric manifestations in temporal lobe epilepsy: a controlled study. *Br J Psychiatry* 1979; 135:411–417.

33. Sengoku A, Yagi K, Seino M, Wada T. Risks of occurrence of psychoses in relation to the types of epilepsies and epileptic seizures. *Folia Psychiatr Neurol Jpn* 1983; 37:221–226.

34. Hermann BP, Chabria S. Interictal psychopathology in patients with ictal fear. *Arch Neurol* 1980; 37:667–668.

35. Schmitz B. Psychosen bei Epilepsie: eine epidemiologische Untersuchung. Thesis, Freie Universität Berlin, 1988.

36. Slater E, Moran PAP. The schizophrenia-like psychoses of epilepsy: relation between ages of onset. *Br J Psychiatry* 1969; 115:599–600.

37. Mellers JD, Adachi N, Takei N, Cluckie A, et al. SPET study of verbal fluency in schizophrenia and epilepsy. *Br J Psychiatry* 1998; 173:69–74.

38. Maier M, Mellers J, Toone B, Trimble M, et al. Schizophrenia, temporal lobe epilepsy and psychosis: an in vivo magnetic resonance spectroscopy and imaging study of the hippocampus/amygdala complex. *Psychol Med* 2000; 30(3):571–581.

39. Flugel D, Cercignani M, Symms MR, Koepp MJ, et al. A magnetization transfer imaging study in patients with temporal lobe epilepsy and interictal psychosis. *Biol Psychiatry* 2006; 59(6):560–567.

40. Kristensen O, Sindrup HH. Psychomotor epilepsy and psychosis. II. Electroencephalographic findings. *Acta Neurol Scand* 1978; 57:370–379.

41. Jensen I, Larsen JK. Mental aspects of temporal lobe epilepsy. *J Neurol Neurosurg Psychiatry* 1979; 42:256–265.

42. Taylor DC. Ontogenesis of chronic epileptic psychoses: a reanalysis. *Psychol Med* 1971; 1:247–253.

43. Bruton CJ. *The neuropathology of temporal lobe epilepsy*. Maudsley Monographs 31. Oxford: Oxford University Press, 1988.

44. Tebartz van Elst L, Baeumer D, Lemieux L, Woermann FG, et al. Amygdala pathology in psychosis of epilepsy: a magnetic resonance imaging study in patients with temporal lobe epilepsy. *Brain* 2002; 125(Pt 1):140–149.

45. Rusch N, Tebartz van Elst L, Baeumer D, Ebert D, et al. Absence of cortical gray matter abnormalities in psychosis of epilepsy: a voxel-based MRI study in patients with temporal lobe epilepsy. *J Neuropsychiatry Clin Neurosci* 2004; 16(2):148–155.

46. Landolt H. Some clinical EEG correlations in epileptic psychoses (twilight states). *Electroencephalogr Clin Neurophysiol* 1953; 5:121.

47. Mula M, Trimble MR, Lhatoo SD, Sander JW. Topiramate and psychiatric adverse events in patients with epilepsy. *Epilepsia* 2003; 44(5):659–663.

48. Mula M, Trimble MR, Yuen A, Liu RS, et al. Psychiatric adverse events during levetiracetam therapy. *Neurology* 2003; 61(5):704–706.

49. Thomas L, Trimble MR, Schmitz B, Ring HA: Vigabatrin and behaviour disorders: a retrospective study. *Epilepsy Res* 25 (1996):21–27.

50. Krishnamoorthy ES, Trimble MR. Mechanisms of forced normalisation. In: Trimble MR, Schmitz B, eds. *Forced Normalisation and Alternative Psychoses of Epilepsy*. Petersfield UK: Wrightson, 1998:192–207.

51. Taylor DC. Factors influencing the occurrence of schizophrenia-like psychosis in patients with temporal lobe epilepsy. *Psychol Med* 1975; 5:249–254.

52. Reutens DC, Savard G, Andermann F, Dubeau F, et al. Results of surgical treatment in temporal lobe epilepsy with chronic psychosis. *Brain* 1997; 120(Pt 11):1929–1936.

53. APA. Diagnostic and statistical manual of mental disorders, 4th ed (DSM-IV): draft criteria. Washington, DC: American Psychiatric Association, 1993.

54. Amann BL, Pogarell O, Mergl R, Juckel G, et al. EEG abnormalities associated with antipsychotics: a comparison of quetiapine, olanzapine, haloperidol and healthy subjects. *Hum Psychopharmacol* 2003; 18(8):641–646.

55. Trimble MR. *Biological psychiatry*. 2nd ed. Chichester: John Wiley & Sons, 1995.

30

Conditioning Mechanisms, Behavior Technology, and Contextual Behavior Therapy

JoAnne C. Dahl
Tobias L. Lundgren

long with the earliest documentation of epileptic seizures, behavioral conditioning mechanisms were noted as a viable means to control seizures. Galen described seizures as a predictable chain of behaviors that could be interrupted by stimulating different parts of the body (1). In 1881, Gowers published a series of case studies showing that behavioral techniques could interrupt seizure development (2). He described specific forms of stimulation, such as putting pressure on and massaging the hand where the patient felt a seizure begin, as well as more general techniques, such as the application of a strong aroma at the beginning of a seizure. In 1857, Brown-Sequard presented case studies in which seizures were successfully aborted using a variety of stimulations, also contingent upon seizure onset (3). In 1931, Jackson wrote that the motor seizure now called "Jacksonian march" (4) could be stopped by vigorous rubbing of the affected limb (5).

These early reports showed an understanding of the value of behavioral techniques in controlling seizures and were conceptualized under the principle of competitive recruitment. This principle holds that seizures arising from hyperexcitable groups of neurons in the brain, when localizable by a specific and identifiable behavioral correlate, can be blocked from progressing by behaviors that competitively recruit relatively normal brain cells, thereby increasing their normal activity and reducing hypersynchronization of the seizure focus.

During the first half of the twentieth century, experimental behaviorists demonstrated that seizures in animals could be elicited and interrupted using conditioning techniques (6–10), consistent with the principle of competitive recruitment. Different forms of behavioral stimulation were found to interrupt seizure progression when applied at the start of the seizure.

Conditioning techniques were subsequently applied to patients. In 1956, Efron reported the case of a jazz singer who consistently experienced seizures as she was about to perform on stage (11). Her seizures could be arrested using second-order conditioning of an olfactory stimulus to a bracelet. Efron first introduced the smell of jasmine, which the patient associated with a calming effect, presumably associated with a decrease in cortical activity. The patient inhaled the jasmine under situations that placed her at high risk of having seizures (specifically, performing on stage) as well as when seizures actually began. When the singer had learned to successfully interrupt seizures using the jasmine, Efron then conditioned the smell of jasmine to a bracelet, and finally to the thought of the bracelet. This study demonstrated that the singer was able to counteract the increase in cortical activity associated with her seizure onset through conditioning, consistent with the principle of competitive recruitment, and it marked the beginning of conditioning as seizure therapy for patients with epilepsy.

Electroencephalographic (EEG) technology further contributed to understanding the effects of conditioning mechanisms on seizures. Forster, for example, used video-EEG over a 30-year period to study conditioning mechanisms involved in reflex epilepsy in children (12). In 1964, he and his coworkers showed that seizure thresholds could be altered by habituation (13). They determined the threshold frequency and intensity by which specific stimuli could trigger seizures in patients with reflex epilepsy. Then, by exposing patients to stimuli at these thresholds over prolonged periods, seizures were habituated, and the patients were no longer sensitive to the seizure-triggering stimuli, resulting in fewer seizures.

Forster further used video-EEG to show that seizures could be extinguished by combining desensitization with competing responses (14). Seizure behaviors were analyzed for patients with reflex epilepsy, who were then exposed to their identified seizure-triggering stimuli and, at the same time, instructed to perform a distracting ritual. These procedures resulted in nearly complete seizure control, along with significant reductions of epileptiform abnormalities on continuous EEG recordings. By 1977, Forster presented similar data from over 30 patients with various forms of reflex epilepsy, demonstrating nearly complete seizure control and reduced epileptiform abnormalities (12).

This chapter reviews several specific forms of behavioral therapy for patients with epilepsy, including their underlying principles, methods, and outcomes.

EEG BIOFEEDBACK

Using EEG biofeedback techniques, operant conditioning mechanisms were shown by two research groups to produce brain rhythms that protected against seizures. These investigators used EEG biofeedback to train patients to normalize their brain wave activity and thereby elevate seizure threshold. Sterman and colleagues published studies from 1970 to 1981 showing the sensory motor rhythm (SMR) was anticonvulsant in cats and patients with epilepsy. After training patients to produce the SMR, they found seizure frequency reductions from 35 to 50% at one-year follow-up (15). Behavioral correlates to the SMR are active inhibition of peripheral motor activity and the mental state described as concentrated alertness.

Birbaumer and colleagues (16, 17) showed that instrumental conditioning of slow cortical potentials (SCP) reduced epileptiform activity. By observing that all organisms have a tendency to seize as the brain fluctuates in cortical activity, they redefined epilepsy as the inability to control cortical excitability. Whereas normal feedback mechanisms within the brain control these transitions

of excitability, these authors reasoned that patients with epilepsy have hyperexcitability of cortical tissue because of a failure of these down-regulating mechanisms, leading to an explosive chain reaction of excitation among neuronal networks, manifesting as a seizure. The specific seizure symptoms depend on where and how much of the network is involved. Treatment with SCP biofeedback is thus designed to train the person with epilepsy to downshift his or her cortical excitability and thereby reduce the risk of a seizure.

SCP treatment is therefore based on a functional analysis of behavior as compared to other biofeedback techniques. Whereas SMR therapy trains the patient to produce a specific antiepileptic brain rhythm to protect the patient in much the same way as drug therapy, SCP training is built on an awareness of the chain of seizure behavior, requiring the patient to generate up- or down-going responses of cortical activity contingent on its baseline level.

THEORY OF CONDITIONING

On the basis of animal research (18), Fenwick theorized a conditioning mechanism underlying seizures and suggested using this mechanism as a basis for the behavioral treatment of epilepsy (19). He suggested that focal seizures occur when restricted populations of neurons surrounding the focus are sufficiently excited, whereas generalized seizures occur when the level of cortical excitability reaches the point at which thalamic recruiting volleys generalize and spread. He further proposed that these epileptogenic activities are not random and do not occur in a vacuum, but rather act in a predictable manner and are influenced by behavior.

Fenwick referred to the animal research of Lockard and Ward (18), which conceptualized the conditioning mechanism underlying the seizure process in terms of what they called group one and group two neurons. Group one neurons were defined as the dysfunctional pacemaker group that consistently fire epileptogenic activity, whereas group two neurons were the partially affected neurons surrounding the group one neurons. Group two neurons mostly behave in a normal fashion but occasionally get recruited by the group one dysfunctional neurons, resulting in epileptogenic activity spreading out and away from the focus (group one neurons). The patient would typically sense the seizure onset when dysfunctional signals passed from group one to group two neurons. Consistent with this model, Lockard and Ward observed that not all monkeys developed seizures after injury to the exact same brain site, though all showed abnormal EEG activity from group one neurons. They speculated that monkeys who reacted with increased activity of group two neurons at the first signs of spreading of the dysfunctional signals counteracted and stopped the spread of the "would be" seizure.

Such observations in the context of this model suggested that damaged neurons predisposed to epilepsy but that the behavioral response to the dysfunction was critical to whether epilepsy actually develops.

BEHAVIOR MEDICINE MODEL OF EPILEPSY

In the behavior medicine model, epilepsy consists of an organic predisposition to seizures, and intrinsic and extrinsic factors that influence the probability of seizure occurrence. Wolf summarized this new paradigm (20):

Epileptic seizures can be triggered by both nonspecific facilitating factors such as sleep withdrawal, fever, or excessive alcohol intake, and specific reflex epileptic mechanisms. These consist of sensory or cognitive inputs activating circumscribed cortical areas or functional anatomic systems that, due to some functional instability, respond with an epileptic discharge. Interruption of seizure activity at the stage of the aura (i.e., locally restricted discharge) also can be achieved by nonspecific (e.g., relaxation or concentration techniques or vagal nerve stimulation) or by specific focus-targeted sensory or cognitive inputs. The latter, again, activate circumscribed cortical areas. Intriguingly, in some patients, the same stimulus can either precipitate or abort a seizure. The response depends on the state of cortical activation: seizure precipitation occurs in the resting condition, and seizure interruption occurs when the epileptic discharge has begun close to the activated area. These relations can be understood on the background of experimental data showing that an intermediate state of neuronal activation is a precondition for the generation of paroxysmal depolarization shifts, whereas a hyperpolarized neuron will remain subthreshold, and a depolarized neuron that already produces action potentials is not recruitable for other activity. Sensory input meeting an intermediately activated pool of potentially epileptic neurons is adequate to produce a seizure. In another condition, the same stimulus can depolarize a neuron pool in the same area sufficiently to block the further propagation of nearby epileptic activity. Understanding these interactions facilitates the development of successful non-pharmaceutical therapeutic interventions for epilepsy.

APPLIED BEHAVIOR ANALYSIS IN THE TREATMENT OF EPILEPSY

The behavior medicine model of epilepsy is based both on the underlying pathophysiology and principles of conditioning. Epilepsy is defined as a predisposition that can be both triggered and inhibited by certain interactions, behaviors, and cognitions. Depending on the baseline "state of cortical excitation," a stimulus can either trigger or inhibit a seizure. Treatment strategies are based on functional analysis and are individualized to help the patient with epilepsy do the following:

- *Predict* the seizure response by discrimination of intrinsic and extrinsic factors associated with seizure onset
- *Prevent* seizure occurrence by applying exposure procedures to "high"-risk situations or activities associated with seizure occurrence
- *Interrupt* or *counteract* an ongoing seizure response by initiating an appropriate "correcting" or competing response
- *Reinforce* himself or herself for doing so

Methods for functional analyses and individualized treatment procedures are presented in a handbook (21).

Prediction of Epileptic Seizures

Discriminating "high risk" factors and early symptoms of seizures allows patients to *predict* the occurrence of seizures. Tools to enhance identification of these factors include seizure diaries, seizure behavior observations, and, if possible, video-EEG recordings. The most reliable way to confirm the identities of the seizure-inducing factors is to confirm how the patient actually responds to what he or she believes are the seizure triggers.

Spector and co-workers found that 88% of patients were reliably able to identify factors that precipitated their seizures (22). Antecedents included specific triggers that enhanced cortical excitation and synchronization in discrete areas of the brain that were uniquely receptive to these particular influences, such as certain light and sound frequencies or visual patterns. On the other hand, triggers could be nonspecific factors that also generally enhanced shifts in neuronal excitation; examples included anticipation, stress, conflict, fear, and physical exertion. Another type of trigger is the physical sensation at the start of the seizure.

Not all seizures begin with signs that are identifiable to the patient. Patients are usually able to recognize the initial symptoms of simple partial and complex partial seizures. The seizure response itself may have been observed by others a number of times and may be on video. In the case of generalized seizures, antecedents may include emotional, physical, or environmental factors.

Several studies show that fear and stress increase the risk for seizures and, consequently, *preventive* treatment studies have targeted these antecedents (22). Several studies have evaluated the effects of relaxation techniques (23, 24) and yoga (25), performed interictally, to reduce stress levels.

Interrupting Ongoing Epileptic Seizures

Interrupting an ongoing seizure has been attempted by most patients with epilepsy, either consciously or by accident (21), resulting in aborting or postponing seizure onset, moving to a safe place, and shortening seizure length. Figures vary, but between 23% and 53% of patients have aborted a seizure (22). Most commonly, patients either increase or decrease cortical activity depending on the upward or downward shift in cortical activity induced by the seizure trigger (21).

The functional analysis helps the patient determine, in each situation, which direction the countermeasure should aim for. If the trigger is characterized by a high cortical excitation, the countermeasure would be a slow transition downward, whereas if the trigger is a drowsy state, the countermeasure would warrant an increase in cortical excitement. A variety of techniques for changing cortical activity are available so that patients can choose an appropriate countermeasure depending on their specific situation (21, 26, 27). Examples of up-going (that is, cortically exciting) countermeasures are whistles, strong smells (for example, a raw onion), strong tastes like fresh ginger, singing, shouting, tactile stimulation with massage or pinching, and jumping up and down. Examples of down-going countermeasures are breathing exercises, muscle relaxation, or focused concentration on a song, a mathematical problem, or a calming picture. Betts and co-workers (28, 29) used aromas to stimulate a general arousal when applied at the time of seizure onset, resulting in an immediate halt to seizure activity. In the case of developmentally challenged individuals, countermeasures can be employed by caretakers to help interrupt seizures.

Seizure triggers and seizure responses constantly change along with the infinite variations of contingencies. Under the seizure behavioral analysis approach, patients are taught the underlying principles and to swiftly apply the appropriate countermeasure at the start of each seizure. They learn that this approach is different conceptually from standard drug therapy. For the latter, epilepsy is seen as an uncontrollable illness with unpredictable seizures, where medication is the only alternative, in contrast to the seizure behavioral analysis approach, which conceptualizes epilepsy as a tendency to seize in which seizures are predictable and controllable.

Treating the Function of Seizures

One of the most difficult parts of the behavioral analysis approach is to understand the *function* of the actual seizure in the life of the patient. At first glance, an epileptic seizure would probably not be viewed as having a function. In fact, when medical professionals use the word "functional" to refer to seizures, they mean psychogenic

nonepileptic seizures. In the operant conceptualization, all epileptic seizures would be called functional since they all "function" or operate on the environment in some way. For example, seizure behavior looks scary or painful to observers, or elicits a range of behaviors towards the person with epilepsy.

Is it possible that seizures could be reinforced by the effects they have on the environment? In a long-term study, a majority of children with refractory seizures did not want to become seizure-free, counter to the wishes of parents, caretakers, teachers, and physicians (30). Children and young people report positive reinforcement from others based on their seizures, such as special privileges or attention, physical contact, being someone special; further, seizures themselves may be stimulating or may induce euphoria. Dostoyevsky describes his seizure experience as follows "the air was filled with a big noise and I tried to move. I felt the heaven was going down upon the earth and that it had engulfed me. I have really touched God. He came into me myself. Yes, God exists. I cried, and I don't remember anything else. You all, healthy people . . . can't imagine the happiness we epileptics feel during the second before our fit . . . I don't know if this felicity lasts for seconds, hours, or months but believe me, for all the joys that life may bring, I would not exchange this one" (31). This positive description shows the complexity of the function of the seizure experience.

Young people and adults also report that seizures may be a means to avoid undesirable situations or to reduce anxiety and tension. Not surprisingly, therefore, the *function* of seizures correlates with social skills. In a long-term study of children with drug-refractory seizures, social skill competency was inversely related to the frequency of seizures occurring in social situations (30). The more developed the social skills, the fewer seizures that occurred in social situations; whereas the less developed the social skills, the more often that children's seizures occurred in specific social settings. Children with poorly developed social skills reported that seizures prompted desirable social consequences such as being held, being seen, and being the center of attention. Seizures that were reported as stimulating were often maintained while nonstimulating seizures were controlled, and seizures that were anxiety-reducing were less likely to respond to conventional anticonvulsant drugs.

This overview of the possible functions of a seizure shows how complicated and sophisticated the functional analysis must be. If the patient's seizures function in a desirable direction or effectively reduces something undesirable, conventional treatment is not likely to work. Still, the issue of function is a difficult one for all treating professionals. Do people choose to have seizures? In our experience, people can influence the probability of a seizure occurring, and once it starts, they can choose to some degree the course it will take. The treating professional should look carefully at what functions the seizures may serve and help the client to find more attractive alternatives.

EVALUATION OF BEHAVIOR TREATMENT OF EPILEPSY

Studies evaluating behavior therapy as a treatment for epilepsy have been reviewed a number of times over the past 30 years. Mostofsky and Balaschak reviewed 60 studies in 1977 (32), Kraft and Poling (1982) added 11 studies to their review of studies from 1960 to 1980 (33), Goldstein reviewed studies published from 1980 to 1990 (34), and, most recently, Cochrane reviewed studies of the psychologic treatment of epilepsy (35). Methodological inadequacies discussed in the early reviews were low numbers of subjects, inadequate randomization, absence of serum anticonvulsant concentrations to confirm medication compliance during treatment phases, lack of objective physiologic measures, and sole reliance on self-rating.

Goldstein reviewed seven studies that used EEG testing, anticonvulsant serum concentration measurements, sufficient numbers of subjects, one-year follow-ups, and appropriate statistical methods (23, 36–40). These studies included measures relevant to cognitive behavior therapy, including seizure diaries to document seizure frequency, duration, situation, response, and consequence. Social skills and coping skills were rated as well. Most dependent measures were tracked over a 10-week baseline, thereby providing the information needed for the seizure behavioral analysis. Treatments were individualized based on the behavioral analysis but also included preventive exercises, discrimination of seizure triggers, training in seizure countermeasures, and contingency management.

The Cochrane review assessed randomized or quasi-randomized studies of one or more types of psychologic or behavior modification techniques (35). Using strict criteria comparable to medical studies, the meta-analysis determined that all the trials were too small and their methodologies inadequate, leading to the conclusion that there was no reliable evidence to support the use of behavior treatments for patients with epilepsy and that further trials were needed.

ACCEPTANCE AND COMMITMENT THERAPY

Acceptance and Commitment Therapy (ACT) is a behavior therapy based on a new theory of language and cognition (41). ACT has been previously evaluated for a number of disorders such as depression, pain (42), and diabetes (43), generally with good outcomes.

ACT and other behavioral approaches for seizure management were studied in patients with refractory seizures in South Africa and India (44). In developing countries such as South Africa and India, the majority of people with epilepsy do not have access to modern anticonvulsant drugs; therefore, inexpensive and assessable alternative treatments are essential. Both studies were randomized, controlled trials and compared ACT and a control condition in South Africa, and ACT and yoga in India. Essentially the same ACT treatment protocol was used in both studies. Participants included adults with frequent, EEG-verified refractory seizures. Treatment consisted of 11 hours of therapy divided between two individual and two group sessions, and additional booster sessions at 6 months and one year. The South African study, conducted at an institution for persons with severe epilepsy, showed a significant reduction in seizure frequency and an increase in quality of life at the one-year follow-up (44).

ACT consists of acceptance, defusion, values, contact with the present moment, committed action, and self as context (45). Behavior management of seizures is typically taught toward the end of the ACT protocol (21). The aim of ACT treatment is to help the client create psychologic flexibility around "stuck places" and establish contact with direct and natural contingencies of one's valued directions.

Acceptance refers to accepting aspects of epilepsy that the patient cannot change. Clients learn to accept their predisposition to seize and the associated fears and negative thoughts and emotions, thereby avoiding "going to war" with their seizures, since this is a war the patient cannot win by fighting. Accepting the risk of having seizures and nonetheless living a full life is a skill that must be learned and practiced. Acceptance can improve seizure frequency, as exemplified by some patients who undergo video-EEG monitoring. In this situation, patients "try" to have seizures, and it is exactly this "trying" or acceptance that usually leads to no seizures, even among patients with very frequent seizures.

Defusion involves creating a distance between the client and his or her thoughts, associations, and rules related to epilepsy. Epilepsy-related thoughts, rules, and feelings of stigmatization are looked at objectively rather than from within. The client learns to use the thinking process more effectively.

Contact with the *present moment* means helping clients to be present with positive reinforcement or the vitality of the "here and now" rather than being engaged in problems of the past or fears about the future. Patients struggling with epilepsy commonly believe that they need to get somewhere else other than where they actually are to begin to live, and that they must be seizure-free before they would be acceptable as a partner or in the work force. Learning to make contact with the here and now gives patients a way to let go of the struggle with their private events and to start creating the life they want.

Self as context is one of the fundamental principles of ACT. Through this process, the client creates a place from which fears, thoughts, and feelings can be looked at. The client *has* epilepsy, but he or she *is not* epilepsy. The client *has* fears but *is not* those fears. Self as context entails a perspective that the contents of life are products of human history. Self as context promotes a skill whereby the client learns that "I" is the constant context that has always been there, observing all experiences in life. From this perspective, the daily life experiences that constantly change appear less threatening. If there is no difference between the client and his or her epilepsy, there will be a struggle and suffering. By contrast, distinguishing self from life experiences allows the patient to put the epilepsy in perspective; epilepsy and seizures will simply be one of the many experiences in the content of a person's life, but not the basis for defining the person.

Values are an important process in ACT, since values provide the motivation necessary to commit to the work of getting back into life. "Values illness" is a term describing the process of giving up important, valued life directions in order to control symptoms. When symptom control becomes a person's main preoccupation, important sources of positive reinforcement are neglected and vitality is lost. The more the patient struggles and organizes his or her life around prevention, avoidance, and control of the seizures, the less time that he or she has to become involved in valued life activities. As the avoidance agenda grows, quality of life diminishes. Contacting constant, valued directions provides a way toward a meaningful and vital life and shows patients how far off course they have veered because of their emphasis on avoiding seizures.

Committed Action is the final process in ACT and entails a public commitment regarding actual steps the client is willing to take here and now to overcome obstacles and reclaim or create the chosen valued life. A committed action in ACT is a step taken toward a valued life, fully present and mindful, regardless of the resistance of private events and fears.

The Treatment Protocol

The six processes in ACT create psychologic flexibility and a space for valued living. The following is an outline of the objectives for the four-session ACT treatment protocol.

Session one focuses on establishing the "life compass." The therapist helps the client experience the discrepancy between how the participant wants to live (valued directions) and how he or she is actually living. Barriers to this desired life and how the patient has previously handled those barriers are examined. Associations and "rules" about the seizures held by the client are mapped out. Typical such rules are "I would like to study, but I have epilepsy," or "I would like to have a partner and a family, but no one wants someone with seizures." These rules are then targeted using the process described above.

Sessions two and three each last three hours and typically consist of six to eight people. The goals are to help participants understand, experience, and practice the concepts of taking steps in valued directions despite the obstacles, seeing thoughts as thoughts and not truths, learning and practicing seizure interruption methods, and making public commitments toward creating the vital life of their choosing. Role-playing allows participants to understand with their intellect but also to experience through practice. The group conducts functional analyses of each participant's seizures and brainstorms possible seizure interruption methods.

The aim of the fourth and final session is to summarize and evaluate how the participant is applying the treatment components, taking steps in the valued direction, defusing less useful behaviors, and using seizure control techniques. New commitments to taking steps in the valued life directions are made.

Outcome Measurements

Dependent variables that can be used to measure the effects of this treatment model are seizure frequency and duration, quality of life, vitality, and experiential avoidance with regard to epilepsy. Seizure frequency and duration are combined in the seizure index, used previously in several behavioral studies (27, 36). Two standardized quality-of-life measures that are used are the World Health Organization Quality Of Life (WHOQOL-bref) (46) and the Satisfaction With Life Scale (SWLS) (47). New instruments developed for this purpose include a variation of the Acceptance and Action Questionnaire (AAQ), called here the AAQEP, and the Bulls-Eye, a measure of vitality. The AAQ has shown good reliability and validity, with test-retest reliability values of 0.89 and 0.92 (Cronbach's alpha) (48). The Bulls-Eye shows a test-retest reliability of 0.86 (Pearson's correlation) (49).

The Bulls-Eye measures participants' functioning level, along with persistence and vitality in actions, and consists of four dartboards. For the first three dartboards, the client is asked to choose a valued direction that he or she would like to improve or move toward (or is not satisfied with). The bull's eye of the dartboard represents 100% vitality of a defined valued direction. Using the first three dartboards, subjects are asked to mark how close they are living in the direction of vitality in that chosen value. The last dartboard asks the clients to rate how often they generally try to follow valued life directions despite difficulties and barriers. The distance between the bull's-eye and the edge of the dartboard is 4.5 centimeters. On the first three dartboards, the measurement is figured by taking the distance between the X placed by the subject and the center of the bull's-eye, and an average distance is calculated. The last dartboard is measured the same way as the first three but is presented as a single measure.

Results

Overall the ACT intervention produced >90% reduction in total amount of time spent seizing from baseline to the one-year follow-up (44). Quality of life also significantly improved for the ACT participants as measured by the WHO measure, which includes psychologic health, physical health, environmental health, and quality of social relationships. Interestingly, improvement was not immediately apparent but was significant at the one-year follow-up, with a very large effect size (Cohen's $d = 1.57$). Not only was the outcome positive, but the model itself was supported. For example, the post-treatment score on the AAQEP and the Bull's-Eye both showed a very large effect in favor of the ACT condition, with effect sizes between 1.95 and 3.23. These processes fully mediated the effect seen one year later both in seizure reduction and—more impressively, because these changes emerged only over time—quality of life. For example, the three process scores at post-treatment accounted for 43 to 53% of the variance in quality-of-life outcomes seen a year later, depending on the specific process examined (50).

SUMMARY

In summary, behavior treatments of epilepsy include both specific techniques that manipulate the seizure process and contextual methods of helping the client relate to his or her epilepsy and seizures in ways that allow for living in desired vital life directions. At the very least, behavioral interventions should be used to complement conventional medical therapies. For patients who prefer a nondrug approach or for others who do not have access to anticonvulsant drugs, behavior treatment, which has the most evidence based support of any of the available alternatives, should be considered.

References

1. Temkin O. *The falling illness.* Baltimore: The Johns Hopkins Press, 1945:36–196.
2. Gowers W. *Epilepsy and other chronic convulsive diseases.* London: Churchill., 1881.
3. Brown-Sequard C. *Researches on epilepsy: its artificial production in animals, and its etiology, nature and treatment in man.* Boston: Clapp, 1857.
4. Eriksson T. Jacksonian march. *Arch Neurol Psychiatry* 1940; 43:429.
5. Jackson JH. *Selected writings on epilepsy and epileptiform convulsions.* Taylor J, ed. London: Hodder and Stoughton; 1931.
6. Gelhorn E. Effects of afferent impulses on cortical suppression areas. *J Neurophysiol* 1947; 10:125–138.
7. Leao A. Spreading depression of activity in the cerebral cortex. *J Neurophysiol* 1944; 7:359–390.
8. Leao A. Pial circulation and spreading depression of activity in cerebral cortex. *J Neurophysiol* 1944; 10:409–414.
9. Leao A. Further observations on spreading depression of activity in cerebral cortex. *J Neurophysiol* 1947; 10:409–414.
10. McCulloch W. Mechanism for the spread of epileptic activation of the brain. *Electroencephalogr Clin Neurophysiol* 1949; 1:19–27.
11. Efron R. Effect of olfactory stimuli in uncinate fits. *Brain* 1956; 79:267–281.
12. Forster F. *Reflex epilepsy: behavior therapy and conditional reflexes.* Springfield, IL: Charles C. Thomas; 1977.
13. Forster F, Ptacek L, Peterson W, Chun R, et al. Stroboscopic-induced seizures altered by extinction techniques. *Trans Am Neurol Assoc* 1964; 89:136.
14. Forster F, Campos G. Conditioning factors in stroboscopic induced seizures. *Epilepsia* 1964; 5:156.
15. Lantz D, Sterman M. Neuropsychological assessment of subjects with uncontrolled epilepsy: effects of EEG feedback training. *Epilepsia* 1988; 29:163–171.
16. Birbaumer N, Lutzenberg W, Rockstroh B. Area specific self-regulation of slow cortical potential in the sagittal midline and its effects on behavior. *Electroencephalogr Clin Neurophysiol* 1992; 84:353–361.
17. Rockstroh B, Birbaumer N, Elbert T, Lutsenberger W. Operant control of EEG, event related and slow potentials. *Biofeedback & Self Regulation* 1984; 9:139–160.
18. Lockard J, Ward JA. Epilepsy: a window to brain mechanisms. New York: Raven, 1980.
19. Fenwick P. The behavioral treatment of epilepsy generation and inhibition of seizures. *Neurol Clinic* 1994; 12:175–202.
20. Wolf P. From precipitation to inhibition of seizures: rationale of a therapeutic paradigm. *Epilepsia* 2005; 46:Suppl 1.15–16.
21. Dahl J. *Epilepsy: a behavior medicine approach to assessment and treatment in children.* Göttingen: Hogref & Huber, 1992.
22. Spector S, Goldstein L, Cull C, Fenwick P. Precipitating and inhibiting epileptic seizures: a survey of adults with poorly controlled epilepsy. London: International League Against Epilepsy, 1994.
23. Tan S, Bruni J. Cognitive-behavior therapy with adult patients with epilepsy: a controlled outcome study. *Epilepsia* 1986; 27:255–263.
24. Pushkarich C, Whitman S, Dell J, Hughes J, et al. Controlled examination of effects of progressive relaxation training on seizure reduction. *Epilepsia* 1992; 33:675–680.
25. Ramaratnam S, Sridharan K. Yoga for epilepsy. In: The Cochrane Library 1. Oxford: Update Software, 1999.
26. Dahl J, Brorson L-O, Melin L. Effects of a broad-spectrum behavioral medicine treatment program on children with refractory epileptic seizures: an 8-year follow-up. *Epilepsia* 1992; 33(1):98–102.
27. Dahl J, Melin L, Brorson LO, Schollin J. Effects of a broad-spectrum behavior modification treatment program on children with refractory epileptic seizures. *Epilepsia* 1985; 26(4):303–309.
28. Betts T. An olfactory countermeasures treatment for epileptic seizures using a conditioned arousal response to specific aromatherapy oils. *Epilepsia* 1995; 36(Suppl 3):130–131.
29. Betts T, Fox C, MacCallum R. Assessment of countermeasures used by people to attempt to control their own seizures. *Epilepsia* 1995; 36(Suppl 3):130.
30. Dahl J, Melin L, Leissner P. Effects of a behavioral intervention on epileptic seizure behavior and paroxysmal activity: a systematic replication of three cases of children with intractable epilepsy. *Epilepsia* 1988; 29(2):172–183.
31. Alajouanine F. Dostoyevski's epilepsy. *Brain* 1963:86; 214–221.
32. Mostofsky D, Balaschak B. Psychobiological control of seizures. *Psychol Bull* 1977; 84:723–750.
33. Kraft K, Poling A. Behavioral treatments of epilepsy, methodological characteristics and problems of published studies. *Appl Res Ment Retard* 1982; 3:151–162.
34. Goldstein L. Behavioral and cognitive behavioral treatments for epilepsy: a progress review. *Br J Clin Psychol* 1990; 29:257–269.
35. Ramaratnam S, Baker GA, Goldstein LH. Psychological treatments for epilepsy. *Cochrane Database Syst Rev* 2003; 4.
36. Dahl J, Melin L, Lund L. Effects of a contingent relaxation treatment program on adults with refractory epileptic seizures. *Epilepsia* 1987; 28(2):125–132.
37. Fried R. Rubin S, Carton R, Fox M. Behavioral control of intractable seizures; self regulation of end tidal carbon dioxide. *Psychosom Med* 1984; 46:315–331.
38. Lindsay W, Baty F. Behavioral relaxation training: exploration with adults who are mentally handicapped. *Ment Handicap* 1986; 15:159–162.
39. Montgomery J, Epsie C. Behavioral management of hysterical pseudo seizures. *Behav Psychother* 1986; 143:34–40.
40. Rosseau A, Hermann B, Whitman S. Effects of progressive relaxation on epilepsy: analysis of a series of cases. *Psychol Rep* 1985; 57:1203–1212.
41. Hayes SC, Barnes-Holmes D, Roche B. *Relational frame theory: a post-Skinner account of human language and cognition.* New York: Plenum Press, 2001.

42. Dahl J, Wilson KG, Nilsson A. Acceptance and Commitment Therapy and the treatment of persons at risk for long-term disability resulting from stress and pain symptoms: a preliminary randomized trial. *Behav Ther* 2004; 35:785–802.

43. Gregg JA. A randomized control effectiveness trial comparing patient education with and without Acceptance and Commitment Therapy. Ph.D. diss., University of Nevada, Reno, 2004.

44. Lundgren T, Dahl J, Melin L, Kies B. Evaluation of Acceptance and Commitment Therapy for drug refractory epilepsy: a randomized trial in South Africa: a pilot study. *Epilepsia* 2006; 47:2173–2179.

45. Lundgren T. A development and evaluation of an integrative health model in the treatment of epilepsy. Master's thesis, University of Uppsala, Sweden, 2004.

46. WHO. WHOQOL-BREF: introduction, administration and generic version of the assessment. Geneva: World Health Organization, Program on Mental Health, 1996.

47. Diener E, Emmons RA, Larsen RJ, Griffin S. The Satisfaction With Life Scale. *J Pers Soc Psychol* 1985; 49:71–75.

48. Hayes SC, Strosahl KD, Wilson KG, Bissett RT, et al. Measuring experiential avoidance: A preliminary test of a working model. *Psychol Rec* 2004; 54:553–578.

49. Lundgren T, ed. Validation of the Bulls-Eye. Presented at the 2nd World Congress of Acceptance and Commitment Therapy and Relational Frame Theory; July 23–28; 2006, London.

50. Dahl J, Lundgren T. Behavior analysis of epilepsy: conditioning mechanisms, behavior technology and the contribution of ACT. *The Behavior Analyst Today* 2005; 6(3):191–202.

31 Personality Disorders and Epilepsy

Michael Trimble

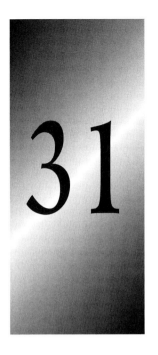

here are few topics in the field of epilepsy research that have attracted more controversy than the association between changes of personality and epilepsy. There are several reasons for this, although most can be traced back to the legacy of Cartesian dualism, which was such a powerful, dishonest, yet seductive backdrop to neuroscience. Although it still remains—like the painful sting of a bee embedded under the skin while the bee itself is dead—ingrained into the thought processes of the lay public and the media, dualism also continues to invade the clinical sciences, and nowhere more in the still-present gap between neurology and psychiatry in many countries.

In the first part of the twentieth century, it was a generally believed that epilepsy was not linked in any direct way with psychiatric problems, although secondary disturbances may have been expected from prolonged use of sedative medications, head injuries, and social stigmatization. In fact, to suggest that epilepsy was anything more than seizures was thought to add to that stigmatization and was thus de facto harmful.

However, amid such theorizing several advances in the neurosciences were being made that bypassed theorists for several years. First, there was a growing understanding of the role of the frontal lobes in regulating behavior, and frontal lobe syndromes, essentially personality disorders, were being described in animals and humans. Second, a temporal lobe syndrome was revealed after bilateral damage to the temporal lobes, which presented as an alteration of personality traits, with calming of emotions, visual agnosis, and alterations of sexual behavior.

This Klüver-Bucy syndrome was later shown to be linked in particular to amygdala damage, whereas an amnestic syndrome followed bilateral destruction of the hippocampi and related structures such as the fornices. Third, and most significantly, a cerebral representation for the emotions was outlined and then elaborated on by Papez, Yakovlev, and MacClean. This rediscovery of Broca's limbic lobe, now viewed as a system for the regulation and expression of the emotions, involved such key structures as the amygdala and the hippocampus. Temporal lobe epilepsy (TLE) was discovered in the clinical setting with the use of the electroencephalograph (EEG), and authors such as Gibbs noted that patients with what was referred to as psychomotor epilepsy were more susceptible to develop psychiatric disorders than those with other epilepsy syndromes; for a more extensive overview and references see Trimble (1).

In the 1960s, Slater and colleagues redefined the interictal psychoses, but it was Geschwind in the 1970s who coined the term "interictal behavior syndrome of TLE" and sparked a controversy that is still ongoing.

253

Interestingly, by this time, Gastaut in France had also described a similar syndrome, and Janz had defined another personality style linked to his syndrome, juvenile myoclonic epilepsy (2–5).

THE GASTAUT-GESCHWIND SYNDROME

It needs to be emphasised that only a minority of patients develop these syndromes, and the full syndrome is not necessarily found in all patients. Some have only some of the features, the full syndrome being seen in less than 10% of those with chronic TLE (6). Some patients display hypergraphia or -religiosity in association with their seizures as a postictal phenomenon, whereas in others it waxes and wanes but is chronic. It may be extinguished by antipsychotic medications if it is seen, as it often is, in association with an interictal psychosis of the schizophrenia-like type. It is probably an all-or-nothing phenomenon, rather than some graded trait, and, as such, is therefore easily missed in small groups of patients.

Bear and Fedio (7) documented 18 traits that were associated with TLE using their inventory (the Bear-Fedio Inventory, or BFI) specifically designed to detect such traits. The authors also noted that patients with right TLE exhibited more emotional traits and tended to deny their negative behaviors, whereas those with a left-sided focus displayed more ideational traits and tended to be more self-critical. The study was criticized, however, for assessing small numbers of patients, and none with other forms of epilepsy, and they did not control for the presence or absence of psychiatric disorder, nor did they specify anticonvulsant medication. Since then, there has been controversy regarding the replication of these findings. Mungas (8) found that the BFI did not differentiate patients with TLE from other neurologic groups but merely reflected the presence or absence of concomitant psychiatric illness. Dodrill and Batzel (9) in a literature review reported that people with epilepsy show more behavioral problems than normal controls and differ from patients with nonneurologic medical problems in that they show more psychotic-like symptoms. Rodin and Schmaltz (10) concluded that the BFI is a general measure of emotional maladjustment but provided, in their view, no support for a specific TLE syndrome. The BFI has also revealed increased traits including humorlessness to occur in patients with frontal lobe epilepsy diagnosed using depth electrodes (11).

Apart from the BFI, most studies that have looked at the issue of personality disorders in patients with epilepsy have used such instruments as the Minnesota Multiphasic Personality Inventory (MMPI) or the Structured Clinical Interview for DSM-IV-TR (SCID)—standardized instruments in psychiatry, but ones that are not attuned to the specific behavioral profile outlined in the interictal

syndrome. Further, such diagnostic manuals as the *Diagnostic and Statistical Manual of Mental Disorders*, 4th Edition (DSM-IV), are of no help in this regard, as this and other well-defined syndromes of epilepsy (e.g., postictal psychosis) will not be found therein.

The characteristics of the Gastaut-Geschwind syndrome include such symptoms as alterations in sexual behaviors, irritability, and viscosity, the latter being a tendency to slow, labored thinking, as if thoughts are emerging from molasses. This sometimes is revealed as circumstantiality, to quote the psychopathologist Frank Fish (12):

> Here thinking proceeds slowly with many unnecessary trivial details but the point is finally reached. The goal of thought is never completely lost and thinking proceeds towards it by an intricate and devious path. This disorder has been explained as the result of a weakness of judgement and egocentricity. It is an outstanding feature of the epileptic personality.

Viscosity appears to be more common in patients with TLE, especially with left or bilateral seizure foci, and is also correlated with duration of epilepsy and left handedness (13). It has been suggested that viscosity may result from impaired linguistic skills.

However, the two most fascinating features of the Gastaut-Geschwind syndrome are hypergraphia and hyperreligiosity.

Hypergraphia

This was first clearly described by Waxman and Geschwind, and refers to the tendency to write excessively and often compulsively (4). They initially discussed seven patients with TLE, all of whom were hypergraphic. The writing of these patients was extensive, and characteristically meticulous, and in four patients the written themes had moral and religious overtones. In a further study, the researchers published three additional cases; one of the patients was reported to have undergone multiple religious conversions. The writing revealed a preoccupation with detail, and a "compulsive quality to much of the written output."

Repetition of words, and often sentences, is seen. Patients are described who wrote long, often detailed descriptions of their lives, and several were producing religious texts, such as the Bible or the Koran. Poetry writing was often a feature. There was often a scrupulous attention to detail, and an associated mood disorder, mainly of euphoria, the latter was often linked to the hypergraphia.

Since these early studies, hypergraphia has been observed in 8% of patients with epilepsy (14) and has been associated with previous psychiatric episodes, emotional maladjustment, computed tomographic (CT) scan abnormalities, and focal epilepsy (especially TLE) (15), along with affective disturbance (especially hypomania) and nondominant foci (16).

The question of the relationship of cerebral laterality to hypergraphia is at present unclear, although at least one report noted an overrepresentation of right-sided foci and an association with episodes of déjà vu. No patient had a left-sided focus for the epilepsy, and a statistically significant excess of right temporal abnormalities was noted. Déjà vu auras are usually driven by a right temporal lobe focus.

Although the relationship of the hypergraphia noted in epilepsy to the ability to produce creative written text for the moment must remain speculative, the phenomenon is obviously the opposite to the effects noted with left-hemisphere lesions, with the subsequent development of aphasia and agraphia.

It has been noted that the content of the writing from patients with epilepsy with hypergraphia often reflects religious or mystical themes. Of fifteen published cases, nine had hyperreligiosity or comparable extensive metaphysical beliefs, and those who see these patients regularly in the clinic, and who ask about such phenomena, recognize the frequent association with the metaphysical.

Religiosity

The "heightened religiosity" of epilepsy has been recognized since the nineteenth century by the French and German alienists (1, 6, 17). Despite this, little attention has been paid to this relationship, although with the growing interest in religious behaviors as a social phenomenon and potential threat to civilization, the study of patients with neurologic and psychiatric disorders and excessive religious feelings seems warranted.

Earlier studies by Bear and colleagues found that "religiosity trait" scores could distinguish between patients with TLE and normal controls and patients with other psychiatric or neurologic conditions including extratemporal focal epilepsy and generalized epilepsy (18). Ecstatic ictal experiences, in some cases accompanied by visions of a religious nature, have been reported in patients with EEG evidence of temporal lobe discharges (17), and sudden religious conversions have been reported in the postictal period, closely related to the first seizure or an increase (or more rarely a decrease) in seizure frequency (19).

Studies Carried Out at the Institute of Neurology. In recent years, further studies specifically examining aspects of religiosity and the often associated hypergraphia in patients with epilepsy have been carried out (20–22). The phenomenology of these states, especially the religiosity, has been evaluated in more detail, as have attempts to further understand the underlying brain associations.

One problem is that measurement of such phenomena as religiosity and hypergraphia is difficult, with few available validated rating scales and mainly a tradition of clinical observation to guide hypotheses. One of the subscales of the BFI relates to religiosity, another to hypergraphia. The scale comes in two versions: one for the patient to fill out, and the other for a caregiver or relative or person who knows the patient well. In the original study of Bear and Fedio, the scoring on the religiosity subscale was greater in patients with temporal lobe epilepsy, even when compared to patients with mixed psychiatric disorders (and no epilepsy). In the study to be described, the Bear-Fedio scale was used, in addition to other scales that assess aspects of individual religious experiences and behavior. We used one scale referred to here as INSPIRIT and another called the Hood Mysticism Scale. The INSPIRIT is a questionnaire that asks about spiritual or religious beliefs and experiences, including time spent on various religious practices, and how close people have felt to powerful forces of one kind or another. There are also direct questions about belief in God and experiences that may have reinforced such beliefs. In our studies this scale was modified to allow for a wider range of religious experiences to be documented than in the original and better descriptions of the nature of them. The Hood scale, which was based on Hood's readings of James's varieties of religious experiences, taps into the quality of them. There are two major factors evaluated by this scale, namely general mystical experience and religious interpretation.

Three experimental groups were defined. The first consisted of twenty-eight people with TLE and a prominent devotion to religion as identified clinically. The second consisted of twenty-two people with TLE who had no religious affiliations, and in the third group were thirty regular churchgoers without known epilepsy. The purpose of the study was to examine in more detail the psychologic profile of those patients with epilepsy and religiosity, and, by comparing them with the other epilepsy sample, to examine the underlying epilepsy variables that may be related to the religious experiences. By examining a group of nonepileptic worshipers, we hoped to capture phenomenological differences between them and our epilepsy sample.

The results of this study were very revealing. First of all, we were able to reconfirm the original findings of Geschwind and his school, and show that the temporal lobe religious group not only, as expected, endorsed the religiosity subscale of the Bear-Fedio scale, but they also revealed other elements of the Gastaut-Geschwind syndrome. This is shown graphically in the accompanying figure (Figure 31-1). Notably, the religious group also scored highly on the subscales of emotionality, philosophical interests, anger and sadness, dependence, and hypergraphia. They were also rated by a significant other

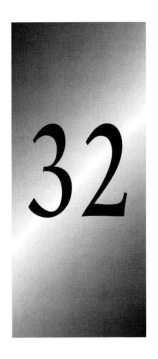

32

Frontal Lobe
Behavioral Disorders

Barbara C. Jobst
Brenna C. McDonald

The frontal lobes are the largest cortical mass of the human brain; their
size distinguishes the human brain
from the brains of related mammals.
Despite significant advances in cognitive neuroscience,
however, many functions and functional networks of the
frontal lobes are still not very well understood.

More than a century ago it was already recognized
that frontal lobe lesions do not necessarily cause impairment of motor function, memory, or speech but may lead
to personality changes. In 1868, Phineas Gage, a rail-
road foreman in Vermont, suffered from severe frontal
lobe damage caused by an iron rod passing through his
head in an explosion. He survived without functional
impairment of his activities of daily living, but it was
noted that he changed from a well-adjusted man to an
irresponsible and convention-neglecting person (1). In
the 1920s, such observations linking the frontal lobes
with behavioral changes led to the development of
frontal lobotomies to modify behavior in psychiatri-
cally ill patients. The procedure was abandoned because
of severe behavioral changes, surgical complications,
and ethical concerns. It became more and more evident,
however, that the frontal lobes are critical to aspects of
human behavior, without necessarily affecting motor
function, overall level of intellect, language, memory,
or other cognitive domains.

Patients with seizures originating in the frontal lobes
have presumably pathologic changes affecting the frontal
lobes, and therefore it seems intuitive that frontal lobe
seizures could lead to behavioral changes similar to those
due to frontal lobe lesions.

This chapter first reviews the functional anatomy
of the frontal lobes and then discusses methods for
assessing frontal lobe dysfunction, neuropsychologic
and neuropsychiatric aspects of frontal lobe epilepsy,
ictal and interictal features, and associated behavioral
disorders.

FUNCTIONAL ANATOMY OF THE FRONTAL LOBES

Anatomically the frontal lobes are frequently subdivided
into the prefrontal cortex and the frontal motor areas
(Figures 32-1 and 32-2) (2). The primary motor area is
located in the precentral gyrus and contains the cortical control of motor function. The supplementary motor
area, on the medial surface of the brain anterior to the
primary motor cortex, is responsible for modulation and
initiation of motor movements. In the language dominant
hemisphere, Broca's area, located laterally anterior to the
primary motor cortex, is critical for expressive language
function.

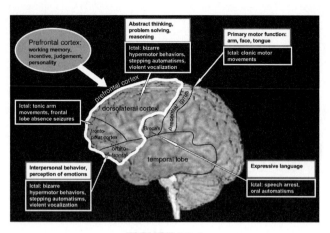

FIGURE 32-1

Functional anatomy of the frontal lobes, lateral view.

All other frontal regions can be summarized as "prefrontal cortex" and include the dorsolateral frontal cortex, the frontopolar regions, the medial and lateral orbitofrontal regions, the medial prefrontal cortex, and the anterior cingulate gyrus (Figures 32-1 and 32-2) (2). The prefrontal cortex is commonly conceptualized as being responsible for "executive functions," including higher-order control of aspects of cognition as well as behavioral regulation. Such "executive" aspects of frontal lobe functioning make a human being a well-adjusted and behaved individual in society and provide man with judgment, incentive, reason, personality, and appropriate behaviors.

Frontal lobe neuronal networks are responsible for response selection/initiation or inhibition to exterior stimuli (3). The prefrontal cortex and its connected neural networks are furthermore responsible for aspects

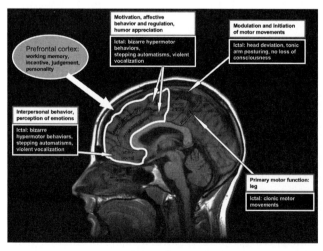

FIGURE 32-2

Functional anatomy of the frontal lobes, medial view.

of attention and working memory. Working memory is the ability to temporarily store information required to carry out complex cognitive tasks online while the information is needed (2).

The dorsolateral frontal cortex is mainly involved in abstract thinking, reasoning, and problem solving. Theory of mind, which is the ability to anticipate and interpret other people's thinking or see things from their point of view in a given situation, has also been associated with the dorsolateral frontal cortex (Figure 32-1) (4). The orbitofrontal cortex is responsible for interpersonal behavior and perception of emotions, and the medial prefrontal cortex and cingulate gyrus have been associated with motivation, affective behavior and regulation, and humor appreciation (Figure 32-2) (4).

ASSESSING FRONTAL LOBE DYSFUNCTION

Neuropsychologic assessment of patients with epilepsy has in the past focused on IQ, memory, and language function, in part because of the emphasis on presurgical evaluation for temporal lobe epilepsy. These patients have traditionally been the largest population receiving comprehensive epilepsy evaluations, including neuropsychologic testing. However, comprehensive neuropsychologic assessment has also always included measures of executive or frontal lobe functioning, which may be more likely to demonstrate deficits in patients with a frontal lobe seizure focus, even when functioning is largely intact in other cognitive domains. This is nicely described by Milner in her report of the case of K. M., who underwent frontal lobe resection at the Montreal Neurological Institute without any change in his IQ (5). Later assessment using the Wisconsin Card Sorting Test, a now commonly used measure of reasoning, problem solving, and concept formation, demonstrated significant abnormalities in executive functions (5).

A wide variety of standardized tests are now used in clinical neuropsychologic practice to assess frontal systems functioning, including measures of attention-related and executive functions (e.g., reasoning, problem solving, response inhibition, concept formation, working memory, vigilance, distractibility, and divided attention; see Table 32-1). In addition, assessment of other core cognitive functions subserved by the frontal lobes, including expressive language and motor skills, is also conducted in any comprehensive neuropsychologic evaluation. Other aspects of neurocognitive functioning thought to rely on the frontal lobes, such as personality and social judgment, still remain difficult parameters to quantify in terms of change over time. Measures of frontal or executive functions targeting particular cognitive subdomains (e.g., reward systems) have been developed for research purposes.

TABLE 32-1
Neuropsychologic Tests of Attention-Related and Executive Functions

Test Name*	Description of Functions Assessed
Wisconsin Card Sorting Test	Reasoning, concept formation, cognitive flexibility, learning from errors
Booklet Category Test	Reasoning, concept formation, cognitive flexibility, learning from errors
Tower Tests (London, Hanoi, Toronto)	Planning, problem solving
Trail Making Tests	Cognitive flexibility, visual scanning and sequencing, psychomotor speed
Paced Auditory Serial Addition Test	Auditory divided attention, working memory
Stroop Color-Word Interference Test	Cognitive flexibility, selective attention, response inhibition
Digit Span (Forward/Backward)	Basic auditory attention, working memory
Continuous Performance Tests	Sustained attention, vigilance, susceptibility to distraction, response inhibition
Twenty Questions Test	Problem solving, concept formation, abstract reasoning, learning from feedback
Cognitive Estimation Tests	Practical judgment, reasoning
Porteus Maze Test	Planning, generation of problem-solving alternatives, learning from errors
Verbal Fluency Tests (Phonemic/Semantic)	Cognitive flexibility, response generation, ability to sustain task effort
Figural Fluency Test	Cognitive flexibility, response generation, ability to sustain task effort

*Integrated test batteries including many of these measures have also been collected and conormed to assess frontal lobe functioning (e.g., Delis-Kaplan Executive Function System, Frontal Assessment Battery).

COGNITION IN FRONTAL LOBE EPILEPSY

The neuropsychologic aspects of frontal lobe epilepsy are not as well studied as other focal epilepsies, particularly temporal lobe epilepsy, although some authors have begun to characterize cognitive outcomes in frontal lobe seizure patients [3, 6]. It has long been noted that intellectual functioning seems to be relatively unaffected in frontal lobe epilepsy whereas executive functioning is often impaired [4, 5]. In two studies in which neuropsychologic findings of patients with unoperated frontal lobe epilepsy were compared to temporal lobe epilepsy patients [3, 6], more significant impairment was noted on certain tests of executive (e.g., tests of conceptualization and estimation ability, cognitive flexibility, working memory span, and response inhibition) and motor (e.g., motor sequencing and coordination) function in the frontal lobe group. Factor analysis showed that motor programming, coordination and response maintenance, and inhibition were more significantly impaired in frontal than in temporal lobe epilepsy [3]. Nevertheless such deficits were not present in about 40% of the patients with frontal lobe epilepsy.

Upton and Thompson [6] suggested there was more significant impairment in left frontal lobe epilepsy than in right frontal lobe epilepsy; but in other studies a reverse trend was found, which has led to the conclusion that there may be no consistent lateralizing cognitive findings in frontal lobe epilepsy [1, 3, 6]. However, motor testing lateralizes seizure onset more reliably than other measures. Rapid bilateral spread of epileptiform activity may contribute to difficulties lateralizing cognitive findings in frontal lobe epilepsy compared to temporal lobe epilepsy [1]. In addition, the importance of rapid propagation of epileptic activity between frontal and temporal regions must be taken into consideration when examining these two epilepsy subtypes, given the high degree of interconnectedness of the frontal and temporal lobes.

Analysis of subgroups of different locations within the frontal lobes is difficult because of insufficient sample size in most studies [1]. The degree to which cognitive performance in patients with frontal lobe epilepsy may differ from that in other neurologic populations with frontal lobe pathology but without seizures has not been systematically studied.

Resective epilepsy surgery may influence cognition in frontal lobe epilepsy, but it also provides an opportunity to study the effects of epilepsy on cognition. Consistent with presurgical findings, patients who underwent frontal lobe resective epilepsy surgery score lower on tests measuring speed or attention, short-term memory, response maintenance or inhibition, and motor coordination, whereas patients with temporal lobe resections may postsurgically improve on such measures [3]. This would suggest that underlying pathology and not epileptiform activity or spread thereof is responsible for the neuropsychologic deficits in patients with frontal lobe epilepsy.

Supplementary motor resections may result in reversible impairment of initiation of behavior. Postsurgically, patients can experience decreased initiation of movement contralateral to the supplementary motor area resection for variable lengths of time. This may include speech inhibition and aphasia (1, 11). It has been suggested that patients with supplementary motor area resections are most susceptible to postsurgical behavioral and cognitive deficits. However, this should not preclude surgery, as these deficits are usually transient (1, 11). Partially targeted frontal lobe resections are less likely to cause postoperative deficits compared to complete lobectomies, in which increased psychomotor slowing has been observed (1).

SOCIAL COGNITION IN FRONTAL LOBE EPILEPSY

Social cognition includes the ability of individuals to interpret the behavior of others and function effectively in their social environment. This includes the ability to be sensitive to the internal states of others and to respond appropriately to that perception, as well as the ability to take another's perspective in a situation. Research suggests that the nondominant frontal and temporal lobes are critical for effective social cognition functioning and regulation of social behavior (8). Farrant et al. tested patients with frontal lobe epilepsy compared to normal controls on a battery of tests of social cognition (4). Humor appreciation and perception of emotional expression were impaired in patients with frontal lobe epilepsy, particularly in terms of perception of anger, fear, and sadness. Such findings have direct clinical implications in terms of social interactions and relationships in frontal lobe epilepsy patients (4). For example, misinterpretation of emotional cues could potentially lead to aggressive behaviors observed in patients with frontal lobe epilepsy. Limitations in humor appreciation can negatively influence social interactions and relationships. No significant group differences were apparent in performance on other tests of social cognition (e.g., theory of mind and faux pas tasks) in the Farrant et al. study, suggesting that social cognition deficits in frontal lobe epilepsy are not reflective of global impairment. Rather, as for cognitive executive functions, it is more likely that specific aspects of social cognition will evidence deficits.

BEHAVIORAL DISORDERS IN FRONTAL LOBE EPILEPSY

Behavioral changes in patients with frontal lobe seizures can be related to multiple causes and occur ictally, postictally, and interictally. Ictal behaviors in frontal lobe epilepsy can be bizarre or subtle and may be mistaken for psychogenic nonepileptic seizures or other psychiatric disease (9). Frontal lobe seizures are often exclusively nocturnal and tend to occur in clusters, causing significant sleep disturbances that can contribute to cognitive and behavioral changes, especially in children. Unusual ictal behaviors such as nonconvulsive status epilepticus and absence status, which is associated with frontopolar and orbitofrontal seizure onset, are reflective of frontal systems dysfunction (e.g., apathy and inattention). Postictal psychosis and impairment of attention and concentration have also been associated with frontal lobe seizures.

Behavioral evaluation of frontal lobe epilepsy patients following epilepsy surgery poses another problem, as behavioral changes could be a result of surgical alteration of brain functioning or a result of improved seizure control. As the frontal lobes are integral to attention-related processes such as working memory, the potential negative impact of antiepileptic medications on these processes cannot be neglected. In addition, epilepsy is associated with social stigma, which can impact social functioning beyond what may be explainable by frontal lobe dysfunction.

Ictal Behaviors in Frontal Lobe Epilepsy

Clonic motor activity is the primary clinical manifestation of seizures originating in the precentral sulcus (9). Typical supplementary motor area seizures consist of head deviation and unilateral tonic arm posturing in a flexed or extended position, without loss of consciousness (9). Very bizarre hyperactive behaviors are characteristic of dorsolateral and orbitofrontal seizures, whereas rocking, jumping, pounding, or bicycling movements are typical for seizures originating in the premotor cortex. Vocalization is frequent, and is often dramatic, including yelling, shouting, or uttering obscenities. Sexual automatisms or pelvic thrusting have also been observed. Frontal lobe hyperactive seizures are brief and there is no loss of consciousness (9). Because of the paucity of electroencephalographic (EEG) abnormalities and because of the often bizarre behavioral manifestations, frontal lobe seizures were often in the past mistaken for symptoms of psychiatric disease, such as psychosis or pseudoseizures.

There is a high incidence of nonconvulsive or absence status (also termed spike-wave stupor) associated with frontal lobe epilepsy (1, 9). In this state patients are partially responsive and do not exhibit any abnormal motor activity. They are able to talk and interact but appear somewhat apathetic and cognitively slow, quite the opposite of the behaviors described previously as typical for brief hyperactive seizures. Absence status can persist for hours or days; it typically presents as a quite sudden behavioral change and may not be recognized as a seizure manifestation.

Postictal Behaviors in Frontal Lobe Epilepsy

Postictal behavior in patients with epilepsy can be quite different from interictal or ictal behaviors. Emotional sequelae, including symptoms of depression and anxiety, have been noted postictally in 45% of patients with refractory partial epilepsy (10), with a median duration of 24 hours. Postictal psychiatric symptoms can also include psychotic features, aggression, neurovegetative symptoms, and hypomania (10). Postictal cognitive changes often include concentration and memory difficulties, as well as potential residual aphasic symptoms in patients with a dominant hemisphere seizure focus. Most of these psychiatric and cognitive abnormalities have been described in unselected patients with partial and generalized epilepsy, or in selected patients with temporal lobe epilepsy. Whether their incidence and occurrence in frontal lobe epilepsy are comparable to those in temporal lobe epilepsy has not been studied systematically. Bilateral independent seizure onset and a cluster of generalized tonic-clonic convulsions are more often associated with postictal psychosis. Preexisting interictal psychiatric disease and a history of psychiatric hospitalization are also risk factors for developing postictal behavioral abnormalities (10).

Interictal Behaviors in Frontal Lobe Epilepsy

Interictal frontal lobe behavioral disorders have complex etiologies. Patients with frontal lobe seizures due to identifiable frontal lobe lesions (e.g., tumor or encephalomalacia) may exhibit behavioral disorders consistent with the lesion location. Patients without clear lesions can exhibit similar disorders, but it is unclear whether these behavioral changes are due to an unidentified lesion, intermittent epileptiform electrical discharges and spread thereof, or frequent seizures.

Patients with epilepsy due to large structural lesions such as tumor, stroke, or posttraumatic encephalomalacia may evidence behavioral disturbances similar to those seen in patients with such brain abnormalities who do not have seizures. Lesions in primary motor cortex can result in weakness and loss of motor coordination, whereas lesions in the supplementary motor area more typically result in a syndrome of loss of motor initiation and planning (11). Orbitofrontal and medial frontal lesions can lead to poor judgment, impulsive behaviors, emotional incontinence, and inability to anticipate the consequences of one's own behavior. Hyperactivity and irritability can be additional features, and patients with orbitofrontal lesions may be unable to learn effectively from experience (i.e., modify their behavior based on negative feedback from the environment). Dorsolateral lesions can result in a contrary syndrome, with apathy, loss of initiative, lethargy, and poor planning.

NEUROPSYCHIATRIC FINDINGS IN FRONTAL LOBE EPILEPSY

Anxiety and mood disorders are the most common psychiatric comorbidities in epilepsy patients across epilepsy subtypes (10), with depressive disorders more common in patients with partial seizures emanating from the temporal or frontal lobes, or in individuals with poorly controlled seizures. Dysfunction of frontal lobe regions has been implicated in behavioral dysfunction and a variety of social impairments, which can vary depending upon the affected frontal subregion. Such behavioral disturbance may therefore be seen in frontal lobe epilepsy and may correlate to some degree with the specific location of epileptogenesis, although the rapid spread of frontal lobe seizures may lead to more generalized frontal lobe–related behavioral disruption. Impulsivity, irritability, disinhibition, hyperactivity, impaired judgment and foresight, and emotional incontinence can be seen following orbital or medial frontal lobe damage, and damage to prefrontal regions may lead to social withdrawal, apathy, lethargy, emotional blunting, insensitivity to social cues and impaired emotion recognition, egocentrism, exhibition of inappropriate affect, and indifference to the opinions of others (4, 8, 13). In addition, the orbital and medial prefrontal cortex and connected circuitry are thought to play a role in addictive behavior, attention-deficit/hyperactivity disorder, and the ability to regulate violent behavior (1). Emotional and behavioral changes associated with frontal lobe epilepsy are receiving increased attention in recent years and are certainly related to alterations in interpersonal interactions. As yet, however, no specific personality types or disorders have been reported to be related to frontal lobe epilepsy, case studies such as that of Phineas Gage notwithstanding. Again, this stands in contrast to temporal lobe epilepsy, in which a particular personality profile has been characterized, although its pervasiveness remains somewhat controversial in the literature. It is also critical to recognize that behavioral or personality changes related to frontal lobe epilepsy, particularly in nonlesional patients, are likely to be less marked than those observed in patients with gross frontal lobe lesions (e.g., tumor), and that seizure frequency is an important covariate to consider when examining neuropsychiatric outcomes in epilepsy.

FRONTAL LOBE BEHAVIORAL DISORDERS IN EPILEPTIC SYNDROMES OTHER THAN LOCALIZATION-RELATED FRONTAL LOBE EPILEPSY

Behavioral abnormalities have also been noted in specific epilepsy syndromes involving the frontal lobe. In benign epilepsy with centrotemporal spikes (Rolandic epilepsy), which involves the primary motor cortex, a negative correlation has been observed between amount of EEG spiking and performance on measures of intellectual ability, short-term memory, and visual perception (i.e., increased epileptiform activity is related to decreased cognitive ability) (12). Patients with juvenile myoclonic epilepsy have been described as "impressionable, unreliable and unable," and have a higher incidence of psychiatric disease compared to the general population (12). It has been suggested that this behavioral profile is related to frontal lobe dysfunction, but this hypothesis warrants further investigation.

There is also evidence for frontal lobe dysfunction in temporal lobe epilepsy (13). The temporal and frontal lobes have strong functional interconnections, and spread of epileptiform activity to the frontal lobes has been hypothesized to be responsible for those deficits. Improvement of frontal lobe function is possible after successful epilepsy surgery in patients with temporal lobe epilepsy, in contrast to patients with frontal lobe epilepsy,

in whom deficits appear more likely to persist postsurgically. Postsurgical seizure control, however, remains the major predictor of improved neuropsychologic function after surgery (7).

CONCLUSION

Studies of cognitive and behavioral changes in frontal lobe epilepsy have been scarce and inconsistent. Although a large battery of tests is available to measure frontal lobe dysfunction, some aspects of frontal lobe function such as personality, incentive, and social interactions remain difficult to quantify. Most studies examining frontal lobe behavioral changes lack a sufficient number of patients to allow consistent and precise localization within the frontal lobes. Further studies, preferably in a multicenter fashion, are necessary to explore frontal lobe behavioral dysfunction in patients with frontal lobe epilepsy as well as in patients with other types of epilepsy.

References

1. Helmstaedter C. Behavioral aspects of frontal lobe epilepsy. *Epilepsy Behav* 2001; 2:384–395.
2. McDonald BC, Flashman LA, Saykin AJ. Executive dysfunction following traumatic brain injury: neural substrates and treatment strategies. *Neurorehabilitation* 2002; 17:333–344.
3. Helmstaedter C, Kemper B, Elger CE. Neuropsychological aspects of frontal lobe epilepsy. *Neuropsychologia* 1996; 34:399–406.
4. Farrant A, Morris RG, Russell T, Elwes R, et al. Social cognition in frontal lobe epilepsy. *Epilepsy Behav* 2005; 7:506–516.
5. Milner B. Aspects of human frontal lobe function. *Adv Neurol* 1995; 66:67–81.
6. Upton D, Thompson PJ. General neuropsychological characteristics of frontal lobe epilepsy. *Epilepsy Res* 1996; 23:169–177.
7. Helmstaedter C, Gleissner U, Zentner J, Elger CE. Neuropsychological consequences of epilepsy surgery in frontal lobe epilepsy. *Neuropsychologia* 1998; 36:681–689.
8. Kirsch HE. Social cognition and epilepsy surgery. *Epilepsy Behav* 2006; 8:71–80.
9. Jobst BC, Siegel AM, Thadani VM, Roberts DW, et al. Intractable seizures of frontal lobe origin: clinical characteristics, localizing signs, and results of surgery. *Epilepsia* 2000; 41:1139–1152.
10. Kanner AM. Recognition of the various expressions of anxiety, psychosis, and aggression in epilepsy. *Epilepsia* 2004; 45(Suppl 2):22–27.
11. Jobst BC, Roberts DW, Thadani VM, Williamson PD. Transient postoperative neurologic deficit after supplementary motor area resection. *Epilepsia*. 2002; 43(Suppl 7):44 (abstract).
12. Besag FM. Behavioral aspects of pediatric epilepsy syndromes. *Epilepsy Behav* 2004; 5(Suppl 1):S3–S13.
13. Shulman M. The frontal lobes, epilepsy, and behavior. *Epilepsy Behav* 2000; 1:384–395.

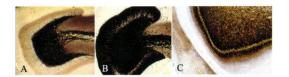

FIGURE 7-2

Control   Latent   Epileptic

Septal

Temporal

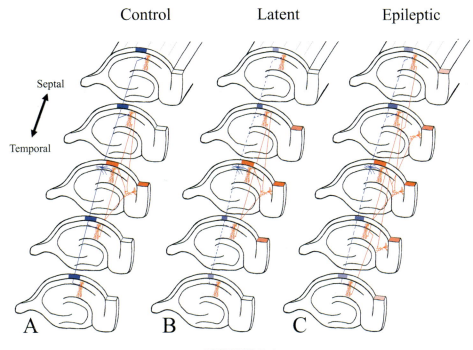

A   B   C

FIGURE 7-4

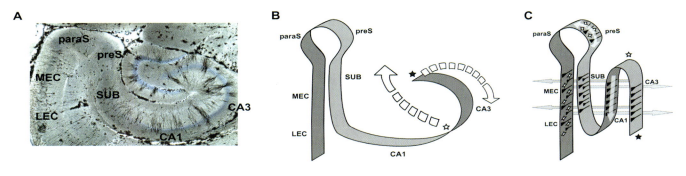

FIGURE 9-2

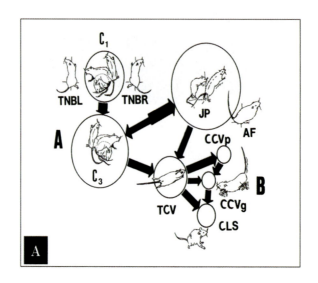

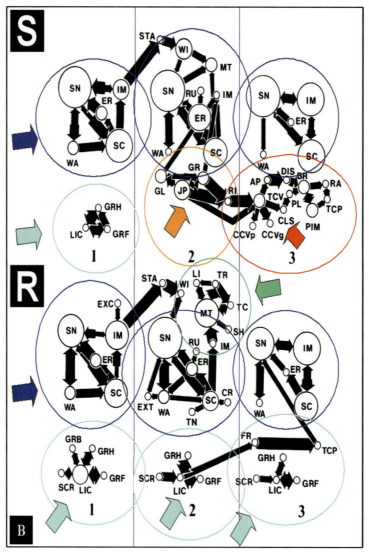

FIGURE 10-1

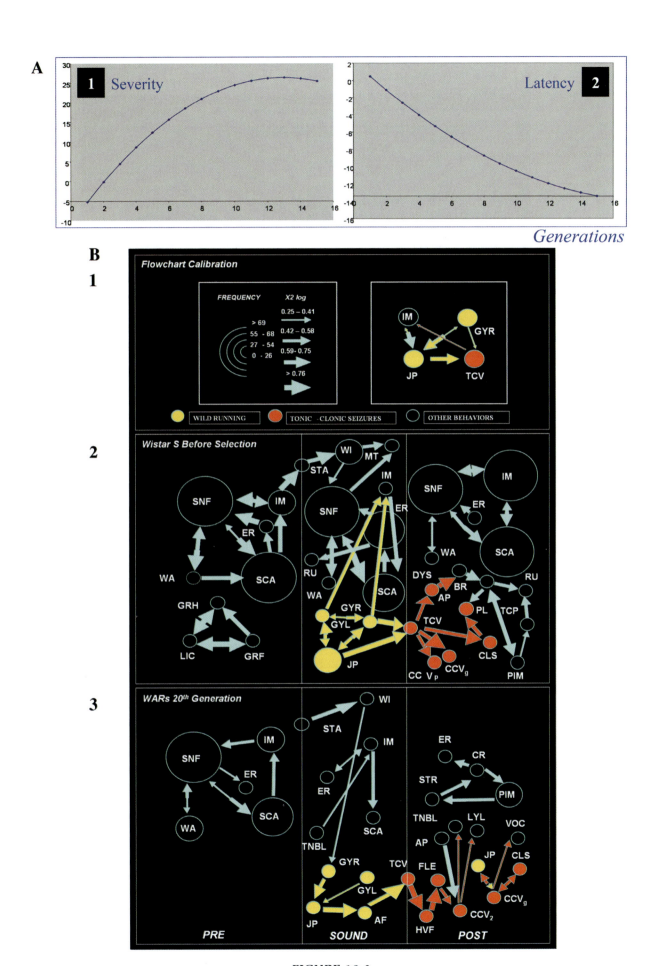

FIGURE 10-2

A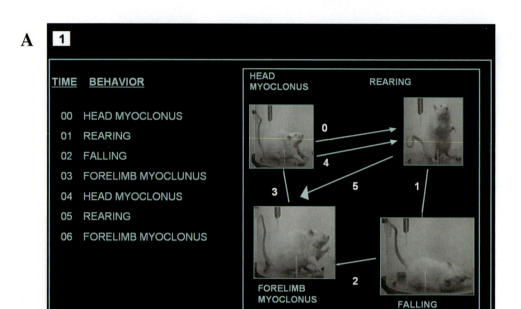

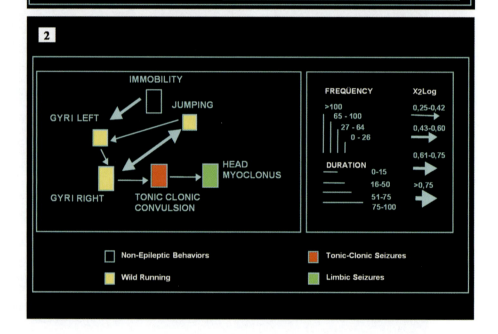

B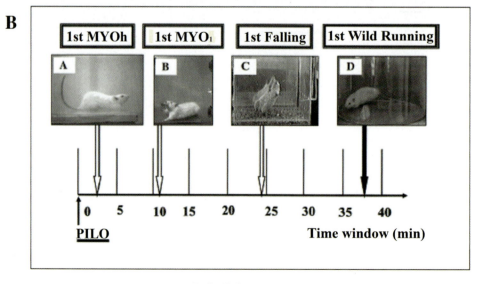

FIGURE 10-3

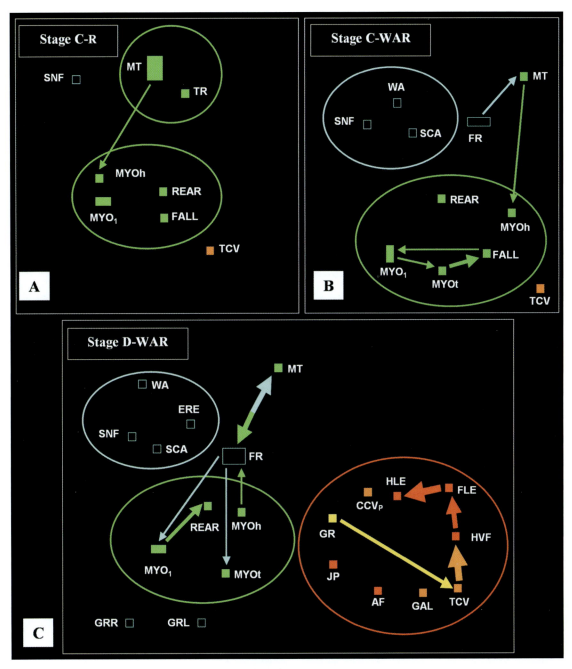

FIGURE 10-4

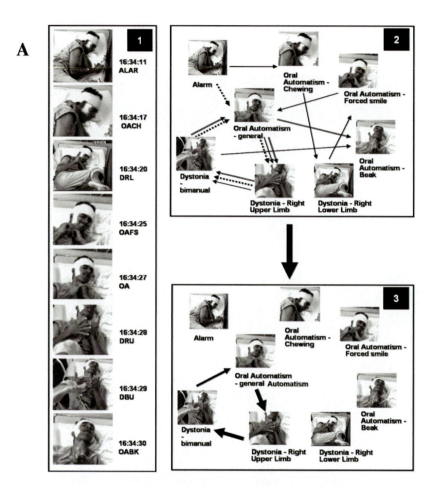

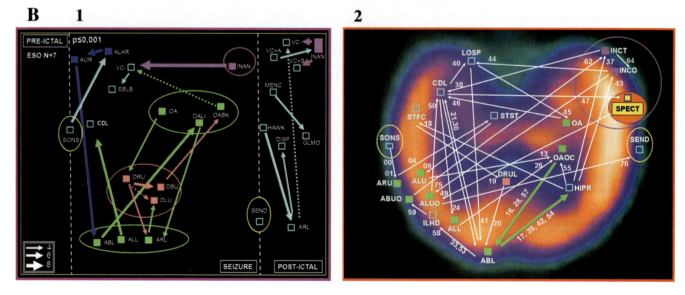

FIGURE 10-5

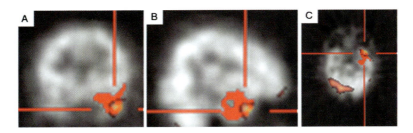

FIGURE 36-2

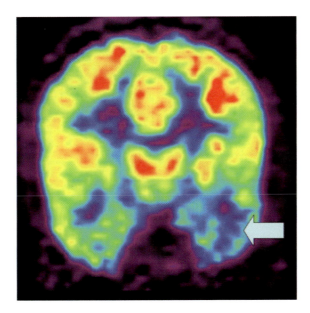

FIGURE 36-3

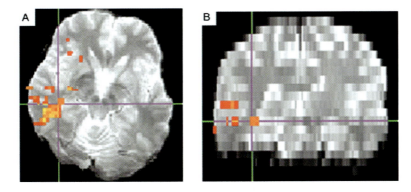

FIGURE 36-5

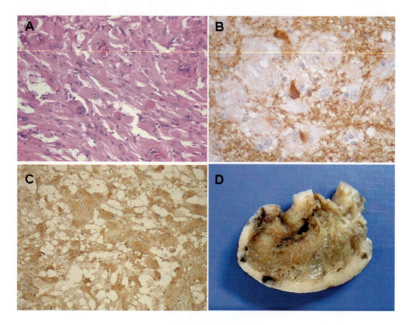

FIGURE 60-2

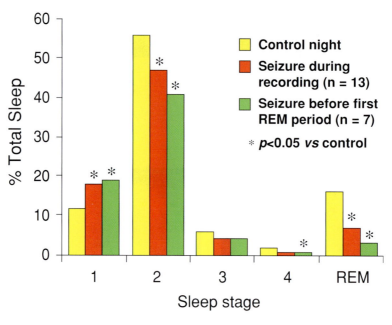

FIGURE 62-1

33

Neurophysiologic Correlates of Psychiatric Disorders and Potential Applications in Epilepsy

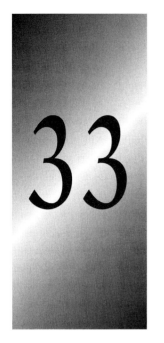

Jonathan J. Halford

A great deal of important research has been done in the field of psychiatry in recent years with various neuroimaging modalities such as functional magnetic resonance imaging (fMRI), positron emission tomography (PET), and single-photon emission computed tomography (SPECT). These new techniques have eclipsed neurophysiologic methods such as electroencephalography (EEG), magnetoencephalography (MEG), and transcranial magnetic stimulation (TMS) because they have improved spatial resolution and the ability to detect changes occurring deep in the brain. (EEG and MEG are more sensitive to signals produced near the brain's surface; TMS affects mainly neurons near the cortical surface.) But neurophysiologic methods may make a comeback for several reasons. First, with the exception of MEG, the other imaging modalities are expensive, while EEG and TMS are relatively economical. No high-field-strength magnets or radioactive materials are needed. Second, EEG, MEG, and TMS have a much higher temporal resolution than any of the other imaging modalities. Third, EEG, and to lesser extent MEG and TMS, are relatively noninvasive, nonthreatening, and easy to administer.

This chapter will briefly explain the most commonly used research methods of neurophysiologic assessment using EEG, MEG, and TMS in subjects with psychiatric disorders, review recent research findings, and suggest avenues for possible application of these methods to the study of psychiatric issues in epilepsy.

QUANTITATIVE EEG: CONVENTIONAL METHODS

Despite skepticism from the conventional EEG community, quantitative EEG (QEEG) continues to be studied as a diagnostic tool for routine psychiatric assessment. In QEEG, several minutes of EEG acquired with multiple channels (usually of nineteen or more electrodes placed on the head in standardized positions) are visually edited for artifacts and analyzed using the fast Fourier transform. This produces an estimate of the quantity of signal at various frequencies (the *power spectral density*) across the entire frequency spectra (the *power spectrum*). The frequency range for analysis has traditionally been separated into four wide frequency bands, including delta (1.5–3.5 Hz), theta (3.5–7.5 Hz), alpha (7.5–12.5 Hz), and beta (12.5–20 Hz). Results from each electrode can be represented as *absolute power* in each band, *relative power* in each band (percentage of power in each channel), *coherence* (a measure of synchronization between activity in two channels), and *symmetry* (the ratio of power in each band between a symmetrical pair of electrodes) (1). Coherence is a frequency-dependent measure of the degree of relatedness between

EEGs recorded over two different brain areas. High EEG coherence between two brain areas indicates that EEG amplitudes at a given frequency and their associated phase angles are correlated across time epochs, suggesting shared activation during a particular task.

Studies have shown QEEG to be useful in differentiating delirium from dementia, in differentiating Alzheimer's disease from controls based on increases in slow activity, and in differentiating various types of dementia. But QEEG is not currently recommended for the evaluation of other psychiatric disorders in clinical practice. Despite optimism by some researchers in the 1990s (1) that QEEG would be useful for psychiatric evaluation if certain standardized QEEG techniques were used, such as the Neurometric Analysis System (2), a lack of consensus as to what abnormalities were characteristic of which psychiatric conditions has cast QEEG's usefulness in doubt.

A good example of this lack of consensus is QEEG studies in patients with depression, which have shown varied results including increased delta and theta absolute spectral power in the right hemisphere, increased right anterior beta activity and reduced theta asymmetry, and no differences between depressed patients and controls. The most common finding in studies of patients with depression is an interhemispheric asymmetry of alpha activity, with increased alpha activity in the right frontal region primarily (3), although one study does not show this (4) and one study shows this asymmetry is present but is different between sexes (5). This alpha asymmetry is thought to represent a trait, because it is also found in adolescent children of depressed mothers and infants of mothers with depressive symptoms (6). This asymmetry in alpha activity in the frontal regions in depressed patients appears to be modestly stable over time, and changes are not associated with changes in depression severity. Studies have also shown decreased alpha activity or decreased delta activity in the right posterior region as well. But no finding in QEEG appears to be sensitive and specific enough to be clinically useful for the diagnosis of depression. This includes QEEG measures during sleep such as short rapid-eye movement (REM) latency, which is present in 30–50% of depressed outpatients and 50–80% of depressed inpatients, but is also present in 20% of normal controls (7). There are also several studies that find QEEG to predict antidepressant treatment response using such measures as increased right frontal alpha activity (8) and reduced REM latency, increased REM density, and decreased sleep efficiency (9).

QEEG is being studied for the evaluation for learning disorders and ADHD, because studies have shown that children and adolescents with these disorders have increased delta and theta activity and decreased alpha and beta activity (1, 10, 11). Studies to confirm that QEEG is definitely useful for diagnosing ADHD are still lacking, however (10). There have been a few QEEG studies in patients with obsessive-compulsive disorder. These studies have shown different and contradictory findings, including an increased frequency of temporal lobe spikes and sharp waves, alpha and delta frequency differences in the temporal regions, increased theta band power and decreased beta band power in the frontotemporal regions, and a decrease of the slow alpha band power.

The QEEG findings in patients with schizophrenia have also been varied and inconsistent. They include the finding of more delta and theta activity and less alpha activity than normal comparison subjects, greater overall absolute theta power, slower mean alpha frequency, and elevated absolute delta and total power in anterior regions than controls, greater slow wave power and slow alpha and fast beta bands, and less alpha power. Two studies have shown that changes in alpha power and theta power in the EEG of schizophrenic patients predict good response to antipsychotic medication (12, 13).

More recent studies in schizophrenic patients using alternative paradigms have produced some interesting findings. One MEG study comparing schizophrenic patients in two states, with and without ongoing auditory hallucinations, showed theta rhythm bursts in the left superior temporal lobe during the auditory hallucinations (14). Studies of EEG coherence during talking and listening have shown decreased frontal-temporal coherence during talking, especially in schizophrenic patients prone to hallucinate (15). This is consistent with other research that suggests that one possible mechanism for auditory hallucinations in schizophrenic patients is that they might mistake their own thoughts or speech for voices. They may mistake their own voice or thoughts for voices because of an abnormality in corollary discharge, the internal sensory feedback that the central nervous system gives itself when it produces a movement or sound.

Overall, QEEG has not been shown to be useful in psychiatry clinical practice. This was confirmed recently by an excellent study of QEEG parameters in a large number of patients with different psychiatric diagnoses, which showed that psychiatric patients, as a whole, showed diffuse decreased delta and theta activity in comparison to controls, but that there were no QEEG findings that could differentiate between various psychiatric diagnoses (16). This is probably due to several technical problems with QEEG including frequent artifact contamination, age and medication effects, subjective choices of analysis epochs, and questionable findings because of the large number of statistical tests that are run (17).

QUANTITATIVE EEG: CORDANCE

A new QEEG measure that is more promising to be useful in psychiatry is EEG *cordance*. Developed by Dr. Andrew Leuchter and coworkers at the University of California at Los Angeles (UCLA), cordance is a complex measure of EEG spectral power derived from resting EEG at each EEG electrode that relates the absolute spectral power to the relative spectral power. Cordance calculations take into account both absolute and relative power because, according to Leuchter and coworkers, brain areas with abnormal function may have low absolute spectral power but elevated relative spectral power in certain frequency bands. Cordance has been shown to have a moderately strong association with cerebral perfusion in normal subjects as measured by PET (18) and SPECT (19).

A small study by Leuchter et al. showed that cordance was decreased in areas of hypometabolism in patients with Alzheimer's disease and above subcortical white matter lesions (19). Another study by Cook et al. has shown decreased theta band cordance in depressed elderly subjects in comparison to normal controls (20). Several studies have shown that responders to antidepressant medication can be distinguished by higher pretreatment frontal theta band cordance (21) and a decrease in prefrontal theta band cordance after antidepressant treatment (22). One recent study also shows that higher pretreatment central cordance predicts response to electroconvulsive therapy (ECT) as well (23). Of particular interest are the studies by this group that show that depressed patients who respond to placebo show markedly different changes in theta band cordance compared to depressed patients who respond to antidepressant medication. The placebo responders show increased prefrontal theta band cordance, but the medication responders show decreased prefrontal theta band cordance (22, 24). Subjects taking antidepressants who have medication side effects have been demonstrated to show different cordance patterns from subjects who experience few side effects (25). All of these studies have been done at UCLA, and these findings have yet to be replicated outside of UCLA. Software to calculate EEG cordance is available by request for free from the UCLA Neuropsychiatric Institute. To our knowledge, EEG cordance has not been measured in epilepsy patients. Besides the obvious application of this QEEG measurement to the assessment of depression in patients with epilepsy, it would be interesting to see whether cordance correlates with temporal lobe hypometabolism as measured by routine fluorodeoxyglucose-positron emission tomography (FDG-PET) scans in partial epilepsy patients.

QUANTITATIVE EEG: SOURCE LOCALIZATION

Finding a solution to the inverse problem—the three-dimensional localization of the sources of voltage fields detected on the scalp—has been a focus for many researchers over the last decade. Some progress in estimating a solution to the inverse problem has been made (1). Multiple methods have been developed, including brain electrical source analysis (BESA), weighted minimum norm estimation, and low-resolution electromagnetic tomography (LORETA). Of the many techniques used when attempting to solve the inverse problem, LORETA is perhaps the most promising (1). LORETA finds a solution to the inverse problem by assuming that neighboring neuronal sources are similarly active (producing a solution with maximal "smoothness"). LORETA is being widely applied in research studies because it has been shown to be optimal compared to other solutions to the inverse problem and because several in vivo studies have provided validation. LORETA may be useful in localizing partial epilepsy (26). LORETA is being applied productively in the analysis of resting EEG (27) and evoked potential studies (28) of psychiatry patients. Studies using LORETA analysis of resting EEG in depressed patients have shown increased beta activity in the right frontal region and increased delta activity in the right temporal region. A recent study showed that the treatment response of depressed subjects to nortriptyline at 4–6 months could be predicted by higher theta activity in the rostral anterior cingulate cortex as measured by LORETA (29). LORETA is available as freeware over the Internet from The KEY Institute for Brain-Mind Research, University Hospital of Psychiatry, Zurich, Switzerland (at http://www.unizh.ch/keyinst/NewLORETA/LORETA01.htm).

QUANTITATIVE EEG: FRONTAL MIDLINE THETA

Theta frequency waves are frequently found throughout the cortex on analysis with quantitative EEG. Theta frequencies are prominent diffusely in the immature brain, during REM sleep, and in various types of cerebral dysfunction. One distinct pattern of focal theta frequency waves is frontal midline theta (FMT) rhythm. In 1972, Ishihara and Yoshi first described FMT rhythm as a train of rhythmic waves, observed at a frequency of 6–7 Hz and 30–60 μV, having a focal distribution with maximum around the frontal midline in the EEG of normal subjects (30). It is associated with cognitive processing, working memory, concentration, and attention, and it may be related to affective functioning.

Frontal midline theta rhythm amplitude is increased during mental tasks, in contrast to the alpha rhythm, which is attenuated during mental tasks. A sustained state of selective attention seems to be a necessary, although not sufficient, condition for the occurrence of FMT. Mental tasks that increase FMT include tasks of orienting, attention, memory, visual searching, and mathematical calculation. Increased attention and arousal cause an increase in FMT, as does increased time pressure during task performance. The amount of FMT varies among human subjects. In some subjects FMT is very prominent, and in others it appears to be absent, based on simple visual observation. FMT varies in amplitude during mental task performance, causing its appearance on EEG to wax and wane. Some researchers have observed that the amplitude of the FMT rhythm shows a periodicity of approximately 40–50 seconds (31). FMT has been localized to the midline prefrontal cortex and anterior cingulate cortex using EEG dipole modeling (32), dual EEG/MEG acquisition with multidipole modeling (33), and MEG with analysis by synthetic aperture magnetometry (SAM) (34). SAM analysis is a method of MEG analysis based on MEG biophysics, neural networks theory, and the general linear model that is capable of producing a three-dimensional estimate of the location of evoked brain activation during most functional imaging stimulus paradigms. SAM analysis, like many newer methods of data analysis being applied in clinical neurophysiology research (such as independent component analysis), does not rely heavily on signal averaging and is therefore able to use the data produced by a large array of sensors (such as many modern MEG sensor arrays) more precisely and efficiently.

Several early studies have reported an association between FMT and epilepsy (35). A more recent study reports that FMT, although possibly being more common in patients with epilepsy, is a nonspecific finding and cannot be used to help make the diagnosis of epilepsy (36). The increase in FMT during cognitive activity was shown in one study not to differ between juvenile subjects with epilepsy and normal controls (37). Overall, the occurrence of frontal midline theta rhythm has not been well studied in the epilepsy population.

There are some studies that report that FMT is decreased in various psychiatric disorders. Increased FMT has been found in subjects with certain personality types such as high extroversion and neuroticism (31). Decreased platelet monoamine oxidase (MAO) activity has been associated with psychiatric disorders including alcoholism, psychopathy, suicidality, and dysthymia (38), and a negative correlation has been found between platelet MAO activity and FMT activity (39). FMT activity was inversely correlated with anxiety based on self-report in one study (31). Patients with anxiety disorders have been found to have low FMT activity, which increases after pharmacological treatment of anxiety with benzodiazepines and tricyclic antidepressants. Increased FMT activity has also been associated with the report of a positive emotional state during meditation. There are many aspects of the FMT rhythm that have not been studied thoroughly, such as its scalp distribution and periodicity. Frontal midline theta may be studied more in the future in psychiatric populations for several reasons. First, evidence from several QEEG data analysis techniques, such as conventional QEEG spectral analysis

and LORETA, shows theta activity abnormalities in the frontal lobes in patients with depression. Second, FMT has a close association with arousal and attention, which are cognitive processes that are commonly affected by psychiatric disorders. Third, FMT is produced mainly in the cingulate cortex, which has been associated with affective processing.

Evoked Potentials: P50

The P50 (or P1) is the first of the mid-latency auditory evoked potentials. (See Figure 33-1 for a diagram of the early and mid-latency auditory evoked potentials.) Although some investigators have reported that the absolute latency and amplitude of the P50 to one single auditory stimulus is abnormal in patients with schizophrenia, most research on the P50 potential has focused on its recovery cycle. In normal subjects a second auditory stimulus following an initial auditory stimulus in less than 1 second (typically in 500 msec) causes a suppression of the P50 evoked potential to the second stimulus by around 50%. This suppression of the second P50 evoked response to paired-pulse stimulation has been reported as abnormal in schizophrenia by many investigators, although some recent investigators have not found this (40). Several studies have shown that this P50 nonsuppression correlates with poor performance on neuropsychologic tests of attention and also correlates with negative symptoms (41, 42).

P50 nonsuppression appears to be a heritable trait present in family members of patients with schizophrenia (43) and is present in individuals who are at high risk for developing schizophrenia because of genetics and

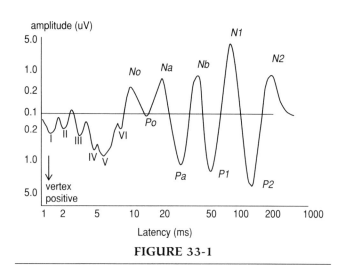

FIGURE 33-1

Short-, middle-, and long-latency auditory evoked potentials. Modified from Barlow HB, Mollon JD. *The Senses.* Cambridge: Cambridge University Press, 1982.

prodromal symptoms (44). Linkage studies of families with P50 nonsuppression have identified chromosome 15 as a probable location for a genetic abnormality (45). Several studies have found abnormalities in the alpha7 neuronal nicotinic acetylcholine receptor subunit gene (*CHRNA7*), a gene on chromosome 15, in subjects with P50 nonsuppression (46), and a preliminary study recently demonstrated that a novel nicotinic agonist improved the P50 suppression abnormality (47).

Although the P50 potential, as detected by EEG, is produced by the auditory cortex in the superior temporal gyrus bilaterally, it is maximally detected at the central vertex, which makes unilateral measurement impossible. But unilateral measurement of this potential is possible using MEG, and this is called the M50 potential. Several MEG studies in patients with schizophrenia have shown M50 suppression on the left side only (48). This is one possible explanation for why some studies of the P50 suppression have not detected abnormalities in schizophrenic patients (since there could be a dilution of the effect of an abnormal potential on the left side on the P50 potential at the vertex by a normal potential from the right side). There is also evidence from a dual EEG/MEG study that the generators of the P50 may be different in schizophrenic patients than in normal controls (49). The M50 suppression abnormality has been correlated with cortical thickness in the primary auditory cortex in one study (50). The nonsuppression of the P50 has been shown to normalize when schizophrenic patients are treated with certain atypical antipsychotics such as clozapine (51). P50 nonsuppression has also been found in bipolar disorder subjects with a history of psychosis (52).

Evoked Potentials: N100

Patients with schizophrenia have been shown to have abnormalities in the auditory N100 potential (also termed N1 potential). The auditory N100 potential is another of the mid-latency auditory evoked potentials (see Figure 33-1) and is generated by the primary and secondary auditory cortices. The amplitude of the N100 has been reported to be decreased in patients with schizophrenia using EEG (53) and MEG (54). The latency of the N100 has also been shown to be prolonged in schizophrenic patients in one study (55). In a study comparing patients with epilepsy to patients with schizophrenia by Ford et al., the N100 amplitude was decreased in patients with schizophrenia but not in patients with epilepsy or in controls (56). This is consistent with a previous study of N100 amplitude in patients with epilepsy (57).

Several recent studies of the N100 in patients with schizophrenia have produced interesting findings using novel paradigms. One study finds that there is an absence of amplitude suppression with paired-pulse stimuli with the M100, similar to M50 and P50 suppression

abnormalities, in patients with schizophrenia (48). One study of the location of the N100 response to different tone frequencies shows that the typical tonotopic pattern of the N100 response is absent in schizophrenic patients (58), suggesting disruption of the primary auditory cortex. Studying the N100 evoked potential while the subject is talking may be another way to study corollary discharge (the dampening effect on the sensory system during self-produced sounds or other stimuli). Normally, the N100 auditory evoked potential produced by a subject who is speaking (evoked by his or her own voice) is decreased in comparison to an N100 auditory evoked potential produced by listening to a playback of his or her own recorded speech. Studies by Ford and colleagues find that this decrease in the N100 amplitude during self-produced sounds is not present in patients with schizophrenia (15), suggesting an abnormality in corollary discharge. To our knowledge, measures of corollary discharge using EEG coherence or the N100 have not been studied in epilepsy patients with interictal psychosis.

Evoked Potentials: Loudness Dependency of the Auditory Evoked Potential (LDAEP)

The loudness dependency of the N1 and P2 mid-latency auditory evoked potentials is being studied as a measure of brain serotonergic neurotransmission and a possible predictor of antidepressant response. The amount that a cortical auditory evoked potential increases as the stimulus loudness increases is its "intensity dependence" or "loudness dependency." Serotonergic neurotransmission is thought to modulate sensory processing in the primary auditory and visual cortices. The highest concentrations and the highest synthesis rates of cortical serotonin have consistently been found in the primary sensory cortices, especially in the primary auditory cortex in the superior temporal gyrus.

It is unclear how to best measure the LDAEP. Many studies simply measure the amplitude difference between the N1 and P2 potentials. This may not be an optimal method, because the auditory evoked potentials are composed of overlapping N1/P2 potentials produced in both the primary and the secondary auditory cortices. Because serotonergic neurotransmission modulates the sensory processing in the primary auditory cortex only (but not the secondary auditory cortex), it is these components produced by the primary auditory cortex that are theoretically best to use in calculating the loudness dependency. But separating out the components produced by primary auditory cortex is not easy. The first attempt to separate out the components produced by primary and secondary cortices was with dipole source analysis (59). A recent study has used LORETA to do this (28). Some researchers believe that measurement of the LDAEP at the central vertex, where the field potentials of both of the primary auditory cortices project, without elaborate analysis techniques such as dipole analysis or LORETA, is sufficient (Gallinat J, email communication to the author, February 1, 2006). Only one study has compared several methods for separating out the signal from the primary auditory cortex for calculating the LDAEP and has concluded that the best means is by using LORETA. The LORETA software can estimate the current density (which is the source for the N1/P2 potential) in the brain regions containing the primary auditory cortex, as specified by Talairach coordinates (28). But further studies are needed to clarify this.

Arguments for the use of loudness dependency of the auditory evoked potential (LDAEP) to study serotonergic function can be drawn from the following studies. The concentration of 5-hydroxyindoleacetic acid (the main metabolite of serotonin) in cerebrospinal fluid (CSF) has been found to correlate negatively with the intensity dependence of sensory evoked potentials (60). Epidural EEG recordings in the primary and secondary auditory cortex of cats show decreased LDAEP in primary auditory cortex with serotonin agonists and increased LDAEP with serotonin antagonists (61). Serotonin agonists (e.g., zimelidine) have been found to reduce that intensity dependence of sensory evoked potentials (62). The neurotrophin brain-derived neurotrophic factor (BDNF) influences the phenotype, structural plasticity, and survival of serotonergic neurons (63). One study has shown a negative correlation between the BDNF serum concentrations and the LDAEP (64). Patients with serotonin syndrome (who are symptomatic because of very high serotonin levels) have extremely low LDAEP (65). Migraine patients may have low serotonin levels between attacks, and the LDAEP has been shown to be elevated in migraine patients between attacks in three studies (64). Abstinent methylenedioxymethamphetamine (MDMA, "ecstasy") users, who have low serotonergic activity, have been shown to have high LDAEP (67). Depressed patients with a history of suicide attempts were shown to have a higher LDAEP in one study (68). Treatment with selective serotonin reuptake inhibitors decreases the LDAEP in normal control subjects (69). Clinical response to treatment with an SSRI has been predicted by higher pretreatment LDAEP in four studies (28, 70–72). LDAEP has been shown to be lower than controls (implying increased serotonogic activity) in patients with schizophrenia (73). This may be a reason why antipsychotic medications with 5-HT2 antagonism, such as atypical antipsychotics, are effective for the treatment of negative symptoms.

But there are also doubts as to whether LDAEP is truly an accurate measure of brain serotonergic activity and whether it is specific for serotonin. Some studies have found that LDAEP correlates with activity in the dopaminergic system as well as the serotonergic system.

Dopamine metabolites in CSF and urine have been found to correlate with LDAEP and in intensity dependence of visual stimuli (74). It has been found that the D1/D2 agonist apomorphine decreased the LDAEP in animals (61), and the LDAEP and the striatal dopamine transporter binding were shown to correlate in one study of patients with obsessive compulsive disorder (75). Also, some studies have produced results that question how accurate a measure of central serotonergic activity the LDAEP is. Studies examining the functional polymorphism in the serotonin transporter gene (5-HTTLPR) have shown both a weaker (76) and a stronger (77) LDAEP in individuals homozygous for the l allele (the allele associated with higher serotonin uptake and central serotonin activity). Also, acute depletion of serotonin availability using tryptophan depletion has been shown in several studies to have no effects (78) or a paradoxical decrease in the LDAEP (79). Those who believe that the LDAEP is a useful measure of serotonergic function have pointed out that the dopaminergic system modulates the serotonergic system in the brainstem, so it is not surprising that they are shown to both effect LDAEP. They also point out the varying methodologies and possible insufficient tryptophan depletion in the tryptophan depletion studies. So the question of whether the LDAEP is a useful measure of brain serotonergic neurotransmission has yet to be answered definitively.

Evoked Potentials: P300

The P300 component of the auditory event-related potential is a positive potential that occurs with an approximate latency of 300 msec after the presentation of novel stimuli embedded among many irrelevant stimuli, to which the subject is required to respond. (This is called an "oddball" paradigm.) Although the cognitive significance of the P300 is still debated, it is thought to be involved in cognitive processing involving attention and working memory, and it is attention dependent. The P300 is related to memory updating and may represent the transfer of relevant information to consciousness. A reduced amplitude of the P300 component of the auditory event–related potential in schizophrenia was first reported 30 years ago (80).

A P300 amplitude reduction, and to a lesser extent latency delay, to the oddball target are fairly consistent findings in neurophysiologic studies of schizophrenia (81), although they have not been found by all researchers (82). The P300 abnormalities are observed mainly in auditory rather than visual paradigms (83), which is consistent with a predominance of auditory rather than visual symptoms in schizophrenia (e.g., hallucinations are primarily auditory). The reduced amplitude of the P300 may be an electrophysiological trait marker of schizophrenia, because it is observed in schizophrenic patients' siblings and other relatives (84) and in high-risk children (85). But studies have also shown the P300 amplitude to be associated with the clinical state of schizophrenic patients, being lower during times of symptom exacerbation (86). Both the P300 amplitude and latency abnormalities increase with illness duration (87), providing evidence that schizophrenia is a neurodegenerative disease. Several studies have shown that the P300 potential field is decreased on the left side in schizophrenic patients (81, 88). The P300 amplitude correlates negatively with disability of daily life in patients with schizophrenia, possibly because it may be associated with thought disorder symptoms (89).

The potential utility of the P300 for diagnosing schizophrenia has been questioned because of a lack of specificity (56). Decreased P300 amplitudes have been found in studies of depression by some (90) but not other investigators (91). A few studies in depressed patients have found prolonged P300 latency (92), but many have not. It is difficult to draw conclusions about P300 abnormalities in depression because of the heterogeneity of patient groups studied, including melancholic depression, geriatric depression, depression with silent cerebral infarction, and medically and nonmedically treated depression. Decreased P300 amplitude has also been found in alcoholics (based mostly on studying the visual P300) and in patients with dissociative disorders, and a prolonged P300 latency has been found in dementia.

Interestingly, a study by Ford et al. (56), examining the P300 in patients with epilepsy and comparing with the P300 in patients with schizophrenia, found that epilepsy patients had a prolonged P300 latency and schizophrenic patients did not. Also, the schizophrenic patients and epilepsy patients with chronic psychotic symptoms had a decreased P300 amplitude, which discriminated them from epilepsy patients without psychotic symptoms (56). This is consistent with previous studies that have shown prolonged P300 latency but normal P300 amplitude in patients with epilepsy (without psychotic symptoms) (57). This is also consistent with studies that show that depressed patients with psychotic features can be discriminated from depressed patients without psychotic features by a lower P300 amplitude (92).

Evoked Potentials: Mismatch Negativity

Mismatch negativity (MMN) is an auditory evoked potential, produced when deviant auditory stimuli occurs infrequently mixed in many standard stimuli (the oddball paradigm), which occurs 150–200 msec after the deviant stimulus. It is thought to be an index of preattentive detection of acoustic changes, which is not attention dependent and is likely generated by multiple regions of the brain including the frontal, temporal, and parietal lobes. A lower-than-normal amplitude of

MMN to pure-tone stimuli has been demonstrated in schizophrenia patients in many studies using EEG (93). A lower MMN amplitude been detected using MEG in most studies (94) but not in a few studies (95) and associated with decreased gray matter volume on MRI measurements of the left planum temporale in one study (96). Abnormal MMN in schizophrenia patients has been shown to be stable over time and correlated with poor functioning (97). A few studies have found that MMN is not abnormal in first-episode schizophrenics but becomes abnormal over time, suggesting that it may be caused by ongoing neuropathological changes (81). Abnormalities in MMN have not been found in relatives of schizophrenic patients (98). MMN abnormalities may be specific for schizophrenia, because they were not found in patients with depression or bipolar disorder in one study (99). To our knowledge, this has not been studied in epilepsy populations.

Evoked Potentials: Contingent Negative Variation

Slow event-related potentials (ERPs) have been studied to a lesser extent than many of those evoked potentials discussed previously. These slow potentials are evoked by auditory or visual stimuli, rise and fall slowly, occur in the range of 100 msec to 550 msec post stimulus, and are thought to modulate the production of mid and late auditory evoked potentials. Of these slow potentials, the contingent negative variation (CNV), also referred to as the "readiness potential," has been studied the most. CNV is a slow cortical ERP, which can be recorded from the scalp between two stimuli in a "go/no-go" task in which a warning stimulus alerts the subject that a second stimulus demanding a response is forthcoming. The CNV appears on the EEG at the midline while the subject is anticipating the second event and preparing for task performance (for example, pressing of a button). Patients with a history of closed head injury and frontal lobe damage show a decreased CNV in comparison to controls (100). Reduced CNV amplitude has been found in patients with schizophrenia and is correlated with negative symptoms in schizophrenic subjects (101). Alcoholic subjects have alterations in the CNV that correlate with neuropsychologic dysfunction (102). In studies of depressed subjects, decreased CNV amplitude and duration have been found by some (103) but not others (104). It is likely that CNV is a measure of selective attention and arousal level and may not be specific to a particular psychiatric disorder. Recent studies of depressed subjects have shown the CNV amplitude to be correlated inversely with severity of depression (105), nonsuppression in the dexamethasone suppression test (106), and suicidal behavior (107). To our knowledge, CNV has not been studied in epilepsy. Whether CNV and other slow potentials will find a role in psychiatric evaluation and management is yet unclear.

Transcranial Magnetic Stimulation

Transcranial magnetic stimulation (TMS) involves the use of handheld coils through which a large amount of electrical current is discharged, producing a brief, strong magnetic field. This magnetic field penetrates the skull, reaches the cerebral cortex, and activates cortical elements without causing significant pain to the subject. TMS is a research tool that is finding increased application in neurology, mostly in studies of cortical motor areas and corticospinal tract conduction. Within the field of psychiatry, TMS is being studied both as a diagnostic tool and as a possible treatment modality for major depression. The use of TMS for treatment of depression involves the administration of repetitive TMS pulses. Many studies have indicated that TMS applied to the prefrontal cortex is beneficial for refractory major depression, although the effect is not large and its efficacy has been questioned by some (108). It does have a better side-effect profile than electroconvulsive therapy. Recent studies in depression using higher-frequency TMS settings have demonstrated better results (109) and suggest that further study is warranted. An improved response time to antidepressant treatment with concurrent TMS treatment in depressed patients has been found by some (110) but not other authors (111). TMS over the left frontotemporal cortex has also been studied for the treatment of medication-refractory auditory hallucinations in schizophrenia, with some studies showing improvement (112) and some studies showing no effect (113). Studies have also shown improvement in negative and depression symptoms in schizophrenics (114). A few studies have found benefit in using TMS to treat other psychiatric disorders such as posttraumatic stress disorder, bipolar disorder, and obsessive compulsive disorder.

For diagnostic purposes in psychiatry, TMS is being used to study neural plasticity, to study cortical connectivity, and most commonly as a noninvasive measure of cortical inhibition (115). To measure cortical inhibition with TMS, one of four paradigms is generally used (116). The first is paired-pulse TMS (ppTMS), in which a subthreshold conditioning pulse precedes a test pulse by 1 to 5 msec, inhibitory interneurons are recruited, and the motor evoked potential (MEP) response is inhibited. (In contrast, if a subthreshold pulse precedes the test pulse by 7 to 20 msec, the MEP response is facilitated.) The second is cortical silent period TMS (CSP), in which motor cortical stimulation superimposed on background electromyographic (EMG) activity results in cessation of EMG activity, producing a silent period. The duration of this silent period represents another measure of cortical inhibition. The third is transcallosal inhibition (TCI),

in which stimulation of the contralateral motor cortex a few milliseconds before stimulation of the ipsilateral motor cortex inhibits the size of the MEP produced by ipsilateral stimulation. The fourth is descending I-wave facilitation. TMS of the human motor cortex results in multiple discharges in the corticospinal tract. The first descending volley is produced by direct neuronal stimulation (D-wave), and this is followed by waves of activation produced through the stimulation of cortical interneurons (I-waves). The facilitation of I-wave activity is assessed using a paired-pulse protocol that involves pairing a suprathreshold first and subthreshold second stimulus (117). Studies have shown that three of these techniques—ppTMS, CSP, and TCI—represent cortical inhibitory phenomena and not other mechanisms such as neuronal refractoriness (118).

Many studies using these TMS paradigms have demonstrated alterations in cortical inhibition in schizophrenia (119). A recent study by Daskalakis et al. showed abnormalities in all three of these TMS measures of cortical inhibition in unmedicated patients with schizophrenia (116). Also, measures of cortical inhibition using TMS have also been noted to be different in patients with schizophrenia after several minutes of TMS stimulation, suggesting altered cortical plasticity (120). But this abnormality in cortical inhibition as measured by TMS does not appear to be specific to schizophrenia because it has also been found in obsessive compulsive disorder, Tourette's disorder, anxiety personality traits, and major depression. Studies using ppTMS and the CSP have shown decreased inhibition in patients with Tourette's disorder (121) and obsessive-compulsive disorder (122). In a study by Wasserman et al., anxiety-related personality traits correlated with decreased cortical inhibition, mainly in men (123). One study in patients with major depression has shown increased cortical inhibition in the left hemisphere and decreased inhibition in the right hemisphere compared to controls (124). Cortical inhibition has been shown to be decreased in studies of poststroke epilepsy (125), posttumor epilepsy (126), and progressive myoclonic epilepsy (127) and increased in studies of generalized epilepsy (128). Two studies in partial epilepsy show mixed results with abnormalities in cortical inhibition based on ppTMS that are sometimes present and that vary between hemispheres (129, 130). No studies have been done to correlate alterations in TMS measures of cortical inhibition with psychiatric symptoms in epilepsy patients.

CONCLUSION

It appears that many of these neurophysiologic analysis techniques and stimulus paradigms hold promise to improve psychiatric patient care by improving diagnostic precision, by predicting treatment response, and by providing new phenotypes for genetic studies. Epilepsy health care providers are in a good position to benefit from and contribute to this growing field because of their access to electrodiagnostic equipment and their familiarity with neurophysiology. But application of these paradigms in clinical practice will not be immediate. Much work must be done to optimize and validate these different diagnostic approaches. Because of the complexity of the central nervous system and the steady improvement in computer technology, there appears to an increasing overabundance of different evoked potentials and neurophysiologic quantitative measures that can be acquired

and calculated. It is exciting that so many neurophysiologic tests have been developed, but the amount of study needed to bring any of these tests into clinical practice is great. It might be better if the researchers in this field would focus on just a few of these neurophysiologic measures and either confirm their clinical usefulness or set them aside. A four-step approach for doing this has recently been outlined in a paper by Boutros et al., using the example of QEEG and ADHD (8). Epilepsy researchers interested in behavioral issues and neurophysiology should consider working with their psychiatry colleagues to form the cooperative efforts needed to bring some of these good ideas into clinical practice.

References

1. Hughes JR, John ER. Conventional and quantitative electroencephalography in psychiatry. *J Neuropsychiatry Clin Neurosci* 1999; 11:190–208.

2. John E, Prichep L, Friedman J, et al: Neurometrics: computer assisted differential diagnosis of brain dysfunctions. *Science* 1988; 293:162–169.

3. Coan JA, Allen JJ. The state and trait nature of frontal EEG asymmetry in emotion. In: Hugdahl K, Davidson RJ, eds. *The Asymmetrical Brain*. Cambridge, MA: MIT Press; 2003:565–615.

4. Reid SA, Duke LM, Allen JJ. Resting frontal electroencephalographic asymmetry in depression: inconsistencies suggest the need to identify mediating factors. *Psychophysiology* 1998; 35:389–404.

5. Miller A, Fox NA, Cohn JF, Forbes EE, et al. Regional patterns of brain activity in adults with a history of childhood-onset depression: gender differences and clinical variability. *Am J Psychiatry* 2002; 159(6):934–940.

6. Dawson G, Frey K, Panagiotides H, Yamada E, et al. Infants of depressed mothers exhibit atypical frontal electrical brain activity during interactions with mother and with a familiar, nondepressed adult. *Child Dev* 1999; 70:1058–1066.

7. Tsuno N, Besset A, Ritchie K. Sleep and depression. *J Clin Psychiatry* 2005; 66: 1254–1269.

8. Deldin PJ, Chiu P. Cognitive restructuring and EEG in major depression. *Biol Psychol* 2005; 70:141–151.

9. Thase ME, Kupfer DJ, Fasiczka AJ, Buysse DJ, et al. Identifying an abnormal electroencephalographic sleep profile to characterize major depressive disorder. *Biol Psychiatry* 1997; 41:964–973.

10. Boutros N, Fraenkel L, Feingold A. A four-step approach for developing diagnostic tests in psychiatry: EEG in ADHD as a test case. *J Neuropsychiatry Clin Neurosci* 2005; 17:455–464.

11. di Michele F, Prichep L, John ER, Chabot RJ. The neurophysiology of attention-deficit/hyperactivity disorder. *Int J Psychophysiol* 2005; 58:81–93.

12. Kikuchi M, Wada Y, Higashima M, Nagasawa T, et al. Individual analysis of EEG band power and clinical drug response in schizophrenia. *Neuropsychobiology* 2005; 51: 183–190.

13. Knott V, Labelle A, Jones B, Mahoney C. Quantitative EEG in schizophrenia and in response to acute and chronic clozapine treatment. *Schizophr Res* 2001; 50(1–2):41–53.

14. Ishii R, Shinosaki K, Ikejiri Y, Ukai S, et al. Theta rhythm increases in left superior temporal cortex during auditory hallucinations in schizophrenia: a case report. *Neuroreport* 2000; 11:3283–3287.

15. Ford JM, Mathalon DH. Corollary discharge dysfunction in schizophrenia: can it explain auditory hallucinations? *Int J Psychophysiol* 2005; 58(2-3):179–189.

16. Coutin-Churchman P, Anez Y, Uzcategui M, Alvarez L, et al. Quantitative spectral analysis of EEG in psychiatry revisited: drawing signs out of numbers in a clinical setting. *Clin Neurophysiol* 2003; 114:2294–2306.

17. Nuwer MR. Clinical use of QEEG. *Clin Neurophysiol* 2003; 114:2225.

18. Leuchter AF, Uijtdehaage SHJ, Cook IA, O'Hara R, et al. Relationship between brain electrical activity and cortical perfusion in normal subjects. *Psychiatry Res* 1999; 90: 125–140.

19. Leuchter AF, Cook IA, Lufkin RB, Dunkin J, et al. Cordance: a new method for assessment of cerebral perfusion and metabolism using quantitative electroencephalography. *Neuroimage* 1994; 1:208–219.

20. Cook IA, Leuchter AF, Uijtdehaage SHJ, Osato S, et al. Altered cerebral energy utilization in late life depression. *J Affect Disord* 1998; 49:89–99.

21. Cook IA, Leuchter AF, Morgan M, Stubbeman WF, et al. Changes in prefrontal activity characterize clinical response in SSRI nonresponders: a pilot study. *J Psychiatr Res* 2005; 39:461–466.

22. Leuchter AF, Cook IA, Witte E, Morgan M, et al. Changes in brain function of depressed subjects during treatment with placebo. *Am J Psychiatry* 2002; 159:122–129.

23. Stubbemann WF, Leuchter AF, Cook IA, Shurman BD, et al. Pretreatment neurophysiologic function and ECT response in depression. *J ECT* 2004; 20:142–144.

24. Leuchter AF, Morgan M, Cook IA, Dunkin J, et al. Pretreatment neurophysiological and clinical characteristics of placebo responders in treatment trials of major depression. *Psychopharmacology* 2004; 177:15–22.

25. Hunter AM, Leuchter AF, Morgan ML, Cook IA, et al. Neurophysiologic correlates of side effects in normal subjects randomized to venlafaxine or placebo. *Neuropsychopharmacology* 2005; 30:792–799.

26. Worrell GA, Lagerlund TD, Sharbrough FW, Brinkmann BH, et al. Localization of the epileptic focus by low-resolution electromagnetic tomography in patients with a lesion demonstrated by MRI. *Brain Topogr* 2000; 12:273–282.

27. Pizzagalli DA, Nitschke JB, Oakes TR, Hendrick AM, et al. Brain electrical tomography in depression: the importance of symptom severity, anxiety, and melancholic features. *Biol Psychiatry* 2002; 52:73–85.

28. Mulert C, Juckel G, Augustin H, Hegerl U. Comparison between the analysis of the loudness dependency of the auditory N1/P2 component with LORETA and dipole source analysis in the prediction of treatment response to the selective serotonin reuptake inhibitor citalopram in major depression. *Clin Neurophysiol* 2002; 113:1566–1572.

29. Pizzagalli D, Pascual-Marqui RD, Nitschke JB, Oakes TR, et al. Anterior cingulate activity as a predictor of degree of treatment response in major depression: evidence from brain electrical tomography analysis. *Am J Psychiatry* 2001; 158:405–415.

30. Ishihara T, Yoshii N. Multivariate analytic study of EEG and mental activity in juvenile delinquents. *Electroencephalogr Clin Neurophysiol* 1972; 33:71–80.

31. Inanaga K. Frontal midline theta rhythm and mental activity. *Psychiatry Clin Neurosci* 1998; 52:555–566.

32. Gevins A, Smith ME, McEvoy LK, Yu D. High-resolution EEG mapping of cortical activation related to working memory: effects of task difficulty, type of processing, and practice. *Cerebr Cortex* 1997; 7:374–385.

33. Asada H, Fukada Y, Tsunoda S, Yamaguchi M, et al. Frontal midline theta rhythms reflect alternative activation of prefrontal cortex and anterior cingulate cortex in humans. *Neurosci Lett* 1999; 274:29–32.

34. Ishii R, Shinosaki K, Ukai S, Inouye T, et al. Medial prefrontal cortex generates frontal midline theta rhythm. *Neuroreport* 1999; 10:675–679.

35. Mokran V, Ciganek L, Kabatnik Z. Electroencephalographic theta discharges in the midline. *Eur Neurol* 1971; 5:288–293.

36. Westmoreland BF, Klass DW. Midline theta rhythm. *Arch Neurol* 1986; 43:139–141.

37. Pellouchoud E, Smith ME, McEvoy LK, Gevins A. Mental effort-related EEG modulation during video-game play: comparison between juvenile subjects with epilepsy and normal control subjects. *Epilepsia* 1999; 40(Suppl 4):38–43.

38. Tripodianakis J, Markianos M, Sarantidis D, Spyropoulou G, et al. Platelet MAO activity in patients with dysthymic disorder. *Psychiatry Res* 1998; 78:173–178.

39. Hashimoto M, Mukasa H, Yamada S, Makamura J, et al. Frontal midline theta and platelet MAO in human subjects. *Biol Psychiatry* 1988; 23:31–43.

40. Johannesen JK, Kieffaber PD, O'Donnell BF, Shekhar A, et al. Contributions of subtype and spectral frequency analyses to the study of P50 ERP amplitude and suppression in schizophrenia. *Schizophr Res* 2005; 78(2-3):269–284.

41. Louchart-de la Chapelle S, Levillain D, Menard JF, Van der Elst A, et al. P50 inhibitory gating deficit is correlated with the negative symptomatology of schizophrenia. *Psychiatry Res* 2005; 136:27–34.

42. Thoma RJ, Hanlon FM, Moses SN, Ricker D, et al. M50 sensory gating predicts negative symptoms in schizophrenia. *Schizophr Res* 2005; 73(2-3):311–318.

43. Clementz BA, Geyer MA, Braff DL. P50 suppression among the relatives of schizophrenia patients. *Schizophr Res* 1997; 24:232.

44. Cadenhead KS, Light GA, Shafer KM, Braff DL. P50 suppression in individuals at risk for schizophrenia: the convergence of clinical, familial, and vulnerability marker risk assessment. *Biol Psychiatry* 2005; 57:1504–1509.

45. Freedman R, Coon H, Myles-Worsley M, Orr-Urtreger A, et al. Linkage of a neurophysiological deficit in schizophrenia to a chromosome 15 locus. *Proc Natl Acad Sci U S A* 1997; 94:587–592.

46. Leonard S, Gault J, Hopkins J, Logel J, et al. Association of promoter variants in the alpha7 nicotinic acetylcholine receptor subunit gene with an inhibitory deficit found in schizophrenia. *Arch Gen Psychiatry* 2002; 59:1085–1096.

47. Olincy A, Harris JG, Johnson LL, Pender V, et al. Proof-of-concept trial of an alpha7 nicotinic agonist in schizophrenia. *Arch Gen Psychiatry* 2006; 63:630–638.

48. Hanlon FM, Miller GA, Thoma RJ, Irwin J, et al. Distinct M50 and M100 auditory gating deficits in schizophrenia. *Psychophysiology* 2005; 42:417–427.

49. Huang MX, Edgar JC, Thoma RJ, Hanlon FM, et al. Predicting EEG responses using MEG sources in superior temporal gyrus reveals source asynchrony in patients with schizophrenia. *Clin Neurophysiol* 2003; 114:835–850.

50. Thoma RJ, Hanlon FM, Sanchez N, Weisend MP, et al. Auditory sensory gating deficit and cortical thickness in schizophrenia. *Neurol Clin Neurophysiol* 2004; 62:1–7.

51. Adler LE, Olincy A, Cawthra EM, McRae KA, et al. Varied effects of atypical neuroleptics on P50 auditory gating in schizophrenia patients. *Am J Psychiatry* 2004; 161:1822–1828.

52. Olincy A, Martin L. Diminished suppression of the P50 auditory evoked potential in bipolar disorder subjects with a history of psychosis. *Am J Psychiatry* 2005; 162:43–49.

53. Ford JM, Mathalon DH, Marsh L. P300 amplitude is related to clinical state in severely and moderately ill schizophrenics. *Biol Psychiatry* 1999; 46:94–101.

54. Clementz BA, Dzau JR, Blumenfeld LD, Matthews S, et al. Ear of stimulation determines schizophrenia-normal brain activity differences in an auditory paired-stimuli paradigm. *Eur J Neurosci* 2004; 18:2853–2858.

55. Boutros NN, Korzyuko O, Oliwa G, Feingold A, et al. Morphological and latency abnormalities of the mid-latency auditory evoked responses in schizophrenia: a preliminary report. *Schizophr Res* 2004; 70(2-3):303–313.

56. Ford JM, Mathalon DH, Kalba S, Marsh L, et al. N1 and P300 abnormalities in patients with schizophrenia, epilepsy, and epilepsy with schizophrenia-like features. *Biol Psychiatry* 2001; 49:848–860.

57. Verlager R, Lefebre C, Wieschemeyer R, Kompt D. Event-related potentials suggest slowing of brain processes in generalized epilepsy and alterations of visual processing in patients with partial seizures. *Cogn Brain Res* 1997; 5:205–219.

58. Rojas DC, Bawn SD, Carlson JP, Arciniegas DB, et al. Alterations in tonotopy and auditory cerebral asymmetry in schizophrenia. *Biol Psychiatry* 2002; 52:32–39.

59. Hegerl U, Juckel G. Intensity dependence of the auditory evoked potentials as an indicator of central serotonergic neurotransmission: a new hypothesis. *Biol Psychiatry* 1993; 33:173–187.

60. von Knorring L, Perris C. Biochemisty of augmenting response of visual-evoked potentials. *Neuropsychobiology* 1981; 7:1–8.

61. Juckel G, Molnar M, Hegerl U, Csepe V, et al. Auditory-evoked potentials as indicator of brain serotonergic activity—first evidence in behaving cats. *Biol Psychiatry* 1997; 41:1181–1195.

62. von Knorring L, Johansson F, Almay B. Augmenting/reducing response in visual evoked potentials in patients with chronic pain syndromes. *Adv Biol Psychiatry* 1980; 4:55–62.

63. Siuciak JA, Boylan C, Fritsche M, Altar CA, et al. BDNF increases monoaminergic activity in rat brain following intracerebroventricular or intraparenchymal administration. *Brain Res* 1996; 710:11–20.

64. Lang UE, Hellweg R, Gallinat J. Association of BDNF serum concentrations with central serotonergic activity: evidence from auditory signal processing. *Neuropsychopharmacology* 2005; 30:1148–1153.

65. Hegerl U, Bottlender R, Gallinat J, Kuss HJ, et al. The serotonin syndrome scale: first results on validity. *Eur Arch Psychiatry Clin Neurosci* 1998; 248:96–103.

66. Afra J, Cecchini AP, Sandor PS, Schoenen J. Comparison of visual and auditory evoked cortical potentials in migraine patients between attacks. *Clin Neurophysiol* 2000; 111:1124–1129.

67. Tuchtenhagen F, Daumann J. High intensity dependence of auditory evoked dipole source activity indicates decreased serotonergic activity in abstinent ecstasy (MDMA) users. *Neuropsychopharmacology* 2000; 22:608–617.

68. Chen TJ, Yu YW, Chen MC, Wang SY, et al. Serotonin dysfunction and suicide attempts in major depressives: an auditory event-related potential study. *Neuropsychobiology* 2005; 52:28–36.

69. Nathan PJ, Segrave R, Phan KL, O'Neill B, et al. Direct evidence that acutely enhancing serotonin with the selective serotonin reuptake inhibitor citalopram modulates the loudness dependence of the auditory evoked potential (LDAEP) marker of central serotonin function. *Hum Psychopharmacol* 2006; 21:47–52.

70. Gallinat J, Bottlender R, Juckel G, Munke-Puchner A, et al. The loudness dependency of the auditory evoked N1/P2-component as a predictor of the acute SSRI response in depression. *Psychopharmacology* 2000; 148:404–411.

71. Paige SR, Fitzpatrick DF, Kline JP, Balogh SE, et al. Event-related potential amplitude/intensity slopes predict response to antidepressants. *Neuropsychobiology* 1994; 30:197–201.

72. Lee TW, Yu YW, Chen TJ, Tsai SJ. Loudness dependence of the auditory evoked potential and response to antidepressants in Chinese patients with major depression. *J Psychiatry Neurosci* 2005; 30:202–205.

73. Juckel G, Gallinat J, Riedel M, Sokullu S, et al. Serotonergic dysfunction in schizophrenia assessed by the loudness dependence measure of primary auditory cortex evoked activity. *Schizophr Res* 2003; 64(2-3):115–124.

74. Von Knorring L, Perris C. Biochemistry of the augmenting/reducing response in visual evoked potentials. *Neuropsychobiology* 1981; 7:1–8.

75. Pogarell O, Tatsch K, Juckel G, Hamann C, et al. Serotonin and dopamine transporter availabilities correlate with the loudness dependence of auditory evoked potentials in patients with obsessive-compulsive disorder. *Neuropsychopharmacology* 2004; 29:1910–1917.

76. Gallinat J, Senkowski D, Wernicke C, Juckel G, et al. Allelic variants of the functional promoter polymorphism of the human serotonin transporter gene is associated with auditory cortical stimulus processing. *Neuropsychopharmacology* 2003; 28:530–532.

77. Strobel A, Debener S, Schmidt D, Hunnerkopf R, et al. Allelic variation in serotonin transporter function associated with the intensity dependence of the auditory evoked potential. *Am J Med Genet B* 2003; 118:41–47.

78. Massey AE, Marsh VR, McAllister-Williams RH. Lack of effect of tryptophan depletion on the loudness dependency of auditory event related potentials in healthy volunteers. *Biol Psychol* 2004; 65:137–145.

79. Kahkonen S, Jaaskelainen IP, Pennanen S, Liesivuori J, et al. Acute tryptophan depletion decreases intensity dependence of auditory evoked magnetic N1/P2 dipole source activity. *Psychopharmacology* 2002; 164:221–227.

80. Roth WT, Cannon EH. Some features of the auditory evoked response in schizophrenics. *Arch Gen Psychiatry* 1972; 27:466–471.

81. Umbricht DS, Bates JA, Lieberman JA, Kane JM, et al. Electrophysiological indices of automatic and controlled auditory information processing in first-episode, recent-onset and chronic schizophrenia. *Biol Psychiatry* 2006; 59:762–772.

82. Meisenzahl EM, Frodl T, Muller D, Schmitt G, et al. Superior temporal gyrus and P300 in schizophrenia: a combined ERP/structural magnetic resonance imaging investigation. *J Psychiatr Res* 2004; 38:153–162.

83. Debruille JB, Schneider-Schmid A, Dann P, King S, et al. The correlation between positive symptoms and left temporal event-related potentials in the P300 time window is auditory specific and training sensitive. *Schizophr Res* 2005; 78(2-3):117–125.

84. van der Stelt O, Lieberman JA, Belger A. Auditory P300 in high-risk, recent-onset and chronic schizophrenia. *Schizophr Res* 2005; 77(2–3):309–320.

85. Friedman D, Vaughan HG, Erlenmeyer-Kimling L. Cognitive brain potentials in children at risk for schizophrenia, preliminary findings. *Schizophr Bull* 1982; 8:514–531.

86. Papageorgiou C, Oulis P, Vasios C, Kontopantelis E, et al. P300 alterations in schizophrenic patients experiencing auditory hallucinations. *Eur Neuropsychopharmacol* 2004; 14:227–236.

87. Wang J, Hirayasu Y, Hiramatsu K, Hokama H, et al. Increased rate of P300 latency prolongation with age in drug-naive and first episode schizophrenia. *Clin Neurophysiol* 2003; 114:2029–2035.

88. Voronkova YA, Lebedeva IS, Gubsky LV, Orlova VA, et al. Subcortical and limbic structures and P300 in schizophrenia. *Hum Physiol* 2005; 31:137–141.

89. Kirihara K, Araki T, Kasai K, Maeda K, et al. Confirmation of a relationship between reduced auditory P300 amplitude and thought disorder in schizophrenia. *Schizophr Res* 2005; 80(2-3):197–201.

90. Kawasaki T, Tanaka S, Wang J, Hokama H, et al. Abnormalities of P300 cortical current density in unmedicated depressed patients revealed by LORETA analysis of event-related potentials. *Psychiatry Clin Neurosci* 2004; 58:68–75.

91. Kaustio O, Partanen J, Valkonen-Korhonen M, Viinamaki H, et al. Affective and psychotic symptoms relate to different types of P300 alterations in depressive disorder. *J Affect Disord* 2002; 71:43–50.

92. Karaaslan F, Gonul AS, Oguz A, Erdinc E, et al. P300 changes in major depressive disorders with and without psychotic features. *J Affect Disord* 2003; 73:283–287.

93. Umbricht D, Krljes S. Mismatch negativity in schizophrenia: a meta-analysis. *Schizophr Res* 2005; 76:1–23.

94. Kircher TT, Rapp A, Grodd W, Buchkremer G, et al. Mismatch negativity responses in schizophrenia: a combined fMRI and whole-head MEG study. *Am J Psychiatry* 2004; 161:294–304.

95. O'Donnell BF, Hokama H, McCarley RW, Smith RS, et al. Auditory ERPs to non-target stimuli in schizophrenia: relationship to probability, task demand, and target ERPs. *Int J Psychophysiol* 1994; 17:219–231.

96. Yamasue H, Yamada H, Yumoto M, Kamio S, et al. Abnormal association between reduced magnetic mismatch field to speech sounds and smaller left planum temporale volume in schizophrenia. *Neuroimage* 2004; 22:720–727.

97. Light GA, Braff DL. Mismatch negativity deficits are associated with poor functioning in schizophrenia patients. *Arch Gen Psychiatry* 2005; 62:127–136.

98. Bramon E, Croft RJ, McDonald C, Virdi GK, et al. Mismatch negativity in schizophrenia: a family study. *Schizophr Res* 2004; 67:1–10.

99. Umbricht D, Koller R, Schmid L, Skrabo A, et al. How specific are deficits in mismatch negativity generation to schizophrenia? *Biol Psychiatry* 2003; 53:1120–1131.

100. Rugg MD, Cowan CP, Nagy ME, Milner AD, et al. CNV abnormalities following closed head injury. *Brain* 1989; 112:489–506.

101. Oke S, Saatchi R, Allen E, Hudson NR, et al. The contingent negative variation in positive and negative types of schizophrenia. *Am J Psychiatry* 1994; 151:432–433.

102. Olbrich HM, Maes H, Valerius G, Langosch JM, et al. Assessing cerebral dysfunction with probe-evoked potentials in a CNV task—a study in alcoholics. *Clin Neurophysiol* 2002; 113:815–825.

103. Heimberg DR, Naber G, Hemmeter U, Zechner S, et al. Contingent negative variation and attention in schizophrenic and depressed patients. *Neuropsychobiology* 1999; 39:131–140.

104. Knott VJ, Lapierre YD. Electrophysiological and behavioral correlates of psychomotor responsivity in depression. *Biol Psychiatry* 1987; 22:313–324.

105. Papart P, Ansseau M, Devoitille JM, Manatanus M, et al. Contingent negative variation and severity of depression. In: Stephanis CN, Rabavilas AD, Soldatos CR, eds. *Psychiatry: A World Perspective*. Amsterdam: Elsevier Science Publishers (Biomedical Division), 1990:402–408.

106. Hemmeter U, Heimberg DR, Naber G, Hobi V, et al. Contingent negative variation and Dex-CRH test in patients with major depression. *J Psychiatr Res* 2000; 34:365–367.

107. Hansenne M, Pitchot W, Moreno AG, Zaldua IU, et al. Suicidal behavior in depressive disorder: an event-related potential study. *Biol Psychiatry* 1996; 40:116–122.
108. Couturier JL. Efficacy of rapid-rate repetitive transcranial magnetic stimulation in the treatment of depression: a systematic review and meta-analysis. *J Psychiatry Neurosci* 2005; 30:83–89.
109. Avery DH, Holtzheimer PE, Fawaz W, Russo J, et al. A controlled study of repetitive transcranial magnetic stimulation in medication-resistant major depression. *Biol Psychiatry* 2006; 59:187–194.
110. Rossini D, Magri L, Lucca A, Giordani S, et al. Does rTMS hasten the response to escitalopram, sertraline, or venlafaxine in patients with major depressive disorder? A double-blind, randomized, sham-controlled trial. *J Clin Psychiatry* 2005; 66:1569–1575.
111. Poulet E, Brunelin J, Boeuve C, Lerond J, et al. Repetitive transcranial magnetic stimulation does not potentiate antidepressant treatment. *Eur Psychiatry* 2004; 19:382–383.
112. Hoffman RE, Gueorguieva R, Hawkins KA, Varanko M, et al. Temporoparietal transcranial magnetic stimulation for auditory hallucinations: safety, efficacy and moderators in a fifty patient sample. *Biol Psychiatry* 2005; 58:97–104.
113. Jandl M, Steyer J, Weber M, Linden DE, et al. Treating auditory hallucinations by transcranial magnetic stimulation: a randomized controlled cross-over trial. *Neuropsychobiology* 2006; 53:63–69.
114. Jandl M, Bittner R, Sack A, Weber B, et al. Changes in negative symptoms and EEG in schizophrenic patients after repetitive transcranial magnetic stimulation (rTMS): an open-label pilot study. *J Neural Transm* 2005; 112:955–967.
115. Daskalakis ZJ, Christensen BK, Fritzgerald PB, Chen R. Transcranial magnetic stimulation: a new investigational tool in psychiatry. *J Neuropsychiatry Clin Neurosci* 2002; 14:406–415.
116. Daskalakis ZJ, Christensen BK, Chen R, Fitzgerald PB, et al. Evidence for impaired cortical inhibition in schizophrenia using transcranial magnetic stimulation. *Arch Gen Psychiatry* 2002; 59:347–354.
117. Ziemann U, Tergau F, Wassermann EM, Wischer S, et al. Demonstration of facilitatory I wave interaction in the human motor cortex by paired transcranial magnetic stimulation. *J Physiol* 1998; 511:181–190.
118. Nakamura H, Kitagawa H, Kawaguchi Y, Tsuji H. Intracortical facilitation and inhibition after transcranial magnetic stimulation in conscious humans. *J Physiol* 1997; 498:817–823.
119. Fitzgerald PB, Brown TL, Marston NA, Oxley TJ, et al. A transcranial magnetic stimulation study of abnormal cortical inhibition in schizophrenia. *Psychiatry Res* 2003; 118:197–207.
120. Oxley T, Fitzgerald PB, Brown TL, de Castella A, et al. Repetitive transcranial magnetic stimulation reveals abnormal plastic response to premotor cortex stimulation in schizophrenia. *Biol Psychiatry* 2004; 56:628–633.
121. Ziemann U, Paulus W, Rothenberger A. Decreased motor inhibition in Tourette's disorder: evidence from transcranial magnetic stimulation. *Am J Psychiatry* 1997; 154:1277–1284.
122. Greenberg BD, Ziemann U, Cora-Locatelli G, Harmon A, et al. Altered cortical excitability in obsessive-compulsive disorder. *Neurology* 2000; 54:142–147.
123. Wasserman EM, Greenberg BD, Nguyen MB, Murphy DL. Motor cortex excitability correlates with an anxiety-related personality trait. *Biol Psychiatry* 2001; 50:377–382.
124. Maeda F, Keenan JP, Pascual-Leone A. Interhemispheric asymmetry of motor cortical excitability in major depression as measured by transcranial magnetic stimulation. *Br J Psychiatry* 2000; 177:169–173.
125. Kessler KR, Schnitzler A, Classen J, Benecke R. Reduced inhibition within primary motor cortex in patients with poststroke focal motor seizures. *Neurology* 2002; 59:1028–1033.
126. Irlbacher K, Brandt SA, Meyer BU. In vivo study indicating loss of intracortical inhibition in tumor-associated epilepsy. *Ann Neurol* 2002; 52:119–122.
127. Manganotti P, Tamburin S, Zanette G, Fiaschi A. Hyperexcitable cortical responses in progressive myoclonic epilepsy. *Neurology* 2001; 57:1793–1799.
128. Macdonell RAL, King MA, Newton MR, Curatolo JM, et al. Prolonged cortical silent period after transcranial magnetic stimulation in generalized epilepsy. *Neurology* 2001; 57:706–708.
129. Werhahn KJ, Lieber J, Classen J, Noachtar S. Motor cortex excitability in patients with focal epilepsy. *Epilepsy Res* 2000; 41:179–181.
130. Cantello R, Civardi C, Cavalli A, Varrasi C, et al. Cortical excitability in cryptogenic localization-related epilepsy: interictal transcranial magnetic stimulation studies. *Epilepsia* 2000; 41:694–704.

VI

EFFECTS OF TREATMENT ON MOOD AND NEUROPSYCHOLOGIC FUNCTION IN ADULTS

34 Cognition

Gholam K. Motamedi
Kimford J. Meador

lthough the majority of patients with epilepsy have normal intelligence, they are more prone to have impaired cognitive performance than age- and education-matched healthy controls. Seizures per se may induce or exacerbate underlying neurocognitive and behavioral dysfunction. However, cognitive disturbances can be present regardless of the state of seizure control. Patients with epilepsy have reduced education, employment level, psychosocial status, and perceived quality of life (QoL) despite optimal seizure control. Independent factors such as seizure type and age of onset, existing neuropathology, psychosocial issues, and untoward effects of treatment may also contribute to patients' cognitive deficits. Although therapeutic interventions may offset the cognitive and behavioral impairment by controlling the seizures, they may cause their own cognitive side effects. Antiepileptic drugs (AEDs) relatively commonly cause such morbidities. Surgical resection of the seizure focus may also induce certain cognitive deficits (1-4).

Because there are no proven effective treatments for cognitive and behavioral impairments in epilepsy, attempts should be made to reduce side effects by using the most appropriate AED and minimizing the dose and number of AEDs. Cognitive side-effect profiles of AEDs must be considered, particularly in extreme age groups.

Any surgical approach should also be tailored when possible to avoid or minimize cognitive deficits (5).

This chapter will focus on the untoward cognitive effects of therapeutic interventions including different medical and surgical treatments in adult patients with epilepsy.

TREATMENT-INDUCED COGNITIVE DYSFUNCTION

Antiepileptic Drug Therapy

Reducing seizure frequency and intensity may offset the negative cognitive effects of AEDs. However, this positive effect might be counteracted by adverse alteration of the underlying physiologic systems involved in neurocognitive function. Therefore, a balance of seizure control and treatment side effects must be sought for each patient. Appropriate management of AED therapy as discussed herein can minimize side effects.

Antiepileptic drugs by virtue of their mechanism of action suppress neuronal excitability and therefore suppress seizures. However, because they exert their effects indiscriminately, neuronal networks involved in maintaining normal cognition may be suppressed as well. Nevertheless, AEDs may have selective effects on different aspects of cognitive function. Reducing the number and dosage of AEDs has been associated with improved cognition, the latter being primarily true when the anticonvulsant level is above the standard therapeutic range. Strategies such as avoiding unnecessary polytherapy, slow initial escalation titration to achieve the lowest effective dose of a single AED, and keeping the drug levels within the therapeutic range lower the chances of cognitive side effects. However, these guidelines may not be applicable to all individuals with refractory epilepsy, in whom seizure control is not achieved without using polytherapy or resection surgery with their untoward side effects. Overall, adverse cognitive and behavioral effects are more common with the older AEDs (especially barbiturates and benzodiazepines) than the newer AEDs, although there are exceptions (e.g., topiramate).

Older-generation AEDs. Cognitive side effects of the older AEDs have been extensively studied. Cognitive effects of carbamazepine, phenobarbital, phenytoin, and primidone in patients with new-onset epilepsy were compared in a parallel study by the Veterans Administration Cooperative Study. There was no consistent pattern across AEDs, and little change in cognition from pre- to post-AED treatment conditions was found (6). Another study by the VA Cooperative Study group found no cognitive differences between carbamazepine and valproate. However, design limitations in these studies may have obscured differences. Further studies have found modest negative cognitive effects for carbamazepine and phenytoin despite few differential effects.

Meador et al. found no differences in the cognitive effects of carbamazepine, phenytoin, and valproate, but worse cognitive performance with phenobarbital. They examined the effects of these older AEDs in healthy volunteers in a double-blind randomized crossover monotherapy study and noted no overall differences between carbamazepine and phenytoin. However, 52% of the variables were significantly worse with AEDs compared to the nondrug conditions. Comparison of phenobarbital, phenytoin, and valproate showed that 32% of the variables were significantly worse for phenobarbital than the other two drugs. Compared to the nondrug conditions, 55% of the variables appeared worse with AEDs. Therefore, phenobarbital had greater untoward cognitive effects, but there were no clinically significant differences between carbamazepine, phenytoin, and valproate (7,8).

Dodrill and Troupin found similar results, that is, no cognitive differences between carbamazepine and phenytoin, after analyzing their data when controlling for AED blood levels (9). Dodrill also addressed the role of duration of treatment on cognitive side effects in a study that examined neuropsychologic performance of patients with epilepsy over a 5-year period. Patients were on stable phenytoin monotherapy, phenytoin with other

AEDs, or AED regimens except for phenytoin. There were no differences found in cognitive performance over time in these patients.

In summary, among the older AEDs, barbiturates and benzodiazepines seem to have the worst cognitive profile, including decreased arousal and deterioration in most areas of cognitive performance. In monotherapy, carbamazepine, phenytoin, and valproate show similar effects to each other on cognitive function including motor speed, attention, response accuracy, and memory. These effects are modest but can be clinically significant. Under certain circumstances such as neurodevelopment or high-demanding cognitive tasks, their side effects might have greater consequences. For patients involved in educational activities or professions that require focused attention or learning, even modest effects could have a serious impact. Clinicians should focus on improving a patient's cognition by achieving better seizure control but at the same time consider the untoward cognitive effects of these AEDs (10).

Some of the old AEDs are known for their positive psychotropic effects. Carbamazepine and valproate are used as mood stabilizers for bipolar disorder and may be helpful for managing impulse control as well. Valproate has been used to treat obsessive compulsive disorder and to prevent panic attacks. Barbiturates and benzodiazepines may help anxiety and insomnia, but can result in adverse psychotropic effects such as hyperactivity, irritability, and depression (11).

Newer-generation AEDs. Side-effect profiles of the newer AEDs have not been fully established yet. Available since the early 1990s, these medications seem to be as effective as the older AEDs in controlling seizures while having overall better side-effect profiles. Multiple studies have suggested more favorable cognitive side-effect profiles for several of the new generation AEDs. Some have been shown to have positive psychotropic effects. For example, lamotrigine can be an effective maintenance treatment for bipolar disorder, particularly to prevent depression. Gabapentin may promote a general sense of well-being regardless of seizure control and therefore might be used in treating mood disturbance (12). These AEDs are reviewed here in the order they were introduced to the market.

Felbamate. Although felbamate is still in limited use because of its potentially fatal hepatic and hematological side effects, there are no formal data on its cognitive effects. Anecdotal reports of felbamate possessing alerting effects and inducing insomnia need further investigation.

Gabapentin. A large double-blind, parallel-group study with dose conversion to monotherapy with gabapentin in patients with epilepsy revealed no cognitive changes compared to the control group, but there were positive changes in adjustment and mood (13). However, a randomized, double-blind, parallel-group study of gabapentin and carbamazepine in healthy volunteers showed greater electroencephalographic (EEG) slowing and cognitive complaints with carbamazepine (14). Other studies have reported contradicting results comparing gabapentin to placebo, including significantly more drowsiness (15). In healthy volunteers gabapentin had minimal effects on cognitive test performance as well as daily and occupational function (16). In nonepileptic rats, gabapentin has less effect on attention compared to benzodiazepines (17).

In a double-blind, randomized crossover design, Meador et al. compared directly the cognitive effects of carbamazepine and gabapentin in healthy subjects. Treatment with gabapentin showed significantly better performance on 26% of the variables compared to carbamazepine. Although both drugs produced some untoward effects compared to the nondrug control, gabapentin produced fewer cognitive effects compared to carbamazepine (18). Using attention/vigilance, psychomotor speed, motor speed, verbal and visual memory, Martin et al. compared gabapentin and carbamazepine in a group of senior adults. Both AEDs induced comparable and mild cognitive effects compared with the nondrug condition, but a better overall tolerability and side-effect profile was seen for gabapentin (19). Mortimore et al. studied the effect of gabapentin on cognition and QoL in epilepsy using a controlled pre- and posttreatment design and found no short-term adverse effects (20).

Lamotrigine. In a study of patients with epilepsy, the cognitive effects of lamotrigine were not different from placebo based on a limited neuropsychologic battery, but the patients' perception of QoL was improved by lamotrigine (21). In healthy adults, lamotrigine has fewer cognitive side effects compared to carbamazepine, phenytoin, and diazepam (22). Meador et al. compared the cognitive and behavioral effects of carbamazepine and lamotrigine in 25 healthy adults using a double-blind, randomized crossover design with two 10-week treatment periods. Forty variables were included in the neuropsychologic test battery. The results showed significantly better performance on more than half of the variables (cognitive speed, memory, mood factors, sedation, perception of cognitive performance, and other QoL perceptions) for lamotrigine (23). In a more recent study, the same researchers compared the cognitive and behavioral effects of lamotrigine and topiramate in healthy adults. Based on an extensive neuropsychologic test battery, adults taking lamotrigine were found to do significantly better using 300-mg daily doses for both drugs (24). In another multicenter, double-blind, randomized, prospective study in

adults with partial seizures, lamotrigine and topiramate were added as adjunctive therapy to carbamazepine or phenytoin. Using standardized measures of cognition, lamotrigine was found to have less cognitive effect than topiramate (25).

Aldenkamp and Baker have reviewed lamotrigine monotherapy and add-on clinical studies to evaluate the impact of lamotrigine therapy on cognitive functioning. The data suggested an equivalent or superior cognitive effect for lamotrigine with a possible secondary positive effect on QoL. Comparing the cognitive and mood effects of low-dose lamotrigine versus valproate and placebo in healthy volunteers via a double-blind, single-dummy, parallel-group design study, the investigators aimed at teasing the effects of lamotrigine from those of better seizure control. Lamotrigine showed a "mood activating" property and improved cognitive activation on simple reaction time measurements compared to placebo and valproate, as well as a more positive subjective report about the impact of the drug (26). In patients with epilepsy, the beneficial effects of lamotrigine on QoL have also been shown by patient perception of psychologic well-being compared to both placebo and carbamazepine (27). Lamotrigine is approved as maintenance treatment for bipolar disorder, in particular to prevent depression.

Investigations of lamotrigine in the developmentally disabled population have indicated seizure reduction rates of up to 50% in some trials (28). It is usually well tolerated in this population; however, its pharmacokinetic profile may be influenced by other AEDs. Brown et al. studied the effects of 12-week, open-label lamotrigine treatment on negative mood and cognition changes in patients receiving corticosteroids and found a significant improvement (29).

Levetiracetam. This new AED, with a novel mechanism of action, has an overall good side-effect profile. Compared to oxcarbazepine and carbamazepine, levetiracetam at therapeutic doses had the least cognitive effects in healthy adults with no effect on motor speed and EEG. A small preliminary study by Neyens et al. showed no significant changes in cognitive performances in patients with chronic epilepsy who were treated with levetiracetam; however, the study was single-blind with only 10 patients and no control group (30). In normal and amygdala-kindled rats, valproate, clonazepam, and carbamazepine, but not levetiracetam, at proper therapeutic doses reduce cognitive (learning) performance (31).

Behavioral problems with levetiracetam have been reported in children and may be seen in adults as well. Cramer et al. reviewed behavioral side effects in adult patients taking levetiracetam in a series of short-term, placebo-controlled studies in epilepsy, cognitive or anxiety disorders, and epilepsy patients observed in long-term trials. Compared to patients taking other AEDs, epilepsy patients taking levetiracetam had a lower incidence of behavioral events. However, these patients had a higher incidence of such side effects compared to patients with cognitive or anxiety disorders treated with levetiracetam (32). It is possible that behavioral findings in these patients are related in part to the seizure disorder itself rather than the AED alone.

Treatment with levetiracetam in a group of patients with temporal lobe epilepsy with and without hippocampal sclerosis did not show any differences in prevalence of cognitive adverse events and depression between the two groups (33). In a recent study in healthy volunteers, levetiracetam in monotherapy produced fewer untoward neuropsychologic and neurophysiologic effects compared to carbamazepine (34).

Oxcarbazepine. Oxcarbazepine is a homologue of carbamazepine and is tolerated slightly better than carbamazepine, phenytoin, and valproate. A double-blind, low-dose, crossover study with healthy volunteers comparing oxcarbazepine to placebo indicated that oxcarbazepine improved performance on a focused attention task and manual writing speed. Oxcarbazepine had a slight stimulant effect on some aspects of psychomotor functioning and improved feelings of alertness, with no effect on long-term memory. However, the low dose used in this study limits any generalization to epilepsy patients (35).

In contrast, a small, randomized, monotherapy, double-blind, parallel-group study of patients with new-onset epilepsy showed no cognitive differences between oxcarbazepine and phenytoin (36). In a small group of healthy volunteers, oxcarbazepine and phenytoin both affected motor speed and reaction time at therapeutic doses; there were no differences between the drugs (37). In newly diagnosed epilepsy patients, oxcarbazepine and carbamazepine, but not valproate and lamotrigine, induced a decrease in the mean alpha frequency (38). In healthy adults, oxcarbazepine was better tolerated and had fewer cognitive and EEG effects than carbamazepine (39).

Tiagabine. A GABA reuptake inhibitor, tiagabine increases the availability of this major inhibitory neurotransmitter. Despite reports of nervousness, difficulty with concentration, depressive mood, and language problems, there are no indications of major cognitive effects during large, randomized, double-blind, add-on, placebo-controlled, parallel-group studies (40). It is advised to titrate the dose up slowly and take it with food to avoid rapid increases in drug level and reduce the risk of side effects. A recent 52-week follow-up study showed no significant differences in cognitive profiles in newly diagnosed patients with epilepsy treated with tiagabine,

newly diagnosed patients with epilepsy treated with carbamazepine, and untreated patients with a single seizure (41).

Topiramate. Topiramate has been associated with language problems, somnolence, psychomotor slowing, and difficulty with memory, particularly at higher doses, in combination with other AEDs, or when rapidly titrated (42). A postmarketing antiepileptic drug survey (PADS) prospectively collected standardized data forms before and during treatment with topiramate for epilepsy. The results showed that psychomotor slowing was the most common complaint, but the majority of patients chose to continue the drug and experienced both a global improvement and better seizure control (43). In healthy volunteers, topiramate has impaired cognitive test performance enough to affect daily and occupational function.

Martin et al. compared gabapentin, lamotrigine, and topiramate in 17 healthy volunteers by using a single-blind, randomized, parallel-group study design (44). The topiramate group developed selective, statistically significant declines on measures of attention and word fluency after acute doses and after 1 month of treatment. Gabapentin and lamotrigine produced no performance changes. This finding may have been due to the faster-than-recommended initial dosage escalation rate for topiramate. Topiramate seems to be better tolerated in the developmentally disabled patients and appears to be particularly effective in patients with refractory Lennox-Gastaut syndrome and those with cognitive disabilities (45). Topiramate has shown some effects on mood stabilization, weight loss, eating disorders, and addiction, but these indications are still under investigation (46).

Comparing the cognitive effects of (slowly introduced) topiramate and valproate as add-on therapy with carbamazepine, Aldenkamp et al. found only one significant difference after a long-term maintenance phase: short-term verbal memory was worse with topiramate (47). Using a moderate-dose escalation rate and higher target doses of the same medications in a similarly designed study, Meador et al. found significant differences on two of twenty-four variables (i.e., Symbol Digit Modalities Test and Controlled Word Association) compared to valproate at the end of the maintenance phase (48). In both of the above studies, the cognitive side effects for topiramate were greater at the end of titration than at the end of maintenance. As noted previously, topiramate has shown greater adverse cognitive effects than lamotrigine in healthy volunteers and epilepsy patients.

Vigabatrin. Vigabatrin is a GABA transaminase inhibitor used outside the United States but not yet approved by the FDA. Its cognitive effects have been extensively studied. Vigabatrin has been reported to produce few adverse effects on cognition or quality of life compared to placebo (49). In one study, vigabatrin added at a dose of 2 g/day to patients' existing AEDs appeared to have no negative impact on attention, mental speed, motor speed, central cognitive processing, and perceptuo-motor performance (50). Controlled clinical trials with vigabatrin have shown serious behavioral side effects in some patients, such as depression and psychosis in 3.4% of adult patients, particularly those with severe epilepsy or a history of psychosis (51); however, other studies have not shown a greater risk for the drug than for other AEDs (52).

Zonisamide. There is little formal neuropsychologic data on zonisamide. It may affect cognitive functions such as acquisition and consolidation of new data. It may have a predilection to affect verbal learning rather than visual-perceptual learning or psychomotor function. Different studies have suggested that zonisamide, in a dose-dependent manner, may affect attention, acquisition, and consolidation of new information. Patients may develop tolerance to the adverse cognitive effects of zonisamide (53).

Pregabalin. Pregabalin has been recently approved for use in the management of partial onset seizures. It has been reported to improve the emotional symptoms of generalized anxiety disorder, but there are limited data available on its neurocognitive effects (54). In healthy volunteers randomized to a double-blind, three-period crossover study, pregabalin at 750 mg/day did not have a significant effect on objective psychometrics (reaction, vigilance, and short-term memory), but it induced subjective sedation (impaired attention and arousal) (55).

Rufinamide. Rufinamide is a potential new AED that is under review by the FDA as an "orphan" drug for Lennox-Gastaut syndrome. In an add-on, multicenter, multinational, double-blind, randomized, placebo-controlled, parallel-study using four different doses of rufinamide, Aldenkamp and Alpherts reported no changes in cognitive testing compared to placebo (56). Although this is promising, rufinamide must be tested further to evaluate its efficiency and side-effect profile.

Epilepsy Surgery

Potential neurocognitive deficits of epilepsy surgery can be minimized by tailoring the resection to the individual patient's condition. The side and site of the resection can influence the risk of deficits following surgery. Temporal lobectomy is the most common type of epilepsy surgery. Left-sided temporal lobectomy may induce verbal memory and learning deficits, and right-sided resections are associated with visual-spatial memory and cognitive declines, although the changes are more consistent for left-sided resections. These potential deficits are affected by the degree of seizure control, level of functioning, and duration of seizure prior to surgery. A large study has shown that the risk of postsurgical verbal memory deficits is greater for standard anterior temporal lobectomy (ATL) and increased in patients with higher preoperative scores, older age, and left-sided resection (57). Patients without hippocampal atrophy and sclerosis are at greater cognitive risk following ATL. Resection of a nonatrophic hippocampus is associated with poorer verbal/visual memory post left ATL, and to a lesser degree, visual-spatial learning deficits post right ATL. Other factors that may predict cognitive deficits after ATL include memory asymmetries on the Wada test and preoperative asymmetry in temporal lobe metabolism as evidenced by positron emission tomography (PET). It has been suggested that right ATL may result in a decline in recalling details of famous past events (retrograde memory). In these patients, defective retrograde memory has been associated with young age at epilepsy onset and polytherapy (58).

In a longitudinal study, Rausch et al. showed both early and late postoperative memory decline in patients with en bloc left temporal lobe resection. Although non-memory scores remained stable over an average follow-up period of 12.8 years, further decreases in verbal as well as visual memory were evident. An initial high memory score and left-sided resection were predictors of verbal memory deficit early after surgery. Higher 1-year postoperative scores were predictors of late memory declines. Despite the possibility of memory loss caused by chronic seizures or aging, patients with left temporal lobectomy may be at risk for a more rapid decline in selective verbal memory skills. Better long-term QoL was associated with both improved seizure control and a better verbal memory skill (59).

Helmstaedter et al. explored the effect of surgery on verbal learning and memory in two groups of elderly epilepsy patients who underwent either selective left-sided amygdalohippocampectomy or anterior two-thirds temporal lobectomy. The results confirmed worsening of verbal learning and memory in both groups, particularly in temporal lobectomy patients. The investigators emphasized the importance of considering memory prognosis, particularly in older patients, given that a negative outcome might accelerate lifetime memory decline in these patients (60). More recently, comparison of medium- and long-term follow-up IQ and memory, and analysis at the individual level, has led to questioning the value of short-term increments in memory scores following temporal lobectomy (61).

Vagus Nerve Stimulation

Vagus nerve stimulation (VNS) is considered for patients with refractory epilepsy who are not considered candidates for resection surgery and for patients with refractory depression. Its mechanism or mechanisms of action remain unclear. It has been suggested that VNS might induce mild cognitive improvement through either better seizure control or other mechanisms. However, this issue remains controversial. A single-arm follow-up study showed no changes in attention, motor, short-term memory, learning, and executive functions at 6 months (62). Findings of another study suggested significant improvement in mood and possibly depression, but not in level of health-related quality of life (HRQoL) at 6 months' follow-up. A longer term follow-up at 24 months of treatment with VNS did not show any negative effects on mood, behavior, cognition, or QoL (63). A literature review did not show any evidence of adverse cognitive effects, but no definite positive effects on cognition either (64). A recent study of ten patients treated with VNS showed impaired cognitive flexibility and creativity, although the results could not be attributed to a general encephalopathy because patients had improved retention and no learning impairment (65).

COGNITIVE DYSFUNCTION IN ELDERLY PATIENTS WITH EPILEPSY

The incidence of new-onset epilepsy is higher among the elderly than younger adults. Elderly patients are more susceptible to the cognitive effects of centrally active drugs for both pharmacokinetic and pharmacodynamic reasons. This susceptibility has been shown for benzodiazepines and barbiturates (66). One study comparing phenytoin and valproate to nondrug baselines reported minimal differences in cognitive effects of these AEDs in elderly patients with epilepsy (67). Nevertheless, given the higher chance of drug interaction and their side effects, the old AEDs, especially the sedating agents, are particularly disadvantageous for elderly patients. However, there are few studies formally assessing the cognitive effects of AEDs in the elderly. A multicenter European study and the recent VA Cooperative Study Trial 428 both examined the effectiveness (i.e., combined efficacy and tolerability) of AED therapy in elderly patients with new-onset epilepsy (68, 69). Both studies found that lamotrigine was better tolerated than carbamazepine. The VA study also found that gabapentin was better tolerated than carbamazepine. The Veterans Affairs Cooperative Trial 428 concluded that lamotrigine or gabapentin were reasonable choices as initial therapy for older patients with newly diagnosed seizures, because the main limiting factor in patient retention was adverse drug reactions and those taking these two AEDs did better than those taking carbamazepine (69).

RECOGNITION AND TREATMENT OF COGNITIVE DYSFUNCTION IN EPILEPSY

The fundamental approach to managing cognitive dysfunction in epilepsy is to control the seizures and, if possible, to use monotherapy at the lowest effective dose. The cognitive profile of the AED should be considered, considering that several of the newer AEDs possess a better cognitive side-effect profile. Clinicians should monitor the patient for cognitive and behavioral side effects. It should be remembered that the patient's subjective perception of cognitive side effects may not correlate well with objective deficits. Thus, other resources to assess for cognitive effects should be considered, such as the opinion of family or friends or objective cognitive testing. Note that a patient's complaint of cognitive side effects may well reflect mood problems because subjective reports of cognitive side effects and mood are highly correlated. Given the high incidence of comorbid depression or other mood disorders in epilepsy, patients should be routinely screened for mood disorders.

The beneficial effect of reducing seizures may offset the adverse cognitive effects of AEDs, at least in part. However, significant improvements in QoL from seizure reduction usually require complete seizure freedom. QoL in patients with epilepsy can be significantly reduced by subtle AED toxicity. Clinicians should bear in mind that increasing AEDs to produce relatively minor reductions in seizure frequency may actually adversely impact the patient's overall QoL. One useful tool to monitor for AED toxicity is the Adverse Events Profile (70).

The presence of overlapping variables complicates the targeted management of cognitive deficits. Therefore, direct treatment of cognitive side effects of epilepsy has been rarely attempted. Recently, pharmacological interventions have been attempted. Donepezil, an anticholinesterase inhibitor at 5–10 mg, improved memory but not attention, visual sequencing, mental flexibility, psychomotor speed, or QoL in eighteen patients with epilepsy. Improvement in memory was not related to changes in attention. The drug was well tolerated except for dizziness and mild gastrointestinal complaints (71). Jia et al. showed that learning and mnemonic impairments induced in pentylenetetrazole-kindled rats were significantly improved by donepezil (72).

Chan et al. showed that low doses of a high-affinity GABA$_B$ receptor antagonist, which fails to treat atypical absence seizure activity, completely reverses the spatial working memory deficit in a rat model of chronic atypical absence seizure (73). This finding suggests that GABA$_B$ receptor antagonists may have a potential for treatment of cognitive impairment in some epilepsy syndromes. These data also suggest that cognitive impairment may be independent of the seizure activity.

An open-label, nonrandomized 3-month study using the stimulant drug methylphenidate in adult patients taking multiple AEDs for partial epilepsy resulted in improved cognition, QoL, and relief from sedation with no increase in seizure frequency (74). There are mixed reports on the effects of VNS on cognition in epileptic patients. Antidepressants, herbal supplements, and non-pharmacological approaches to treat cognitive deficits in epilepsy have been tried.

Another option to treat behavioral problems in patients with seizures is psychopharmacology; however, this should not substitute for attempts to control the seizures or to treat any underlying conditions. Despite the controversial possibility of decreasing the seizure threshold, tricyclic antidepressants and selective serotonin reuptake inhibitors (SSRIs) are used successfully to treat depression and anxiety in patients with epilepsy. Some SSRIs (fluoxetine, paroxetine, fluvoxamine, and, to a lesser degree, sertraline) are inhibitors of the cytochrome P450 enzyme system, which in turn may increase phenytoin, carbamazepine, and valproate levels. Haloperidol has little effect on seizure threshold, but antipsychotic agents such as chlorpromazine and clozapine are not recommended for use in children with psychosis because of the possibility of increased seizures. Despite this risk, clozapine has been reported not to clinically affect seizure threshold; in fact, Langosch and Trimble treated six children with epilepsy and severe psychosis with clozapine with no increase in seizures in three of them and substantial reduction of seizures in the other three (75).

CONCLUSIONS

Patients with epilepsy are more likely to suffer from cognitive and behavioral deficits compared to the general population. These deficits are multifactorial in etiology ranging from biological factors such as seizure type, underlying neuropathology, age of onset, a variety of psychosocial problems, and untoward effects of treatment. The risk of neurocognitive burden from epilepsy may even start before birth in children of women with epilepsy due to in utero exposure to AEDs.

Although epilepsy per se may cause or exacerbate an underlying cognitive impairment, the underlying etiology is commonly a major contributing factor. While treating seizures is necessary and by itself may resolve or alleviate the cognitive deficits of the disease, it may also add to the adverse cognitive and behavioral problems experienced by patients with epilepsy. The major therapeutic modalities (i.e., AEDs and resection surgery) carry some potential cognitive risks. Although AED-induced deficits are reversible, other deficits may not be remediable or even avoidable. Currently there are no effective treatments available for cognitive deficits of epilepsy. Therefore, surgical and medical treatment of epilepsy must be tailored to the individual patient with the potential risks in mind. Clinicians should be aware of these risks, particularly potential cognitive effects of AEDs, to avoid or minimize any negative consequences of the treatment.

References

1. Meador KJ. Cognitive effects of epilepsy and of antiepileptic medications. In: Wyllie E, ed. *The Treatment of Epilepsy. Principles and Practice.* 4th ed. Philadelphia: Lippincott Williams & Wilkins, 2005:1215–1226.
2. Sillanpaa M, Jalava M, Kaleva O, Shinnar S. Long-term prognosis of seizures with onset in childhood. N Engl J Med 1998; 338(24):1715–1722
3. Jokeit H, Ebner A. Effects of chronic epilepsy on intellectual functions. *Prog Brain Res* 2002; 135:455–463.
4. Motamedi GK, Meador KJ. Antiepileptic drugs and memory. *Epilepsy Behav* 2004; 5: 435–439.
5. Motamedi G, Meador K. Epilepsy and cognition. *Epilepsy Behav* 2003; 4(Suppl 2): 25–38.
6. Smith DB, Mattson RH, Cramer JA, Collins JF, Novelly RA, Craft B. Results of a nation-wide Veterans Administration Cooperative Study comparing the efficacy and toxicity of carbamazepine, phenobarbital, phenytoin, and primidone. *Epilepsia* 1987; 28 Suppl 3: S50–58.
7. Meador KJ, Loring DW, Moore EE, Thompson WO, et al. Comparative cognitive effects of phenobarbital, phenytoin and valproate in healthy subjects. *Neurology* 1995; 45: 1494–1499.
8. Meador KJ, Loring DW, Abney OL, Allen ME, et al. Effects of carbamazepine and phenytoin on EEG and memory in healthy adults. *Epilepsia* 1993; 34:153–157.
9. Dodrill CB, Troupin AS. Neuropsychological effects of carbamazepine and phenytoin: a reanalysis. *Neurology* 1991; 41:141–143.
10. Gilliam FG, Fessler AJ, Baker G, Vahle V, et al. Systematic screening allows reduction of adverse antiepileptic drug effects: a randomized trial. *Neurology* 2004; 62:23–27.
11. Ettinger AB, Kanner AM, eds. *Psychiatric Issues in Epilepsy. A Practical Guide to Diagnosis and Treatment.* Philadelphia: Lippincott Williams & Wilkins, 2001.
12. Meador KJ. Cognitive and memory effects of the new antiepileptic drugs. *Epilepsy Res* 2006; 68:63–67.
13. Please supply reference for the first study described in Treatment-Induced Cognitive Dysfunction, Antiepileptic Drug Therapy, Newer-generation AEDs, Gabapentin, 1st paragraph.
14. Please supply reference for the second study described in Treatment-Induced Cognitive Dysfunction, Antiepileptic Drug Therapy, Newer-generation AEDs, Gabapentin, 1st paragraph.
15. Please supply reference for the third study described in Treatment-Induced Cognitive Dysfunction, Antiepileptic Drug Therapy, Newer-generation AEDs, Gabapentin, 1st paragraph.
16. Please supply reference for the fourth study described in Treatment-Induced Cognitive Dysfunction, Antiepileptic Drug Therapy, Newer-generation AEDs, Gabapentin, 1st paragraph.
17. Please supply reference for the fifth study described in Treatment-Induced Cognitive Dysfunction, Antiepileptic Drug Therapy, Newer-generation AEDs, Gabapentin, 1st paragraph.
18. Please supply reference for the Meador et al. study described in Treatment-Induced Cognitive Dysfunction, Antiepileptic Drug Therapy, Newer-generation AEDs, Gabapentin, 2nd paragraph.
19. Martin R, Meador K, Turrentine L, Faught E, et al. Comparative cognitive effects of carbamazepine and gabapentin in healthy senior adults. *Epilepsia* 2001; 42:764–771.
20. Please supply reference for the Mortimore et al. study described in Treatment-Induced Cognitive Dysfunction, Antiepileptic Drug Therapy, Newer-generation AEDs, Gabapentin, 2nd paragraph.
21. Please supply reference for the first study described in Treatment-Induced Cognitive Dysfunction, Antiepileptic Drug Therapy, Newer-generation AEDs, Lamotrigine, 1st paragraph.
22. Please supply reference for the second study described in Treatment-Induced Cognitive Dysfunction, Antiepileptic Drug Therapy, Newer-generation AEDs, Lamotrigine, 1st paragraph.
23. Meador KJ, Loring DW, Ray PG, Murro AM, et al. Differential cognitive and behavioral effects of carbamazepine and lamotrigine. *Neurology* 2001; 56:1177–1182.
24. Meador KJ, Loring DW, Vahle VJ, Ray PG, et al. Cognitive and behavioral effects of lamotrigine and topiramate in healthy volunteers. *Neurology* 2005; 64(12): 2108–2114.
25. Please supply reference for the last study described in Treatment-Induced Cognitive Dysfunction, Antiepileptic Drug Therapy, Newer-generation AEDs, Lamotrigine, 1st paragraph.
26. Please supply reference for the Aldenkamp and Baker study described in Treatment-Induced Cognitive Dysfunction, Antiepileptic Drug Therapy, Newer-generation AEDs, Lamotrigine, 2nd paragraph.

27. Please supply reference for the other study described in Treatment-Induced Cognitive Dysfunction, Antiepileptic Drug Therapy, Newer-generation AEDs, Lamotrigine, 2nd paragraph.

28. Please supply reference for the first study described in Treatment-Induced Cognitive Dysfunction, Antiepileptic Drug Therapy, Newer-generation AEDs, Lamotrigine, 3rd paragraph.

29. Please supply reference for the Brown et al. study described in Treatment-Induced Cognitive Dysfunction, Antiepileptic Drug Therapy, Newer-generation AEDs, Lamotrigine, 3rd paragraph.

30. Neyens LG, Alpherts WC, Aldenkamp AP. Cognitive effects of a new pyrrolidine derivative (levetiracetam) in patients with epilepsy. *Prog Neuropsychopharmacol Biol Psychiatry* 1995; 19:411–419.

31. Please supply reference for the rat study described in Treatment-Induced Cognitive Dysfunction, Antiepileptic Drug Therapy, Newer-generation AEDs, Leviracetam, 1st paragraph.

32. Please supply reference for the Cramer et al. study described in Treatment-Induced Cognitive Dysfunction, Antiepileptic Drug Therapy, Newer-generation AEDs, Leviracetam, 2nd paragraph.

33. Please supply reference for the first study described in Treatment-Induced Cognitive Dysfunction, Antiepileptic Drug Therapy, Newer-generation AEDs, Leviracetam, 3rd paragraph.

34. Please supply reference for the second study described in Treatment-Induced Cognitive Dysfunction, Antiepileptic Drug Therapy, Newer-generation AEDs, Leviracetam, 3rd paragraph.

35. Please supply reference for the study described in Treatment-Induced Cognitive Dysfunction, Antiepileptic Drug Therapy, Newer-generation AEDs, Oxcarbazepine, 1st paragraph.

36. Aikia M, Kalviainen R, Sivenius J, Halonen T, et al. Cognitive effects of oxcarbazepine and phenytoin monotherapy in newly diagnosed epilepsy: one year follow-up. *Epilepsy Res* 1992; 11:199–203.

37. Please supply reference for the study of oxcarbazepine and phenytoin in healthy volunteers described in Treatment-Induced Cognitive Dysfunction, Antiepileptic Drug Therapy, Newer-generation AEDs, Oxcarbazepine, 2nd paragraph.

38. Please supply reference for the study of the effect of oxcarbazepine and 3 other meds on alpha rhythm in newly diagnosed epilepsy patients described in Treatment-Induced Cognitive Dysfunction, Antiepileptic Drug Therapy, Newer-generation AEDs, Oxcarbazepine, 2nd paragraph.

39. Please supply reference for the study of oxcarbazepine vs. carbamazepine in healthy volunteers described in Treatment-Induced Cognitive Dysfunction, Antiepileptic Drug Therapy, Newer-generation AEDs, Oxcarbazepine, 2nd paragraph.

40. Please supply reference for at least one of the large studies described in Treatment-Induced Cognitive Dysfunction, Antiepileptic Drug Therapy, Newer-generation AEDs, Tiagabine.

41. Please supply reference for the 52-week follow-up study described in Treatment-Induced Cognitive Dysfunction, Antiepileptic Drug Therapy, Newer-generation AEDs, Tiagabine.

42. Please supply reference for at least one of the studies described in Treatment-Induced Cognitive Dysfunction, Antiepileptic Drug Therapy, Newer-generation AEDs, Topiramate, 1st paragraph.

43. Please supply references for the PADS described in Treatment-Induced Cognitive Dysfunction, Antiepileptic Drug Therapy, Newer-generation AEDs, Topiramate, 1st paragraph.

44. Martin R, Kuzniecky R, Ho S, Hetherington H, et al. Cognitive effects of topiramate, gabapentin, and lamotrigine in healthy young adults. *Neurology* 1999; 52: 321–327.

45. Please provide reference for the results about topiramate in disabled patients described in Treatment-Induced Cognitive Dysfunction, Antiepileptic Drug Therapy, Newer-generation AEDs, Topiramate, 2nd paragraph.

46. Please provide reference for the last claim in Treatment-Induced Cognitive Dysfunction, Antiepileptic Drug Therapy, Newer-generation AEDs, Topiramate, 2nd paragraph.

47. Please provide reference for the Aldenkamp et al. study described in Treatment-Induced Cognitive Dysfunction, Antiepileptic Drug Therapy, Newer-generation AEDs, Topiramate, 3rd paragraph.

48. Meador KJ, Loring DW, Hulihan JF, Kamin M., et al. Differential cognitive and behavioral effects of topiramate and valproate. *Neurology* 2003; 60(9):1483–1488.

49. Please provide reference for the study comparing vigabatrin to placebo described in Treatment-Induced Cognitive Dysfunction, Antiepileptic Drug Therapy, Newer-generation AEDs, Vigabatrin.

50. Please provide reference for the study of 2 g/day vigabatrin added to existing AEDs described in Treatment-Induced Cognitive Dysfunction, Antiepileptic Drug Therapy, Newer-generation AEDs, Vigabatrin.

51. Please provide reference for the trial showing behavioral side effects described in Treatment-Induced Cognitive Dysfunction, Antiepileptic Drug Therapy, Newer-generation AEDs, Vigabatrin.

52. Please provide reference for study showing no greater risk for vigabatrin than other AEDs, described in Treatment-Induced Cognitive Dysfunction, Antiepileptic Drug Therapy, Newer-generation AEDs, Vigabatrin.

53. Please provide reference(s) for the statements in Treatment-Induced Cognitive Dysfunction, Antiepileptic Drug Therapy, Newer-generation AEDs, Zonisamide.

54. Please provide references for the study of pregabalin in generalized anxiety disorder described in Treatment-Induced Cognitive Dysfunction, Antiepileptic Drug Therapy, Newer-generation AEDs, Pregabalin.

55. Please provide references for the study of pregabalin in healthy volunteers described in Treatment-Induced Cognitive Dysfunction, Antiepileptic Drug Therapy, Newer-generation AEDs, Pregabalin.

56. Please provide reference for the Alderkamp (that should be Aldenkamp, right?) and Alpherts study described in Treatment-Induced Cognitive Dysfunction, Antiepileptic Drug Therapy, Newer-generation AEDs, Rufinamide.

57. Please provide reference for the study described in Treatment-Induced Cognitive Dysfunction, Epilepsy Surgery, 1st paragraph (unless it's covered by Lah et al. 2006).

58. Lah S, Lee T, Grayson S, Miller L. Effects of temporal lobe epilepsy on retrograde memory. *Epilepsia* 2006; 47:615–625.

59. Please provide reference for the study by Rausch et al. described in Treatment-Induced Cognitive Dysfunction, Epilepsy Surgery, 2nd paragraph.

60. Helmstaedter C. Neuropsychological aspects of epilepsy surgery. *Epilepsy Behav* 2004; 5(Suppl 1):S45–S55.

61. Engman E, Andersson-Roswall L, Samuelsson H, Malmgren K. Serial cognitive change patterns across time after temporal lobe resection for epilepsy. *Epilepsy Behav* 2006; 8:765–772.

62. Please provide reference for the single-arm follow-up study described in Treatment-Induced Cognitive Dysfunction, Vagus Nerve Stimulation.

63. Please provide reference for the longer-term follow-up described in Treatment-Induced Cognitive Dysfunction, Vagus Nerve Stimulation.

64. Please provide reference for the literature review described in Treatment-Induced Cognitive Dysfunction, Vagus Nerve Stimulation.

65. Please provide reference for the study showing impaired cognitive flexibility in 3 patients described in Treatment-Induced Cognitive Dysfunction, Vagus Nerve Stimulation.

66. Please provide reference for the study of benzodiazepines and barbiturates described in Cognitive Dysfunction in Elderly Patients with Epilepsy.

67. Please provide reference for the study of phenytoin and valproate described in Cognitive Dysfunction in Elderly Patients with Epilepsy.

68. Please provide reference for the multicenter European study described in Cognitive Dysfunction in Elderly Patients with Epilepsy.

69. Please provide reference for the VA Cooperative Study Trial 428 described in Cognitive Dysfunction in Elderly Patients with Epilepsy.

70. Please provide reference for the Adverse Events Profile mentioned in Recognition and Treatment of Cognitive Dysfunction in Epilepsy, 2nd paragraph.

71. Please provide reference for the first study described in Recognition and Treatment of Cognitive Dysfunction in Epilepsy, 3rd paragraph.

72. Please provide reference for the Jia et al. study described in Recognition and Treatment of Cognitive Dysfunction in Epilepsy, 3rd paragraph.

73. Please provide reference for the Chan et al. study described in Recognition and Treatment of Cognitive Dysfunction in Epilepsy, 4th paragraph.

74. Please provide reference for the methylphenidate study described in Recognition and Treatment of Cognitive Dysfunction in Epilepsy, 5th paragraph.

75. Langosch JM, Trimble MR. Epilepsy, psychosis and clozapine. *Hum Psychopharmacol* 2002; 17:115–119.

35 Mood

Marco Mula
Josemir W. Sander

Antiepileptic drugs (AEDs) have several mechanisms of action likely to be responsible for their antiseizure activity but also for their effect on mood and behavior (Table 35-1). In general terms, the psychotropic effects of AEDs can be broken down into those that are positive and those that are negative. Our knowledge about negative psychotropic properties of AEDs is still limited, without standardized or defined diagnostic criteria. With respect to the older generation of AEDs—that is, drugs available before the 1990s, such as barbiturates, phenytoin, carbamazepine, and valproate—there are no systematic data; whereas for the newer AEDs, there are data from drug trials in which behavioral manifestations are not systematically reported. Thus, the psychopathological nature of psychiatric side effects of AEDs, as well as their severity, time course, and relationship to seizure activity, remain incompletely understood.

MECHANISMS FOR PSYCHIATRIC SIDE EFFECTS OF ANTIEPILEPTIC DRUGS

In a review of the positive and negative psychotropic effects of antiepileptic drugs, it was suggested that two categories of compounds could be identified on the basis of their predominant psychotropic profile (1). On the one hand, sedating drugs are characterized by side effects such as fatigue, cognitive slowing, and weight gain and usually augment gamma-aminobutyric acid (GABA) inhibitory neurotransmission. On the other hand, there are activating drugs with anxiogenic and antidepressant properties that attenuate glutamate excitatory neurotransmission. In the first group are drugs such as barbiturates, valproate, gabapentin, tiagabine, and vigabatrin, and in the second group are felbamate and lamotrigine. Topiramate is likely to have a mixed profile (Figure 35-1). Although this proposed paradigm is straightforward, in patients with epilepsy the scenario is more complicated. The psychotropic effects of the AEDs may be related to direct and indirect mechanisms. The first mechanisms represent the main properties of the drug and can be easily predicted using the theoretical framework previously described. At the same time, AED-related psychopathology may also derive from the interaction between the drug and the underlying epileptic process (Table 35-2). Some phenomena, such as forced normalization (see Chapter 29 on psychosis and forced normalization) or postictal psychosis, may be pharmacologically driven, but they are not related to the AEDs per se; they occur exclusively in patients with epilepsy and are related to other variables such as the severity of the disease

TABLE 35-1
Mechanisms of Action of Antiepileptic Drugs

	VOC Na BLOCKADE	GABA INCREASE	SELECTIVE GABA_A POTENTIATION	DIRECT CL FACILITATION	VOC Ca BLOCKADE	OTHER ACTIONS
BDZ	−	−	++	−	−	−
CBZ	++	?	−	−	+ (L)	+
ETX	−	−	−	−	++(T)	−
PHB	−	+	+	++	?	+
PHT	++	−	−	−	?	+
VPA	?	+	−	−	+ (T)	++
FLB	++	+	+	−	+(L)	+
GBP	−	?	−	−	++ (N, P/Q)	?
LTG	++	+	−	−	++ (N, P/Q, R, T)	+
LEV	−	?	+	−	+ (N)	++
OXCBZ	++	?	−	−	+ (N, P)	+
PGB	−	−	−	−	++ (N, P/Q)	−
TGB	−	++	−	−	−	−
TPM	++	+	+	−	+ (L)	+
GVG	−	++	−	−	−	−
ZNM	++	?	−	−	++ (N, P, T)	+

+ = Secondary action; ++ = primary action; − = not described; ? = controversial;
VOC = voltage opened channel; in brackets the calcium channel subtype.
BDZ = benzodiazepines; CBZ = carbamazepine; ETX = ethosuximide; PHB = barbiturates; PHT = phenytoin; VPA = valproate; FLB = felbamate; GBP = gabapentin; LTG = lamotrigine; LEV = levetiracetam; OXCBZ = oxcarbazepine; PGB = pregabalin; TGB = tiagabine; TPM = topiramate; GVG = vigabatrin; ZNM = zonisamide.

or the presence of abnormalities in the limbic system. Furthermore, the concept that the mechanisms underlying the control of seizures are strictly interlinked with the control of mood and its polarity is suggested by the occurrence of psychopathological states with vagus nerve stimulation or after epilepsy surgery.

NEGATIVE EFFECTS OF ANTIEPILEPTIC DRUGS ON MOOD

Mood disorders are the most common psychiatric comorbidity in patients with epilepsy, but they often remain unrecognized and untreated (2). It is well known that the presence of depression in patients with refractory epilepsy is one of the most important variables to have an impact on the quality of life, even more than seizure frequency and severity (3). Among the potential neurobiological and psychosocial determinants, epilepsy variables such as the epilepsy syndrome or the seizure type (temporal lobe epilepsy and partial seizures), severity (depression increases with increased seizure severity), frequency (either increased or decreased), and AED treatment have been associated with depression. However, probably only a few variables are relevant concerning depressive symptoms exacerbated by AED therapy, including

GABA neurotransmission, folate deficiency, polytherapy, the presence of hippocampal sclerosis, forced normalization, and a past history of affective disorders.

Several studies have suggested a link between depression and treatment with barbiturates (primidone or phenobarbital). Old open studies comparing primidone with carbamazepine showed that, over time, patients were clinically more depressed on a regimen of primidone and less so on carbamazepine (4). Subsequently, other authors using a double-blind crossover design and evaluating patients with standardized clinical instruments have replicated these findings. In children with epilepsy taking barbiturates, a conduct disorder resembling an attention deficit hyperactivity disorder has been described. Moreover, irritability and aggressive behavior are side effects often seen in patients with mental retardation (4).

Some of the newer AEDs, including vigabatrin, tiagabine, and topiramate, have been linked with depression as a treatment-emergent adverse effect (Table 35-3).

Vigabatrin has been the most extensively studied, largely as a result of being the first of the newer compounds to be introduced to clinical practice. In some patients the onset of depression was linked with a dramatic control of seizure frequency (probably a form of forced normalization), whereas in others it was unrelated to this; on the

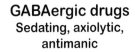

GABAergic drugs
Sedating, axiolytic,
antimanic

Anti-glutamatergic drugs
Activating, axiogenic,
antidepressant

Barbiturates,
Benzodiazepines, Valproate,
Vigabatrin, Tiagabine,
Gabapentin

Topiramate

Felbamate
Lamotrigine

Levetiracetam ?
Pregabalin ?

FIGURE 35-1

Classification of anticonvulsant drugs according to their psychotropic properties.

whole, however, it appeared to be more common in patients with a past history of depression. Thus, in the series reported in the literature, at least 50% of cases usually reported previous episodes of an affective disorder (5).

It is of interest that those AEDs that seem associated more with depression share a potentiation of the inhibitory neurotransmission mediated by the benzodiazepine-GABA receptor. In psychiatric practice, it is known that benzodiazepines can provoke depressive symptoms, and withdrawal can provoke a depressive illness. This observation is not easy to explain but has been used as further evidence for a GABAergic hypothesis of depression. A number of clinical observations and experimental studies have shown that GABAergic mechanisms are involved in the pathogenesis of depression.

Topiramate is usually considered an AED with a mixed profile, but its GABAergic properties are probably prominent, and data from studies of functional neuroimaging showed that treatment with topiramate was associated with the onset of depression and a significant augmentation in GABAergic inhibitory neurotransmission. Previous clinical studies also showed that depression is one of the main treatment-emergent adverse events during topiramate therapy (6). It was observed that relevant risk factors were a rapid titration schedule of the drug, a past psychiatric history, and probably a more severe form of epilepsy as suggested by the association with seizure frequency and the presence of tonic-atonic seizures. Interestingly we also noted that cotherapy with lamotrigine was a significant protective factor, suggesting some antidepressant properties of this AED (6).

In the pathogenesis of AED-induced depressive symptoms, a relevant role is played by the limbic structures. There is growing evidence in the literature that depression might be linked to small hippocampal volumes, and this association has been described in patients with epilepsy but also in patients without epilepsy with a major depressive disorder. Our group demonstrated that patients with temporal lobe epilepsy and hippocampal sclerosis were more prone to developing depression during therapy with topiramate than patients with temporal lobe epilepsy and normal magnetic resonance imaging (MRI), matched for starting dose and titration schedule of topiramate. Although patients with hippocampal sclerosis

---

TABLE 35-2
Mechanisms for Psychiatric Side Effects of Antiepileptic Drugs in Patients with Epilepsy

DIRECT (DRUG-RELATED)

• Mechanism of action of the drug
• Drug toxicity
• Drug withdrawal

INDIRECT (EPILEPSY-RELATED)

• Forced normalization phenomenon
• Postictal syndromes
• Affective symptoms in patients with hippocampal sclerosis

TABLE 35-3
Psychotropic Effects of Anticonvulsants

	NEGATIVE	POSITIVE
BARBITURATES	Depression, hyperactivity	Anxiolytic, hypnotic
Phenytoin	Encephalopathy	
Ethosuximide	Behavioral abnormalities, psychosis	
Carbamazepine – Oxcarbazepine		Mood stabilizing, antimanic
Valproate	Encephalopathy	Mood stabilizing, antimanic, (anxiolytic)
Felbamate	Depression, anxiety, irritability	(Increased attention and concentration)
Lamotrigine	Insomnia, agitation	Mood stabilizing, antidepressant
Vigabatrin	Depression, aggression, psychosis	
Topiramate	Depression, psychomotor slowing, psychosis	Antibulimic in binge eating disorders (mood stabilizing)
Gabapentin	Behavioral problems in children	(Anxiolytic)
Zonisamide	Agitation, depression, psychoses	
Tiagabine	Depression (non–convulsive status epilepticus)	
Levetiracetam	Irritability, emotional liability	
Pregabalin		Anxiolytic

are more likely to be affected by a more severe form of epilepsy, in which treatment resistance and polytherapy can be present, the regression analysis showed that only hippocampal sclerosis and not the AED regimen was a predictive factor for depression (7).

Another issue of interest is folate deficiency. Patients receiving several AEDs are reported to have low serum, red cell, or cerebrospinal fluid (CSF) folate levels. This deficit appears greater in patients with epilepsy who also show psychopathology, and it is known that folic acid plays a crucial role in several important central nervous system transmethylation reactions and is linked to monoamine metabolism. It is interesting that anticonvulsants with a positive impact on mood and behavior, such as carbamazepine or lamotrigine, have minimal effects on folate levels.

POSITIVE EFFECTS OF ANTIEPILEPTIC DRUGS ON MOOD

AEDs are used extensively in psychiatric practice for a broad spectrum of psychiatric disorders, especially bipolar disorders, and some are well known to stabilize mood. Since its introduction into the clinical management

of epilepsy, carbamazepine has been reported to have psychotropic properties. Over time, several controlled studies have been carried out comparing the effects of carbamazepine in acute mania with placebo, lithium, or neuroleptics. These studies have shown that carbamazepine is equivalent to lithium in many cases, and that the time course of the antimanic effect is a little slower than with neuroleptics but equivalent to lithium (8). This is relevant for those patients who are refractory to lithium and require an alternative. Carbamazepine has also been shown to be an effective treatment for the prophylaxis of bipolar disorder, controlled studies suggesting that patients with an unstable bipolar disorder with rapid fluctuations (rapid cyclers) do better on carbamazepine or a combination of carbamazepine and lithium.

Valproate has been used in manic episodes, depressive episodes, and for maintenance therapy of bipolar disorder; the strongest supporting evidence is for acute mania (8). There is possibly an effect in behavioral problems associated with affective lability, aggression, and impulsivity across a range of different clinical contexts, but currently, controlled studies are available mainly for bipolar depression.

Some of the new AEDs (e.g., tiagabine) have failed to show any efficacy in primary psychiatric disorders,

TABLE 35-4
Clinical Guideline Recommendations for Antiepileptic Drugs in Bipolar Disorder

		CBZ	GBP	LTG	OXC	VPA
APA	Acute mania/mixed mania	+	−	−	+	+
	Acute bipolar depression	−	−	+	−	−
	Acute rapid cycling	−	−	+	−	+
	Maintenance	+	−	+	+	+
BAP	Acute mania/mixed mania	+	−	−	−	+
	Acute bipolar depression	−	−	+	−	+
	Rapid cycling	−	−	+	−	+
	Maintenance	+	−	+	+	+

APA = American Psychiatric Association; Hirschfeld et al. Practice Guideline for the Treatment of Patients with Bipolar Disorder (Revision). *Am J Psychiatry* 2002;159(Suppl 4):1–50.
BAP = British Association of Psychopharmacology; Goodwin GM. Evidence-based guidelines for treating bipolar disorder: recommendations from the British Association for Psychopharmacology. *J Psychopharmacol* 2003;17:149–173.
CBZ = carbamazepine; GBP = gabapentin; LTG = lamotrigine; OXC = oxcarbazepine; VPA = valproate.

whereas others (e.g., topiramate) may have adjunctive uses, such as weight loss in the management of weight gain as a side effect of atypical antipsychotics or in comorbid eating disorders (9). The data on the effects of oxcarbazepine on psychiatric disorders are limited and definitely less conclusive than those regarding carbamazepine. Oxcarbazepine, however, seems to be less effective than lithium, but as effective as carbamazepine, in acute mania; but oxcarbazepine is probably better tolerated than carbamazepine. The lack of efficacy of gabapentin in bipolar disorders has emerged from controlled studies that failed to detect such an effect (8).

During clinical trials in the development of lamotrigine as an AED, it was observed that it had antidepressant properties. The cumulative results of the studies so far provide evidence that lamotrigine is effective in the management of the depressed phase of bipolar disorder type II and in the long-term stabilization of mood in patients with rapid cycling bipolar disorder (Table 35-4).

Pregabalin is probably the most interesting molecule of the newest compounds. Controlled studies have demonstrated that it is better than placebo in anxiety disorders such as generalized anxiety disorder (8).

Data currently published suggest an important role for AEDs in psychiatric disorders, but it is difficult to extrapolate from these studies in psychiatric patients directly to patients with epilepsy. It would clearly be very useful to know whether drugs have a positive influence on the psychic status of patients with epilepsy beyond their influence on seizure activity. However, there is little scientific evidence for this; most of the studies are uncontrolled and based on quality-of-life parameters rather than on a formal psychiatric evaluation. The use of a drug as both an antiepileptic and an antidepressant or mood stabilizer should be an important option for rational pharmacotherapy in patients with uncontrolled epilepsy and comorbid psychiatric disorders. Further studies are required.

Lamotrigine is the only compound recently investigated as a psychotropic agent in patients with epilepsy. Several blind studies have shown significant improvement in quality-of-life outcomes when lamotrigine is compared to carbamazepine or valproate, but studies addressing the specific issue of depression are lacking (4). An open study reported a significant antidepressant effect of lamotrigine in thirteen patients with uncontrolled epilepsy and depression. In two different studies from our group, we observed that lamotrigine significantly reduced the occurrence of psychopathology during therapy with topiramate (6) or levetiracetam (10). All of these studies taken together suggest a possible role of lamotrigine as an antidepressant or mood stabilizer in those patients with uncontrolled epilepsy and depressive symptoms.

VAGUS NERVE STIMULATION AND MOOD

Several studies with different methodological approaches have demonstrated that vagus nerve stimulation (VNS) may bilaterally activate a wide range of brain regions: the nucleus of the solitary tract and brainstem regions in its vicinity, the thalamus, hypothalamus, amygdala, hippocampus, and isocortex. The regions are particularly relevant in the context of both epileptogenesis and neuropsychiatric disorders. The details of activation remain somewhat obscure because different studies report slightly different effects regarding possible lateralization of the activations obtained; but a dose-dependent enhancement effect of VNS on retention and recognition performance in animals and patients with epilepsy has been demonstrated, showing the functional impact of these activations.

The Food and Drug Administration approved VNS for the treatment of drug-resistant epilepsy in 1997, and the European Community did so in 1994. Reports from the early randomized controlled trials on VNS for epilepsy treatment (E03, E05) suggested improved quality of life in a majority of patients, with 50–60% of patients reporting that their quality of life had improved in the 14-week period since implantation. Subsequently, several small studies and an international, randomized, multisite outcome study evaluated the effect of VNS on mood in patients with epilepsy using specific mood outcome measures from standardized psychiatric rating scales; but the majority of studies were too small to definitely prove the specificity of the effect and to exclude a placebo effect (11).

In patients with depression but without epilepsy, the role of VNS in the regulation of mood seems to be much clearer than in patients with depression and epilepsy. The first studies conducted involved patients with very severe forms of depression resistant to at least two antidepressant medications. Because the disorders were very severe and chronic, a substantial placebo effect was very unlikely to occur. Some of these studies showed a response rate of up to 40% in the acute phase, with an apparent continued improvement for 2 years. However, controlled studies in a similar patient population showed no significant benefit for low current stimulation. VNS is now available as a treatment for chronic or recurrent depression in several countries. The Food and Drug Administration recently approved VNS in patients who have not responded to four or more adequate antidepressant treatments. Strong anti-anxiety effects have also been demonstrated in depressed patients. Further studies in anxiety disorders are ongoing.

This treatment modality may be a possibility for combination therapy for epilepsy and psychiatric disorders without concerns of adverse effects due to drug-drug interactions. However, VNS, like other antiepileptic modalities, is also associated with the onset of psychiatric side effects, especially those that are based on indirect mechanisms such as the forced normalization phenomenon or postictal states.

CONCLUSIONS

Among the psychiatric adverse effects of AEDs, a variety of behavioral problems are the most commonly reported, followed by depression, with psychosis being a relatively rare though severe complication. Several factors are implicated in their occurrence, and the risk is likely to be linked to severity of epilepsy, polytherapy, rapid titration, and high dosages of the drugs. It is important to identify a clinical phenotype more at risk of developing psychopathology, to inform patients and their families and to make sure that the patients at risk are seen frequently. In general terms, a previous psychiatric history or a familial predisposition and a diagnosis of mesial temporal lobe epilepsy are associated with a high risk of psychopathology. Hippocampal sclerosis makes the risk higher for affective symptoms such as depressed mood and mental slowing.

In clinical practice, patients presenting with depression and epilepsy should always have their anticonvulsant therapy reviewed, and polytherapy should be avoided when possible. In individuals with uncontrolled epilepsy and a previous history of episodic psychopathology, especially a psychosis, the aim of complete seizure control should be carefully approached.

Antiepileptic drugs may be used in epilepsy or as psychotropic drugs or mood stabilizers at the same time, tailoring the appropriate therapy in relation to the psychic status of the patient.

References

1. Ketter TA, Post RM, Theodore WH. Positive and negative psychiatric effects of antiepileptic drugs in patients with seizure disorders. *Neurology* 1999; 53(Suppl 2): S53–S67.
2. Gaitatzis A, Trimble MR, Sander JW. The psychiatric comorbidity of epilepsy. *Acta Neurol Scand* 2004; 110:207–220.
3. Boylan LS, Flint LA, Labovitz DL, Jackson SC, et al. Depression but not seizure frequency predicts quality of life in treatment resistant epilepsy. *Neurology* 2004; 62:258–261.
4. Schmitz B. The Effects of Antiepileptic Drugs on Behavior. Trimble MR, Schmitz B, eds. In: *The neuropsychiatry of epilepsy*. Cambridge: Cambridge University Press, 2002:241–255.
5. Thomas L, Trimble M, Schmitz B, Ring H. Vigabatrin and behaviour disorders: a retrospective survey. *Epilepsy Res* 1996; 25:21–27.
6. Mula M, Trimble MR, Lhatoo SD, Sander JW. Topiramate and psychiatric adverse events in patients with epilepsy. *Epilepsia* 2003; 44:659–663.
7. Mula M, Trimble MR, Sander JW. The role of hippocampal sclerosis in topiramate-related depression and cognitive deficits in people with epilepsy. *Epilepsia* 2003; 44:1573–1577.
8. Spina E, Perugi G. Antiepileptic drugs: indications other than epilepsy. *Epileptic Disord* 2004; 6:57–75.
9. Mula M, Cavanna AE, Monaco F. Psychopharmacology of topiramate: from epilepsy to bipolar disorder. *Neuropsychiatric Disease and Treatment* 2006; 2(4):475–488.
10. Mula M, Trimble MR, Yuen A, Liu RS, et al. Psychiatric adverse events during levetiracetam therapy. *Neurology* 2003; 61:704–706.
11. Elger CE, Hoppe C. Vagus nerve stimulation and mood. Trimble MR, Schmitz B, eds. In: *The Neuropsychiatry of Epilepsy*. Cambridge: Cambridge University Press, 2002:283–295.

EPILEPSY SURGERY

36 Presurgical Evaluation for Epilepsy Surgery

Manjari Tripathi
Satish Jain

majority of persons with epilepsy do well on antiepileptic drugs (AEDs). However, there are about 30–40% of persons with epilepsy who continue to have seizures despite the best intention of treatment even with the latest AEDs (1). It is this subset that must be identified and considered for an expedited and exhaustive evaluation for the possibility of a surgical cure of their seizures.

Medical intractability can be defined as a situation in a given person who has received an accurate diagnosis of epilepsy (nonepileptic seizures being ruled out) and, despite an adequate trial of appropriately selected and dosed AEDs, continues to have seizures, which thus results in serious impairment of the person's health or quality of life.

The prevalence of medically intractable epilepsy is not precisely known, but it has been estimated at about 5% to 10% of the epilepsy population (2). As many as 100,000 to 180,000 persons in the United States are estimated to have medically intractable epilepsy. Estimates from the incidence of epilepsy also suggest that at least 5,000 persons with epilepsy would go on to have medical intractability each year. Predictors of intractability are mental retardation, high initial seizure frequency, remote symptomatic etiology, and poor short-term treatment outcome (3). A history of infantile

spasms, earlier age of seizure onset, and status epilepticus have also been implicated as risk factors (4). Thirty percent of those whose seizures fail to improve with treatment during the first year, versus 4% of those whose seizures respond, eventually have uncontrolled seizures in the years to follow, hence the control of seizures in the first year of therapy may give a clue to who should be investigated further (5).

Persistent seizures undermine psychosocial, educational, and occupational opportunities and development of an individual (6). Numerous studies have demonstrated quality-of-life impairment in these persons (7). In addition, there is always the issue of unpredictability, injuries, and sudden death. Persons with epilepsy have a 23 times higher risk of sudden death than the general population. The risk is high, at around 1:200 person-years, or between 0.5% and 1.5% per year, in persons with medically intractable epilepsy (8, 9).

WHOM TO EVALUATE?

Patients considered for presurgical evaluation should typically meet the following two criteria: (1) disabling seizures that have not been controlled by adequate trials of appropriate AEDs without adverse side effects, and (2) clinical, neuroimaging, or electroencephalographic

(EEG) evidence of an epileptogenic brain region that may be safely resected (10, 11), or, if no focal region is responsible, the seizures are disabling enough to warrant a palliative surgical procedure.

WHEN TO EVALUATE?

Seizure recurrence in a person within the first few years of therapy would be the appropriate time at which to decide to investigate. Ideally anyone not responding to an appropriate AED (two having been tried) in adequate doses should be evaluated.

HOW TO EVALUATE?

It is mandatory to proceed in a systematic manner in the presurgical delineation of the epileptogenic zone. Noninvasive methods must be used to their fullest available potential before an invasive procedure. The various techniques utilized for the same are listed in Table 36-1. The list is not exhaustive, and new noninvasive techniques are being developed and coming into use. These are discussed individually in the following subsections.

Neurologic History, Seizure Semiology, and Examination

The process starts with identification of the seizure semiology by history. A careful history taking is the first and most important step in the evaluation of an intractable seizure disorder. The profile of a patient's ictus can be defined by the following ten-point system: (1) a sequential description of the seizure episodes, usually given by eyewitnesses. An aura or warning should always be asked for. (2) Age of onset. (3) Etiology or risk factors, including history of febrile seizures, head injury, encephalitis, perinatal factors, and so on. (4) Seizure frequency. (5) Seizure-aggravating and -alleviating factors. (6) Compliance with medication. (7) Psychologic factors. (8) Impact of seizures. (9) Family history. (10) Effect of prior and current AED treatments (seizure outcome, the best AEDs so far, doses used, and side effects experienced).

Knowledge and recognition of semiological lateralizing signs during seizures is an important component of the presurgical evaluation and adds further information to the electrophysiological monitoring by a video-EEG (VEEG) (12). The lateralizing and localizing value of the semiology correlates well with the cortical representation of various functions; hence these should be examined in microscopic and meticulous details (13). Table 36-2 illustrates the various localizing features of different phenomena in order of their localizing accuracy. The list of lateralizing features increases over time as more and more observations are validated.

Interictal EEG

Interictal EEG recording is a noninvasive tool that is invaluable in evaluating patients with intractable epilepsy. Cascino et al. (14) performed a very elegant study and came to the conclusion that unilateral interictal EEG discharges correlated well with the findings of ipsilateral temporal lobe atrophy and a good surgical outcome. The routine EEG almost invariably records only interictal epileptiform activity in patients with intractable epilepsy, and this identifies the irritative zone in patients with partial seizures. The irritative zone may correspond to the site of seizure onset, but it does not always approximate the size of the critical epileptogenic brain region. The relatively short duration of the routine EEG provides only a limited sample of interictal activity. Serial EEGs or prolonged interictal studies may increase the likelihood of recording epileptiform abnormalities. The consensus of previous studies suggests that interictal epileptiform abnormalities may be a good index of the epileptogenic temporal lobe. Interictal discharges, however, may incorrectly lateralize the epileptic temporal lobe in 10–20% of patients. The presence of unilateral anterior temporal lobe spikes is also a predictor of favorable operative outcome. The lateralizing value of the scalp-recorded ictal EEG is also better in patients with temporal lobe epilepsy (TLE) and unilateral temporal lobe spikes (15). In extratemporal lesions and epileptogenic zones the interictal EEG may have a lower yield; however, some studies have demonstrated that when comparing the EEG foci with the

---

TABLE 36-1
Techniques Used to Localize the Primary Epileptogenic Zone

a. Neurologic history, seizure semiology, and examination
b. Interictal EEG
c. Video-EEG monitoring
d. High-resolution MRI and additional protocols
e. Ictal and interictal SPECT
f. PET
g. Simultaneous EEG and fMRI
h. MEG
i. Coregistered multimodality imaging and electrophysiology
j. Intracranial EEG and cortical stimulation
k. Neuropsychologic testing
l. Sodium amobarbital test (Wada test)

TABLE 36-2

The Localizing and Lateralizing Value of Seizure Semiology

SEMIOLOGY	LATERALIZING VALUE	SYMPTOMATOGENIC ZONE
Ictal dysphasia and aphasia	100% dominant	Impairment of language areas
Unilateral dystonic posturing	100% contralateral	Activation of basal ganglia, temporal lobe epilepsy (TLE)
Hemifield visual aura	100% contralateral	Brodmann areas 17–19 and adjacent areas, occipital lobe epilepsy
Version	100% contralateral	Brodmann areas 6 and 8, frontal lobe epilepsy (FLE)
Automatisms with preserved consciousness	100% nondominant	Unknown, TLE
Postictal palsy	93% contralateral	Possible exhaustion or inhibition of Brodmann areas 4 and 6
Postictal nose wiping	92% ipsilateral	Unknown, TLE
Tonic activity	89% contralateral	SMA, possibly also Brodmann area 6, the anterior cingulate gyrus, FLE
Figure of 4 sign	89% contralateral	SMA or prefrontal areas
Unilateral sensory aura	89% contralateral	Brodmann areas 1, 2, and 3
Clonic activity	83% contralateral	Brodmann areas 4 and 6, FLE
Unilateral ictal eye blinking	83% ipsilateral	Unknown
Ictal speech	83% nondominant	Impairment of areas other than those involved in language production
Ictal vomiting	81% nondominant	Nondominant lobe and Papez circuit
Ictal spitting	75% nondominant	Central autonomic network involvement

lesions shown by magnetic resonance imaging (MRI), the same location of the interictal foci was found in 68.4% (16). What is interesting is that this modality of investigation, when combined with functional MRI (fMRI), is now an increasingly utilized research tool in the presurgical evaluation of intractable epilepsy.

Video-EEG (VEEG) Monitoring

With VEEG monitoring, video images of the patient's seizure are recorded and analyzed with simultaneous EEG signals. When contemplating epilepsy surgery as a potential treatment of intractable epilepsy, VEEG monitoring should be performed to record seizure episodes and to confirm their concordance with the historical, routine EEG and MRI data. Recording of seizures also allows the clinician to confirm that the patient's habitual seizures are fully evaluated and documented. It is not rare for VEEG monitoring to uncover psychogenic nonepilepsy seizures or to detect seizures that arise from areas other than the presumed site.

The number of recorded seizures required for localization of the surgical focus varies from patient to patient. At least five seizures from the same brain location need to be recorded to achieve a 95% chance of not encountering a seizure that comes from another location. Theoretically

about twenty seizures may have to be recorded to exclude independent bilateral seizure onsets, but this may not be practically feasible (17). The average duration of monitoring required to record about five seizures has been shown to be 6 to 7 days (18). Fortunately, two to five recorded seizures may be sufficient in many patients with surgically remediable epilepsy.

Magnetic Resonance Imaging

An epilepsy-protocol MRI has become a necessity in the presurgical evaluation of patients with intractable epilepsy. The MRI readily reveals the common substrates of mesial temporal sclerosis (MTS), cortical dysplasias, and cavernous hemangioma, and so forth. The optimal technique in adult patients with partial epilepsy must include coronal or oblique-coronal images using T1-weighted and T2-weighted sequences. The most common imaging alteration in an adult with intractable partial epilepsy is medial temporal lobe atrophy with a signal intensity change (19). Fluid-attenuated inversion recovery (FLAIR) sequences increase the sensitivity and must be performed. The lesion often appears as a signal change in these patients. High-resolution diffusion tensor imaging (DTI) identifies lateralizing abnormalities of the hippocampus in patients with a normal MRI; another exciting area of research is the postictal DTI in which diffusion measurements could help lateralize the seizure focus (20, 21). Magnetization-prepared rapid gradient echo (MP-RAGE) and DTI are also helpful in locating cortical dysplasias and identifying lesions when conventional imaging studies are negative.

Hippocampal volumetric measurement helps to identify the side of lesion in patients with MTS (22). In one study, volumetry revealed unilateral damage in 77% of the patients, T2-relaxometry in 64%, and spectroscopy in 53%. Volumetry and T2-relaxometry (not spectroscopy) were associated with a 1-year postoperative outcome with volumetry predicting outcome correctly in 100% of the cases, whereas T2-relaxometry classified 96.4% of patients with hippocampal sclerosis (23). Proton magnetic resonance spectroscopy (^{1}H-MRS) has been shown to be a reliable indicator of the side of seizure origin in patients with medial temporal lobe epilepsy. This can be done by revealing a reduction in N-acetylated compound (NA) concentrations or abnormalities in the creatine (Cr)/NA or NA/choline ratios. There is also an observed elevation of glutamine (Glx) levels together with reductions in N-acetyl aspartate (NAA) (Figure 36-1) levels probably consistent with the hypothesis of epilepsy-related excitotoxicity as a possible underlying mechanism. The underlying pathogeneses for the metabolic changes are likely to be complex and may relate to focal neuronal loss, gliosis, or a functional alteration intimately associated with the frequency of seizure activity. A meta-analysis of various studies analyzing the lateralizing value in the preoperative evaluation of patients demonstrated a positive predictive value in all patients with ipsilateral MRS creatine/NA compounds ratio abnormality for good outcome, which was 82%

Glx/NAA=1.4   Glx/NAA=0.59

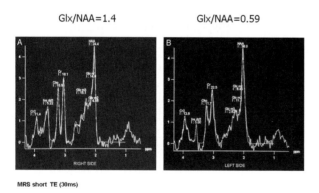

MRS short TE (30ms)

FIGURE 36-1

Elevation of glutamine (Glx) levels together with reductions in N-acetyl aspartate (NAA) result in a higher Glx/NAA ratio on the right side by magnetic resonance spectroscopy (MRS). (Courtesy of Dr. S. B. Gaikwad, Department of Neuroradiology, AIIMS, Delhi.)

in patients with an ipsilateral MRS abnormality when compared to patients with bilateral MRS abnormalities. Data for MRI-negative patients were conflicting. MRS, to date, still remains a research tool with clinical potential. Further studies limited to nonlocalized ictal scalp EEG or MRI-negative patients are required for validation of its usefulness in patients (24).

Individuals with a normal MRI have substrate-negative epilepsies. The anatomical localization of the epileptogenic zone in these individuals commonly involves the neocortex and may be extrahippocampal. Studies with 3-tesla MRI scans may improve the diagnostic yield of structural neuroimaging in patients with focal cortical dysplasias and substrate-negative epilepsies especially by tractography studies. Phased-array surface coil studies would improve clinical decision making in about 38% of patients (25).

To obviate the need or to minimize the extent of intracranial implantation, several advances have been made to help delineate the surgical focus. The major advances are in the areas of functional imaging and coregistration of multimodal images. Functional neuroimaging refers to the imaging of electrophysiological, metabolic, biochemical, or perfusion disturbances around the epileptogenic region. These are discussed herein.

Single-Photon Emission Computed Tomography (SPECT)

SPECT is an important noninvasive technique for peri-ictal imaging in patients with intractable partial epilepsy syndromes being considered for epilepsy surgery. Ictal SPECT studies are superior to interictal images in localization-related epilepsy. SPECT studies involve cerebral blood flow imaging using radiopharmaceuticals such as technetium-99m-hexamethylpropylene amine oxime (^{99m}Tc-HMPAO). These studies produce a "photograph" of the peri-ictal cerebral perfusion pattern that was present soon after the injection. The SPECT images can be acquired up to 4 to 6 hours after the termination of the seizure, so the individual patient can recover from the ictus before being transported to the nuclear medicine facility. Focal hypoperfusion in the region of the epileptogenic zone is often found in interictal SPECT. However, this has a low sensitivity and a relatively high false-positive rate in patients with TLE and a low yield in patients with extratemporal seizures. Ictal SPECT studies show hyperperfusion (26, 27). However, both interictal and ictal SPECT must be done in a given patient so that both can be compared to each other for subtraction ictal SPECT coregistered to interictal SPECT (SISCOS) (Figure 36-2). The spatial resolution of SPECT, however, remains low. There are now methods to enhance this, which will be discussed.

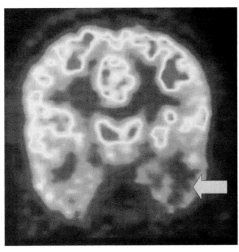

FIGURE 36-2

SISCOS showing left anterior temporal uptake in a patient with cortical dysplasia. Also note the contralateral cerebellar diaschisis. (Courtesy of Dr. C. S. Bal, Department of Nuclear Medicine, AIIMS, Delhi.) See color section following page 266.

Positron Emission Tomography (PET)

PET is another functional neuroimaging study that may be useful in identifying a localization-related abnormality in the presurgical planning of patients with intractable partial epilepsy. However, this investigation may not be available in all centers, and it is costly. It is also logistically difficult to perform ictal PET, unlike ictal SPECT. The most common study used in the evaluation of intractable partial epilepsy is the ^{18}F-deoxyglucose (FDG)-PET. Temporal lobe epilepsies are probably best evaluated by this modality (Figure 36-3) because the yield is highest (sensitivity 90%, with a false lateralization in 1–2%). Unfortunately, PET is less useful in patients with neocortical or extratemporal epilepsy, especially if there is no substrate seen by MRI. Other novel tracer studies may also be useful in localization. Central benzodiazepine receptors (BZDR) and central opiate receptors can be identified with ^{11}C-flumazenil PET and ^{11}C-carfentanil PET, respectively. Focal BZDR decreases and increases, or decreased selected opiate receptor activity, may

be present in patients with substrate-directed pathology. The hippocampal pathological abnormalities may be intimately associated with both epileptogenesis and the development of comorbidity. Abnormalities in excitatory and inhibitory neurotransmitter systems have been implicated in medial temporal lobe epilepsy. Another PET tracer, alpha-^{11}C-methyl-L-tryptophan (AMT), has also been shown to be potentially useful in the assessment of patients with intractable epilepsy (28, 29).

Magnetoencephalography (MEG)

The difference between signals recorded by MEG versus those recorded by EEG is that the skull and the tissue surrounding the brain affect the magnetic fields measured by MEG much less than they affect the electrical impulses measured by EEG. The advantage of MEG over EEG is therefore greater accuracy owing to the minimal distortion of the signal. This allows for more usable and reliable localization of brain function. To generate a signal that is detectable, approximately 50,000 active neurons are needed. Because current dipoles must have similar orientations to generate magnetic fields that reinforce each other, it is often the layer of pyramidal cells in the cortex, which are generally perpendicular to its surface, that give rise to measurable magnetic fields. Furthermore, it is often bundles of these neurons located in the sulci of the cortex, with orientations parallel to the surface of the head, that project measurable portions of their magnetic fields outside of the head. MEG picks up this electrical epileptiform activity in the brain and is a useful diagnostic tool for neocortical and frontal seizure foci. Various studies show that MEG source imaging (MSI), coregistered with anatomical imaging, can help to delineate epileptic activity (Figure 36-4) and yields

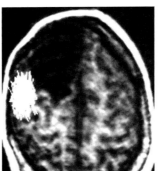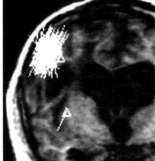

FIGURE 36-3

FDG-PET in the same patient (Fig. 36-2) shows left temporal hypoperfusion. (Courtesy of Dr. C. S. Bal, Department of Nuclear medicine, AIIMS, Delhi.) See color section following page 266.

FIGURE 36-4

MSI of a patient with refractory frontal lobe seizures (sequela to an abscess at birth) with MEG showing a cluster in the remnant of the secondary motor area (SMA); patient is seizure free for 5 years following EcoG-guided resection. (Courtesy of Dr. G. Mathern, Pediatric Epilepsy Surgery Program at University of California at Los Angeles, California, United States.)

localizing information with a high positive predictive value in epilepsy surgery candidates, who typically may require invasive monitoring (30–32).

Multimodality Imaging

Subtraction Ictal Single-photon Emission Tomography Coregistered to MRI (SISCOM). SISCOM represents a recent innovation in neuroimaging. It essentially gives a better anatomical representation to the SPECT focus, hence overcoming its limitations. The interictal image is subtracted from the ictal image to derive the difference (subtraction) in cerebral blood flow related to the epileptogenic zone. Images with intensities of more than two standard deviations are coregistered onto the structural MRI. SISCOM findings have been shown to correlate with the operative outcome. SISCOM may also be used in the determination of where to place intracranial EEG electrodes (33). The sensitivity of SISCOM in detecting an abnormal focus in a group of patients with complex epilepsy was twice that of the conventional method (88% vs. 39%). In this group of mostly nonlesional epilepsy patients, presence of a concordant SISCOM focus independently predicted excellent postsurgical outcome, whereas MRI did not. Data also show that the SISCOM can localize extratemporal seizure foci and identify patients who are more likely to benefit from surgery, even when the MRI is negative for a structural lesion. A SISCOM abnormality can be demonstrated in nearly 80% of patients with intractable nonlesional extratemporal epilepsy. When this extratemporal SISCOM focus is resected, about 55% to 60% will experience excellent seizure control, whereas extratemporal nonlesional epilepsy without the use of SISCOM typically results in only 25% to 40% with an excellent postsurgical outcome (34).

FDG-PET Coregistered to MRI. Recent studies have demonstrated the usefulness of coregistering the FDG-PET to MRI especially in the recognition of temporal and extratemporal epileptogenic zones (35, 36).

fMRI/EEG. fMRI and EEG performed simultaneously (SEM) is another emerging research tool for monitoring interictal as well as ictal discharges and their associated blood oxygen level dependent (BOLD) changes during MRI studies (Figure 36-5). This new modality is a marriage of the benefits of both investigations—that is, the high temporal resolution and sensitivity to epileptic abnormalities of EEG and the high spatial resolution and noninvasive localization of cerebral metabolic change of fMRI (37–39). Concordance of the findings on this technique does exist with intracranial EEG recordings (40). In the coming years this modality will offer another easy noninvasive method for presurgical evaluation.

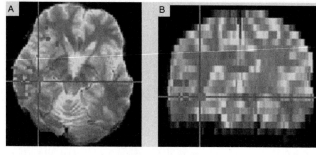

FIGURE 36-5

fMRI/EEG of a patient with refractory musicogenic epilepsy showing right temporal BOLD signal changes occurring at the onset of the ictus. (Courtesy Dr. J. Stern, University of California at Los Angeles Seizure Disorder Center, UCLA, Los Angeles, California, United States.) See color section following page 266.

Intracranial EEG Recording

With the advent of multimodality noninvasive monitoring in patients with intractable epilepsy the utilization of intracranial EEG monitoring is declining; however, this must be performed until most of the recently-developed modalities are validated (41). It is usually performed when extracranial scalp VEEG recording shows indeterminate seizure onset or multifocal or discordant onsets; the MRI is normal, has multiple lesions, or has a dual pathology; and the standard noninvasive procedures disclose results that are inconclusive or in conflict with each other. The percentage of patients who require intracranial electrode implantation varies between centers, but about 5% to 20% of temporal surgery candidates and 40% to 70% of extratemporal surgery candidates require the procedure (42). Persons having the epileptogenic zone in and around eloquent cortex also require either extraoperative or intraoperative stimulation to map areas so as not to cause a postoperative deficit. The only drawback of these procedures is that they are invasive and have potential complications associated with them (43). The choice of placing grids or depths depends on the hypothesis formulated regarding the possible site of origin of these seizures during the phase I evaluation with noninvasive methods. Invasive evaluation comprises the phase II of the presurgical evaluation.

Other semi-invasive methods such as sphenoidal and foramen ovale placements can be performed, but these have a limited sampling area and can be applied only in select patients in whom the epileptogenic area is postulated to be temporal; hence, only in a few patients do they avert the need for invasive recordings. These electrodes also increase the specificity of the interictal EEG (44, 45).

Intraoperative Electrocorticography (ECoG)

Intraoperative electrocorticography (ECoG) is used in many surgeries to guide the extent of resection. The procedure is particularly needed in resection of nonlesional extratemporal brain regions (46).

Neuropsychologic Assessment

Comprehensive neuropsychologic testing is indicated for most patients with intractable epilepsy. It is necessary to assess the cognitive, functional, and motor abilities before surgery. Further, it is essential to counsel patients regarding the deficits that could develop following surgery based on the impact this would have on their quality of life (47). Neuropsychologic evaluation differs from other methods used to localize cerebral lesions in that it involves application of a specified battery and performance on the same. These tests sample a wide variety of cognitive abilities, analyzing mainly language proficiency, visuospatial skills, and memory. Testing of memory is crucial in the investigation because of the common involvement of the temporal lobes in epileptogenesis. Different aspects of learning and memory are tested, and measures sensitive to the same should be included. Appraisal of frontal lobe function is another important prelude to surgery in this area. The battery used would depend on the ease, validity, and standardization for that specific population. Cognitive functions sampled typically include "intelligence" (IQ tests), attention, language skills, visuospatial abilities, "executive skills," and other abilities associated with frontal lobe function, and learning and memory. Thus, the assessment samples vary widely among a variety of functions, providing a comprehensive picture of an individual patient's performance. Thus, neuropsychologic tests can be used in lateralizing and localizing the seizure focus for epilepsy surgery through assessment of function of each area of the brain.

Some patients who have been selected for epilepsy surgery also undergo pre- and postsurgical visual field and language examinations. The indication for these tests depends on the location and the extent of the surgery planned. All neocortical resections involving the temporal, parietal, and occipital regions would require a formal visual field test. Presurgical language function assessment is also performed when the presumed site of surgery is in the vicinity of the language area. Peroperative awake craniotomy and mapping of the eloquent cortex is done in cooperative patients to prevent postoperative deficits (48).

Intracarotid Amobarbital Test (The Wada Test)

While in Montreal, Juhn Wada developed a test designed to definitively confirm hemispheric lateralization and dominance of speech in candidates for surgical treatment of epilepsy. The Wada test predicts the ability of the brain to sustain speech function and verbal learning after epilepsy surgery and is performed by injecting amobarbital into the internal carotid artery on the side to be resected. The anesthetic drug temporarily paralyzes the hemisphere injected. It helps in the assessment of whether the contralateral hemisphere can sustain critical cognitive and language functions, and if the hemisphere undergoing the operation could lose some cerebral function after surgery. It has also been used to predict postsurgical amnesia in that those who had failed performed significantly worse following surgery and hence are at higher risk of memory deficits. The Wada test is also useful in predicting laterality of seizure focus in candidates for temporal lobectomy.

This procedure is now in its sixth decade and, despite its invasive character, is still a routine in most centers for determining the lateralization of language and memory before epilepsy surgery. Although the technique is a gold standard, it does have certain drawbacks. The dosage of amobarbital varies, and latencies between injection and stimulus presentation and latencies between injection of one side and the other also vary from center to center. Language is tested by using several language tasks (e.g., word generation or counting, comprehension, naming, repetition, and reading). The exact procedure and how to interpret the findings vary between centers and also depends on the experience of the psychologist and the team. Stimuli for memory testing are either presented first and then followed by a distracting stimulus to be recalled during amobarbital injection, or alternatively, a given number of stimuli are presented during anesthesia and must be recollected after the effect of amobarbital has worn off. The first method may be misleading because transient language impairment may limit the performance. This is also true for the second method, in which high verbal contents of stimuli may result in falsely high failure rates. About 60% of centers present stimuli within the first 3 minutes; whereas other centers wait with the testing for 3 minutes, to overcome an initial period of confusion, particularly when the language-dominant hemisphere is injected. Bilateral testing is done in 80% of centers but not always.

Among the new techniques available, fMRI is one of the most promising alternatives to the Wada test. This noninvasive method has several advantages, including the possibility of mapping relevant areas within the hemispheres and being able to prolong examination time in case of discordant results. Many fMRI studies have focused on correlations with the intracarotid amobarbital procedure as the gold standard and found an agreement of about 90%. More important, recent studies have demonstrated a significant correlation between presurgical fMRI testing and postsurgical outcome for fMRI activations in frontal language areas. In a few studies, prediction for outcome is higher for fMRI than for the intracarotid amobarbital procedure. However, further refinements regarding the paradigms and analysis procedures in fMRI are needed to improve the contribution of fMRI for presurgical assessment (49, 50).

Other noninvasive techniques such as optical imaging are also under evaluation.

CONCLUSION

The decision of whether to try another AED or to initiate epilepsy surgery evaluation should be individualized by weighing various factors. Whether two or more than two AEDs should be tried before evaluation for surgical consideration depends on the probability of excellent outcome after epilepsy surgery relative to that with further AED trials and the impact of uncontrolled seizures on the patient's quality of life and the associated psychosocial and occupational factors (51, 52). Ultimately,

all patients whose seizures are incapacitating and intractable should undergo noninvasive presurgical evaluation to determine whether epilepsy surgery is an appropriate treatment option. It is very important that this evaluation be conducted as soon as epilepsy becomes, or has the potential to become, medically refractory. The most compelling reason to consider presurgical evaluation from the patient's perspective, however, is to enable the patient to lead a normal independent life, have the capability to drive, and have a normal social and vocational life. Other potential benefits for many individuals include the reduction of mood dysfunction, arresting cognitive decline, and reducing medication burden and toxicity.

With careful patient selection after performing a gamut of exhaustive investigations, all of which help in identifying the epileptogenic zone enabling epilepsy surgery, it is possible to achieve a life free of seizures for many patients.

References

1. Kwan P, Brodie MJ. Early identification of refractory epilepsy. *N Engl J Med* 2000; 342:314–319.
2. Hauser W. The natural history of drug resistant epilepsy: epidemiologic considerations. *Epilepsy Res Suppl* 1992; 5:25–28.
3. Sillanpaa M. Remission of seizures and predictors of intractability in long-term follow-up. *Epilepsia* 1993; 34(5):930–936.
4. Berg A, Levy S, Novotny E, Shinnar S. Predictors of intractable epilepsy in childhood: a case-control study. *Epilepsia* 1996; 37:24–30.
5. Camfield P, Camfield C. Antiepileptic drug therapy: When is epilepsy truly intractable? *Epilepsia* 1996; 37(Suppl 7):S60–S65.
6. Schachter S, Shafer P, Murphy W. The personal impact of seizures: correlations with seizure frequency, employment, cost of medical care, and satisfaction with physician care. *J Epilepsy* 1993; 6:224–227.
7. Baker GA, Nashef L, van Hout BA. Current issues in the management of epilepsy: the impact of frequent seizures on cost of illness, quality of life, and mortality. *Epilepsia* 1997; 38(Suppl 1):S1–S8.
8. Ficker D, So E, Shen W, Annegers J, et al. Population-based study of the incidence of sudden unexplained death in epilepsy. *Neurology* 1998; 51:1270–1274.
9. Racoosin JA, Feeney J, Burkhart G, Boehm G. Mortality in antiepileptic drug development programs. *Neurology* 2001; 56:514–519.
10. Engel J Jr. Surgery for seizures. *N Engl J Med* 1996; 334:647–652.
11. Engel J Jr, Wiebe S, French J, Sperling M, et al. Practice parameter: temporal lobe and localized neocortical resections for epilepsy. Report of the Quality Standards Subcommittee of the American Academy of Neurology, in Association with the American Epilepsy Society and the American Association of Neurological Surgeons. *Neurology* 2003; 60:538–547.
12. Serles W, Caramanos Z, Lindinger G, Pataraia E, et al. Combining ictal surface-electroencephalography and seizure semiology improves patient lateralization in temporal lobe epilepsy. *Epilepsia* 2000; 41:1567–1573.
13. Loddenkemper T, Kotagal P. Lateralizing signs during seizures in focal epilepsy. *Epilepsy Behav* 2005; 7:1–17.
14. Cascino GD, Trenerry MR, So EL, Sharbrough FW, et al. Routine EEG and temporal lobe epilepsy: relation to long-term EEG monitoring, quantitative MRI, and operative outcome. *Epilepsia* 1996; 37:651–656.
15. Steinhoff BJ, So NK, Lim S, Luders HO. Ictal scalp EEG in temporal lobe epilepsy with unitemporal versus bitemporal interictal epileptiform discharges. *Neurology* 1995; 45:889–896.
16. Degen R, Ebner A, Lahl R, Bartling S, et al. MRI and EEG findings in surgically treated patients with partial seizures due to neuronal migration disorders, their relations to each other and to surgery outcome. *Acta Neurol Scand* 2003; 108:309–318.
17. Haut S, Legatt A, O'Dell C, Moshe S, et al. Seizure lateralization during EEG monitoring in patients with bilateral foci: the cluster effect. *Epilepsia* 1997; 38:937–940.
18. Todorov A, Lesser R, Uematsu S, Yankov Y, et al. Distribution in time of seizures during presurgical EEG monitoring. *Neurology* 1994; 44:1060–1064.
19. Jackson GD, Berkovic SF, Tress BM, Kalnins RM, et al. Hippocampal sclerosis can be readily detected by magnetic resonance imaging. *Neurology* 1990; 40:1869–1875.
20. Salmenpera TM, Simister RJ, Bartlett P, Symms MR, et al. High-resolution diffusion tensor imaging of the hippocampus in temporal lobe epilepsy. *Epilepsy Res* 2006; 71(2-3):102–106.

21. Diehl B, Symms MR, Boulby PA, Salmenpera T, et al. Postictal diffusion tensor imaging. *Epilepsy Res* 2005; 65:137–146.
22. Jack CR, Sharbrough FW, Twomey CK, Cascino GD, et al. Temporal lobe seizure: lateralization with MR volume measurements of the hippocampal formation. *Radiology* 1990; 175:423–429.
23. Goncalves Pereira PM, Oliveira E, Rosado P. Relative localizing value of amygdalo-hippocampal MR. *Epilepsy Res* 2006; 69:147–164.
24. Willmann O, Wennberg R, May T, Woermann FG, et al. The role of 1H magnetic resonance spectroscopy: meta-analysis in pre-operative evaluation for epilepsy surgery. *Epilepsy Res* 2006; 71(2-3):149–158.
25. Knake S, Triantafyllou C, Wald LL, Wiggins G, et al Grant PE. A prospective study. 3T phased array MRI improves the presurgical evaluation in focal epilepsies: *Neurology* 2005; 65:1026–1031.
26. Henry TR, Babb TL, Engel J Jr, Mazziotta JC, et al. Hippocampal neuronal loss and regional hypometabolism in temporal lobe epilepsy. *Ann Neurol* 1994; 36:925–927.
27. McNally KA, Paige AL, Varghese G, Zhang H, et al. Localizing value of ictal-interictal SPECT analyzed by SPM (ISAS). *Epilepsia* 2005; 46:1450–1464.
28. Sata Y, Matsuda K, Mihara T, Aihara M, et al. Quantitative analysis of benzodiazepine receptor in temporal lobe epilepsy: [125I]iomazenil autoradiographic study of surgically resected specimens. *Epilepsia* 2002; 43:1039–1048.
29. Juhasz C, Chugani DC, Muzik O, Shah A, et al. Alpha-methyl-L-tryptophan PET detects epileptogenic cortex in children with intractable epilepsy. *Neurology* 2003; 60:960–968.
30. Oishi M, Kameyama S, Masuda H, Tohyama J, et al. Single and multiple clusters of magnetoencephalographic dipoles in neocortical epilepsy: significance in characterizing the epileptogenic zone. *Epilepsia* 2006; 47:355–364.
31. Fischer MJ, Scheler G, Stefan H. Utilization of magnetoencephalography results to obtain favourable outcomes in epilepsy surgery. *Brain* 2005; 128(Pt 1):153–157.
32. Knowlton RC, Elgavish R, Howell J, Blount J, et al. Magnetic source imaging versus intracranial electroencephalogram in epilepsy surgery. A prospective study. *Ann Neurol* 2006; 59:835–842.
33. So EL. Integration of EEG, MRI and SPECT in localizing the seizure focus for epilepsy surgery. *Epilepsia* 2000; 41(Suppl 3):S48–S54.
34. O'Brien TJ, So EL, Mullan BP, Hauser MF, et al. Subtraction ictal SPECT co-registered to MRI improves clinical usefulness of SPECT in localizing the surgical seizure focus. *Neurology* 1998; 50:445–454.
35. Chandra PS, Salamon N, Huang J, Wu JY, et al. FDG-PET/MRI coregistration and diffusion-tensor imaging distinguish epileptogenic tubers and cortex in patients with tuberous sclerosis complex: a preliminary report. *Epilepsia* 2006; 47:1543–1549.
36. Knowlton RC. The role of FDG-PET, ictal SPECT, and MEG in the epilepsy surgery evaluation. *Epilepsy Behav* 2006; 8:91–101.
37. Stern JM. Simultaneous electroencephalography and functional magnetic resonance imaging applied to epilepsy. *Epilepsy Behav* 2006; 8(4):683–692.
38. Stern JM, Tripathi M, Akhtari M, Korb A, et al. Musicogenic seizure localization with simultaneous EEG and functional MRI (SEM). *Neurology* 2006; 66(Suppl 2):90.
39. Sands SF, Akhtari M, Tripathi M, Stern JM. Real-time EEG during functional MRI. *Neurology* 2006; 66(Suppl 2):361.
40. Benar CG, Grova C, Kobayashi E, Bagshaw AP, et al. EEG-fMRI of epileptic spikes: concordance with EEG source localization and intracranial EEG. *J Neuroimaging* 2006; 30:1161–1170.

41. Whiting P, Gupta R, Burch J, Mota RE, et al. A systematic review of the effectiveness and cost-effectiveness of neuroimaging assessments used to visualise the seizure focus in people with refractory epilepsy being considered for surgery. *Health Technol Assess* 2006; 10:1–250.

42. Schiller Y, Cascino GD, Sharbrough FW. Chronic intracranial EEG monitoring for localizing the epileptogenic zone: an electroclinical correlation. *Epilepsia* 1998; 39:1302–1308.

43. Hamer HM, Morris HH, Mascha EJ, Karafa MT, et al. Complications of invasive video-EEG monitoring with subdural grid electrodes. *Neurology* 2002; 58:97–103.

44. Velasco TR, Sakamoto AC, Alexandre V Jr, Walz R, et al. Foramen ovale electrodes can identify a focal seizure onset when surface EEG fails in mesial temporal lobe epilepsy. *Epilepsia* 2006; 47:1300–1307.

45. Sperling MR, Guina L. The necessity for sphenoidal electrodes in the presurgical evaluation of temporal lobe epilepsy: pro position. *J Clin Neurophysiol* 2003; 20:299–304.

46. Bautista R, Cobbs M, Spencer D, Spencer S. Prediction of surgical outcome by interictal epileptiform abnormalities during intracranial EEG monitoring in patients with extrahippocampal seizures. *Epilepsia* 1999; 40:880–890.

47. Sanyal SK, Chandra PS, Gupta S, Tripathi M, et al. Memory and intelligence outcome following surgery for intractable temporal lobe epilepsy: relationship to seizure outcome and evaluation using a customized neuropsychological battery. *Epilepsy Behav* 2005; 6:147–155.

48. Mueller WM, Morris GL 3rd. Intraoperative and extraoperative identification of eloquent brain using stimulation mapping. *Neurosurg Clin North Am* 1993; 4:217–222.

49. Medina LS, Bernal B, Dunoyer C, Cervantes L, et al. Seizure disorders: functional MR imaging for diagnostic evaluation and surgical treatment—prospective study. *Radiology* 2005; 236:247–253.

50. Benke T, Koylu B, Visani P, Karner E, et al. Language lateralization in temporal lobe epilepsy: a comparison between fMRI and the Wada Test. *Epilepsia* 2006; 47:1308–1319.

51. Vickrey BG, Hays RD, Engel J Jr, Spritzer K, et al. Outcome assessment for epilepsy surgery: the impact of measuring health-related quality of life. *Ann Neurol* 1995; 37:158–166.

52. McLachlan RS, Rose KJ, Derry PA, Bonnar C, et al. Health-related quality of life and seizure control in temporal lobe epilepsy. *Ann Neurol* 1997; 41:482–489.

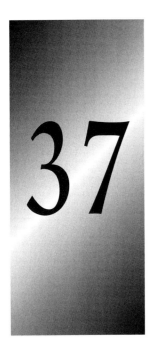

37 Neuropsychologic Outcomes after Epilepsy Surgery in Children

J. Helen Cross

onsideration and referral for epilepsy surgery is now relatively routine in the management of children with drug-resistant epilepsy. Key to any presurgical evaluation as to whether this may be an option is not only whether seizures arise from one area of the brain, but also the risk of functional consequence should that area be removed. The rate of cognitive and behavior problems in this group of children is high, and expectations of parents often include major improvements in these domains. Previously, any indication of likely benefit was derived from data translated from adult studies. and often inappropriately because the populations and underlying pathologies/procedures concerned were represented in different proportions. This aside, increasing data are now available for review from pediatric populations. Such data, however, require interpretation alongside consideration of what may be the natural history of the condition should surgery not be performed.

THE NATURAL HISTORY OF COGNITIVE DEVELOPMENT IN CHILDREN WITH EPILEPSY

The ultimate cognitive outcome of children with epilepsy will depend on a range of variables, including age of onset of epilepsy, extent and side of lesion, pathology, medication, and environmental factors. Seizures, however, are thought to have a major impact on early developmental progress; the term "epileptic encephalopathy" has been adopted for the condition whereby neurodevelopmental impairment is related to ongoing epileptic activity and therefore could be seen to be potentially reversible. The neurodevelopmental outcome of some of the more severe epileptic encephalopathies appears to be improved in those cases where seizure control has been achieved, and parents regularly report an improved state of awareness and learning during periods of relative seizure control. With an aim, therefore, of cessation of seizures from early surgery, it could be presumed that this may lead to improved developmental outcome. Such outcome has been more difficult to demonstrate, not least because of the difficulty in carrying out longitudinal studies, following children from presentation to long term postoperative review, either practicably or with consistent standardized neuropsychologic assessment spanning all age groups, not to mention the lack of data to suggest the natural history of these children with or without surgery by which to compare (1). Traditionally adult data have been transferred to presume what may or may not happen in children, but with differing ranges of procedures and pathologies, and the certain degree of plasticity that is presumed to exist in childhood, this is not entirely appropriate.

Early-onset epilepsy has a major impact on cognition. Cogntive outcome in children with congenital hemiplegia (and consequently damage of the contralateral hemisphere) at 6 years is not significantly different from that of normal controls. However, this is not the case should they present with epilepsy prior to five years of age; IQ is significantly lower at six years of age compared to normal controls or hemiplegic children without epilepsy (2). In addition, the rate of cognitive dysfunction in those coming to surgery is high. Vasconcellos et al. reviewed 100 consecutive children coming to resective surgery for epilepsy and showed that children were more likely to have an IQ <70 if seizure onset was less than two years of age (3). This was unrelated to the underlying pathology. A further series of children with temporal lobe epilepsy presenting for temporal resection showed 57% with intellectual dysfunction and also showed a high degree of correlation with age of onset of epilepsy, seen in 82% of children with seizure onset under the age of one year (4). A key question remains as to whether early cessation of seizures can have positive impact on neurocognitive development. Longitudinal studies of children with long-standing epilepsy suggest a decline with time in intelligence or developmental quotient (IQ), a measure of ability relative to normal peers. A drop, therefore, indicates that a gap is widening between those being assessed and normal peers—it does not imply a loss of skills. A stable IQ score therefore suggests maintenance of the learning trajectory, which may not otherwise have been achieved in children where seizure control is not seen.

NEURODEVELOPMENTAL ASSESSMENT

To be accurate in statements about neurodevelopmental progress, it is important to ensure appropriate standardized assessments. The problem we have is that there is no such standardized test that covers all age groups. The developmental age, as opposed to the chronological age, of the child will be important at the time of assessment. Neurodevelopmental assessment and the monitoring of gains with time in the very young are especially important. Many studies have relied on parental report of educational progress. Although this can give a general judgment of how a child may be progressing, it is very subjective and highly related to the degree of awareness and behavior. Parental expectation may also heavily influence such a judgment. The Vineland adaptive behavior scales are often reported, because they are easily applied (not necessarily by a neuropsychologist), can be used thoughout all ages, and provide scores in several domains. They are also administered by interview and therefore can be administered over a telephone. Subtle changes in certain areas, however, will not be determined, in particular in the area of speech and language. The Wechsler

scales are the most detailed but are lengthy to administer and score. By necessity, funding is often available only to administer such at specific time points, if at all, and in some may be available longitudinally only within the context of research programs. Such scales are also not adapted to children under 3 years; the Bayley scales are often used to this age but are not directly comparable. More specifically, when considering longitudinal review of children, the key questions to be addressed first need to be considered before deciding which tests are most likely and when (over a certain period of time) to answer such questions. Concerns aside as to how any benefit from surgical intervention may be determined, the study of children pre- and postoperatively can lead to insights with regard to models of outcome of intellectual function and brain plasticity, and hence such study is important.

DOES EPILEPSY SURGERY HAVE AN IMPACT?

Infantile Spasms

Infantile spasms as part of West syndrome, associated with hypsarrhythmia on electroencephalogram (EEG) and developmental plateau, remain one of the more severe epileptic encephalopathies, with a high rate of long-term morbidity. The rate of subsequent mental retardation is high, with medically treated studies quoting normal developmental outcome in only 9–28% of infants, highly dependent on etiology. However, there is also some evidence that an early response to treatment leads to better developmental outcome. Surgical intervention with resection of unilateral abnormal tissue, whether detected on flurodeoxyglucose (FDG) positron emission tomography (PET) or magnetic resonance imaging (MRI), led to an apparent improved developmental outcome, as measured by Vineland adaptive behavior scales, up to 2 years postsurgery, with 50% achieving a developmental quotient >50 at this stage (5). Subsequent analysis of a further cohort undergoing surgery has revealed developmental outcome to be higher the shorter the duration of spasms prior to surgery (6). Although there is no comparable longitudinal group with which to compare directly, the results suggest a better neurodevelopmental outcome for those in whom surgery was undertaken compared to those medically treated, and all children with unilateral lesions as an underlying etiology to spasms should undergo early evaluation for surgery.

Hemisyndromes

Children requiring hemisphere disconnection procedures for management of their epilepsy have, on the whole, a pre-existent hemiplegia in association with underlying congenital pathology, whether a malformation of cortical development or ischemic insult. Such children make up around one-third of pediatric epilepsy surgery series. A small number have what may be classed as a progressive pathology—namely, Sturge Weber syndrome (in which the underlying pial angioma may be congenital but hemiplegia and epilepsy are progressive in nature) and Rasmussen syndrome. When children are assessed for hemispherectomy, the determination of cerebral lateralization is paramount for an indication of the likely impact of the procedure on intellectual functions as well as on speech and language. In those with congenital hemiplegia, and consequently presumed abnormality of the contralateral hemisphere, the early onset of epilepsy is likely to have resulted in dominance of the normal hemisphere, left or right, in cognitive and language development. Later-onset pathologies, such as acquired stroke or Rasmussen encephalitis, may show a variable degree of relocalization of function dependent on the age, duration of illness, and hemispheric dominance.

The largest study published to date assessing postoperative neuropsychologic outcome following hemispherectomy reports results on 71 children, split into three groups dependent on etiology: cortical dysplasia, Rasmussen encephalitis, and vascular abnormalities, including stroke (7). Little change was seen as a group between pre- and postoperative scores in any of the three groups, although the cortical dysplasia group had considerably lower IQ preoperatively than the other two groups and consequently a significantly lower IQ postoperatively. However, it was also evident that the group of children undergoing surgery for developmental malformations had a significantly lower age of onset of epilepsy (<12 months) than the other groups, which is likely, as suggested from other studies, to have had a significant impact on outcome. Our own study of 33 patients undergoing hemidisconnection (in the majority, functional hemispherectomy) showed similar findings (8). Most studies report little longitudinal change in IQ following hemidisconnection procedures, although a "significant" change is regarded as at least 15 IQ points (2SD), and this would be a measure of increased rate of progress relative to peers. Some report gains, and a very few report loss. This result implies that any decline or arrest of intellectual function took place prior to surgery, although cessation of seizures may have led to maintained trajectory as opposed to a decline.

It is likely that comparative studies of children who did or did not undergo surgery are required over a much longer duration of follow-up to determine the relative merits of surgery on developmental outcome, although even limited studies available suggest that seizure outcome and age at surgery are likely to influence this.

Lateralization of dominance with regard to speech and language is of primary importance to be aware of the likely effect of hemidisconnection on these faculties.

The assumption is taken that early (congenital) pathology associated with onset of epilepsy under five years results in language development in the contralateral hemisphere. Psychologists have used this premise along with handedness and dichotic fused-word tests to predict likely language outcome. Recent data have suggested, however, that left-to-right shifts in language dominance are more likely to occur in patients who have lesions encroaching on the left hippocampus (9), while the efficacy and speed with which reorganization is achieved may also be dependent on frequency, severity, and spread of seizures. This may be particularly relevant in children with later-onset Rasmussen encephalitis, where timing of the hemidisconnection syndrome may intimately be dependent on the degree to which relocalization of function has taken place. Often in Rasmussen encephalitis of the dominant hemisphere a discussion may be undertaken as to whether waiting will lead to more likely relocalization, or whether relocalization may be enforced by performing the surgery earlier in the natural history. Small studies have shown that recovery of language to a limited, communicative degree may, however, take place with relatively late surgery (10).

Focal Epilepsy

Much data have been acquired in adults with regard to outcome following temporal lobectomy, the most common procedure performed in this population for hippocampal sclerosis. Despite temporal resection making up about one-quarter of procedures in children, the range of pathologies and preoperative cognitive ability remains much wider. It is only relatively recently that data on outcome in children have become available, especially more representative data. When children were originally considered for this procedure, it was on the basis of adult criteria, which included normal cognitive ability. It is now apparent that cognitive ability will not influence likelihood of seizure freedom and therefore should not preclude consideration for surgery.

Early data from children undergoing temporal lobectomy suggested little overall risk to cognitive function. A multicenter study in the United States accumulated data from 43 children who underwent left temporal resection and 39 right and showed no significant reduction in cognitive status for either group (11). Analysis of individual scores showed a small percentage to have either a decline or improvement in verbal or nonverbal functioning. As indicated previously, however, children were selected on the basis of adult criteria, and all children included in the study had a full scale IQ (FSIQ)>69. Gleissner et al. more recently asked the question whether children recovered better than adults from memory deficits as a consequence of temporal lobe surgery, matching children for comparison with adults for pathology, onset of epilepsy, side of surgery, and type of surgery (12). This study showed that only children, rather than adults, undergoing left resections, recovered verbal learning capacity, reaching preoperative levels at 12 months following surgery. Children undergoing right resection showed improvement in visual memory, in contrast to adults, who showed deterioration.

There is relatively little information with regard to neurodevelopmental outcome following resective procedures of other areas of the brain. In general, reports are of heterogeneous groups with small numbers of individual procedures. Studies that have reported temporal versus extratemporal epilepsy have shown gains in attention, processing speed, memory, and bimanual coordination. In general, further impairments are not demonstrated following surgery; moreover, no change in intellectual functioning overall is demonstrated (13). A recent study of preschool children coming to focal resection between the ages of 3 and 7 years (16 temporal, 9 frontal, 18 multilobar, and 7 hemispherectomy) showed, at 12 months following surgery, 82% to be functioning at a similar level to preoperatively (14). Notably, development was delayed in 84% coming to surgery. Two to three years postsurgery, 29 out of 40 (72%) performed at their preoperative levels, whereas a further eight showed significant gains >15 IQ points from preoperatively. This suggests that developmental gains may accumulate over a longer period and do not necessarily become evident in early postoperative months. This has implications for when postoperative outcome is assessed. Duration of epilepsy was the only predictor of long term cognitive change; children with shorter intervals between onset of epilepsy and surgery had greater gains in developmental quotient. However, in this study, seizure outcome did not significantly contribute to the prediction of postoperative cognitive change.

CONCLUSION

The rate of intellectual disability is high in children with symptomatic focal epilepsy coming to surgery. Despite the difficulties in obtaining longitudinal studies in pediatric epilepsy, there is increasing evidence that neurodevelopmental trajectory is at least maintained postoperatively and, in a significant minority, improved. Outcome is most likely to be related to underlying pathology and seizure load—data to date do not support seizure outcome as being influential on ultimate outcome. Careful preoperative evaluation is required, however, whatever the age or etiology, in order that appropriate risks can be determined and realistic expectations outlined. No promise can be made of improvement in cognitive ability, even in the event of seizure freedom, and this requires careful exploration with parents prior to any surgical decision being made.

References

1. Cross JH, Jayakar P, Nordli D, Delalande O, et al. Proposed criteria for referral and evaluation of children with epilepsy for surgery. *Epilepsia* 2006; 47:952–959.
2. Muter V, Taylor S, Vargha-Khadem F. A longitudinal study of early intellectual development in hemiplegic children. *Neuropsychologia* 1997; 35:289–298.
3. Vasconcellos E, Wyllie E, Sullivan S, Stanford L, et al. Mental retardation in pediatric candidates for epilepsy surgery: the role of early seizure onset. *Epilepsia* 2001; 42:268–274.
4. Cormack F, Cross JH, Vargha Khadem F, Baldeweg T. The development of intellectual abilities in temporal lobe epilepsy. *Epilepsia* 2007; 48:201–204.
5. Asarnow RF, LoPresti C, Guthrie D, et al. Developmental outcomes in children receiving resection surgery for medically intractable infantile spasms. *Dev Med Child Neurol* 1997; 39:430–440.
6. Jonas R, Asarnow RF, LoPresti C, Yudovin S, et al. Surgery for symptomatic infant-onset epileptic encephalopathy with and without infantile spasms. *Neurology* 2005; 64:746–750.
7. Pulsifer M, Brandt J, Salorio CF, Vining EP, et al. The cognitive outcome of hemispherectomy in 71 children. *Epilepsia* 2004; 45:243–254.
8. Devlin AM, Cross JH, Harkness W, Chong WK, et al. Clinical outcomes of hemispherectomy for epilepsy in childhood and adolescence. *Brain* 2003; 126:556–566.
9. Liegeois F, Connelly A, Cross JH, Gadian DG, et al. Language dominance in children with early lesions of the left hemisphere. *Brain* 2004; 127:1229–1236.
10. Boatman D, Freeman J, Vining E, et al. Language recovery after left hemispherectomy in children with late onset seizures. *Ann Neurol* 1999; 46:579–586.
11. Westerveld M, Sass K, Chelune GJ, et al. Temporal lobectomy in children: cognitive outcome. *J Neurosurg* 2000; 92:24–30.
12. Gleissner U, Sassen R, Schramm J, Elger CE, et al. Greater functional recovery after temporal lobe epilepsy surgery in children. *Brain* 2005; 128:2822–2829.
13. Lendt M, Gleissner U, Helmstaedter C, Sassen R, et al. Neuropsychological outcome in children after frontal lobe epilepsy surgery. *Epilepsy Behav* 2002; 3(1):51–59.
14. Freitag H, Tuxhorn I. Cognitive function in preschool children after epilepsy surgery: rationale for early intervention. *Epilepsia* 2005; 46:561–567.

38

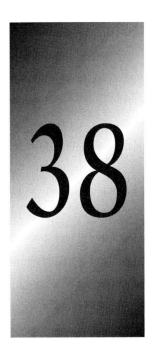

Neuropsychologic Outcomes after Epilepsy Surgery in Adults

Sallie Ann Baxendale

S urgical treatment for epilepsy is a viable treatment option for up to 10% of adults with medically intractable seizures. Initially developed in the 1930s, the surgical option is not new, but the development of the concept of surgically remediable epilepsy syndromes in the early 1990s means that surgery is no longer viewed as a last resort. Today patients do not necessarily have to exhaust the entire canon of antiepileptic drugs before they consider the surgical option. Indeed, some epilepsy experts have suggested that best clinical practice requires the identification of suitable patients as early as possible in the course of their seizure disorder to circumvent the development of many of the social and cognitive problems associated with chronic epilepsy.

Two-thirds of the adults who go through epilepsy surgery undergo an anterior temporal lobectomy or an amygdalohippocampectomy. This bias is reflected throughout the remainder of this chapter. Extratemporal neocortical resections and lesionectomies make up the majority of the other surgical procedures in adults with epilepsy. Limbic resections are typically associated with high success rates: up to 75% of patients being rendered seizure-free postoperatively; with some improvement in seizure frequency typically seen in 90% of cases. The chances of becoming seizure-free following an extratemporal resection are somewhat lower at around 40–50%, dependent upon the underlying pathology, but worthwhile improvements in seizure frequency are still

seen in 80% of patients, making the surgical option a very attractive proposition for a large number of people with otherwise limited treatment alternatives.

However, although epilepsy surgery may offer a viable treatment opportunity for many patients, the procedures are not without risk to neuropsychologic function. This chapter examines the neuropsychologic outcomes associated with epilepsy surgery in adulthood. The remainder of the chapter is divided into three parts. The first part examines the historical background of neuropsychologic assessment in epilepsy surgery and outlines the ways in which neuropsychologic outcomes are measured today. The second part examines the pre-, peri-, and postoperative factors that influence neuropsychologic outcome following resection of the mesial temporal lobe structures. The third part of the chapter examines neuropsychologic outcome following other surgical procedures and offers a summary of the discussion, drawing some conclusions for current clinical practice.

ASSESSING NEUROPSYCHOLOGIC OUTCOME

Historical Background

The assessment of neuropsychologic function following epilepsy surgery has a long history and dramatic origins (1). In October 1953, William Scoville presented the case of

H.M. to a meeting of surgeons. H.M. had undergone the bilateral removal of his mesial temporal structures in a last-ditch, experimental attempt to control his disabling seizures six weeks previously. Scoville reported that the extensive bilateral hippocampal resection had resulted in no marked physiologic or behavior changes

> with the exception of a very grave, recent memory loss, so severe as to prevent [H.M.] from remembering the location of the rooms in which he lives, the names of his close associates or even the way to the toilet.

H.M.'s profound memory deficits never resolved and came to be known as the mesial temporal lobe amnesic syndrome. To this day H.M. stands as a grim testament to the potentially devastating neuropsychologic hazards of epilepsy surgery. In a careful reading of the historical literature it is particularly disturbing to realize that H.M was not the first to undergo a bilateral temporal lobe resection or the first to develop a profoundly dense amnesic syndrome as a result, but the effects of the surgery on previous patients were assessed solely in terms of seizure frequency or change in psychiatric state, with apparently nobody recognizing the profound changes in memory function in the mainly institutionalized patients. This sorry tale serves as a salutary reminder to epilepsy surgery services today to ensure the ongoing holistic assessment of "outcome" to ensure that patients are able to make a truly informed decision regarding the surgical option.

H.M.'s misfortune triggered the involvement of neuropsychologists in epilepsy surgery programs, and they continue to play a vital role today. Whereas recognition of the profound neuropsychologic consequences effectively consigned the bilateral temporal lobectomy to the archives of disasters in medical history, the unilateral removal of the mesial temporal lobe structures continued to offer a viable treatment option for patients with medically intractable seizures. Over the following three decades, the careful examination of the neuropsychologic deficits associated with a right or left temporal lobectomy—research dominated by Brenda Milner and her colleagues at the Montreal Neurological Institute—led to the development of the material specific model of memory function. Whereas amnesic syndromes were rare following a unilateral temporal lobectomy, patients who underwent a left or dominant temporal lobe resection typically showed deficits in the learning and recall of verbal material postoperatively. Although the finding was less consistent, patients who underwent a right or nondominant temporal lobectomy tended to show deficits in the learning and recall of visual material. These deficits were also seen to a lesser degree in preoperative patients, and the identification of these patterns began to be used to localize seizure foci in the preoperative evaluation of potential surgical patients. The wide acceptance of the material specific

model of temporal lobe memory function meant that postoperative neuropsychologic outcome was primarily understood to be a function of the laterality of seizure focus and the extent of the surgical section.

In the 1990s the material specific model of temporal lobe memory function began to be criticized on a number of counts. In 1995, Chelune (4) introduced the concept of hippocampal adequacy versus functional reserve in the determination of postoperative neuropsychologic outcome. He argued that neuropsychologic outcome following the removal of mesial temporal lobe structures depended on both the functional reserve of the contralateral structures left in situ and the adequacy, or functional integrity, of the structures that had been removed.

In addition to the consideration of bilateral function in the assessment of neuropsychologic outcome following surgery, the research literature in the 1990s revealed that the way in which memory was tested appeared to play an important role in the extent of the deficit observed. Many postoperative deficits were task-specific and highly dependent upon the demands of the task employed.

The recognition of surgically remediable epilepsy syndromes in the 1990s meant that many more people with epilepsy became "eligible" to be considered for surgery (3). Prior to the 1990s only a minority of surgical candidates were in full-time employment, and many were exceedingly disabled by very frequent seizures. Indeed the frequency and severity of the seizures were a factor in the surgical decision-making process in many centers. In the face of frequent, life-threatening seizures and no other medical solutions, the possible neuropsychologic outcome of surgery had a lower weighting in the surgical decision-making process for many patients operated on in previous decades. However, as the surgical option has been extended to far greater numbers of people with epilepsy, many of whom are in full-time employment and who may experience only a relatively small number of seizures a year, the consideration of the possible neuropsychologic deficits associated with the surgery has a significant weighting and may frequently tip the balance when it comes to weighing the potential costs against the possible benefits of the surgical option.

Partly in response to this need, and partly in response to the recognition of task-specific demands in the definition of postoperative memory deficits, the 1990s saw a move away from the use of experimental cognitive tasks in the assessment of epilepsy surgery patients toward the application of standardized clinical tests of learning and recall, such as the Wechsler Memory Scales, the Rey Osterrieth Figure Recall task, the California Verbal Learning Task, and the Rey Auditory Verbal Learning task in the United States, and their national equivalents in other parts of the world.

The development and application of reliable change indices (RCIs) for these standardized clinical measures ensured the reliable detection and reporting of postoperative changes in cognitive function (8). With the acceptance of an "industry standard" in the definition of postoperative decline, clinicians have begun to turn their attention to the prediction of neuropsychologic outcome in an attempt to ensure that prospective surgical patients in the new millennium have as much information as possible regarding all aspects of outcome following surgery, enabling them to make as informed a decision as possible regarding this elective treatment.

TEMPORAL LOBE EPILEPSY SURGERY

Neuropsychologic concerns following a standard or selective temporal lobe resection focus primarily on memory function, although general intellect and language functions are also routinely assessed pre- and postoperatively in most centers. Changes in general intellectual function (IQ) are rare postoperatively, although some patients may experience a mild improvement in overall function if they had excessive subclinical electroencephalographic (EEG) activity preoperatively. Postoperative changes in language function are common in patients who have undergone a dominant temporal lobe resection, and they most frequently manifest themselves as word-finding difficulties, which can occasionally be quite pronounced in the acute postoperative period.

Approximately one-third of patients experience a postoperative decline in memory function following a temporal lobe resection. The side of the surgery interacts with a number of other factors to determine the nature and extent of the decline. For the majority of patients, preoperative memory deficits remain, but no further deterioration is evident. Memory function improves in up to 1 in 7 patients postoperatively.

Postoperative neuropsychologic outcome depends upon the interaction of a number of different pre-, peri-, and postoperative factors (7) (see Table 38-1). Some

TABLE 38-1

Influential Factors in Neuropsychologic Outcome Following Temporal Lobe Resection

FACTORS	CHARACTERISTICS ASSOCIATED WITH POSTOPERATIVE DETERIORATION IN VERBAL MEMORY	MEASUREMENTS
PREOPERATIVE FACTORS		
Age at Surgery	Older	Quantifiable: years
Gender	Males	Categorical: male/female
IQ	Lower IQ	Quantifiable: Wechsler Intelligence Scales
Clinical features	Discordance with MTLE syndrome	Qualitative: multidisciplinary assessment
	Absence of unilateral temporal slow waves	Categorical: Interictal EEG data
Age at onset	Older	Quantifiable: years
Underlying pathology	Absence of HS or mild HS	Quantifiable: via MRI hippocampal volumes and T2 relaxometry (and verifiable via histopathological analysis).
	Presence of cortical dysplasia	Categorical: yes/no
Functional integrity of the proposed resected tissue	Good	Inferred; via baseline neuropsychologic tests, IAP scores and functional imaging data
Functional integrity of the contralateral structures	Poor	Inferred; via baseline neuropsychologic tests, IAP scores and functional imaging data
SURGICAL FACTORS		
Laterality	Left or dominant hemisphere resection	Categorical: right/left or dominant/nondominant
Surgical procedure (Equivocal evidence)	? greater extent of lateral resection	Categorical: surgical procedure
	? greater extent of mesial resection	Quantifiable via postoperative MRI measurements
POSTOPERATIVE FACTORS		
	No postoperative improvement in seizure frequency	Categorical: Engel classifications

of these factors can be directly measured and are easily quantified, for example the age of the patient at the time of the surgery. Other factors can be measured only indirectly; for example, the functional integrity of the hippocampus can be inferred via baseline neuropsychologic tests, performance on the intracarotid amobarbital procedure (IAP), and functional magnetic resonance imaging (fMRI) studies.

Preoperative Factors: Patient Characteristics

The demographic, clinical, and neuropsychologic characteristics of patients prior to surgery have a very significant impact on their likely neuropsychologic outcome following temporal lobe epilepsy surgery.

The age of the patient at the time of surgery is an influential factor in determining the nature and extent of postoperative memory function (6). Group studies have consistently shown that older patients are more likely to experience a postoperative decline in memory function. Cortically represented learning and data acquisition skills appear to be particularly sensitive to age-related factors, with surgical patients over the age of 30 most at risk of a decline in verbal learning. Postoperative changes in consolidation and retrieval of information appear to be more resistant to the effects of age at the time of surgery. Nevertheless, chronic temporal lobe epilepsy is associated with progressive memory impairment, and surgery, particularly if unsuccessful, accelerates this decline. The stepwise decline in memory function effected by a dominant temporal lobe resection is therefore of particular concern for older patients in their 50s and 60s who may be considering surgery.

There is some evidence to suggest that gender may play a small part in neuropsychologic outcome following a temporal lobe resection. Males appear to be more susceptible to a postoperative decline in verbal memory function than females. This does not appear to be due to physiologic differences in hippocampal pathology; rather, females tend to be more efficient in using memory-enhancing strategies, such as semantic clustering. These strategies are unaffected by surgery. There is limited evidence in the literature to suggest that patients with higher IQs are less likely to experience a significant postoperative decline in memory function. It is possible that the same mechanism—the ability to use effective memory strategies—underpins this occasional finding.

It is unsurprising that one of the most potent and consistently reported predictors of postoperative decline in memory function is preoperative level of function. The better memory function is prior to surgery, the more likely the patient is to experience a postoperative decline in function. In common parlance, the more you have to lose, the more likely you are to lose it.

Clinical Features

The clinical history, ictal semiology, and underlying pathology also have a significant impact on neuropsychologic outcome. Generally speaking, the more a patient's profile conforms to the "classic" unilateral mesial temporal lobe epilepsy syndrome, the higher the patient's chances of becoming seizure-free postoperatively. A good postoperative outcome in terms of seizure control is associated with a history of a prolonged febrile convulsion, the onset of habitual seizures in childhood, clear-cut unilateral hippocampal sclerosis evident on the MRI scan (with an absence of cortical dysplasia), concordant ictal and interictal EEG data with clearly lateralizing ictal features, and no history of status epilepticus. Although there are some inconsistencies in the literature, a recent meta-analysis found that long-term memory outcome is related to seizure outcome (11). The factors associated with a good postoperative seizure outcome are therefore indirectly related to long-term memory outcome following temporal lobe epilepsy surgery, and many of these factors, such as a later onset of habitual seizures, qualitative and quantitative MRI indices of pathology, and EEG data, have been individually correlated with neuropsychologic outcome in the literature.

The duration of the seizure disorder per se does not appear to have a direct influence on neuropsychologic outcome when the effects of age of seizure onset and age at the time of surgery are controlled for.

Pathology

The type and extent of the pathology underlying the seizure focus in temporal lobe epilepsy patients has a very significant impact on postoperative neuropsychologic function. The presence of hippocampal sclerosis (HS) is a protective prognostic factor against a postoperative decline in memory function (2). Generally speaking, the greater the extent of preoperative hippocampal volume loss evident on MRI, and subsequently verified as HS histopathologically, the less likely the patient will be to experience a postoperative decline in memory function. This is in large part because patients with extensive unilateral HS already tend to have impaired memory function preoperatively. The presence of HS does not appear to be a protective factor in people with intact preoperative memory function, and some patients with very severe HS can be at risk of postoperative memory decline if they have useful function to lose preoperatively.

The other important caveat to note is the presence of bilateral HS. Bilateral HS usually signals decreased functional reserve in the contralateral structures and is associated with poor memory function before and after both right and left temporal resections.

Postoperative deterioration is not confined to memory function in patients without HS. These patients are also at higher risk of significant declines in confrontation naming and verbal conceptual ability following a dominant temporal lobectomy, although verbal memory remains the most substantial area of decline. Unlike their HS counterparts, postoperative neuropsychologic outcome in patients without HS appears to be independent of seizure outcome.

Standardized temporal lobe resections for the removal of tumors within the temporal lobe that also include the excision of the hippocampus are typically associated with postoperative memory deficits, regardless of the tumor type. Whatever the primary pathology, the presence of cortical dysplasia, even in areas far removed from the operative site, is associated with a poorer postoperative outcome in terms of both seizure control and cognitive function.

Surgical Factors

Although it is by no means the be-all and end-all, the laterality of surgery remains an important determinant of postoperative neuropsychologic outcome. While deficits in verbal memory are more commonly seen following a dominant temporal lobe resection, up to one in five right or nondominant temporal lobe resection patients also demonstrate significant postoperative declines on tests of verbal learning and recall. Postoperative declines on analogous tasks involving visual material are also seen in both right and left groups, although they are less reliably detected (12) and are often less salient for the patients, unless their occupation/lifestyle imposes a heavy reliance on visual memory skills.

Within the customary surgical limits, the mesial or lateral extent of a standardized temporal lobe resection does not appear to have a significant impact on postoperative memory function, although patients who undergo a full resection are more likely to be seizure-free postoperatively or require reoperation. Serial postoperative scans suggest that the hippocampal remnant left in situ following surgery undergoes significant volume loss over the first few postoperative months, with a concomitant decline in memory function.

There is much debate in the literature about the relative merits of a standardized en-bloc temporal lobe resection (STLR) verses a selective amygdalohippocampectomy (SAH) in terms of neuropsychologic outcome (5). Whereas early studies suggested significantly lower neuropsychologic deficits following the selective procedure, the results from subsequent trials have put in question whether there are any real differences between the two. Comparisons between the two procedures can be complicated by patient selection, whereby those with more diffuse seizure foci may be more likely to be offered the more extensive resection. Postoperative MRI studies have suggested that there may be more secondary damage to the temporal lobe after SAH than was initially recognized. The collateral damage to cortical tissues adjacent to the surgical approach, evident in postoperative MRI signal changes, has been associated with deficits in both verbal and visual memory following SAH. Fluorodeoxyglucose positron emission tomography (PET) studies have also demonstrated hypometabolism in temporal structures left in situ following SAH. Although some of the inconsistencies in the literature may relate to individual surgical skill, it is also possible that an SAH results in a disconnection of the preserved cortex, giving a similar functional outcome to a standardized resection, as both types of resection interrupt a circuit likely to be essential for normal storage and retrieval of information.

Postoperative Factors

Postoperative neuropsychologic outcome is a dynamic entity. Deficits seen three months after surgery may have resolved nine months later. Longitudinal follow-up studies suggest that postoperative changes stabilize two years after the surgery for the majority of patients. However, the presence of ongoing seizures can result in an ongoing deterioration of function. All postoperative patients have an elevated lifetime risk of the development of a permanent amnesic syndrome if the contralateral hippocampus left in situ following surgery is damaged, either gradually by ongoing seizure activity or abruptly following an episode of status epilepticus. These risks are considerably higher for the 10% of patients who do not experience a significant improvement in seizure frequency postoperatively.

Predicting Postoperative Function

Many of the factors discussed thus far have been studied in univariate designs. However, they all interact to shape the nature and extent of postoperative neuropsychologic deficits in temporal lobe epilepsy patients. Some, such as laterality of the seizure focus and preoperative level of function, are more potent predictors of postoperative function than others. However, these factors can be pooled in multivariate study designs, and logistic regression models can be used to combine quantitative and categorical data to assess the relative contribution of each factor. The models created can then be used to create individual predictions of neuropsychologic outcome based on each candidate's unique preoperative data and characteristics. Multicenter collaboration and a very large sample size would be needed to examine the relative contribution of all of the factors that have been associated with postoperative neuropsychologic outcome in the literature to date. However, a number of centers have published logistic regression equations combining the preoperative data from multidisciplinary investigations (9). These models are being used as a rational basis for the counseling of prospective patients regarding their probable neuropsychologic outcome following surgery.

There is a lively debate within the literature at present as to whether data from the IAP is useful in the prediction of postoperative neuropsychologic outcome. The IAP scores are one of the most direct measures of the functional integrity and reserve of the mesial temporal lobe structures and have been shown to predict postoperative memory and seizure outcome. However, the IAP is an invasive test. The relatively small added value of IAP scores in these models calls into question the role of the IAP in predicting memory outcome when adequate data from noninvasive procedures are available. If IAP data are available, it makes sense to use them; however, it may not be clinically or ethically justified for a patient to undergo an IAP just to provide data to predict memory decline. Data from PET studies, fMRI, and proton chemical shift imaging (CSI) spectroscopy are also being used in the prediction of postoperative outcome with some success in unilateral study designs.

The prediction of neuropsychologic outcome will never be perfect. We often have only indirect, or relatively insensitive, measures of many of the important variables that shape the nature and level of postoperative memory function. In addition, there will always be other factors that we cannot measure or predict. There is also much evidence to suggest that subjective memory complaints bear little relation to objective measures of memory postoperatively. Nevertheless, these approaches are providing invaluable information for patients and their families when they come to assess the potential risks and benefits of this elective surgical procedure.

OTHER SURGICAL PROCEDURES

Extra-temporal surgical resections of lesions or areas of dysplasia can also be conducted solely for the relief of medically intractable epilepsy. The resections tend to be individually tailored, and the neuropsychologic outcome very much depends on side, site, and type of the resection, with language and memory functions a particular concern if the proposed surgery involves or borders on eloquent frontal cortex. fMRI paradigms can be very helpful in alerting surgeons to the potential dangers of the resection, and awake craniotomies with intraoperative assessment of language and memory can be performed to minimize the risks.

A corpus callosotomy (CC) can be an effective procedure for a small minority of patents with very disabling generalized seizures. Seizure outcome does not appear to be related to the extent of the resection once 50–66% of the callosum is divided, but a complete callosotomy carries the risk of disconnection syndrome. The postoperative risk for neuropsychologic deficits following a CC does not appear to be influenced by atypical language representation or other unusual patterns of cognitive organization.

Another standardized procedure for medically intractable epilepsy is the transcallosal surgical resection of hypothalamic harmatoma (HH). As with most other surgical procedures, a complete resection of the lesion gives the best results, but memory difficulties are common in the early postoperative period. These resolve for most patients, and both patient and family reports of the impact of surgery on cognitive and behavioral functions are generally favorable.

A new surgical procedure, multiple subpial transection (MST) to the hippocampus, has recently been proposed as an alternative to the standard en bloc resection or SAH in patients with mesial temporal lobe epilepsy (10). Preliminary reports of the procedure on 21 cases suggest good seizure control and minimal neuropsychologic changes. However, more cases will need to be reported to confirm the efficacy and to explore full neuropsychologic advantages of this new technique.

CONCLUSIONS

Outcome is no longer considered simply in terms of seizure control following epilepsy surgery. The neuropsychologic risks of surgery are now well recognized and very much part of the pre- and postoperative evaluation process. Over the last two decades, we have moved from a narrow focus on seizure laterality to a far broader consideration of how the side of surgery interacts with a range of demographic, clinical, neurophysiologic, and neuropsychologic factors to shape the nature and extent of postoperative cognitive deficits. These factors, originally identified in retrospective studies of large surgical cohorts, are now being used to identify those patients most at risk of a postoperative memory decline and form the rational basis for preoperative counseling at the bedside. Each patient's distinctive preoperative characteristics can be used to create a unique prediction of the patient's likely postoperative outcome, on a number of measures. fMRI paradigms and other innovative techniques are on the threshold of providing even more accurate measures of functional and structural integrity, which, once integrated into these models, will hopefully provide even greater accuracy. Although the neuropsychologic risks of epilepsy surgery remain, our continued efforts in this area will ensure that patients are able to make as informed a decision as possible regarding this elective procedure.

References

1. Baxendale S. Amnesia in temporal lobectomy patients: historical perspective and review. *Seizure* 1998; 7(1):15–24.

2. Bell BD, Davies KG. Anterior temporal lobectomy, hippocampal sclerosis, and memory: recent neuropsychological findings. *Neuropsychol Rev* 1998; 8(1):25–41.

3. Cascino GD. Surgical treatment for epilepsy. *Epilepsy Res* 2004; 60(2-3):179–186.

4. Chelune GJ. Hippocampal adequacy versus functional reserve: predicting memory functions following temporal lobectomy. *Arch Clin Neuropsychol* 1995; 10(5):413–432.

5. Clusmann H, Schramm J, Kral T, Helmstaedter C, et al. Prognostic factors and outcome after different types of resection for temporal lobe epilepsy. *J Neurosurg* 2002; 97(5):1131–1141.

6. Grivas A, Schramm J, Kral T, von Lehe M, et al. Surgical treatment for refractory temporal lobe epilepsy in the elderly: seizure outcome and neuropsychological sequels compared with a younger cohort. *Epilepsia* 2006; 47(8):1364–1372.

7. Hamberger MJ, Drake EB. Cognitive functioning following epilepsy surgery. *Curr Neurol Neurosci Rep* 2006; 6(4):319–326.

8. Hermann BP, Seidenberg M, Schoenfeld J, Peterson J, et al. Empirical techniques for determining the reliability, magnitude, and pattern of neuropsychological change after epilepsy surgery. *Epilepsia* 1996; 37(10):942–950.

9. Lineweaver TT, Morris HH, Naugle RI, Najm IM, et al. Evaluating the contributions of state-of-the-art assessment techniques to predicting memory outcome after unilateral anterior temporal lobectomy. *Epilepsia* 2006; 47(11):1895–1903.

10. Shimizu H, Kawai K, Sunaga S, Sugano H, et al. Hippocampal transection for treatment of left temporal lobe epilepsy with preservation of verbal memory. *J Clin Neurosci* 2006; 13(3):322–328.

11. Tellez-Zenteno JF, Dhar R, Hernandez-Ronquillo L, Wiebe S. Long-term outcomes in epilepsy surgery: antiepileptic drugs, mortality, cognitive and psychosocial aspects. *Brain* 2007; 130(Pt 2):334–345.

12. Vaz SA. Nonverbal memory functioning following right anterior temporal lobectomy: a meta-analytic review. *Seizure* 2004; 13(7):446–452.

39

Psychiatric Outcomes after Epilepsy Surgery in Adults

Kristina Malmgren

There are many issues to take into account when considering the literature on psychiatric outcomes after epilepsy surgery (see Table 39-1). Published series have widely varying study populations. Since postoperative psychiatric morbidity is related to preoperative psychiatric morbidity, selection of patients is an issue. In some centers but not in others, psychiatric disorders, and especially psychosis, have been considered a contraindication to epilepsy surgery (1). The absence of such a selection bias at a tertiary referral center does not preclude the possibility of a referral bias, since physicians may not consider, or hesitate to refer for presurgical investigation, patients with both epilepsy and psychiatric disorders.

GENERAL ISSUES

Most of the literature on adults is concerned with psychiatric morbidity after temporal lobe resections, and there is surprisingly little data concerning patients who have undergone frontal lobe resections or other procedures. Interestingly, the literature on psychiatric disorders after resective neurosurgery for diagnoses other than epilepsy is very sparse, and it is therefore not possible to try to find out whether part of the short-term postoperative psychiatric morbidity is related to the neurosurgical procedure per se.

Some studies are retrospective, based on patient files and without a preoperative psychiatric baseline. Follow-up periods vary widely and are in some studies cross-sectional, grouping together patients with a follow-up of less than a year with patients who have been followed for several years. Ideally, psychiatric follow-up of patients in epilepsy surgery programs should be prospective and longitudinal, with a preoperative assessment and structured follow-up—something that has been discussed and recommended for many years but still is often lacking.

The methodology of the psychiatric evaluation differs between studies. While some investigators use only screening instruments (especially for depression and anxiety), others use structured psychiatric interviews and include information from family members (and sometimes from medical personnel) as a basis for formal psychiatric diagnoses. Although rating scales typically tap self-perceived psychiatric symptoms during a brief period, structured psychiatric interviews may ascertain lifetime as well as current psychiatric diagnoses. Several authors have pointed out the difficulties in applying current diagnostic systems such as the *Diagnostic and Statistical Manual of Mental Disorders* (DSM) or the International Statistical Classification of Diseases and Related Health Problems (ICD) (2–4). These diagnostic systems are especially unsatisfactory in the classification of organic psychosyndromes, which are commonly present in patients with neurologic disorders in general and

---

TABLE 39-1

*Issues to Consider in the Evaluation of
Psychiatric Outcomes Following Epilepsy Surgery
in Adults*

Study population
Selection of epilepsy surgery candidates (referral bias
    versus selection bias)
Surgical procedures (temporal versus frontal lobe or
    other extratemporal resections)
Number of patients

Study design
Retrospective versus prospective studies
Cross-sectional versus longitudinal studies
Follow-up period

Psychiatric evaluation
Screening instruments versus structured psychiatric
    interviews
Weaknesses in current diagnostic systems for psychiatric
    disorders

---

with epilepsy in particular. (In DSM-IV the chapter on organic mental disorders from the earlier DSM versions has been omitted.) This has led to suggestions of new diagnostic entities specific to epilepsy, but other diagnostic systems have been used also (5, 6). The International League Against Epilepsy (ILAE) is therefore developing a classification of neuropsychiatric disorders associated with epilepsy (see Chapter 24).

This chapter will focus on affective disorders, psychotic disorders, and organic psychosyndromes before and after epilepsy surgery in adults. An attempt will be made to differentiate the psychiatric outcomes for patients after temporal lobe resections and after other resection types (often grouped together as extratemporal resections). Finally, the implications of our current knowledge for counseling and postoperative management will be discussed.

AFFECTIVE DISORDERS

Anxiety Disorders

In studies of affective disorders in patients with epilepsy, most of the attention has been focused on depression, despite the fact that anxiety is common and may be equally disabling. In a recent systematic review, Beyenburg et al. point out that it is unclear whether current diagnostic instruments for anxiety are adequate in epilepsy populations, and they also emphasize the diagnostic problems, given that anxiety may also be an ictal or a postictal phenomenon. They conclude that the prevalence of anxiety symptoms is higher in patients with epilepsy than in the general population or in patients with several chronic

medical disorders but that anxiety disorders often go unrecognized and untreated (2) (see also Chapter 27).

Preoperative Anxiety Disorders

Patients with temporal lobe epilepsy. The prevalence of anxiety disorders reported in candidates for epilepsy surgery varies across studies. Also, many surgical series focus on depression and do not mention anxiety disorders. In Taylor's study from 1972 of patients treated with temporal lobe resection, 7 of the 100 patients (7%) were reported in the subgrouping of neuroses to be anxious preoperatively (7). Jensen did not specify anxiety but reported 7/74 patients (9.5%) to have a neurosis before temporal lobe resection (8). In more recent studies anxiety disorders were found by Manchanda et al. in 10% of 231 temporal lobe patients undergoing presurgical assessment (9), by Ring et al. in 18% of 60 patients (10), and by Wrench et al. in 23% of 43 patients (11). In these studies clinical interviews constituted the core of the psychiatric assessment. In the multicenter study by Devinsky et al., 24.7% of 360 patients (322 of whom underwent temporal lobe resections) were found to have an anxiety disorder preoperatively using the Beck Anxiety Inventory, while interviewer-based ratings were somewhat lower (17.5%) (12).

Patients with extratemporal epilepsy. Patients undergoing resective procedures other than temporal lobectomy have been included only in a minority of studies, and in several of these studies patients are lumped into an "extratemporal" group because of small numbers. In the study by Manchanda et al., 16.3% of 43 extratemporal patients were diagnosed with anxiety disorders (9), similar to 18% of 17 patients in the study by Wrench et al. (11). In the study by Devinsky et al., 38/360 patients (10.6%) underwent resections outside the temporal lobe. Results are not reported separately for these patients, but the authors state that there was no relationship prior to surgery between presence or absence of anxiety and the location of the surgery (12).

Prevalence and Course of
Postoperative Anxiety Disorders

Patients with temporal lobe epilepsy. Taylor mentions only "improvement" in the anxious patients at follow-up (7). In more recent studies, a few have longitudinally studied the patients postoperatively and found an early increase in anxiety disorders, which to a great extent had remitted at 3 months. In the study by Ring et al., 42% of the patients had a generalized anxiety disorder 6 weeks after surgery versus 10% after 3 months (10). Wrench found that 42% of the patients had an anxiety disorder at 1 month versus 24% at 3 months postoperatively (11). Devinsky found a drop to 10% in self-reported anxiety (data available for 261 patients constituting 72.5% of the sample) at three months postoperatively. Two years after surgery the self-administered and interviewer-based ratings were similar (9.4% and 10.4% respectively) (12).

Most studies have found no relationship between the laterality of resection and postoperative anxiety disorders (10, 11; for more references see 12) or between obtained seizure control and rates of postoperative anxiety even if the study with the largest sample size found a trend toward diminished anxiety in seizure-free patients (12).

Patients with extratemporal epilepsy. In the study by Wrench et al., 6% of the 17 extratemporal patients had an anxiety disorder at 1 month postoperatively, which was significantly less than for the temporal lobectomy group, versus 17% at 3 months (11). Devinsky et al. do not report psychiatric outcomes separately for these patients but state that there was no relationship between anxiety at the 2-year follow-up and the location of the surgery (12).

Obsessive-Compulsive Disorder

In a recent study, 14.5% of 62 patients with temporal lobe epilepsy were diagnosed with obsessive-compulsive disorder (OCD) compared to 1.2% of healthy controls. Only one of nine patients had an earlier OCD diagnosis, and the authors conclude that OCD may be under-diagnosed in patients with epilepsy (13).

In epilepsy surgery candidates, Taylor reported that 4/100 patients had obsessional features preoperatively (7). In more recent literature, epilepsy surgery has been reported to result in improvement of symptoms; for references see (14). In one study five patients with mesial temporal lobe epilepsy and obsessive traits were identified in an epilepsy surgery series, the size of the sample, however, not being stated. Two of these five patients developed an OCD within two months of the surgical intervention (14).

Depressive Disorders

Depression is the most frequent comorbid psychiatric disorder in epilepsy, with a reported lifetime prevalence between 6% and 30% in population-based studies, increasing to up to 50% in patients in specialized epilepsy centers. The lack of more precise incidence and prevalence data is attributed to differences in methodology and sample populations but also to underreporting of symptoms and underdiagnosis by clinicians; for references see (3). Depression may also be an ictal or a peri-ictal (pre- or postictal) phenomenon, which may again complicate diagnosis. The clinical presentation of interictal depressive disorders can be identical to that in patients who do not have epilepsy, but several authors have pointed out that in a proportion of epilepsy patients there are difficulties in applying current diagnostic systems (3, 5). A general (not epilepsy-specific) relationship between specific anatomic substrates and mood has been suggested along two axes: anterior versus posterior and left versus right.

Several studies suggest that the farther anterior the lesion, the more profound effect it may have on mood. Other studies suggest hemispheric asymmetry for mood, with lesions in the left hemisphere more often being associated with depression. However, there are also studies that have failed to find any relationship between a lesion site along either of the two axes and mood disorders; for discussion and references see (15).

Preoperative Depressive Disorders

Patients with temporal lobe epilepsy. Taylor reports that 17 out of 100 patients (17%) were depressed preoperatively (7). In more recent studies, depressive disorders were found by Manchanda et al. in only 3% of 231 temporal lobectomy candidates (9), by Ring et al. in 21% of 60 patients (10), and by Wrench et al. in 33% of 43 patients preoperatively (11). In the multicenter study by Devinsky et al., 22.1% of 360 patients were found to have a depressive disorder preoperatively using the Beck Depression Inventory, and interviewer-based presurgical ratings for depression were similar (22.3%) (12).

Patients with extratemporal epilepsy. In the study by Manchanda et al., only 4.7% of 43 extratemporal patients were diagnosed with mood disorders (9), in contrast to 54% of the 17 patients in the study by Wrench et al. (11). In the study by Devinsky et al., 38/360 patients (10.6%) underwent resections outside the temporal lobe, and the authors found no relationship prior to surgery between presence or absence of depression and the location of the surgery (12).

Prevalence and Course of Postoperative Depressive Disorders

Patients with temporal lobe epilepsy. Taylor does not report changes in rates of depression specifically (7). In more recent studies the early postoperative increase in anxiety disorders has not been paralleled by a similar early increase in depression. In the study by Ring et al., 24% of the 60 patients were depressed 6 weeks after surgery, versus 38% after 3 months (10). Wrench et al. found 26% of their 43 patients to be depressed 1 month postoperatively, versus 30% at 3 months (11). Devinsky et al. report lower levels of postoperative depression, with a drop in the percentage of self-reported depressive symptoms 3 months after surgery to around 10% (data available for 259 patients, amounting to 72.3% of the sample) and the rate of depression was 11.7% two years postoperatively (12). Although many studies have investigated a possible relationship between the laterality of resection and postoperative depressive disorders, most investigators have not found evidence for such a relationship; for references see (12). Devinsky et al. confirmed earlier findings that the greatest predictive factor for postoperative depression was preoperative depression (6, 12), and also confirmed that depressive symptoms were significantly less frequent in seizure-free patients (8.2%) than in patients with persisting seizures (17.6%); for references see (12).

Patients with extratemporal epilepsy. In the study by Wrench et al., none of the 17 patients was depressed one month after surgery, which was significantly less than for the temporal lobectomy group. Three months postoperatively 17% were depressed (11). In the study by Devinsky et al., results are not reported separately for extratemporal patients, but no relationship between depression at the 24-month follow-up and the location of the surgery was reported.

In a study by Suchy and Chelune, changes in self-reported mood pre- to postsurgery (mean follow-up 7.3 months after surgery), assessed by the Beck Depression Inventory (BDI), was examined in 15 right frontal, 15 left frontal, 15 right temporal, and 15 left temporal lobectomy patients. In this study temporal lobectomy patients were matched to frontal lobectomy patients, and overall, self reported mood improved following surgery, irrespective of seizure control. The authors found no significant effects of laterality or location on the BDI scores, although frontal patients showed more extreme changes in mood in either direction than temporal patients. Also, patients with left frontal surgery appeared to be at a slightly greater risk for being depressed than the other patient groups (15).

Manic Disorders

Hypomanic and manic episodes in patients with epilepsy are rare, and earlier reports have mainly been case studies; for references see (16). In a recent retrospective study, 16 patients were identified with new-onset mania after temporal lobectomy (12 right-sided and 4 left-sided resections) in a series of 415 consecutive patients (3.9%). These patients were compared with a control group of 16 patients who did not experience any mood problems within the first year after temporal lobectomy and a group of 30 patients who experienced depression within the first postoperative year. The manic episodes were usually transient, and all but one case remitted within 1 year from onset (16).

PSYCHOTIC DISORDERS

There is no consensus on the classification of psychotic syndromes associated with epilepsy, and current diagnostic systems are unsatisfactory (4, 17). Psychoses may also be ictal, postictal, or interictal. Epidemiological data are scarce, but the overall evidence suggests that schizophrenia-like psychosis is 6–12 times more likely to occur in patients with epilepsy than in the general population (4). Many studies have reported a relationship between schizophrenia-like psychosis and temporal lobe epilepsy, and evidence points toward an association between mediobasal rather than neocortical temporal lobe abnormalities and psychosis. A preponderance of left-sided pathology has been suggested in patients with schizophrenia-like psychosis, but there are problems with available data, and the laterality issue remains undecided; for references see (1, 4, 17, 18).

Interictal Psychosis and Epilepsy Surgery

One of the main issues in the literature on epilepsy surgery and psychosis has been whether to operate on patients with chronic interictal psychosis. Data from early surgical series were summarized by Trimble, who pointed out that selection criteria varied between centers and that the number of patients with preoperative psychiatric disorders was, for example, far greater in the early Guy's Maudsley series than in the Montreal series (1). Taylor described 16 patients out of 100 as psychotic preoperatively (16%), four of whom had lost their psychosis at follow-up (7). In the Danish series 11/74 patients (15%) were psychotic before temporal lobe resection, and postoperatively one patient was reported to have a normal psychiatric status, five were improved, while five were unchanged (8). It has often been assumed that disturbed behavior will prevent adequate preoperative evaluation, and this, together with the observation that the psychosis usually does not improve or may even be exacerbated after surgery, has led many epilepsy centers to reject these patients from their surgical programs purely on psychiatric grounds (19). Trimble has commented that: "Whether or not this is justified is not clear in the sense that it might still be considered better to be psychotic without seizures than to be psychotic with them" (17). More recently, several case series have been published demonstrating the feasibility of presurgical evaluation and temporal lobe resection in patients with chronic psychosis. Reutens et al. reported on five patients from the Montreal Neurological Institute with the dual diagnosis of chronic psychosis and intractable epilepsy who underwent temporal lobe resection (three left- and two right-sided) uneventfully, and in whom seizure cessation led to several benefits despite persisting psychosis (20). Marchetti et al. reported comparable experiences in six patients (21).

De Novo Psychosis after Epilepsy Surgery

In Taylor's series 7/100 patients developed psychosis postoperatively (7), and the corresponding number in the Danish series was 9/74 patients (12%) (8). Summing figures from different series, Trimble wrote in 1992 that paranoid or schizophrenia-like psychoses were shown to develop in 3.8 to 35.7% of cases, with a mean of 7.6%. No clear predictors of which patients were at risk of developing psychosis were identified, and there was no agreement in the literature on the relationship to seizure control. However, where laterality could be established, it was right-sided in over 60%; for references see (1). In most but not all of the later studies, the proportion of patients developing de novo psychosis is lower: in the study by Leinonen et al. from Kuopio, 3/57 patients (5.3%) developed de novo psychosis after temporal lobe resection, two after right and one after left-sided resections (22); in the study by Malmgren et al. one of 70 patients (1.4%) developed a psychosis after a right-sided resection (6), Koch-Stoecker reports de novo psychosis in 4/100 patients (4%) without mentioning side of resection (23), and Devinsky reports 4/360 (1.1%) patients with de novo psychosis postoperatively, two after right-sided and two after left-sided resections (12).

Not only de novo interictal psychosis but also de novo postictal psychosis after epilepsy surgery has been described. In the report by Manchanda et al., 4/298 patients (1.3%) developed postictal psychosis de novo after right-sided temporal lobectomy (24). In the study by Christodoulou et al., 3/282 (1.1%) patients developed de novo postictal psychosis, two after a left-sided selective amygdalohippocampectomy and the third after a right-sided temporal lobectomy (25).

ORGANIC PSYCHOSYNDROMES

Taylor pointed out in 1987 that "Psychiatrists and psychologists ought to notice that the traits of aggressiveness, rudeness, stickiness, meanness, meticulousness, irritability, and so on which are regarded as personality traits are probably not personality traits but components of an organic psychosyndrome" (18).

The current diagnostic systems are even more unsatisfactory in the classification of organic psychosyndromes than in the classification of other psychiatric disorders, and different diagnostic approaches have been utilized.

Blumer and coworkers have defined an interictal dysphoric disorder that they do not discuss in terms of organic psychosyndrome but that has the following characteristics: "a pleomorphic and intermittent affective–somatoform disorder with at least three of eight symptoms: depressive mood, anergia, irritability, pain, insomnia, euphoric mood, fear and anxiety." In their study of 44 patients with temporal lobe epilepsy, 57% were diagnosed with a dysphoric disorder before surgery. Postoperatively 39% of their 44 temporal lobectomy patients experienced either de novo psychiatric complications or exacerbation of preoperative dysphoric disorder. All psychiatric complications occurred in the first two postoperative months. They also found that preoperatively four of six frontal lobectomy patients (67%) had a

dysphoric disorder, in contrast to five out of six patients (83%) postoperatively (5).

Although they do not discuss these symptoms in terms of organic psychopathology, Ring et al. state that during the course of their study they noted emotional lability in many patients postoperatively (10). Pursuing this issue in a subsequent study, the same group found a relation between the amount of tissue removed and the emotional lability. They interpret these findings as showing "that affective lability is basically a subtle organic brain syndrome that is directly associated with the cerebral insult of surgery," and they discuss the problems of using the present classificatory systems such as ICD-10 or DSM-IV in epilepsy patients (26).

Malmgren et al. (6) used the diagnostic system of Lindqvist and Malmgren for diagnosis of organic psychosyndromes in their longitudinal study of psychiatric morbidity after epilepsy surgery. This system is based on a psycho-physiologic theory and assumes that the brain reacts in a limited number of ways to different injuries (27). The organic disorders within the Lindqvist-Malmgren system relevant to the study were the astheno-emotional disorder and the emotional-motivational blunting disorder (26). The symptoms of the astheno-emotional disorder include concentration difficulties, especially problems with upholding sustained attention; mental fatigability; memory difficulties, which are mainly secondary to the attentional deficit; irritability; and emotional lability. The astheno-emotional disorder has also been studied in patients with normal pressure hydrocephalus and in patients with subarachnoidal hemorrhage, and the diagnostic entity is related to several earlier constructs, especially Bonhoeffer's "emotional-hyperaesthetic weakness state"; for references see (6).

The emotional-motivational blunting disorder is better known under its traditional label "frontal lobe syndrome" and mainly includes emotional and motivational flattening with a varying degree of effect on behavior, ranging from inactivity and lack of spontaneity to shallow euphoria and thoughtless and unrestrained behavior. However, an etiologically neutral name is to be preferred, since the same syndrome occurs, for example, with mesolimbic and hypothalamic lesions. At the time of presurgical evaluation 27/70 patients (39%) had either of these diagnoses (6).

Within the first postoperative year almost half of the patients (49%) showed symptoms of the astheno-emotional disorder, with no difference between the 53 temporal lobectomy patients and the 16 patients who had had extratemporal (mainly frontal) resections. The presence of an astheno-emotional disorder prior to surgery was shown to be an independent risk factor for developing postoperative anxiety or depression disorder. The emotional-motivational blunting disorder was significantly more common in the extratemporal patients

(38%), and when present, it existed preoperatively in all but worsened postoperatively in a few.

In a study of personality disorders (according to DSM-III-R, axis I and axis II) as predictors of severe postsurgical psychiatric complications (defined as necessitating admission to a psychiatric hospital) in patients undergoing temporal lobectomy for epilepsy, Koch-Stoecker found that 61/100 patients had some kind of personality disorder preoperatively (23). Such a diagnosis was shown to be an independent risk factor for a severe postoperative psychiatric illness within two years after surgery. The author argues that the personality disorders represent individually formed expressions of mental vulnerability and that this vulnerability reduces the patients' capacity to handle life stressors, regardless of whether these stressors are physical or mental, thus increasing the risk of psychiatric disorders.

SUMMARY AND CONCLUSIONS

Psychiatric disorders are common in patients with pharmaco-resistant epilepsy who are considered for epilepsy surgery. In early series, as many as 87–92% of the patients had a psychiatric disorder preoperatively (7, 8), whereas in more recent series the corresponding percentages range between 47% (9) and 57% (5, 11). The discrepancies may be related both to differences in selection criteria and to varying methodology for ascertainment of psychiatric diagnoses. Anxiety and depression are the most common psychiatric diagnoses and are probably also often underdiagnosed (2, 3). Several longitudinal studies have demonstrated an increase in anxiety, but not in depression, during the first months after epilepsy surgery, after which the anxiety diminishes (10, 11). No clear relationship has been disclosed between postoperative anxiety and depressive disorders and side or site of resection (11, 12). Several studies have shown that the greatest predictive factor for postoperative anxiety and depressive disorders is a history of anxiety or depression (6, 12). One large study has shown depressive symptoms to be less frequent, two years after epilepsy surgery, in seizure-free patients than in patients with persisting seizures, and there was a similar but weaker trend toward diminished anxiety in seizure-free patients (12). Surprisingly few studies have included patients who have undergone resections other than temporal lobe resections. Apart from one study in which there was no early postoperative rise in anxiety in extratemporal patients (11), differences in the rates of postoperative anxiety and depression have not been disclosed between patients after temporal or extratemporal resections (6, 11, 12). Many factors, psychologic as well as physiologic, may interact in the causation of mood disorders in epilepsy patients (2, 3). It is also likely that multiple mechanisms contribute to the postoperative improvement

in depression and anxiety disorders. These may include elimination of seizures by removal of dysfunctional limbic areas, improved sense of self-control, reduced fear of seizures, and reduced antiepileptic drug burden.

Schizophrenia-like psychosis is 6–12 times more likely to occur in patients with epilepsy than in the general population. It is associated with temporal lobe epilepsy and more specifically with mediobasal abnormalities (4). A preponderance of left-sided pathology has been suggested in patients with schizophrenia-like psychosis, but the laterality issue remains undecided (1, 4, 17, 18). There is a longstanding discussion whether to operate on patients with epilepsy and chronic interictal psychosis or not. It has often been assumed that disturbed behavior will prevent evaluation, and this, together with the observation that the psychosis does not improve after surgery, has led many centers not to offer these patients presurgical evaluation (1, 19). However, several recent case series have demonstrated that presurgical evaluation and temporal lobe resection can be feasible and rewarding in patients with chronic interictal psychosis (20, 21).

De novo psychosis after temporal lobectomy seems to be less common in more recent series (6, 12, 22, 23) than in earlier ones (7, 8), and no clear predictors have been identified. Recently de novo postictal psychosis has been reported in two case series (24, 25).

Organic psychosyndromes are common in epilepsy patients (7), but current diagnostic systems (ICD and DSM) are even more unsatisfactory in the classification of organic psychosyndromes than in the classification of other psychiatric disorders. Therefore, different diagnostic approaches have been used, which leads to difficulties in comparing studies. Several studies have shown that organic psychosyndromes (whether interictal dysphoric disorder, emotional lability, astheno-emotional disorder, or personality disorder) may exacerbate in the early postoperative period (5, 6, 10, 23). Presence of an organic psychosyndrome may also be an independent risk factor for developing postoperative anxiety or depression disorder (6) or more in general for a severe postoperative psychiatric illness requiring hospitalization (23).

Despite the high frequency of psychiatric disorders in epilepsy patients, prospective studies of pharmacological therapy are lacking. However, available data suggest that patients respond well to standard psychopharmacological drugs, but still many patients go untreated (2, 3). The reasons for this include underdiagnosis, but also concern on the part of psychiatrists that antidepressant treatment, for example, may worsen the seizure situation in patients with severe epilepsy. Pharmacological treatment also needs to be supplemented with other measures, such as support from the comprehensive epilepsy team or psychotherapy. The presurgical psychiatric evaluation is indispensible, not only to diagnose and treat ongoing psychiatric disorders but also to identify predictors of postoperative psychiatric morbidity, which is of importance also in the counseling process and in the planning of postoperative support and rehabilitation efforts. Still, a preoperative psychiatric assessment is not included in all epilepsy surgery programs, and one of the reasons for this may be communication problems as suggested by Kanner: "If the goal of any presurgical evaluation is to recognize all postsurgical risks, why are psychiatric evaluations not performed in all patients? Clearly, the arguments against the inclusion of a psychiatric evaluation as part of any presurgical evaluation are another example of poor communication between neurologists and psychiatrists" (28). Improved collaboration between epileptologists and psychiatrists is a necessity, both in order to improve diagnosis and clinical management of patients pre-and postoperatively and in order to further our knowledge. Hopefully a consensus on classification of psychiatric disorders in patients with epilepsy will also facilitate further prospective and longitudinal studies of pre-and postoperative psychiatric morbidity in epilepsy surgery candidates. Studies also need to include patients subjected to other resection types than temporal lobe resections, where data is clearly lacking.

References

1. Trimble MR. Behaviour changes following temporal lobectomy, with special reference to psychosis. *J Neurol Neurosurg Psychiatry* 1992; 55:89–91.
2. Beyenburg S, Mitchell AJ, Schmidt D, Elger CE, et al. Anxiety in patients with epilepsy: systematic review and suggestions for clinical management. *Epilepsy Behav* 2005; 7:161–171.
3. Kanner AM. Depression in epilepsy: prevalence, clinical semiology, pathogenic mechanisms, and treatment. *Biol Psychiatry* 2003; 54:388–398.
4. Sachdev P. Schizophrenia-like psychosis and epilepsy: the status of the association. *Am J Psychiatry* 1998; 155(3):325–336.
5. Blumer D, Wakhlu S, Davies K, Hermann B. Psychiatric outcome of temporal lobectomy for epilepsy: incidence and treatment of psychiatric complications. *Epilepsia* 1998; 39(5):478–486.
6. Malmgren K, Starmark J-E, Sjöberg-Larsson C, Ekstedt G, et al. Non-organic and organic psychiatric disorders in patients after epilepsy surgery. *Epilepsy Behav* 2002; 3:67–75.
7. Taylor DC. Mental state and temporal lobe epilepsy: a correlative account of 100 patients treated surgically. *Epilepsia* 1972; 13:727–765.
8. Jensen I, Larsen JK. Mental aspects of temporal lobe epilepsy: follow-up of 74 patients after resection of a temporal lobe. *J Neurol Neurosurg Psychiatry* 1979; 42:256–265.
9. Manchanda R, Schaefer B, McLachlan RS, Blume WT, et al. Psychiatric disorders in candidates for surgery for epilepsy. *J Neurol Neurosurg Psychiatry* 1996; 61:82–89.
10. Ring HA, Moriarty J, Trimble MR. A prospective study of the early postsurgical psychiatric associations of epilepsy surgery. *J Neurol Neurosurg Psychiatry* 1998; 64(5):601–604.
11. Wrench J, Wilson SJ, Bladin PF. Mood disturbance before and after seizure surgery: a comparison of temporal and extratemporal resections. *Epilepsia* 2004; 45(5):534–543.
12. Devinsky O, Barr WB, Vickrey BG, Berg AT, et al. Changes in depression and anxiety after resective surgery for epilepsy. *Neurology* 2005; 65(11):1744–1749.
13. Monaco F, Cavanna A, Magli E, Barbagli D, et al. Obsessionality, obsessive-compulsive disorder, and temporal lobe epilepsy. *Epilepsy Behav* 2005; 7:491–496.
14. Kulaksizoglu IB, Bebek N, Baykan B, Imer M, et al. Obsessive-compulsive disorders after epilepsy surgery. *Epilepsy Behav* 2004; 5(1):113–118.
15. Suchy Y, Chelune G. Postsurgical changes in self-reported mood and composite IQ in a matched sample of patients with frontal and temporal lobe epilepsy. *J Clin Exp Neuropsychol* 2001; 23(4):413–423.
16. Carran MA, Kohler CG, O'Connor MJ, Bilker WB, et al. Mania following temporal lobectomy. *Neurology* 2003; 61(6):770–774.
17. Trimble MR. The psychoses of epilepsy. New York: Raven Press; 1991.
18. Taylor DC. Psychiatric and social issues in measuring the input and outcome of epilepsy surgery. In: Engel J Jr, ed. *Surgical Treatment of the Epilepsies*. New York: Raven Press; 1987:485–503.
19. Glosser G, Zwil AS, Glosser DS, O'Connor MJ, et al. Psychiatric aspects of temporal lobe epilepsy before and after anterior temporal lobectomy. *J Neurol Neurosurg Psychiatry* 2000; 68(1):53–58.
20. Reutens DC, Savard G, Andermann F, Dubeau F, et al. Results of surgical treatment in temporal lobe epilepsy with chronic psychosis. *Brain* 1997; 120:1929–1936.
21. Marchetti RL, Fiore LA, Valente KD, Gronich G, et al. Surgical treatment of temporal lobe epilepsy with interictal psychosis: results of six cases. *Epilepsy Behav* 2003; 4:146–152.
22. Leinonen E, Tuunainen A, Lepola U. Postoperative psychoses in epileptic patients after temporal lobectomy. *Acta Neurol Scand* 1994; 90(6):394–399.
23. Koch-Stoecker S. Personality disorders as predictors of severe postsurgical psychiatric complications in epilepsy patients undergoing temporal lobe resections. *Epilepsy Behav* 2002; 3(6):526–531.
24. Manchanda R, Miller H, McLachlan RS. Post-ictal psychosis after right temporal lobectomy. *J Neurol Neurosurg Psychiatry* 1993; 56(3):277–279.
25. Christodoulou C, Koutroumanidis M, Hennessy MJ, Elwes RD, et al. Postictal psychosis after temporal lobectomy. *Neurology* 2002; 59(9):1432–1435.
26. Anhoury S, Brown RJ, Krishnamoorthy ES, Trimble MR. Psychiatric outcome after temporal lobectomy: a predictive study. *Epilepsia* 2000; 41(12):1608–1615.
27. Lindqvist G, Malmgren H. Organic mental disorders as hypothetical pathogenetic processes. *Acta Psychiatr Scand* 1993; 88(Suppl 373):5–17.
28. Kanner AM. When did neurologists and psychiatrists stop talking to each other? *Epilepsy Behav* 2003; 4:597–601.

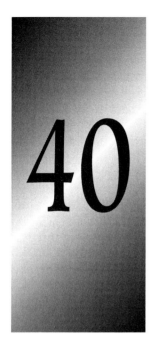

40 Indicators of Psychosocial Adjustment and Outcome after Epilepsy Surgery

Sarah J. Wilson
Joanne Wrench
Michael M. Saling
Peter F. Bladin

CORE CHALLENGES OF EPILEPSY SURGERY

The neurosurgical treatment of intractable complex partial seizures now constitutes a routine procedure in many tertiary epilepsy centers, including the Comprehensive Epilepsy Program of the Austin Hospital in Melbourne, Australia. Our program has considered the longitudinal assessment of surgical outcome to be paramount in informing ongoing clinical practice within the program. In assessing outcome, our research team has focused on two core challenges of epilepsy surgery, namely, (1) to effect a successful medical outcome entailing significant seizure reduction or complete seizure relief with minimum neurologic and neuropsychologic comorbidity, and (2) to translate this outcome into the daily life of the patient to allow the benefits of medical success to be realized. This may entail the removal of restrictions previously imposed by chronic epilepsy and the experience of psychosocial change for the patient and the family.

From more than 15 years of longitudinal follow-up, our team has found that the second core challenge of epilepsy surgery may be just as difficult to achieve as the first, and carries the added risk of potentially undermining the entire surgical enterprise (1). From the perspective of the clinical team, meeting the second core challenge requires a detailed understanding of the neurobiological

basis of the patient's thinking and behavior and how this relates to the psychosocial functioning of the individual and the family. It includes an intricate understanding of both patient and family perceptions of epilepsy and its associated effects, as well as expectations accompanying surgery. From the perspective of the patient, the second challenge often involves learning how to "become well" and engage in new thinking and health behaviors that may be underpinned by intrapsychic change. The degree to which patients achieve this significant task is tied to their perceptions of surgical success (1).

The implication is that predicting a patient's postoperative psychosocial functioning is clinically important for ensuring a successful outcome. This prediction is not just dependent on one variable, namely, postoperative seizure frequency, as initially proposed by a health-related quality-of-life approach. Rather, predicting a patient's ability to meet the second core challenge of epilepsy surgery is complex and requires an appreciation of the interactions between neurobiological and psychosocial factors (1). Given this complexity, our program has adopted a multidisciplinary approach that is embodied in the Seizure Surgery Follow-up and Rehabilitation Program. This program includes a range of pre- and postoperative assessments of patients and their families, which also serve as a means of conducting extensive follow-up research (1). The present chapter provides a review of key concepts and findings that have arisen from this research that are relevant to meeting the second core challenge of epilepsy surgery.

THE NECESSITY OF ANTICIPATING PSYCHOSOCIAL ADJUSTMENT

Prior to surgery, the notion of equilibrium provides a useful heuristic for the balance that exists between the demands of intractable complex partial seizures and the level of psychosocial functioning of the patient and the family. This equilibrium can be considered to reflect patient and family perceptions of what is achievable in the context of intractable seizures, providing a significant source of variability across patients. Surgical intervention disrupts this equilibrium, typically bringing a new set of expectations for daily life that are based on the assumption of seizure freedom. Thus, after surgery the patient undergoes a process of adjustment to reestablish psychosocial equilibrium, ideally in the absence of seizures and their associated psychosocial effects (2). As noted, this adjustment process can be complex and include intrapsychic change, which varies in the sequence and rate of change across individuals (3). Ultimately this heterogeneity reflects the way in which individual patients come to terms with the reality of their outcome, in light of their expectations and the psychosocial effects previously attributed to seizures. These attributions are influenced by health and illness perceptions that are embedded within the psychosocial and cultural context of the patient. In meeting the second core challenge of epilepsy surgery, a key issue for the clinical team is to understand this individual process of adjustment and to predict those patients at risk of adjustment difficulties so that appropriate support services can be provided.

Describing the Nature of Psychosocial Adjustment

At a fundamental level, the process of psychosocial adjustment is based on a very simple but elegant assumption that the majority of patients are chronically ill before surgery and are rendered almost immediately well after surgery. Despite increasing medical sophistication to effect this dramatic transition, less emphasis has been placed on understanding the nature of the adjustment process that accompanies it and how that impacts on outcome. Thus, our early work focused on describing essential features of the adjustment process as reported by patients and their families, using a qualitative, phenomenological approach (4). This approach identified a constellation of regularly occurring psychosocial features that appeared to arise as a manifestation of the dramatic transition from chronically ill to well. These features can be classified into four key domains and constitute a syndrome, namely, the "burden of normality" (see Figure 40-1).

The phenomenology of the burden of normality principally reflects the patient's experience of the second core challenge of epilepsy surgery. At a broad level, it encapsulates issues such as "Who am I now that I don't have my epilepsy?" and "Can I meet the challenges of living a seizure-free life?" (2) The degree to which individuals report adjustment issues partly reflects the extent to which epilepsy has formed part of their identity and the perceived level of psychosocial disablement it has caused (5). A recent comparative study with cardiac surgery patients clearly illustrated the importance of such precursory features, with the occurrence of symptoms of the burden of normality significantly associated with illness chronicity prior to surgery (6).

Stated another way, chronic illness can have powerful effects on self-identity, producing a heightened focus on health and increased psychologic distress, whereas good health tends to be taken for granted (7). In this sense, the task of becoming well involves downplaying the role of health in self-identity, potentially bringing other facets of identity into focus. Where epilepsy has played a dominant role or been detrimental to the development of these other facets, grief for the loss of epilepsy may be salient, including a perceived "lack of excuses" (for example, in work or social identity). Also salient, there may be increased self-expectations and a sense of pressure to prove "normality" in these other domains, often in an attempt to make up for "lost years." These psychologic phenomena can lead to observable changes in the patient's behavior, either reported as "overdoing it" or "shirking" new responsibilities. They may also challenge family relationships, for example, downplaying the role of health in identity may downplay the role of the caregiver, with ensuing conflict over the patient's level of independence. Alternatively, increased expectations on the part of family and friends may be placed on the individual, with an associated decrease in postoperative support. Not surprisingly, all of these changes may be accompanied by the report of significant alterations in mood, notably postoperative anxiety and depression.

Considered in this way, identity reconceptualization is a central feature of the burden of normality, epitomizing the transition from chronically ill to well. In other words, it appears fundamental to the experience of many of its symptoms. Two case vignettes have been included to provide examples of the way in which patients might present with symptoms of the burden of normality following surgery. These vignettes highlight that patients can report symptoms in varying degrees and at different time points post surgery, depending on the patient's personal history, coping abilities, and psychosocial context. This likely accounts for the finding that patients

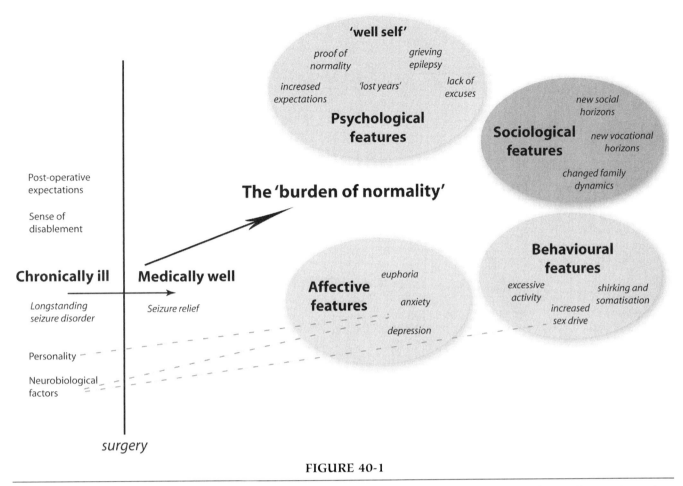

FIGURE 40-1

Essential features of the process of adjustment constitute a psychosocial syndrome, the burden of normality, as the patient adapts to being well.

rendered seizure-free do not automatically perceive their surgery as successful or show immediate improvements in psychosocial functioning (1).

Capturing Individual Adjustment Trajectories

Given the variability in adjustment issues reported by patients post surgery, measures that average across individuals at a given time point seem somewhat misplaced. Thus, more recently our work has focused on depicting postoperative adjustment at an individual level with a view to identifying markers of psychosocial outcome. To this end, we used a mathematical modeling technique that is capable of identifying individual patient profiles or adjustment trajectories, as well as subgroups of patients who share similar outcome trajectories. In particular, the technique models specific features of postoperative adjustment at given time points to allow trajectories associated with good or poor outcomes to be identified in individuals and subgroups of patients (3).

This method indicated that a range of trajectories can ultimately lead to good psychosocial adjustment and outcome, including the experience of early adjustment difficulties. In contrast, the presence of early postoperative mood disturbance, specifically anxiety, served as a marker of poor longer term outcomes, whereas resolution of early anxiety was associated with good outcomes (see Figure 40-2).

The influence of mood on postoperative outcome has been broadly demonstrated in the research literature, and in our own work has been shown to influence the patient's perception of surgical success independent of seizure outcome (1). Postoperative mood disturbance is also associated with increased hospital readmission and utilization of outpatient services after surgery when compared to seizure recurrence (1). Taken together, these findings suggest that to detect patients at risk of poor longer term psychosocial outcomes, attention should also be focused on identifying factors associated with early postoperative mood disturbance.

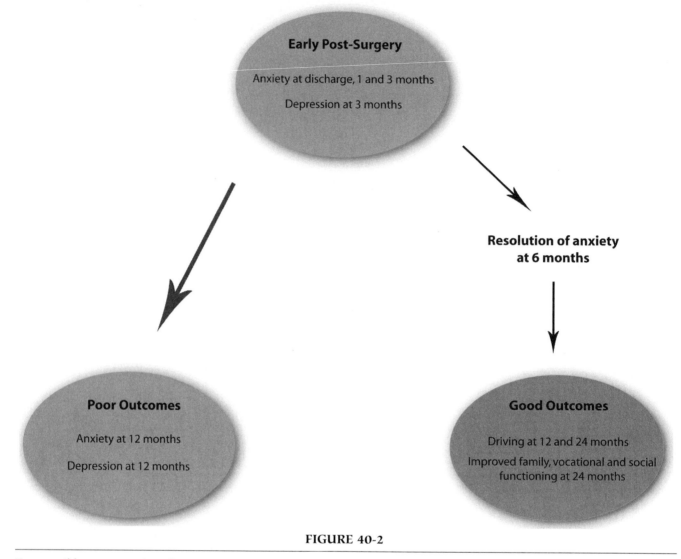

FIGURE 40-2

Two possible postoperative adjustment trajectories with early unresolved mood disturbance serving as a marker of poor longer term psychosocial outcome.

MARKERS OF POSTOPERATIVE MOOD DISTURBANCE

To identify markers of postoperative mood disturbance, both neurobiological and psychosocial factors need to be taken into account. For example, we have recently found that early mood disturbance after epilepsy surgery is more commonly reported by patients undergoing temporal resections as opposed to resections outside the temporal lobe (so-called extratemporal resections) (8). Specifically, temporal patients were more likely to report early postoperative anxiety, particularly at the 1-month review. This was also the case for postoperative depression, despite extratemporal patients reporting an increased lifetime prevalence of depression before surgery (see Table 40-1). Many of the temporal lobe cases constituted de novo depression, compared to a complete absence of de novo depression in the extratemporal group. As such, in addition to psychosocial adjustment issues encapsulated by the burden of normality, neurobiological factors appear to place temporal lobe patients at increased risk of mood disturbance early after surgery. This likely reflects the removal, deafferentation, or disruption of limbic system structures within the brain after temporal resection.

Neurobiological Markers: The Role of Limbic System Structures

In delineating the role of limbic system structures in postoperative mood disturbance, we recently measured the volume of the hippocampus in each temporal lobe

TABLE 40-1

Percentage of Temporal and Extratemporal Patients with Depression and Anxiety Before and Early After Epilepsy Surgery

	TEMPORAL ($n = 43$)	EXTRATEMPORAL ($n = 17$)
Preoperative history of anxiety (%)	23	18
Postoperative anxiety (%)		
Discharge	12	6
One month	42	6*
Three months	24	17
Preoperative history of depression (%)	33	53
Postoperative depression (%)		
Discharge	17	12
One month	26	0*
Three months	30	17

*$p < 0.05$.

from the preoperative magnetic resonance imaging (MRI) scans of patients undergoing mesial temporal, nonmesial temporal, and extratemporal resections, and neurologically matched controls (9). This showed a negative association between the size of the hippocampus contralateral to the side of surgery and the occurrence of early postoperative mood disturbance, specifically depression in patients undergoing mesial temporal lobe resections (see Figure 40-3). In these patients the effect was most pronounced for those experiencing seizure recurrence, but was also evident for those developing de novo depression independent of seizure recurrence. In other words, a smaller contralateral hippocampus preoperatively provides a potential marker of vulnerability to early postoperative mood disturbance in mesial temporal patients, highlighting the importance of neurobiological markers of postoperative adjustment.

The significance of preoperative neurobiological markers has also been demonstrated for changes in sexual functioning following surgery. Improved sexual functioning is included in the phenomenology of the burden of normality, as patients commonly attribute it to improved confidence to establish new sexual relationships without the "awkwardness" of their medical symptoms (10). We have also found that amygdala volume serves as a preoperative structural marker of this change in temporal resection patients (11). Specifically, patients reporting improved sexuality following temporal lobe resection had a significantly larger preoperative amygdala contralateral to the site of their surgery than patients reporting a sexual decrease, no change, or controls. The implication of these findings is that neurobiological and psychosocial factors may interact to shape the patient's psychosocial outcome trajectory, pointing to the potential utility of neurobiological markers for informing preoperative counseling

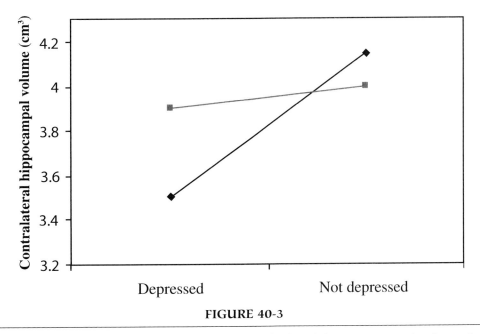

FIGURE 40-3

Preoperative contralateral hippocampal volume serves as a marker of vulnerability to postoperative depression following mesial temporal resection (diamond group, mesial temporal resection; square group, nonmesial temporal resection).

CASE VIGNETTE 2

Making Up for Lost Time

Case 2 is a 36-year-old female who underwent left anterior temporal lobectomy for intractable complex partial seizures. She had a history of a febrile illness, followed by the onset of complex partial seizures in infancy. She experienced a period of seizure freedom in childhood. Preoperative MRI showed left hippocampal sclerosis. Her psychiatric history included a 2-week inpatient stay for depression following status epilepticus in her late 20s. She also suffered from long-standing, intermittent dysthymic symptoms and chronic feelings of low self-esteem, which she ascribed to the restrictions imposed on her life by epilepsy. She had a monozygotic twin who, she felt, exemplified the reality of what she had been denied because of epilepsy.

Six weeks post surgery, case 2 was noted to be anxious and depressed. She was suffering from headaches almost daily and complaining bitterly about her memory. She stated that her family did not understand the stress of epilepsy or the operation, and that she was finding the recovery phase difficult. She reported an inability to cease work around the farm on which she lived with her partner. She engaged in relatively intense physical activity for 12 to 16 hours per day accompanied by poor sleep, fatigue, and lowered mood. Her "inability" to cease work was ascribed to a desire to make up for all the time she had lost because of her epilepsy, including periods of hospitalization. This belief was further fueled by her partner, who felt that surgery was unnecessary and unlikely to be successful.

Four months post surgery, case 2 experienced two generalized tonic-clonic seizures in the context of excessive outdoor work in conditions of extreme heat. These seizures confirmed the partner's belief of the futility of surgery and led to a catastrophic reaction by case 2. She became severely depressed and contemplated suicide, believing her surgery to have failed. Ongoing treatment using a combination of antidepressants and cognitive behavior therapy showed resolution of her symptoms by 24 months post surgery, at which time she had been seizure-free for 20 months.

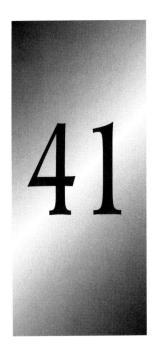

The Myth of Silent Cortex and the Morbidity of Epileptogenic Tissue: Implications for Temporal Lobectomy

Orrin Devinsky
Charles Kyriakos Vorkas

We review three commonly held myths regarding temporal lobe epilepsy (TLE): (1) that TLE is a static disorder with minimal morbidity and mortality, (2) that epileptogenic tissue impairs only the functions of the seizure focus, and (3) that the temporal lobe contains areas of nonfunctional, "silent" cortex.

Chronic TLE can cause progressive structural and cognitive or behavioral complications. Aside from the seizure focus, primary epileptogenic cortex may have a deleterious influence on distant brain areas, impairing the functions of these areas that lie outside the focus. Removing this "nociferous" cortex and reducing the antiepileptic drug (AED) burden can improve cognitive or behavioral and metabolic function in areas remote from the resection. Anterior temporal lobectomy (ATL) often removes functional tissue that may or may not be epileptogenic. Because normal brain does not contain functionless, "silent" areas, ATL can have negative as well as positive cognitive or behavioral consequences. To improve the outcomes of focal cortical resections for seizure control, we need to better define functional and nociferous cortex and more clearly understand their boundaries and interactions.

ATL is the most common epilepsy surgery. We can partially predict the memory and naming deficits

after ATL (1, 2) and advise patients that mood and anxiety problems will often improve (3), but the risk factors for other postoperative cognitive or behavioral disorders remain poorly defined. When we counsel potential ATL patients and make decisions about the extent of resection, the definition and delineation of functional and dysfunctional areas become critical. For example, a standard ATL often involves resection of functional areas (e.g., temporal pole neocortex) separate from the seizure focus. Better understanding of functional neuroanatomy can help improve neurosurgical patients' risk–benefit profiles.

A series of critical questions must be considered in resective operations: (1) Are any functions performed by tissue in the epileptogenic focus? (2) If yes, what are the functions, where are these functional areas located, and how well will other areas compensate for the loss of that tissue? (3) How are the boundaries of the epileptogenic focus defined, and how wide a margin around the focus, (4) if any, should be resected for complete seizure control? Does the epileptogenic focus impair the function of adjacent or distant areas? (5) Are there epileptogenic areas outside the primary focus in which resection may improve cognitive or behavioral function?

Of these five questions, we usually consider only the first three, as we have yet to develop the tools needed to assess the latter two. For the first two questions, in

ATL patients, language and memory functions are the focus of attention. Emotion, visual recognition and learning, topographic memory and orientation, music, sexual, and other functions are rarely considered. Similarly, studies on emotional function are often limited to assessments of mood and anxiety, whereas social function is rarely addressed (4). In many cases, patients may not report emotional and social issues, which are more apparent to family members, friends, coworkers, and teachers (5). The third question is outside the scope of this chapter. Our current methods are crude for defining the minimal tissue resection required for full seizure control or a resection that balances the benefits of reduced seizure burden with functional deficits. The last two questions address the murky topic of nociferous cortex. Are there areas outside the seizure focus that become more functional when the epileptogenic cortex is resected or disconnected? If so, how do we define the extent of this phenomenon after surgery? Can we predict it before surgery?

The concept of nociferous cortex was introduced by Penfield and Jasper (6), who described an aggressive child whose behavior improved dramatically after hemispherectomy: "Among patients who have large areas of abnormality in one hemisphere, abnormal behavior may appear, together with advancing mental retardation. The behavioral abnormality is often a more important complaint than the seizures themselves. Radical complete excision may correct the abnormal behavior, stop the seizures, and allow improvement in the patient's mental state." There is evidence that more restricted epileptogenic foci can also be nociferous. For example, right-sided ATL improved verbal memory (7), as well as metabolic functions remote from the operative site. Further, preoperative depression and anxiety often resolve after ATL (8, 9).

TEMPORAL LOBE EPILEPSY: MORBIDITY AND MORTALITY OF A PROGRESSIVE DISORDER

Chronic epilepsy can produce progressive structural and functional impairment. Hippocampal atrophy is associated with epilepsy duration. Recurrent status epilepticus or tonic-clonic seizures are associated with progressive atrophy in the ipsilateral (most prominent) and contralateral hippocampus, and the ipsilateral thalamus (10). Cerebral, cerebellar, and white matter atrophy correlates with intellectual disability, duration of epilepsy, and status epilepticus (11). Hippocampal neuronal density and dendritic spine density remote from the seizure focus are also reduced (10).

Metabolic imaging studies reveal evolving changes in TLE. There is a progressive uncoupling of metabolism and blood flow. Metabolic abnormalities, often extending beyond the seizure focus, increase with epilepsy duration. Temporal and extratemporal metabolic abnormalities may improve after ATL (10).

The duration and severity of epilepsy are associated with increased frequency and magnitude of cognitive and psychiatric disorders. Cross-sectional neuropsychologic studies correlate epilepsy duration with mental deterioration. Cognitive dysfunction is more severe in patients with a greater seizure burden. In patients with refractory epilepsy, depression occurs in approximately 50%, with suicidal ideation in nearly 20% (12), and psychosis is 6- to 12-fold more frequent, correlating with the duration and severity of epilepsy. Recurrent bouts of postictal psychosis may progress to chronic interictal psychosis (10).

The morbidity and mortality of epilepsy are mainly due to seizures, which can cause injuries such as dislocated shoulders, broken teeth, and burns, or death from drowning or vehicle accidents (13). Other causes of mortality are sudden, unexplained death in epilepsy patients (SUDEP), suicide, and status epilepticus (13). The rate of SUDEP (per 1000 patient-years) in patients with refractory epilepsy ranges from 4.5 in patients who undergo vagus nerve stimulator (VNS) implantation to 13.7 in patients with recurrent seizures after epilepsy surgery (14). Over a decade, SUDEP can occur in more than 5% of patients with severe refractory epilepsy. Suicide rates are increased as much as 25-fold in patients with TLE (13).

THE MYTH OF SILENT CORTEX

The myth that the normal brain contains functionless "silent" areas arose from the leading holistic theory of brain function, which posited a near-equipotentiality of cortical regions outside the sensorimotor regions. Data from resection, disconnection, and electrical stimulation was misinterpreted to fit that model. The concept of silent cortex—truly nonfunctional areas that, when removed, could be fully compensated for by other areas—was consistent with the tenets of gestalt, holistic psychology and neurology, in which the majority of brain was considered to support general intellectual functions. This view was concordant with the prevailing notion of a general intelligence factor underlying the IQ. Brain areas were often considered expendable. Frontal lobotomy emerged from the holistic view of redundant cortex and supported the concept of silent cortex. The remarkable absence of intellectual changes after large frontal and other cortical resections was more apparent than real, illustrated by the tragedy of prefrontal lobectomies. The greatest error was reliance on the existing tests to assess function. Standardized evaluations available in the 1940s and 1950s were relatively insensitive. Also, in some patients, cerebral tissue was likely nonfunctional or dysfunctional from structural or epileptogenic abnormalities. Findings from these patients could not be transferred to those without these abnormalities (e.g., psychiatric patients). Further, an apparent lack or disturbance of function could have had additional causes: (1) resection of nociferous cortex or reduction of AEDs after ATL can balance negative outcomes, (2) minor deficits are obscured by poor test sensitivity or test-retest effects of cognitive testing, and (3) neural plasticity can allow for other cortical areas in the functional network to partially compensate for a deficit.

Lack of recognized changes after major disconnective surgery and lack of responses to electrical stimulation supported the concepts of redundant and silent cortex. Initially, callosotomies were considered to have no behavioral complications. The two cases of severe alien hand syndrome after thirty callosotomies were mistakenly attributed to psychologic factors (15). Early studies found that, except for sensorimotor areas, electrical stimulation in patients evoked no subjective or objective effects. Stimulation of the anterior frontal cortex produced "neither a seizure nor a conscious experience" (16). The concept of silence was introduced by the observation that "a strange silence follows stimulation anterior to the somatic motor zone" (17). The absence of stimulus-induced symptoms and observed deficits after resections of association cortex fostered the false view that many brain areas go unused and that certain cortical or subcortical regions and white matter tracts have little functional value. These myths reflected existing bias as well as the insensitivity of clinical and neuroscientific tools, not brain function.

The myth of silent cortex is not merely a historical curiosity; it contributes to ongoing misconceptions. Modern epileptologists often refer to language and sensorimotor areas as "eloquent," relegating, by implication, other areas to a lower functional or "noneloquent" status, which in turn implies a "license to resect." Extensive resections that include these "noneloquent" areas may control seizures, and the benefits may far outweigh potential small negative consequences. Yet, functional considerations are often minimized with the removal of areas such as the temporal poles and right frontal lobe, which contribute to social and emotional cognition. These critical psychosocial factors are poorly assessed by standard testing (4, 10).

The concept of silent, functionless cortex is denied by the evolutionary costs of increased cortical size, as well as by functional imaging studies. Large, complex, and energy-consuming brains evolved in circumstances in which needed resources were rare and variably distributed. Natural selection factors intensively limited cortical volume and aggressively selected against nonessential tissue, making large-brained mammals rare (18).

TEMPORAL LOBE STRUCTURAL-FUNCTIONAL RELATIONS: IMPLICATIONS FOR ATL

White Matter

The role of white matter in normal and pathological states is often underappreciated. White matter forms the infrastructure for synthesis and synchronization of neural systems. As mammalian and primate neocortex evolved, white matter increased at an exponential rate of 1.32 times the volume of neocortical gray matter (18). Research on temporal lobe function and epilepsy focuses on neurons, although white matter is also critical. White matter lesions may influence epileptogenicity by affecting the hypersynchrony underlying the epilepsy network, and may also impair function in areas adjacent to and remote from the seizure focus. Recent studies show that chronic TLE is associated with abnormalities in ipsilateral and contralateral temporal and extratemporal white matter. Further, impaired informational processing speed and efficiency correlate with decreased white matter volume in TLE patients. The effects of ATL white matter resection on cognitive and behavioral functions are poorly defined. After ATL, we cannot easily differentiate the effects of gray matter from the effects of white matter lesions in the subcortical region and temporal stem. In primates, selective anterior temporal stem lesions impair certain anterograde memory functions (e.g., delayed match-to-samples), but most are spared (10).

Cognitive and behavioral disorders may result from disconnection syndromes and secondary neuronal loss from white matter lesions that can cause disconnection and trans-synaptic degeneration. Similarly, when the neuron's nucleus dies, axonal loss follows. Secondary neuronal loss occurs in regions that are strongly connected with resected cortex or severed tracts. Temporal lobe lesions cause transneuronal degeneration. Temporal lobectomy or infarction can cause atrophy of the ipsilateral fornix, mammillary body, hypothalamus, mammillothalamic tract, and the anterior thalamic nucleus. In TLE patients, magnetic resonance imaging (MRI) shows transneuronal degeneration effects in the fornix and mammillary bodies and contralateral cerebellum (10). The naming and verbal memory deficits occurring after left-sided ATL may partly result from disconnection and trans-synaptic degeneration. Reduced plasticity may render older subjects more susceptible to the direct and secondary effects of brain surgery. Older age and later onset of epilepsy in ATL patients is associated with accelerated postsurgical memory decline (19).

Medial Temporal Lobe

The Amygdala. Amygdala lesions are associated with impairments in emotional perception, memory, and expression (primarily of negative valence, such as fear and anger). Damage to the amygdala and its forward projections interferes with accurate emotional and psychophysical reactions to social cues, and hampers the use of these reactions to modulate behavior (4). Inputs to this system occur in the temporal regions, where sensory information travels forward and upward into frontal regions for higher level analysis, response planning, and response execution. Social cognition depends primarily on the frontal lobes, although the amygdala and other temporal regions play an important role as well. Thus, ATL may directly or indirectly affect higher-order social behavior, either by lesioning neocortical and limbic temporal connections with frontal regions or by removing the influence of epileptiform activity on frontal regions (4).

ATL impairs the acquisition of conditioned fear, and left-sided ATL impairs memory for emotionally arousing verbal material. Increased sexual drive after ATL correlates with the size of the contralateral (preserved) amygdala. Smell is diminished in the nostril ipsilateral to the ATL. Recognition of scary music is impaired after ATL on either side. Preserved recognition of happy and sad music in ATL subjects suggests that the amygdala, not the auditory association cortex, contains the critical lesion for the deficit in recognizing scary music (10). Prosody perception is impaired with bilateral amygdala lesions, although other cortical regions are also involved in this function (4).

Pathological activation of the amygdala in TLE may contribute to anxiety, irritability, mood disorders, and paranoia. After ATL, depression and anxiety often improve, although new psychiatric problems may develop (3, 9). Removing the dysfunctional amygdala may improve hyposexuality. Conversely, resecting the normal amygdala may impair normal emotion and cause behavioral problems, including emotional flattening or lability, depression, anxiety, mania, or selective loss of emotional responsiveness (10).

The Hippocampus.   ATL in the dominant hemisphere impairs verbal memory to some extent in nearly 40% of patients (2). Predictors of postoperative verbal memory decline are (1) dominant hemisphere resections, (2) MRI findings other than unilateral mesial temporal sclerosis (MTS), (3) relatively preserved preoperative immediate or delayed verbal memory function, and (4) intact memory on the intracarotid amobarbital test in the hemisphere with the seizure focus. Dominant-hemisphere surgery has the strongest association ($p < 0.0001$), and the preoperative verbal memory, the weakest ($p < 0.05$) (2). Verbal memory deficits are predicted on MR spectroscopy by high right-sided and low left-sided preoperative values or low values in the left temporal lobe before right-sided ATL (20).

The intracarotid amobarbital test and preoperative neuropsychologic data help predict amnesia, but the interpretation of test results varies between centers, and individual patient outcomes are hard to predict. Some patients fail this test but have no memory decline postoperatively. Others who fail the test and undergo an operation sparing the hippocampus and parahippocampal gyrus can still have clinically significant memory loss. Even when the intracarotid amobarbital test results are abnormal on both sides, ATL may be performed without detriment to memory. However, considerable individual heterogeneity exists for memory outcome, even in patients with hippocampal sclerosis. Patients with normal hippocampi or mild hippocampal sclerosis are at greatest risk for broad verbal memory deficits and naming impairments after left-sided ATL, but many with moderate to severe hippocampal sclerosis can also have verbal memory loss, mainly for retrieval (10).

After nondominant ATL (usually on the right side), verbal memory may improve, but visual and spatially encoded memories may be impaired. Right-sided ATL mildly impairs the perception of complex patterns but more severely affects retention of the perceived material. Recent work suggests that the right anterior temporal cortex is specialized for perception of facial emotion and plays a role in emotional modulation. Another model suggests that the hemispheres are specialized for the valence of emotion perceived, with negative emotions associated with the right hemisphere and positive ones with the left (4). The right hemisphere is also associated with self-identity.

Learning novel faces and recognizing negative facial emotions are reduced after right-sided ATL. Right-sided ATL also impairs recognition of famous faces, and left-sided ATL impairs naming of famous faces (10). Somatoform disorders may emerge after right ATL (4). Patients who had right ATL were less able to recognize negative facial emotions, although those with early-onset TLE and right MTS also have difficulties matching face to emotion name, especially fear (21). It is unclear whether ATL affects facial emotion perception or recognition to a greater extent than does the underlying epilepsy (4).

Lateral and Basal Temporal Cortex

Primary Auditory and Auditory Association Cortex.   Patients with left auditory cortex lesions are impaired on tasks involving temporal information perception, but unimpaired on tasks involving perception of spectral information, whereas patients with right hemisphere auditory cortex lesions have the opposite impairments. Lesion and functional imaging studies in humans suggest a specialization of function linked to right auditory cortical areas for processing of pitch and pitch direction, and that the left auditory cortex is more extensively activated in response to rapid frequency transitions of speechlike stimuli or tones. The nondominant temporal cortex has a major role in the perception of emotional prosody (4).

Right-sided ATL causes greater impairment in tone discrimination and recall of rhythmic patterns than left-sided ATL. Right temporal lobe lesions, but not right-sided ATL, may impair the comprehension of emotional prosody. Voice discrimination is impaired by right temporal lobe lesions, and voice recognition by right parietal lobe lesions. The ability to distinguish two famous voices (declarative knowledge) may be impaired by left temporal lobe lesions, but recognition of personally familiar voices is usually preserved. Although the recognition of familiar voices seems to depend on intact right inferior and lateral parietal cortex, the discrimination of individual voices may be impaired with lesions of either temporal lobe. The effects of ATL on voice discrimination have not been systematically studied (10).

Multimodal Auditory Association Cortex. Wernicke's aphasia and receptive amusia, even in partial forms, are rare after ATL. Receptive language comprehension and associative verbal fluency may improve after dominant ATL, possibly owing to removal of nociferous anterior temporal lobe cortex, which improves Wernicke's area function. Comprehension may be mildly impaired after left-sided ATL, especially when speech is presented rapidly. Multiple subpial transections through Wernicke's area can cause paraphasias and mild deficits in comprehension (10).

Basal Temporal Language Area. Electrical stimulation of the left basal temporal language area produces language dysfunction. In approximately one-third of patients, stimulation of the fusiform gyrus (60% of affected electrodes), the inferotemporal gyrus (30%), and the parahippocampal gyrus (10%) interfered with language function (22). The functions most severely affected were usually receptive language, spontaneous speech, and passage reading. The dominant basal temporal area may link visual association cortex with comprehension and reading areas superiorly and naming areas anteriorly, serving visual associative, naming, and receptive language functions.

A quantitative and controlled analysis showed significantly greater impairment in confrontation naming after basal temporal language area resections (23). Other language functions were not affected. This area may be included in ATLs performed at many epilepsy centers, even if mapping identifies language functions. Resection of this area, as with the temporal pole, may contribute to naming deficits after dominant ATL (10).

Visual Association Cortex. The posterolateral temporal lobe neocortex has the higher-order visual association cortex. The fusiform and lingual gyri contain the visual pattern template area, including the region that recognizes facial images and stores facial memories. The right temporal lobe is dominant for visuospatial processing, and transient prosopagnosia can rarely complicate right posterior temporal lobectomy. Right-sided ATL, resecting both medial memory and basal visual areas, can impair the learning of novel faces and recognition of famous faces.

The specialized color area (V8/V4) analyzes the wavelength of light and computes color constancy. Unilateral fusiform and adjacent anterior basal occipital lesions can produce achromatopsia, which typically affects the contralateral hemifield or upper quadrant, although patients are often unaware of the deficit. Bedside testing can easily identify achromatopsia, although the frequency of partial achromatopsia after ATL is unknown.

The temporal lobe supports two forms of topographic orientation: using environmental features as landmarks and learning new geographic routes. The fusiform, lingual, and parahippocampal gyri learn and store environmental features (landmarks) that aid spatial navigation. These regions are activated during functional MRI studies when a subject perceives buildings but not objects or faces. Bilateral or right-sided lesions in these areas can cause landmark agnosia, in which patients lose their way because they cannot identify specific environmental features despite preserved spatial knowledge. In contrast, patients with anterograde amnesia can navigate familiar environments, but cannot learn new environments after damage to the right parahippocampal gyrus, which impairs route learning. After right-sided ATL, topographic and episodic memory for navigation, scene recognition, and map drawing are mildly impaired (24).

Temporal Pole. Temporal pole lesions in monkeys disrupt social behavior, reducing affiliative behavior and leading to social isolation. In humans, the limbic temporal pole (BA 38) has naming, sensory, and emotional functions. In functional studies, it is activated while recalling proper names, detecting a familiar stimulus, analyzing auditory stimuli, and learning new visual patterns (25). In a positron emission tomographic (PET) study of ATL patients, naming people did not activate the frontotemporal network needed to retrieve proper nouns. The nondominant temporal pole is activated by processing abstract words, perceiving sad faces, and experiencing anger. The temporal poles, as well as the orbitofrontal gyri, are activated during recall of emotionally traumatic events (10).

The temporal pole may be involved pathologically in some cases of TLE and is resected in standard ATL. Some patients with cryptogenic TLE show increased T2 signal in temporal pole white matter, with a loss of gray–white matter demarcation, suggesting atrophy. Some deficits after ATL may partly result from resection of the pole: impaired recall of individuals' names, names of other living things, words acquired in late childhood and adulthood, and infrequently used words. Linking faces with names may be especially impaired. Lesions of the left temporal pole or the middle and inferior temporal gyri (BA 21, 22) can impair recall of specific names. In general, the more anterior a dominant temporal lobe lesion, the greater the impairment for retrieval of unique names of places, persons, and objects. In contrast, lesions of the posterior and inferior temporal lobes (BA 20, 21) impair retrieval for common, nonunique nouns, but not for unique entities. Temporal pole resection, together with amygdala resection, may contribute to positive and negative behavioral effects of ATL (4, 10).

CONCLUSION

In counseling patients about the effects of ATL, both positive and negative effects should be considered. The most important benefit is seizure control, although many patients can also experience improvements in mood, anxiety, and cognition. These benefits may be enhanced by reductions in antiepileptic and psychotropic medications. The potential benefits of resecting nociferous cortex remain difficult to define, apart from the potential improvement in memory function after nondominant

ATL. Seizure freedom after surgery correlates with improved quality of life and mental health (3).

The negative effects should also be reviewed. In addition to risks related to the neurosurgical procedure, the potential effects of resecting functional tissue should be discussed and individualized based on a synthesis of data from the presurgical evaluation. Defining the location of the seizure focus and functional tissue is critical in counseling patients. The effects of surgery on language and memory functions are most often discussed and those for which we have the most data to base our discussions. However, a major goal for the future is to better define the cognitive and behavioral consequences of ATL, as well as its social and emotional risks and benefits. Studies on social and emotional changes after epilepsy surgery are few, often based on retrospective data, and focused on depression and anxiety. The spectrum of social and emotional function and dysfunction is much wider, however, and we need to develop better tools to study the psychosocial outcomes of epilepsy surgery. Functional and nociferous cortex can both affect cognitive, social, and emotional functions. Epilepsy surgery would likely be safer and more beneficial if we could better define the boundaries between functional, dysfunctional but nonharmful, and dysfunctional and nociferous areas in our patients.

*R*eferences

1. Davies KG, Bell BD, Bush AJ, Hermann BP, et al. Naming decline after left anterior temporal lobectomy correlates with pathological status of resected hippocampus. *Epilepsia* 1998; 39:407–419.
2. Stroup E, Langfitt J, Berg M, McDermott M, et al. Predicting verbal memory decline following anterior temporal lobectomy (ATL). *Neurology* 2003; 60:1266–1273.
3. Spencer SS, Berg AT, Vickrey BG, et al. Initial outcomes in the Multicenter Study of Epilepsy Surgery. *Neurology* 2003; 61:1680–1685.
4. Kirsch HE. Social cognition and epilepsy surgery. *Epilepsy Behav* 2006; 8:71–80.
5. Wilson SJ, Bladin PF, Saling MM, Pattison PE. Characterizing psychosocial outcome trajectories following seizure surgery. *Epilepsy Behav* 2005; 6:570–580.
6. Penfield W, Jasper HH. Epilepsy and the functional anatomy of the human brain. Boston: Little, Brown, 1954:841–842.
7. Mayanagi Y, Watanabe E, Nagahori Y, Nankai M. Psychiatric and neuropsychological problems in epilepsy surgery: analysis of 100 cases that underwent surgery. *Epilepsia* 2001; 42(Suppl 6):19–23.
8. Glosser G, Zwil AS, Glosser DS, et al. Psychiatric aspects of temporal lobe epilepsy before and after anterior temporal lobectomy. *J Neurol Neurosurg Psychiatry* 2000; 68:53–58.
9. Devinsky O, Barr WB, Vickrey BG, et al. Changes in depression and anxiety after resective surgery for epilepsy. *Neurology* 2005; 65:1744–1749.
10. Devinsky O. The myth of silent cortex and the morbidity of epileptogenic tissue: implications for temporal lobectomy. *Epilepsy Behav* 2005; 7:383–389.
11. Hermann B, Seidenberg M, Bell B, et al. The neurodevelopmental impact of childhood-onset temporal lobe epilepsy on brain structure and function. *Epilepsia* 2002; 43:1062–1071.
12. Boylan LS, Flint LA, Labovitz DL, et al. Depression but not seizure frequency predicts quality of life in treatment-resistant epilepsy. *Neurology* 2004; 62:258–261.
13. Fukuchi T, Kanemoto K, Kato M, et al. Death in epilepsy with special attention to suicide cases. *Epilepsy Res* 2002; 51:233–236.
14. Sperling MR, Feldman H, Kinman J, Liporace JD, et al. Seizure control and mortality in epilepsy. *Ann Neurol* 1999; 46:45–50.
15. Akelaitis AJ. Studies on the corpus callosum: IV. Diagnostic dyspraxia in epileptics following partial and complete section of the corpus callosum. *Am J Psychiatry* 1945; 101:594–599.
16. Penfield W, Jasper H. Highest level seizures. *Res Publ Assoc Res Nerv Mental Dis* 1946; 26:252–271.
17. Penfield W. Some observations on the cerebral cortex of man. *Proc R Soc London B Biol Sci* 1947; 134:329–347.
18. Allman J. Evolving brains. New York: Freeman, 1999.
19. Helmstaedter C, Kurthen M, Lux S, et al. Chronic epilepsy and cognition: a longitudinal study in temporal lobe epilepsy. *Ann Neurol* 2003; 54:425–432.
20. Incisa della Rocchetta A, Gadian DG, Connelly A, et al. Amnesia after unilateral temporal lobectomy: a case report. *Epilepsia* 1994; 35:757–763.
21. Meletti S, Benuzzi F, Rubboli G, et al. Impaired facial emotion recognition in early-onset right mesial temporal lobe epilepsy. *Neurology* 2003; 60:426–431.
22. Shaffler L, Luders HO, Morris HH 3rd, et al. Anatomic distribution of cortical language sites in the basal temporal language area in patients with left temporal lobe epilepsy. *Epilepsia* 1994; 35:525–528.
23. Krauss GL, Fisher R, Plate C, et al. Cognitive effects of resecting basal temporal language areas. *Epilepsia* 1996; 37:476–483.
24. Spiers HJ, Burgess N, Maguire EA, et al. Unilateral temporal lobectomy patients show lateralized topographical and episodic memory deficits in a virtual town. *Brain* 2001; 124:2476–2489.
25. Devinsky O, D'Esposito M. Neurology of cognitive and behavioral disorders. Contemporary neurology series. Vol. 68. New York: Oxford University Press, 2004.

VIII

PEDIATRIC AND
ADOLESCENT EPILEPSY

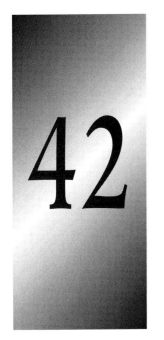

Behavioral Aspects of Pediatric Epilepsy Syndromes

Frank M.C. Besag

The International League Against Epilepsy (ILAE) classification lists over 40 epilepsy syndromes and related conditions (1), many of which start in childhood. In the past, the emphasis has been on the outcome in terms of seizure control. However, there has been an increasing recognition of the value of the syndrome classification with regard to other factors, particularly cognition and behavior. In some of these cases daytime epileptiform discharges or the nighttime abnormalities of continuous spike waves during slow-wave sleep (CSWS)/electrical status epilepticus of slow-wave sleep (ESES) may play a role. The behavioral aspects of the epilepsies of childhood and adolescence have been reviewed in recent publications (2–4). The purpose of this chapter is to provide a summary of the current knowledge of some of the pediatric epilepsy syndromes and to indicate how this might influence clinical practice in the treatment of epilepsy in children and teenagers.

WEST SYNDROME

West syndrome consists of infantile spasms, learning disability, and hypsarrhythmia on the electroencephalogram (EEG). The spasms are flexor, mixed flexor-extensor, or

extensor. Onset is generally under 12 months, typically between 3 and 7 months. West syndrome may be either cryptogenic or symptomatic, that is, secondary to an identifiable cause. Mental retardation is common in the syndrome, having been reported in more than 70% of cases (5).

The cognitive and behavioral changes at the onset of the syndrome are often striking. Guzzetta (6) has recently discussed the suggestion that visual problems may underlie some of the behavioral changes seen early in the syndrome. Previous publications have reported a high rate of behavioral problems, including autism, particularly in children who also have tuberous sclerosis (7). Thirteen percent of those with cryptogenic spasms were said to have remained autistic. In another report, for those who also had tuberous sclerosis, 58% remained autistic (8). The fascinating report by Bolton et al. (9) has indicated that autism is more likely to occur in children with tuberous sclerosis who had infantile spasms and, in addition, had temporal lobe tubers.

A characteristic feature of West syndrome is the gross EEG abnormality of hypsarrhythmia. It is hardly surprising that children with such a major disturbance in the EEG also have poor cognitive function and behavioral disturbance. The implication of this is that eliminating the hypsarrhythmia should be associated with a marked improvement in cognitive function and consequently might be associated with a marked improvement in behavior. Reports of both surgical and medical treatment appear to confirm this. Chugani et al. (10) investigated babies with West syndrome using positron emission tomography. In some of the subjects this revealed local cortical abnormalities that could be removed surgically. In several such cases this surgery was followed by marked improvement or normal development. Jambaque et al. (11) treated children with tuberous sclerosis and West syndrome using vigabatrin. Those whose infantile spasms came under control not only had a significant increase in mental score but also showed an improvement in behavior, despite continuing partial seizures.

DRAVET SYNDROME OR SEVERE MYOCLONIC EPILEPSY IN INFANCY

In Dravet syndrome, seizure onset is in the first year of life, usually with febrile convulsions or generalized clonic seizures, followed by myoclonic, partial, or typical absence seizures, or a combination of two or all three, between 2 and 3 years. The seizures may be prolonged. Initially the EEG does not usually show paroxysmal abnormalities, but recordings within the second year of life show interictal generalized spike-wave complexes or generalized polyspike waves or both. Delayed development is usually seen in the second year, and unsteadiness is also generally present.

A recent longitudinal study of twenty-one children with this syndrome has confirmed the pattern of normal early development followed by severe cognitive impairment and marked slowing or stagnation between 1 and 4 years of age (12). Behavioral problems are said to be common, which is not surprising in view of the marked loss of skills in previously normal children. In a follow-up study of 53 cases, Caraballo and Fejerman (13) diagnosed hyperactivity in 45 (85%) and autism in 2 (3.5%). Casse-Perrot et al. (14) found that behavioral problems were generally present in this syndrome and that interpersonal relationships rarely exceeded the developmental level of 2 years of age. The behaviors described included hyperactivity, "psychotic-type relationships," and autistic traits. They also commented that all the children had periods of "lesser excitation" during which they could relate better with others. This variability, at some stage during the evolution of the syndrome, might suggest that the epilepsy itself was affecting behavior in a "state-dependent" way. Dravet originally reported resistance to antiepileptic medication, but the report by Nieto-Barrera et al. (15) indicated that 56% of 18 patients aged 2–22 years had a seizure reduction of more than 50% with topiramate; 3 were seizure-free. Atypical absence seizures were particularly responsive to treatment. This report included no cognitive or behavioral assessment. Such assessments

should be considered mandatory in future studies, which should also include serial EEGs. Ceulemans et al. (16) have recommended treatment with the combination of topiramate and valproate. The finding that this syndrome may be associated with de novo mutations in the *SCN1A* gene (17) adds interest to the debate about whether the cognitive and behavioral deterioration reflect some underlying neurodegenerative condition or are the effect of the epilepsy itself.

LENNOX-GASTAUT SYNDROME

Seizure onset is generally between 1 and 9 years with a peak at 3 to 5 years of age. Multiple seizure types occur, including brief tonic, atonic, myoclonic, and atypical absence seizures. Some emphasize the essential role of axial tonic seizures in the definition. The EEG is abnormal with diffuse slow spike-wave discharges in the waking record and usually fast rhythms of around ten cycles per second in sleep. Seizures are generally resistant to treatment. The prognosis both in terms of seizure control and learning ability is often poor. Many cases are symptomatic, and perhaps 40% follow West syndrome.

Despite the fact that Lennox-Gastaut syndrome is associated with major cognitive and behavioral problems, there is very little published work on the behavioral aspects of this syndrome. A diagnosis of primary autism was made in nine children with this syndrome by Boyer and Deschatrette (18). In a large, long-term study of 338 patients who were followed into adulthood, Roger et al. (19) reported that 62.4% had an unfavorable outcome and that 20.4% had fairly rare partial seizures and neurologic or psychiatric symptoms. Septien et al. (20) reported two children with Lennox-Gastaut syndrome who had a frontal behavioral syndrome with hypokinesia, distractibility, aggressiveness, and alexithymia. In an examination of the neuropsychologic features of this syndrome, Kieffer-Renaux et al. (21) found that in the first year of the seizure disorder behavioral problems were frequent, including hypokinesia, with inability to pursue an activity for more than a few minutes. Autistic or psychotic features were present in some of the patients. General major slowing of intellectual function and impairment of motor speed were also noted. On long-term follow-up, there was perseverative behavior, slowness, and apathy.

The current author has questioned the use of terms such as "apathy" to describe the people with Lennox-Gastaut syndrome, because the frequency of the epileptiform discharges implies that inability to engage with activities is more likely than an unwillingness to do so (3). It is also perhaps not surprising that some children whose functioning is impaired by frequent seizures and frequent epileptiform discharges respond in an irritable way when demands are made of them. The use of polypharmacy in an attempt to control the difficult-to-treat seizures is another likely cause of both of the apparent apathy and the behavioral problems in some of the children. In particular, benzodiazepines have often been used, and these are notorious for causing behavioral problems in children.

Lennox-Gastaut syndrome is another childhood epilepsy syndrome in which early, effective treatment might significantly improve the cognitive and behavioral outcome. Some of the newer antiepileptic drugs (AEDs), such as lamotrigine, appear promising in this regard (22). It is also interesting, in this context, to note the behavioral improvements reported by Aldenkamp et al. (23) in sixteen children treated with vagus nerve stimulation (VNS), twelve of whom had Lennox-Gastaut syndrome. The subgroup that responded best in terms of seizure control were those with the highest mental age and highest social function at baseline. These patients were reported to be more "easy to handle" and "less tense" with an improvement in mood and a decreased tendency for behavior disorders. However, the most prominent improvements were seen in the group in which VNS had no apparent effect on seizure frequency; this subgroup had more independent behavior, mood improvement, and fewer symptoms of a pervasive developmental disorder. The implication is that the VNS might have reduced the frequency of the epileptiform discharges, although a direct effect on mood might also have explained these results. Further prospective studies with EEG monitoring are required.

Septien et al. (20) found that the behavior of two patients who had an anterior two-thirds corpus callosotomy in the early teenage years improved, in terms of frontal-lobe syndrome, within 2 months of the surgery.

There have also been reports of deterioration in behavior with treatment. However, these reports are subject to several confounding factors, discussed elsewhere (24), including the "release phenomenon" that can occur when a person with severe disabling epilepsy is suddenly enabled by a sharp reduction in seizure frequency but has not yet learned how to use this new-found ability in ways that are socially acceptable.

BENIGN CHILDHOOD EPILEPSY WITH CENTROTEMPORAL SPIKES (BECTS)/ ROLANDIC EPILEPSY

The age of onset is 3 to 13 years with a peak at around 9 years. Brief hemifacial seizures, typically occurring on waking from sleep or in sleep, consist of unilateral paresthesiae of the tongue, lips, gums, and inner cheek, unilateral tonic, clonic, or tonic-clonic seizures involving the face, lips, tongue, and pharyngeal and laryngeal muscles, causing speech arrest, drooling, and saliva pooling. The seizures occur with retained consciousness. Some seizures generalize into tonic-clonic seizures. The EEG shows typical centrotemporal spikes. There are no neurologic lesions. In the past it has been stated that there are no neurologic deficits. The EEG becomes normal, and the seizures stop, during the teenage years.

The syndromes discussed earlier in this chapter often have a very poor outcome in terms of seizure control, cognition, and behavior. In contrast, BECTS has traditionally been associated with a good outcome: seizure control by the mid-teenage years and no neurologic, cognitive, or behavioral problems. However, there is now a considerable body of evidence demonstrating that the epileptiform discharges may have an effect on cognition/behavior and that this syndrome lies on a spectrum with CSWS/Landau-Kleffner syndrome. The evidence for this point of view has been highlighted by several articles in a recent symposium (25–27). These studies have also reviewed the range of cognitive/behavioral problems that have been reported, including verbal learning, speech, and oromotor deficits; fine motor and visuomotor disability; and transient dysgraphia.

Weglage et al. (28) found that forty children with BECTS had significantly impaired IQ, visual perception, and short-term memory, compared to forty control children matched for age, sex, and socioeconomic status. It is of particular interest that deficits in IQ were significantly correlated with the frequency of EEG spikes and not with the frequency of seizures. Croona et al. (29) found significantly lower scores on neuropsychologic testing on seventeen children, aged 7–14 years, compared to controls. Although the teachers did not notice any difference in function and behavior between the two groups, the parents of the children with BECTS recognized greater difficulties with concentration, temper, and impulsiveness. Giordani et al. (30) carried out brief psychometric screening on 200 children aged 4–13 years with BECTS before they entered a trial on gabapentin. Because their parents had agreed for them to enter a drug trial, this was a selected group, possibly with more severe epilepsy or other problems than those in the general population with BECTS. There was some evidence for selective cognitive and behavioral problems. The subjects performed worst on a test of verbal attention, with the next lowest score being on visual attention. The scores for all seizure groups were within the average range for intellect and memory, but the simple partial seizure group performed relatively worse on verbal learning. They concluded that the overall variability and pattern of performance suggested a relative weakness in attention. Al-Twajri and Shevell (31) compared two groups of children with Rolandic epilepsy. In group 1 there was seizure control with one drug or no medication, and in group 2 two AEDs were needed for seizure control. The difference in the frequency of comorbid conditions, including tics, attention-deficit hyperactivity disorder, and learning disability, almost reached statistical significance ($p = 0.06$). Metz-Lutz and Filippini (27) have pointed out that atypical EEG features, particularly a slow-wave focus or asynchronous spike-wave foci were associated with poorer overall cognitive performance from the onset of BECTS. This again raises the question of whether children with a poorer outcome have abnormal brains from the outset, resulting in both greater EEG abnormality and more cognitive impairment or whether the greater EEG abnormality is responsible, at least in part, for the poorer cognitive outcome.

Two major issues arise from the studies of BECTS. The first is the role of brief daytime epileptiform discharges in affecting cognition/behavior, and the second is the role of CSWS in some children with BECTS in causing temporary or permanent cognitive/behavioral problems. With regard to the first issue, in the past it was considered unfashionable to pay too much attention to treating EEG abnormalities; this was considered to be "EEG cosmetics." However, there has been a growing realization that, in many cases, epileptiform discharges may affect cognition and behavior. Although it remains true to say that the EEG should never be treated and that it is only clinical problems in the patient that should be treated, the work of Binnie et al. (32) and others has highlighted the importance of searching for cognitive and behavioral changes that might be related to epileptiform discharges. When the latter are detected, treatment may be more than justified. The recent book by Deonna and Roulet-Perez (2) provides many clinical examples of how such treatment has been of benefit. With regard to the second issue, the recognition that BECTS lies on a spectrum with CSWS implies that any child with BECTS who develops unexpected cognitive or behavioral problems should have overnight EEG monitoring. If CSWS is detected, it should be treated and careful follow-up with serial EEG monitoring should be arranged.

LANDAU-KLEFFNER SYNDROME—ACQUIRED EPILEPTIC APHASIA

This syndrome generally presents after language acquisition but before 6 years of age with verbal auditory agnosia and may be followed by auditory agnosia for environmental sounds as well. Expressive language is affected, probably as a consequence of the auditory agnosia, and the child may become mute. EEG abnormalities include spikes and spike-wave discharges, which may be multifocal but tend to occur in the temporal regions. Unilateral or bilateral 1–3-Hz spike-wave discharges occur. The nighttime EEG typically shows electrical status epilepticus of slow-wave sleep (ESES), implying that at least 85% of slow-wave sleep is occupied by spike-wave discharges. Around 30% of the children with this syndrome do not present with seizures, although the EEG abnormalities are present. The seizures tend to resolve by the early- to mid-teenage years. The progress of language development is very variable. Language may recover spontaneously, require treatment, or remain permanently impaired.

It is not surprising that behavioral problems occur in association with the loss of speech abilities in children who were previously able to understand and communicate normally. Aggression, sleep disorders, hyperkinesia, and autism have all been described in association with this syndrome. Many of the reports are of single case studies or small case series. Several of these have been summarized in a recent review (3). There have also been several papers and reviews discussing the relationship between autism, epileptiform discharges, and Landau-Kleffner syndrome (33, 34). This subject has been reviewed by Deonna and Roulet-Perez in their recent book (2). In other reports in which language disturbance in association with epilepsy has been studied, it is not clear whether all the children met the criteria for Landau-Kleffner syndrome. Shinnar et al. (35) prospectively identified 177 children with language regression and stated that most (88%) met the criteria for autism or had autistic features. They emphasized the need for early identification and treatment.

Landau-Kleffner syndrome is interesting because it raises a number of issues. Although this is an epilepsy syndrome, it is said that between one-fourth and one-third of the children who have Landau-Kleffner syndrome do not appear to have clinical seizures. This implies that long-standing definitions of epilepsy, which depend on the presence of clinical seizures, might need to be challenged. The second issue that is of particular interest is that Landau-Kleffner syndrome is perhaps the most dramatic model of an epilepsy syndrome in which the epileptiform discharges appear not only to affect cognition and behavior but also to cause permanent damage if they are allowed to continue. The approach to the management of Landau-Kleffner syndrome has changed dramatically over recent years. Older publications suggested that treatment was of value only in controlling the seizures and would have no effect on language function. Recent publications have emphasized the importance of early effective treatment. Medical treatments include steroids, sodium valproate, benzodiazepines, sulthiame, and intravenous immunoglobulin. Surgical treatment with multiple subpial transection can be of great value when medical treatment has failed. The study by Robinson et al. (36) revealed that in their series, no child who had ESES for more than 2 years had a normal language outcome. It is anticipated that the sooner effective treatment is started, the less likely it will be that long-term cognitive and behavioral problems will occur. This raises the question of when surgical intervention should be considered. The outcome of this syndrome is very variable: some children recover spontaneously whereas others have permanent language deficits, which may be severe. If surgery is carried out too early, it may have been unnecessary; but if it is carried out too late, the child may be left with serious problems that could have been avoided.

OTHER SYNDROMES INVOLVING ESES OR CSWS

The ILAE classification also lists a childhood epilepsy syndrome entitled "epilepsy with continuous spike-and-waves during slow-wave sleep (other than LKS)." The definition states the following (37):

> There is a constant and severe deterioration in neuro-psychological functions associated with the disorder, and language capacity can be particularly affected. Patients also may show a profound decrease in intellectual level, poor memory, impaired temporospatial orientation, reduced attention span, hyperkinesis, aggressive behaviour, and even psychosis. . . . Motor impairment, in the form of dyspraxia, dystonia, ataxia, or unilateral deficit, has been emphasized as one of the outstanding disturbances occurring in this syndrome. . . . There is a strict association between the pattern of neuropsychological derangement and the location of the interictal focus. A deterioration of language is observed in cases showing the predominance of paroxysmal abnormalities over one or both temporal regions, whereas a mental deterioration and an autistic behavior evoking a frontal lobe syndrome has been described in children exhibiting interictal frontal foci or clear cut anterior predominance of the discharges. On the other hand, causative factors for motor impairment in the form of dyspraxia, dystonia, ataxia, or unilateral deficit observed in some children during the period of continuous spikes and waves during slow sleep would be a predominant involvement of motor areas by continuous spike-wave activity and the appearance of negative myoclonus during wakefulness.

The prominence of autistic features in association with CSWS has been emphasized by several workers (33, 34). The classification of a specific acquired frontal syndrome with CSWS has also been suggested (38).

Early-onset benign childhood occipital epilepsy, also called early-onset benign childhood seizures susceptibility syndrome with occipital or extraoccipital spikes or Panayiotopoulos syndrome, usually has a very good outcome but an atypical type may also occur with mild impairment of scholastic performance, with or without ESES (26).

Saltik et al. (39) found that several clinical features indicated the development of ESES in a group of sixteen children with idiopathic partial epilepsies. These features included an increase in seizure frequency, addition of new types of seizures, appearance of cognitive or behavioral changes, or a progression in EEG abnormalities. Behavioral and psychiatric problems occurred in 81% (13 of 16), including anxiety, depression, distractibility,

hyperactivity, impulsivity, and being easily frustrated. After remission of the ESES, three of the thirteen patients had an excellent recovery, one was diagnosed as having the Landau-Kleffner syndrome, and nine patients performed better but did not achieve premorbid levels.

It is particularly important to note that children who deteriorate in terms of their cognition and behavior may do so because of CSWS without necessarily having prominent language impairment. If a child's behavior deteriorates and this is associated with the onset of cognitive or neurologic problems, there is a strong argument for requesting overnight EEG monitoring, unless another cause can be found.

JUVENILE MYOCLONIC EPILEPSY (JANZ SYNDROME)

The classical triad in this syndrome consists of myoclonic seizures, particularly affecting the upper limbs, worst soon after waking; absence seizures; and generalized tonic-clonic seizures on awakening. Approximately one-third are photosensitive. The EEG shows polyspike-wave complexes and irregular spike-wave discharges, usually with a frequency of more than three per second. The age of onset is usually considered to be from 12 to 18 years in most cases, but some patients may have absence seizures in childhood that are not recognized as the beginning of the syndrome.

This is another syndrome that is often associated with a good prognosis. However, the original publication by Janz and Christian (40), more recently updated by Janz (41), pointed out that many patients had attractive but unstable, suggestible, unreliable, and rather immature personalities, often resulting in inadequate social adjustment. Reintoft et al. (42) confirmed some of these characteristics in thirty-three patients and found a trend toward social maladjustment, although this was not statistically significant. Perini et al. (43) found that the rate of psychiatric disorder in eighteen people with juvenile myoclonic epilepsy (JME) in their study was 22%. Devinsky et al. (44) tested frontal lobe function in fifteen patients with JME who had a normal IQ and found that their performance was variable, with some patients showing marked impairment and others none. Concept formation/abstract reasoning and mental flexibility, cognitive speed and planning, and organization were particularly affected. Janz has pointed out that the neurophysiology, neuropsychology, and neuroimaging findings all suggest frontal lobe dysfunction in JME.

The epileptic myoclonus in this syndrome is usually most marked in the first hour or so after waking, and this corresponds to frequent polyspike or spike-wave epileptiform discharges in the EEG. In the light of this, it might be predicted that people with JME would function poorly in the morning. This prediction is in keeping with the recent finding by Pung and Schmitz (45) that, in contrast to people with temporal lobe epilepsy, subjects with JME tended to feel better later in the day. These factors might have implications for the timing of neuropsychologic testing; people with JME might function less well first thing in the morning and better later in the day.

CONCLUSION

Although the aim of epilepsy treatment has traditionally been seizure freedom, it could be argued that ongoing cognitive and behavioral difficulties are more likely to affect the prospects of an individual than ongoing seizures. An understanding of when these problems are likely to occur and how to avoid or treat them is clearly of major importance to the clinician and the patient. The patterns of these difficulties that are likely to be associated with specific syndromes are now beginning to emerge. However, much of the published work is still confined to individual case studies or small series, often with no validated behavioral measures. Apart from the need to carry out carefully designed prospective studies, perhaps the most important points emerging from the information available so far are that epileptiform discharges during both daytime and nighttime (especially CSWS) can affect cognition or behavior and that early effective treatment with medication or surgery can sometimes improve outcome greatly.

References

1. Engel J Jr; International League Against Epilepsy (ILAE). A proposed diagnostic scheme for people with epileptic seizures and with epilepsy: report of the ILAE Task Force on Classification and Terminology. *Epilepsia* 2001; 42:796–803.
2. Deonna T, Roulet-Perez R. Cognitive and behavioural disorders of epileptic origin in children. Cambridge, UK: Mac Keith Press/Cambridge University Press, 2005.
3. Besag FM. Behavioral aspects of pediatric epilepsy syndromes [review]. *Epilepsy Behav* 2004; 5(Suppl 1):S3–S13.
4. Gobbi G, Schmitz B, Cornaggia C, Brown S, et al., eds. Cognitive and behavioral outcomes of epileptic syndromes. *Epilepsia* 2006; 47(Suppl 2).
5. Jambaque I, Mottron L, Chiron C. Neuropsychological outcome in children with West syndrome. In: Jambaque I, Lassonde M, Dulac O, eds. *Neuropsychology of Childhood Epilepsy*. New York: Kluwer Academic/Plenum Publishers, 2001:175–183.
6. Guzzetta F. Cognitive and behavioral outcome in West syndrome. *Epilepsia* 2006; 47 (Suppl 2):49–52.
7. Riikonen R, Amnell G. Psychiatric disorders in children with earlier infantile spasms. *Dev Med Child Neurol* 1981; 23:747–760.
8. Hunt A, Dennis J. Psychiatric disorder among children with tuberous sclerosis. *Dev Med Child Neurol* 1987; 29:190–198.
9. Bolton PF, Park RJ, Higgins JN, Griffiths PD, et al. Neuro-epileptic determinants of autism spectrum disorders in tuberous sclerosis complex. *Brain* 2002; 125(Pt 6):1247–1255.
10. Chugani HT, Shewmon DA, Shields WD, Sankar R, et al. Surgery for intractable infantile spasms: neuroimaging perspectives. *Epilepsia* 1993; 34:764–771.
11. Jambaque I, Chiron C, Dumas C, Mumford J, et al. Mental and behavioural outcome of infantile epilepsy treated by vigabatrin in tuberous sclerosis patients. *Epilepsy Res* 2000; 38:151–160.
12. Wolff MD, Casse-Perrot C, Dravet C. Severe myoclonic epilepsy of infants (Dravet syndrome): natural history and neuropsychological findings. *Epilepsia* 2006; 47(Suppl 2):45–48.
13. Caraballo RH, Fejerman N. Dravet syndrome: a study of 53 patients. *Epilepsy Res* 2006; 70S:S231–S238.
14. Casse-Perrot C, Wolf M, Dravet C. Neuropsychological aspects of severe myoclonic epilepsy in infancy. In: Jambaque I, Lassonde M, Dulac O, eds. *Neuropsychology of Childhood Epilepsy*. New York: Kluwer Academic/Plenum Publishers, 2001:131–140.
15. Nieto-Barrera M, Candau R, Nieto-Jimenez M, Correa A, et al. Topiramate in the treatment of severe myoclonic epilepsy in infancy. *Seizure* 2000; 9:590–594.
16. Ceulemans B, Boel M, Claes L, Dom L, et al. Severe myoclonic epilepsy in infancy: toward an optimal treatment. *J Child Neurol* 2004; 19:516–521.
17. Claes L, Ceulemans B, Audenaert D, Smets K, et al. De novo SCN1A mutations are a major cause of severe myoclonic epilepsy of infancy. *Hum Mutat* 2003; 21:615–621.
18. Boyer JP, Deschatrette A. [Convulsive autism or Lennox-Gastaut syndrome? Apropos of 9 cases of primary autism associated with Lennox-Gastaut syndrome]. [French]. *Neuropsychiatrie de l Enfance et de l Adolescence* 1980; 28:93–100.
19. Roger J, Remy C, Bureau M, Oller-Daurella L, et al. [Lennox-Gastaut syndrome in the adult]. [French]. *Rev Neurol (Paris)* 1987; 143:401–405.
20. Septien L, Giroud M, Sautreaux JL, Brenot M, et al. [Effects of callosotomy in the treatment of intractable epilepsies in children on psychiatric disorders]. [French]. *Encephale* 1992; 18:199–202.
21. Kieffer-Renaux V, Kaminska A, Dulac O. Cognitive deterioration in Lennox-Gastaut and Doose epilepsy. In: Jambaque I, Lassonde M, Dulac O, eds. *Neuropsychology of Childhood Epilepsy*. New York: Kluwer Academic/Plenum Publishers, 2001:185–190.
22. Motte J, Trevathan E, Arvidsson JF, Barrera MN, et al. Lamotrigine for generalized seizures associated with the Lennox-Gastaut syndrome. Lamictal Lennox-Gastaut Study Group. *N Engl J Med* 1997; 337:1807–1812.
23. Aldenkamp AP, van der Veerdonk SHA, Majoie HJM, Berfelo MW, et al. Effects of 6 months of treatment with vagus nerve stimulation on behaviour in children with Lennox-Gastaut syndrome in an open clinical and nonrandomised study. *Epilepsy Behav* 2001; 2:343–350.
24. Besag FMC. Behavioural effects of the new anticonvulsants. *Drug Saf* 2001; 24:513–536.
25. Stephani U, Carlsson G. The spectrum from BCECTS to LKS: the Rolandic EEG trait—impact on cognition. *Epilepsia* 2006; 47(Suppl 2):67–70.
26. Gobbi G, Boni A, Filippini M. The spectrum of idiopathic Rolandic epilepsy syndromes and idiopathic occipital epilepsies: from the benign to the disabling. *Epilepsia* 2006; 47(Suppl 2):62–66.
27. Metz-Lutz MN, Filippini M. Neuropsychological findings in Rolandic epilepsy and Landau-Kleffner syndrome. *Epilepsia* 2006; 47(Suppl 2):71–75.
28. Weglage J, Demsky A, Pietsch M, Kurlemann G. Neuropsychological, intellectual, and behavioral findings in patients with centrotemporal spikes with and without seizures. *Dev Med Child Neurol* 1997; 39:646–651.
29. Croona C, Kihlgren M, Lundberg S, Eeg-Olofsson O, et al. Neuropsychological findings in children with benign childhood epilepsy with centrotemporal spikes. *Dev Med Child Neurol* 1999; 41:813–818.
30. Giordani B, Caveney AF, Laughrin D, Huffman JL, et al. Cognition and behavior in children with benign epilepsy with centrotemporal spikes (BECTS). *Epilepsy Res* 2006; 70:89–94.
31. Al-Twaijri WA, Shevell MI. Atypical benign epilepsy of childhood with rolandic spikes: features of a subset requiring more than one medication for seizure control. *J Child Neurol* 2002; 17:901–904.
32. Binnie CD, de Silva M, Hurst A. Rolandic spikes and cognitive function. *Epilepsy Res* 1992; Suppl 6:71–73.
33. Tuchman R. Treatment of seizure disorders and EEG abnormalities in children with autism spectrum disorders. *J Autism Dev Disord* 2000; 30:485–489.
34. Deonna T, Roulet E. Autistic spectrum disorder: evaluating a possible contributing or causal role of epilepsy. *Epilepsia* 2006; 47 (Suppl 2):79–82.
35. Shinnar S, Rapin I, Arnold S, Tuchman RF, et al. Language regression in childhood. *Pediatr Neurol* 2001; 24:183–189.
36. Robinson RO, Baird G, Robinson G, Simonoff E. Landau-Kleffner syndrome: course and correlates with outcome. *Dev Med Child Neurol* 2001; 43:243–247.
37. Tassinari CA, Volpi L, Michelucci R. Electrical status epilepticus during slow sleep. http://www.ilae-epilepsy.org/Visitors/Centre/ctf/electric_stat_slow_sleep.cfm. Accessed 27 April 2007.
38. Roulet PE, Davidoff V, Despland PA, Deonna T. Mental and behavioural deterioration of children with epilepsy and CSWS: acquired epileptic frontal syndrome. *Dev Med Child Neurol* 1993; 35:661–674.
39. Saltik S, Uluduz D, Cokar O, Demirbilek V, et al. A clinical and EEG study on idiopathic partial epilepsies with evolution into ESES spectrum disorders. *Epilepsia* 2005; 46:524–533.
40. Janz D, Christian W. Impulsiv-Petit mal. *Dtch Z Nervenheilk* 1957; 176:346–386.
41. Janz D. The psychiatry of idiopathic generalized epilepsy. In: Trimble M, Schmitz B, eds. *The Neuropsychiatry of Epilepsy*. Cambridge, UK: Cambridge University Press, 2002:41–61.
42. Reintoft H, Simonsen N, Lund M. A controlled sociological study of juvenile myoclonic epilepsy. In: Janz D, ed. *Epileptology*. Stuttgart: Thieme, 1976:48–50.
43. Perini GI, Tosin C, Carraro C, Bernasconi G, et al. Interictal mood and personality disorders in temporal lobe epilepsy and juvenile myoclonic epilepsy. *J Neurol Neurosurg Psychiatry* 1996; 61:601–605.
44. Devinsky O, Gershengorn J, Brown E, Perrine K, et al. Frontal functions in juvenile myoclonic epilepsy. *Neuropsychiatry, Neuropsychology, & Behavioral Neurology* 1997; 10:243–246.
45. Pung T, Schmitz B. Circadian rhythm and personality profile in juvenile myoclonic epilepsy. *Epilepsia* 2006; 47(Suppl 2):111–114.

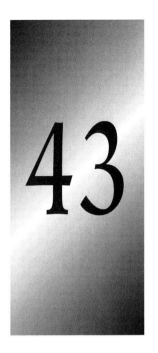

43 Psychiatric Aspects of Epilepsy in Children

David W. Dunn
Joan K. Austin

E pilepsy in childhood is a pervasive disorder that includes not only seizures but also significant effects on cognition, behavior, and quality of life. These later problems can become even more disruptive than seizures for the child with epilepsy. The purpose of this chapter is to review the behavioral and emotional complications of epilepsy in childhood. Autistic disorder and attention deficit hyperactivity disorder (ADHD) are covered in Chapters 56 and 57, respectively, and will be only briefly mentioned in this chapter.

Epidemiological studies have shown that psychiatric problems are common in children with epilepsy. In England, two separate epidemiological studies conducted over 30 years apart found a remarkably similar prevalence of emotional and behavioral difficulties (1, 2). In both studies more than half of the children with both epilepsy and additional neurologic problems had psychiatric problems, and one-fourth of the children with uncomplicated epilepsy suffered from behavioral problems. In comparison, psychiatric problems were noted in 11–12% of children with chronic illnesses not involving the central nervous system and in 6–9% of healthy controls. A similar survey conducted in the United States reported behavioral problems in 31% of children with seizures, 21% of children with heart disease, and 8.5% of controls (3).

Similarly, studies of children seen in university-based epilepsy clinics have documented the increased prevalence of psychiatric difficulties in this population and have determined the specific psychiatric diagnoses found in children with epilepsy. Caplan et al. (4) reported a greater than 50% rate of psychopathology in children 5–16 years of age with complex partial or absence seizures. They noted disruptive behavior disorders alone or comorbid with mood or anxiety disorders in more than one-third of patients, and mood or anxiety disorders in more than one-fourth of children. Symptoms of thought disorder were found in 10% of the children with complex partial seizures. Evaluating children with epilepsy 9–14 years of age, we found that one-third had ADHD, one-fifth a disruptive behavior disorder (oppositional defiant disorder or conduct disorder), and one-third an anxiety disorder. One in twenty had a depressive disorder, although in another study of older adolescents, one-fourth had symptoms of depression.

Although behavioral and emotional problems are common, the recognition of behavioral difficulties has been a problem. Ott et al. (5), in a study from a university-based epilepsy clinic, found that 61% of the children with epilepsy had evidence of a psychiatric disorder using *Diagnostic and Statistical Manual of Mental Disorders*, 4th edition (DSM-IV) criteria. However, only 33% of the children had received any mental health care. Similarly, Ettinger et al.

(6) noted that one-fourth of the children and adolescents in their comprehensive epilepsy clinic had symptoms of depression, yet none were receiving treatment.

RISK FACTORS FOR PSYCHIATRIC PROBLEMS IN CHILDREN WITH EPILEPSY

Epilepsy is a heterogeneous disorder and thus it should be expected that there are multiple risk factors for psychiatric problems (7). These risk factors include demographic, neurologic, seizure-related, treatment-based, family, and individual variables.

Demographic factors are only weakly predictive of psychiatric problems. Gender has been an inconsistent predictor. Some studies have found more problems in boys, others no difference by gender, and one more problems in girls with poorly controlled seizures. Age of seizure onset seems to be a better predictor of cognitive problems than of behavioral difficulties Age of the child may be a significant factor, however, with more depression found in adolescents than in younger children with epilepsy.

Neurologic variables are one of the most consistent predictors. Children with additional neurologic deficits have a higher prevalence of psychiatric disorders. Autistic disorder and the pervasive developmental disorders are most commonly associated with intellectual disability and epilepsy. These children also have more evidence of disruptive behavior disorders and, in adolescence, lower self-esteem. Quality-of-life surveys generally show that children with epilepsy and intellectual disability have impairment beyond the additive effects of two chronic disorders. Even in children with epilepsy and normal intelligence, language impairment has been associated with psychopathology.

Seizure type and syndrome are weak predictors of psychiatric problems, particularly after controlling for intellectual ability. The increased prevalence of behavioral problems in the children with the symptomatic or cryptogenic epilepsies is probably better attributed to intellectual disability or seizure frequency and severity than to specific seizure type or syndrome. Adults with complex partial seizures may have more emotional problems, but in children, seizure type has not been a consistent predictor of psychopathology.

Antiepileptic drugs (AEDs) are possible contributors to behavioral problems (8). Surveys have found psychiatric side effects in 2–15% of patients on AEDs. Behavioral side effects were more common with the older sedative AEDs such as the barbiturates or benzodiazepines. Topiramate, one of the newer AEDs, has been associated with attention problems and slow processing. The prevalence of behavioral side effects seems to be lower with the newer AEDs than with older medications. However, individual hypersensitivity to any of the AEDs may result in behavioral side effects. Higher doses of AEDs and polypharmacy have been associated with behavioral problems, but the association is complicated by the severity of the underlying seizure disorder.

Family factors are associated with psychiatric problems in the child with epilepsy. In particular, the quality of the relationship between the child and the parents has been most consistently associated with behavioral problems in children with epilepsy (9). Studies of children with chronic seizures also have found that the parent-child relationship has been more strongly associated with behavioral problems than has any epilepsy-related factor. Impact of seizures on the family should be monitored. A consistent finding in our studies has been the positive effect of family mastery. The children in families that are organized, cooperative, and confident in their ability to handle the challenge of epilepsy are least likely to experience behavioral difficulties.

SPECIFIC PSYCHIATRIC DIAGNOSES IN CHILDREN WITH EPILEPSY

The specific psychiatric disorder seen in children with epilepsy will depend on several factors. In comparison to children seen in the community, children treated in a comprehensive epilepsy clinic are more likely to have behavioral problems because children with comorbidity are more often referred to specialty clinics. Children with epilepsy and intellectual disability are at increased risk for autistic spectrum disorders. ADHD and the disruptive behavior disorders most often present in the preschool and elementary school years. Depression, bipolar disorder, and suicidal ideation are more likely to occur in adolescents. Although anxiety may be seen at any age, separation anxiety is more often a disorder of the younger child, and panic disorder occurs in the adolescent.

The disruptive behavior disorders include ADHD, oppositional defiant disorder (ODD), and conduct disorder. Symptoms of ADHD, covered in detail in Chapter 57, are found in one-third of children with epilepsy, and ADHD probably is the most common psychiatric disorder found in the elementary school age child with seizures (10). Oppositional defiant disorder is characterized by defiance, anger, and irritability. Conduct disorder is a repetitive pattern of behavior that includes major violations of standards, such as stealing, property destruction, and assault. The prevalence of these disorders in children with epilepsy is less well established than the prevalence of ADHD in children with epilepsy. In our clinical series of children 9–14 years of age, we found ODD in 21% and conduct disorder in 18%. The large epidemiological study from England (2) reported conduct disorder in 24% of children with complicated epilepsy and 17% of children with uncomplicated epilepsy. In comparison, the general population prevalence of ODD and conduct disorder range from 2% to 16%.

Additional central nervous system damage and intractable seizures are risk factors for disruptive behavioral disorders in children with epilepsy. Seizure type has not been a consistent factor, although involvement of the basal frontotemporal region has been postulated to be a factor in adults with epilepsy and aggression. Treatment with sedative AEDs has resulted in hyperactivity, irritability, and aggression. In children with intellectual disability, there are case reports of aggression after treatment with gabapentin. Family factors may be particularly important. A family history of disruptive behavior disorder, chaotic or dysfunctional families, and parental separation or divorce has been associated with ODD and conduct disorder in children with epilepsy.

Depressive disorders are one of the most frequent complications of epilepsy in children and adolescents (11). Studies of all pediatric age groups find a prevalence of 10–30% and studies restricted to adolescents with epilepsy show that one-fourth experience symptoms of depression. Depression also frequently goes unrecognized. As one example, in a university-based epilepsy clinic, 26% of the children and adolescents reported symptoms of depression and yet none had received a prior diagnosis of mood disorder (6).

Risk factors for depression in children with epilepsy include both those factors associated with depression in children without epilepsy and those specific for the child with epilepsy. In the general population, there is an interaction between genetic and environmental factors. A positive family history accounts for much of the variance in transmission of depression. In addition, maternal depression adversely affects the maternal-child relationship and family functioning. Other important risk factors are death of a parent, trauma or abuse, and chronic illness. Recent studies have shown an interaction between a genetic variant in serotonin transporter gene and stressful life events that convey an increased vulnerability to depression. There may be specific risk factors associated with epilepsy. Adults with frontal or temporal localization–related epilepsies reportedly have an increased risk of depression. However, studies in children have not found a consistent association between seizure type or syndrome and depression. Children with more frequent seizures appear to be at increased risk, but this may be a nonspecific association with a chronic illness. In adults with epilepsy, depression has been associated with barbiturates, tiagabine, topiramate, and vigabatrin.

Both depression and suicidal ideation have been reported in children treated with barbiturates. Family dysfunction is a significant factor in depression and may be exacerbated by the stress or the stigma associated with epilepsy. The child or adolescent with a negative attitude toward illness and an external or unknown locus of control has been found to be at increased risk for depression.

Depression and suicide attempts may also be risk factors for seizures (12). Although the mechanism is not known, this might be an effect of alterations in monoaminergic neurotransmitters or possibly neurologic effects of changes in stress hormones.

Depression in children and adolescents may differ from that seen in adults. Children are more often irritable and angry than sad. They have frequent somatic complaints such as headaches or stomachaches. Adolescents may have a reactive form of depression and will appear happy when spending time with friends but may not have the energy or motivation to seek out companionship. Withdrawal and avoidance of previously enjoyed activities is another clue for the diagnosis of depression. Children with depression, including those with epilepsy, frequently have comorbid psychiatric disorders. Caplan et al. (13) found that anxiety or disruptive behavior disorders were present in two-thirds of the children with depression and epilepsy. An atypical depression with brief episodes, irritability, and anger has been described in adults with epilepsy but not in children or adolescents. Postictal symptoms of depression also have been reported in approximately 50% of adults with intractable partial epilepsy, but similar information is not available in children and adolescents.

Bipolar disorder has received little attention in the clinical studies of children with epilepsy. In a large community-based survey of adults with epilepsy, Ettinger et al. (14) noted a prevalence of bipolar disorder of 8.1%, more than twice that found in adults with asthma or diabetes mellitus, or healthy controls. No information exists for prevalence rate in children. Salpekar et al. (15) found 38 pediatric patients with both epilepsy and bipolar disorder identified retrospectively in a review of 5 years of clinic records from a large university-based pediatric epilepsy clinic.

The limited information on bipolar disorder in children with epilepsy may be partially due to continuing controversy about the diagnostic criteria for childhood bipolar disorder. Children with recurrent depression and mania lasting at least 4–7 days are relatively uncommon. A broader definition of juvenile bipolar disorder is currently being used by many researchers. Children with this disorder have a chronic condition with severe irritability, mood lability, and hyperarousal. Older reports of hyperkinetic syndrome in children with epilepsy listed symptoms of irritability, mood lability, and hyperactivity that might fit this broad definition of childhood bipolar disorder. A more recent study described combined anxiety, depression, and disruptive behavior in 4.7% of the children. Some of these children might be considered

reduction in aggression. The effects of SSRIs are more variable, with some children improving and others worsening. For the child with epilepsy, AEDs are an obvious first choice. Stimulants and atomoxetine are probably safe with little or no effect on seizure threshold, although an occasional child with more intractable seizures may have an increase in seizure number with stimulants. Atypical antipsychotics should be added only when the aggression is severe and nonresponsive to behavioral therapies and first-line medications.

Pharmacological treatment of anxiety and depression is similar. The SSRIs are used most commonly (19). There are good double-blind placebo-controlled trials showing the effectiveness of these agents for anxiety in both children and adolescents. The response of depression to SSRIs in children has been less robust, although adolescents seem to respond as well as adults to these agents. Open-label trials of sertraline and citralopram for adults with epilepsy and depression have demonstrated effectiveness and safety. A concern in children and adolescents is the potential of adverse psychiatric side effects of the SSRIs. An increase in suicidal ideation and self-injurious behaviors has been reported in children and adolescents receiving antidepressant therapy. This may be the result of activation occurring early in the course of treatment. Another psychiatric side effect of the SSRIs has been apathy.

Treatment of bipolar disorder in children and adolescents with epilepsy may benefit from the effect of AEDs on both epilepsy and bipolar disorder (15). Currently divalproex sodium, carbamazepine, and lamotrigine have been shown to be effective in the treatment of both epilepsy and bipolar disorder. Although no controlled trials exist for children with epilepsy and bipolar disorder, a retrospective chart review found better clinical global impression of improvement (CGI-I) ratings in children with both disorders who received monotherapy with these three agents plus oxcarbazepine.

Treatment of psychotic disorder is dependent on the etiology of psychosis (19). Psychosis due to nonconvulsive status epilepticus requires treatment of seizures, whereas psychosis secondary to introduction of a new AED necessitates discontinuation of the drug. In most other situations, psychosis requires antipsychotic medication. Lowering of the seizure threshold occurs with chlorpromazine and clozapine, suggesting that these agents should be avoided. The negative effect of haloperidol on seizure control seems to be negligible, and open-label trials of risperidone have found no increase in seizure frequency. The major adverse effects of haloperidol are extrapyramidal movement disorders, and those of risperidone are weight gain and metabolic problems.

CONCLUSION

Psychiatric disorders are commonly associated with epilepsy in children. Disruptive behavior disorder, depression, and anxiety may each be found in about one-fourth to one-third of children with epilepsy. These problems can be a major stress for families and children. Children at most risk are those with additional neurologic damage, more intractable seizures, and dysfunctional families. Assessment is critical because too many children with epilepsy have unrecognized psychiatric problems. Although data on interventions are limited, treatment should consist of a combination of education, counseling, and, in more severe impairment, psychotropic medications.

References

1. Rutter M, Graham P, Yule W. A neuropsychiatric study in childhood. London: Mac Keith Press, 1970.
2. Davies S, Heyman I, Goodman R. A population survey of mental health problems in children with epilepsy. *Dev Med Child Neurol* 2003; 45:292–295.
3. McDermott S, Mani S, Krishnaswami S. A population-based analysis of specific behavior problems associated with childhood seizures. *J Epilepsy* 1995; 8:110–118.
4. Caplan R, Arbelle S, Magharious W, et al. Psychopathology in pediatric complex partial and generalized epilepsy. *Dev Med Child Neurol* 1998; 40:805–811.
5. Ott D, Siddarth P, Gurbani S, et al. Behavioral disorders in pediatric epilepsy: unmet psychiatric need. *Epilepsia* 2003; 44:591–597.
6. Ettinger AB, Weisbrot DM, Nolan EE, et al. Symptoms of depression and anxiety in pediatric epilepsy patients. *Epilepsia* 1998; 39:595–599.
7. Dunn DW, Austin JK. Behavior issues in pediatric epilepsy. *Neurology* 1999; 53:S96–S100.
8. Loring DW, Meador KJ. Cognitive and behavioral effects of epilepsy treatment. *Neurology* 2001; 42(Suppl 8):24–32.
9. Rodenburg R, Meijer AM, Deković M, Aldenkamp AP. Family predictors of psychopathology in children with epilepsy. *Epilepsia* 2006; 47:601–614.
10. Dunn DW, Austin JK, Harezlak J, Ambrosius WT. ADHD and epilepsy in childhood. *Dev Med Child Neurol* 2003;45:50–54.
11. Plioplys S. Depression in children and adolescents with epilepsy. *Epilepsy Behav* 2003; 4:S39–S45.
12. Hesdorffer DC, Hauser WA, Olafsson E, Ludvigsson P, et al. Depression and suicide attempt as risk factors for incident unprovoked seizures. *Ann Neurol* 2006; 59:35–41.
13. Caplan R, Siddarth P, Gurbani S, Hanson R, et al. Depression and anxiety disorders in pediatric epilepsy. *Epilepsia* 2005; 46:720–730.
14. Ettinger AB, Reed ML, Goldberg JF, Hirschfeld RMA. Prevalence of bipolar symptoms in epilepsy vs other chronic health disorders. *Neurology* 2005; 65:535–540.
15. Salpekar JA, Conry JA, Doss W, et al. Clinical experience with anticonvulsant medication in pediatric epilepsy and comorbid bipolar spectrum disorder. *Epilepsy Behav* 2006; 9:327–334.
16. Jones JE, Hermann BP, Barry JJ, Gilliam FG, et al. Rates and risk factors for suicide, suicidal ideation, and suicide attempts in chronic epilepsy. *Epilepsy Behav* 2003; 4:S31–S38.
17. Vazquez B, Devinsky O. Epilepsy and anxiety. *Epilepsy Behav* 2003; 4(Suppl 4): S20–S25.
18. Williams J, Steel C, Sharp GB, et al. Anxiety in children with epilepsy. *Epilepsy Behav* 2003; 4:729–732.
19. Kanner AM, Dunn DW. Diagnosis and management of depression and psychosis in children and adolescents with epilepsy. *J Child Neurol* 2004; 19(Suppl 1):S65–S72.
20. Caplan R, Siddarth P, Bailey CE, et al. Thought disorder: a developmental disability in pediatric epilepsy. *Epilepsy Behav* 2006; 4:726–735.
21. Myers K, Collett B. Rating scales. In: Weiner JM, Dulcan MK, eds. *Textbook of Child and Adolescent Psychiatry*. 3rd ed. Washington, DC: American Psychiatric Publishing, 2004:149–163.
22. Dunn DW, Austin JK. Differential diagnosis and treatment of psychiatric disorders in children and adolescents with epilepsy. *Epilepsy Behav* 2004; 5:S10–S17.
23. Alldredge BK. Seizure risk associated with psychotropic drugs: clinical and pharmacokinetic considerations. *Neurology* 1999; 53:S68–S75.

44

Behavioral and Psychiatric Effects in Patients with Multiple Disabilities

Michael Kerr
Seth A. Mensah

P eople with multiple disabilities can face many barriers toward reaching the goal of a fulfilling life. Behavioral and psychiatric disturbances are common, and the additional presence of epilepsy poses further challenges to the quality of life of the individuals and their families and to care providers. This chapter will explore directly our understanding of these disturbances, potential causes, and assessment. Last, we will discuss key management issues that affect clinical epilepsy management directly.

No population is, of course, unique; however, it is the presence of speech and communication difficulties in this subgroup of patients with epilepsy that presents a challenge in the assessment and management of any behavioral and psychiatric disturbance. Clinicians are required to modify their diagnostic approach to the patient's cognitive level and communication skills, a challenge that persists throughout the patient's lifespan.

DEFINITIONS

This area is particularly beset by definitional difficulties, reflecting international variance and the trend for terminology to become dated and recognized as pejorative. Our approach to this issue is to use the term *people with multiple disabilities* (PWMD) as a pragmatic approach to

a population that, in general, is easily recognized within epilepsy services. Although not an official term, it is used to reflect a population with functional difficulties across the domains of intellectual capacity, communication, and frequently mobility. In general terms in pediatric care, this will be the population subsumed in the United States within the term *mental retardation*. In the adult population it again encompasses this group, but those with brain injury acquired outside the developmental period, such as trauma, may be included in addition.

People with multiple disabilities exhibit a wide range of characteristics but share the following in common: limited speech and communication, difficulty in basic physical mobility, tendency to forget skills through disuse, trouble generalizing skills from one situation to another, and a need for support in major life activities.

DESCRIBING AND MEASURING BEHAVIORAL AND PSYCHIATRIC DISTURBANCE

Some reflection on the definition of psychologic and behavioral disturbance is necessary, because the usual classification systems rely on a level of communication not present in PWMD to distinguish subtle features of psychopathology. Although the application of psychiatric classification may work well, behavioral abnormality is more complex. Table 44-1 shows a range of studies

TABLE 44-1

Summary Table of Classification of Behavioral and Psychiatric Disturbance

AUTHOR/STUDY	RATING SCALE	BEHAVIOR & PSYCHOPATHOLOGY
Brown et al. (15)	Aberrant Behavior Checklist	37%: overall problematic behavior • 6%: conduct problem • 12%: shy/inactive • 6%: hyperactive • 6%: social withdrawal with agitation • 4%: undifferentiated behavior disturbance • 3%: autistic-like behavior
Reid (16)		• Affective disorder • Schizophrenic disorder • Dementing syndrome • Autistic spectrum disorder • Hyperkinetic syndromes • Neurotic disorder • Conduct disorder • Personality disorder
Rutter et al. (17) (IOW study)	Rutter Scale	• Hyperactivity • Rage • Antisocial behavior • Schizophrenia-like psychosis
Lund (13)	Modified for mental retardation version of Feighner's criteria and DSM-III criteria	27%: overall psychiatric disorder • 10.9%: generic behavior disorder category • 5%: psychoses of uncertain type • 3.6%: dementia • 3.6%: early childhood autism • 2%: neurosis • 1.7%: affective disorder • 1.3%: schizophrenia
Lewis et al. (9)	Developmental behavior checklist	Findings: no significant increase in epilepsy group vs. nonepilepsy group • Disruptive • Self-absorbed • Communication disturbance • Anxiety • Social relating • Antisocial
Eyman et al. (18)		• Hyperactivity • Aggression • Problems with speech • Difficulties with eating/dressing
Capes and Moore (19)		Particularly increased: • Hyperactivity • Aggression • Withdrawal
Steffenberg et al. (20)	Handicap, Behavior and Skills Schedule Childhood Autism Rating Scale Autistic Behavior Checklist Asperger Syndrome Diagnostic Checklist Global/Social and Occupational Function Assessment Scales	59%: at least one psychiatric diagnosis • 31%: self-injurious behavior • 27%: autistic disorder • 11%: autistic-like condition • 7%: ADHD • 3%: Asperger syndrome • 3%: autistic traits • 3%: overanxious disorder • 1%: stereotypy/habit disorder • 1%: elective mutism • 1%: conduct disorder • 1%: chronic motor tic disorder

exploring pathology in PWMD; of interest are the high rates of disorder as a baseline independent of the presence of epilepsy and the changing definitions of behavioral abnormalities. With such a range of populations, diverse sampling methods, and ever-changing definitions, epidemiological studies are difficult.

Prevalence of Epilepsy in PWMD

Prevalence is most affected by sampling because this correlates highly with the level of intellectual disability. The prevalence of epilepsy in PWMD ranges from 6% to 60%, with the rate being 6% to 41% in population-based studies. Of the general epilepsy population, 25% (1) to 31–41% (2, 3)) are considered to have intellectual disability. By the age of 10, the prevalence of epilepsy in PWMD is estimated to be 15%. Prevalence is also affected by the underlying etiology of the PWMD. Table 44-2 shows prevalence figures by sample including within certain known causes of multiple disabilities.

Prevalence of Behavior and Psychologic Disorder

Figures for the presentation of behavioral disturbance differ greatly by place of residence and population sampled; yet a range of prevalence from 50% to 60% seems to be reasonable. Of individuals with multiple disabilities, an estimated 40–70% have psychologic disorders.

The impact of seizure disorder on the prevalence of psychologic disturbance has provided contrasting information. The classical, and still definitive, epidemiological survey, the Isle of Wight study, showed within the pediatric population a correlation between evidence of brain damage and psychologic disturbance that was further reinforced by the addition of epilepsy.

It has been reported by some researchers (Lund [4]) that the prevalence of psychiatric disturbance increases with increasing seizure frequency in populations of people with intellectual disability. There was a prevalence of psychiatric disturbance of 56% in the active epilepsy group compared with 26% in those in remission in one study (4). In contrast other studies report no demonstrable epilepsy-associated increase in behavioral and psychiatric disturbance in this population (Corbett [5, 6]; Deb and Hunter [7, 8]; Espie et al. (9); and Lewis et al. [10]).

THE CAUSATION OF BEHAVIORAL AND PSYCHOLOGIC MORBIDITY

Understanding the potential causation of behavioral and psychologic morbidity is central to assessment and the formation of management plans.

Behavioral Phenotypes

Since the initial description of self-injurious behavior in the Lesch–Nyhan syndrome, further patterns of behavior, such as those associated with conditions such as Prader–Willi syndrome and Williams syndrome, have also been identified (see Figure 44-1). The increasing recognition of behavioral characteristics or "behavior phenotypes"—a characteristic pattern of motor, cognitive, linguistic, and social abnormalities, which is consistently associated with a biological disorder—has further developed the understanding of genetic influences on behavior.

Pharmacological Mechanisms

The potential impact of drugs on behavior in PWMD is, of course, a major concern to individuals and caregivers alike. Therefore, the assessment of potential drug effect is a key clinical competency when managing epilepsy in PWMD. Although much of the assessment, as we will discuss later, is one of objective information gathering, ideally the clinician will be guided by high-quality scientific information. Many case study and case series reports exist for the novel antiepileptic drugs (AEDs), suggesting their impact on behavior. However, direct randomized, controlled trial evidence for a negative impact on behavior from AEDs is what is needed but is rare. Where it does exist, it is hampered by a lack of valid outcome measures and relates to the more novel AEDs. Interpretation of the trial of add-on lamotrigine versus placebo in Lennox-Gastaut showed very little apparent impact on behavior (11). This study used high-quality behavioral and quality-of-life measures, and the absence of a negative impact of medication use in such a difficult population is noteworthy. Similar data were reported in a study with topiramate conducted by Sachdeo et al. (12). Although this study used less well-validated outcome measures, it did show an increase in reported behavioral disturbance (topiramate 21% vs. control 10%). A more recent placebo-controlled add-on study of topiramate in PWMD by Kerr et al. (13) showed no significant behavior deterioration when compared to controls as measured by the Aberrant Behavior Checklist.

An assessment of data from the relatively few trials in PWMD would suggest that there exist no data to confirm specific drug effect on behavior as measured, although trials are often of short duration and outcome measures poor. Notwithstanding this, the studies tend to show a side-effect distribution in PWMD similar to that in the general population. Behavior change as a direct result of side effects experienced by people unable to communicate them may, of course, be present.

Physical Illness and Pain

There is increasing evidence that PWMD with and without epilepsy experience a high morbidity, reduced life

TABLE 44-2
Prevalence of Epilepsy

SYNDROME	PREVALENCE	STUDY
Mental Retardation		
Mild (IQ 50–70)	6%	Lhatoo and Sander (1)
	15%	Ross and Peckham (21)
Moderate (IQ 35–49)	20–25%	Sillanpää (2)
Severe (IQ < 50)	24%	Lhatoo and Sander (1)
	30%	Lhatoo and Sander (1); Steffenberg et al. (20)
Profound (IQ < 20)	50%	Sillanpää (2)
		Lhatoo and Sander (1); Corbett (4, 5)
Cerebral palsy		
• Across lifespan	5–40%	Fryers and Russell (22)
• At age 17 or more cumulative risk:	9%	Forsgren (23)
• At age 5	28%	Goulden et al. (24), Lhatoo and Sander (1)
• At age 10	31%	Goulden et al. (24), Lhatoo and Sander (1)
• At age 22	38%	Goulden et al. (24), Lhatoo and Sander (1)
Down syndrome		
• Across lifespan	5–10%	Appleton (25)
• Children	1.4%	Tatsuno et al. (26)
• Age >35	12.2%	Veall (27)
Fragile X	25%	Wisniewski et al. (28)
	30–40%	Appleton (25)
Tuberous sclerosis	>60%	Hunt (29)
	80–90%	Sillanpää and Lähdetie (30)
Sturge-Weber syndrome	>70%	Bebin and Gomez. (31)
Lennox-Gastaut syndrome	Up to 90%	Aicardi (32)
West syndrome	Up to 90%	Aicardi (32)
Autistic spectrum disorder	30%	Melville and Cameron (32)
Autism		
• With mild mental retardation	5%	Melville and Cameron (33)
• With profound mental retardation	50%	Melville and Cameron (33)
PWMD with:		
Serious visual problems	10–30%	Fryers and Russell (22)
Hearing problems	Up to 5%	Fryers and Russell (22)
Serious problems with speaking	60–85%	Fryers and Russell (22)

expectancy, increased health care utilization, and poorer access to health delivery and promotion services compared with the general population (14).

The cognitive impairment and communication difficulties present in these patients result in an inability to report or adequately describe their symptoms or the distress caused by physical disorders. Symptoms of physical illness, often unidentified or misdiagnosed, may therefore manifest as behavioral and psychiatric disturbance.

Sensory stimuli such as loud noises, crowds, and bright lights, which usually pose no discomfort to cog-nitively intact individuals, can cause extreme distress to PWMD.

Socioenvironmental Mechanisms

Socioenvironmental mechanisms considered to be etiological in the behavioral and psychiatric disturbances in people with multiple disabilities and epilepsy include (1) self-stimulation, (2) social attention, (3) escape from aversive demands, and (4) obtaining access to tangible rewards. Table 44-3 highlights these areas.

PRADER-WILLI SYNDROME
Behavioral Characteristics: Neonates feed poorly (often tube-fed) and are described as hypotonic or "floppy." Overeating becomes apparent in childhood and continues into adulthood. Adults have delayed satiation of appetite. Food stealing and consumption of "unpalatable" (pet, frozen, rotting) food is not uncommon. Outbursts of temper, mood abnormalities, self-injury through skin-picking, and some other maladaptive behaviors occur more frequently than among people of the same age and sex with equivalent cognitive impairments. Repetitive speech and persistent questioning may reflect relative deficits in processing information presented aurally. Affective disorders and psychotic symptoms have been reported, sometimes with a clinical picture resembling cycloid psychoses with much greater frequency among the older disomy subtype. Obsessional and compulsive behaviors similar to those of normal childhood occur relatively frequently.

WILLIAMS SYNDROME
Behavioral Characteristics: Typical behavioral characteristics include overfriendliness, generalized anxiety, attentional problems, and hyperacusis. Visuospatial skills tend to be more severely impaired than language related skills, but auditory memory and face processing skills appear to be relatively intact. Social disinhibition and inappropriate friendliness are typical in children with Williams syndrome, and these characteristics can give rise to significant problems as adults. Mental health problems, especially related to anxiety, are also frequently reported in adults.

Adapted from http://www.ssbp.co.uk/files/syndromes (Society for the Study of Behavioural Phenotypes).

FIGURE 44-1

Behavioral phenotypes.

Epilepsy Mechanisms

There is very strong evidence for an increased prevalence of emotional disturbance in individuals with epilepsy who do not have multiple disabilities, but finding a similar link with PWMD and epilepsy has been much harder. Epidemiological evidence does not support such a population link in adults or in children. Deb and Hunter (7, 8) showed an underlying prevalence of behavioral disorder of 52.5% in patients with epilepsy and PWMD, and 58% in the non-epilepsy population. Lewis and colleagues (10), in an epidemiologically defined population of children with multiple disabilities, reported no difference in causality of behavior and emotional disturbance between those with and without epilepsy. Work by Lund (4) and other researchers, however, has shown that aggression and self-injury were associated with frequent seizures and polytherapy.

Control-Related Behavioral Change

One area of individual impact commonly arising in practice is that of an improvement in an individual's seizures seemingly leading to deterioration in behavior (see Chapter 29 on psychosis and forced normalization).

It is rare to confirm such an association when detailed recordings are obtained; however, this "paradoxical normalization" can occur, and the underlying mechanisms may be similar to those seen in the clinical phenomenon of forced normalization.

Behaviors Associated with Seizures. Peri-ictally and interictally related behavioral and psychiatric disturbance is widely described in the medical literature.

Preictal psychiatric disturbance in PWMD presents as changes in affect and behavior, unprovoked irritability, and poor frustration tolerance—symptoms that often resolve after the ictus. Ictal psychiatric phenomena, which may be too complex or strange for the patient with multiple disabilities to verbalize or conceptualize, are extremely rare and may present as confusional episodes and may be associated with nondirected aggressive behavior. Postictal psychosis is the best recognized postictal disorder in PWMD. There is usually a nonpsychotic period that ranges from a few hours to up to 1 week after a cluster of generalized tonic-clonic seizures and may often present as episodes of delirium consisting of confusional states associated with agitation, some clouding of the level of consciousness, bizarre behavior, and sleep disturbances. These episodes may last from a few hours to up to 1 month, and may remit spontaneously or their resolution may be aided by low doses of neuroleptic agents (see Chapter 29 on psychosis and forced normalization). Psychiatric disorders in PWMD, however, are most frequently seen interictally. Interictal psychosis may be difficult to separate from postictal psychosis and should be suspected in the presence of bizarre behavior. Insomnia also usually occurs early in a psychotic process. Verbal patients may be able to voice paranoid delusions and

TABLE 44-3
Stressors that May Trigger Behavioral Problems

TYPE OF STRESSOR	EXAMPLES
Transitional phases	Change of residence, new school or work place, altered route to work Development landmarks (e.g., going into puberty, achieving majority)
Interpersonal loss or rejection	Loss of parent, caregiver, friend, roommate Breakup of romantic attachment Being fired from a job or suspended from school
Environmental	Overcrowding, excessive noise, disorganization Lack of satisfactory stimulation Reduced privacy in congregate housing School or work stress
Parenting and social support problems	Lack of support from family, friends, or partner Destabilizing visits, phone calls, or letters Neglect Hostility Physical or sexual abuse
Stigmatization because of physical or intellectual problems	Taunts, teasing, exclusion, being bullied or exploited
Frustration	Due to inability to communicate needs and wishes Due to lack of choices about residence, work situation, diet Because of realization of deficits

Source: Expert Consensus Guideline Series: Treatment of Psychiatric and Behavioral Problems in Mental Retardation (34).

acknowledge hallucinations, but many patients with multiple disabilities may be unable to verbalize their positive symptoms or conceptualize them as a mental experience. Negative symptoms may present as loss of cognitive function or regression.

The recognition of interictal depressive and anxiety disorders may be difficult in PWMD for reasons mentioned earlier in this chapter. Patients experiencing these disorders may appear withdrawn and increasingly isolated, may refuse to participate in individual and group activities, may appear more irritable, and may be more prone to violent outbursts. Anxiety disorders may be suspected when patients suddenly refuse to be left alone (e.g., sleep in their own room) and are unwilling to participate in their usual activities. Many PWMD adapt to a specific routine and environment, and so any deviation from such routines may trigger marked anxiety and aggressive behavior as a way of resisting the changes. In such situations, behavioral strategies may be sufficient to reestablish their baseline behavior. However, identification of symptoms such as changes in appetite, early night insomnia, middle night or early morning awakening, or excessive somnolence may suggest an underlying endogenous psychiatric process. Attention deficit hyperactivity disorder is relatively frequent among pediatric PWMD and is among the earliest psychiatric disturbances

reported in patients with epileptic encephalopathies such as Landau-Kleffner syndrome and in autistic children. Its diagnosis is usually self-evident.

ASSESSMENT OF BEHAVIORAL OR PSYCHIATRIC DISORDERS IN THE CONTEXT OF EPILEPSY MANAGEMENT

The clinician working with PWMD and epilepsy is likely to be required to address the need for assessment in two relatively distinct areas. The first is as part of a diagnostic process in which a behavioral event must be differentiated as to whether it reflects an ictal phenomenon; the second will arise within the process of epilepsy treatment and, in the main, reflects a need to understand a behavior in the context of treatment. Recognition of the potential etiological mechanisms highlighted earlier can be helpful. Skills needed outside of usual epilepsy competencies include psychologic assessment of the functions of behavior and psychiatric assessment of PWMD.

Differentiating Epilepsy and Behavior

The process of such differentiation is, in essence, no different from that in any other epilepsy context—a clear witness history, examination, and appropriate additional investigations. As in any other epilepsy context, the full range of differential diagnosis exists including nonorganic disorders such as nonepileptic attack disorder (NEAD) and conversion disorders through to cardiac and endocrinologic disorders. The diagnosis must be based on positive evidence of epilepsy rather than a default to behavior disorder.

Most important is the diagnostic confusion that arises where the potential ictal phenomenon is one of rage or acute behavioral outburst. In this case, progress to video electroencephalograph (EEG) monitoring would be the definitive diagnostic process; however, the behavior disorder itself may militate against successful participation in investigation. In such situations clinicians must focus on a process of obtaining both objective descriptors of behavior and more detailed psychologic assessment of the behavior to differentiate it from other nonepilepsy-determined behaviors.

This involves primarily a good-quality clinical history with emphasis on the temporal sequence of events and the temporal relationship between onset of behavioral and psychiatric disturbance and seizure activity, supplemented where possible with video recording. Following an accurate description of the behavior, the next stage is an attempt to understand the behavior through functional analysis, which aims to delineate the purpose of the behavior. This is particularly important where doubt exists.

Frequently in complex cases, assessment will need a multiprofessional approach. This is particularly so for the clinic-based practice because some of the determinants of non-epilepsy-related behaviors will lie in the individual's environment and quality of care provision. So services with skills to assess such environments such as psychology, nursing, and social care may need to be involved.

Behavior in the Context of Epilepsy Treatment

It is likely that the most common clinical scenario arises during epilepsy management when the professional is called upon to assess the relative impact of epilepsy and its treatment on a particular behavioral disturbance. Most frequently this question focuses on potential impact of AEDs on behavior. As we have discussed, the relative evidence for AED effect is low whereas the evidence for preexisting social, genetic, and cognitively determined factors is high. A structured approach is recommended as we have shown in Figure 44-2. Of this, the primary aim is to (1) identify and define the apparent behavior abnormality and its chronological history, (2) assess the association with seizures, (3) assess the association with treatment, (4) assess underlying mechanisms, and (5) investigate as appropriate.

TREATMENT APPROACHES

The key treatment competencies are (1) defining a care plan, (2) exploring epilepsy or treatment-related causations, and (3) advising others on potential impacts of psychotropic interventions.

Defining a Care Plan

Because of the potential for PWMD to slip between clinical services, it is particularly important that the epileptologist is clear about the issue as to whether the behavior appears linked to epilepsy or its treatment or is believed to be independent of it. Such clarity will help nonepilepsy services provide the appropriate support and not expect solutions from the epileptologist, which will not be forthcoming. Thus, a care plan is essential. In cases in which there is no epilepsy-related causation, such a plan should (1) identify the reasons why epilepsy has been excluded as an etiological mechanism, (2) comment on future epilepsy management, and (3) offer support if the clinicians have concerns over how their management approaches may impact on epilepsy. Where epilepsy-related mechanisms are implicated, the clinician should highlight the approaches to this problem (see following) and also request appropriate support for the behavioral problem from other care services.

Exploring Epilepsy or Treatment-Related Causations

When a seizure-related mechanism is suspected, the management plan should be one of a continued search for optimal seizure control. When identifiable postictal behaviors are found, it will be worth formulating specific plans for these behaviors, including the use of benzodiazepines to modify the seizures.

When treatment-related factors are suspected, such as a drug effect, then a risk assessment must be performed as to the potential risk of drug reduction. This is relatively simple when the AED appears to have had no effect on the seizures, but it is much more difficult when significant seizure control has been achieved. In such cases the risks of withdrawal must be documented, communicated, and balanced with the risks from the behavior. Where the implicated AED has gained seizure freedom or dramatic success, it will be worth exploring treatments for the behavior or psychologic disturbance before discontinuing the AED.

Advising Others on Potential Impacts of Psychotropic Interventions

Psychotropic medication usage is high in this population. Much of this is for behavioral intervention rather

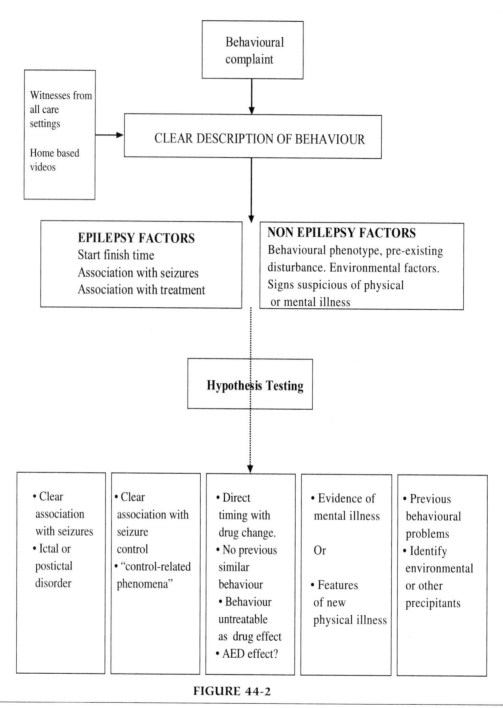

FIGURE 44-2

The assessment of behaviour in the setting of epilepsy management.

than the specific control of recognized psychiatric illness. Professionals are often using medications off-label and will need to follow professional guidance and standards in this setting.

Notwithstanding the indication, the potential impact of psychotropic medication on seizure frequency will muddy the clinical waters and is worth reviewing. All antidepressants and antipsychotic drugs have been reported to cause seizures in people without epilepsy, and

the identified factors for this observation include (1) high plasma serum concentrations, (2) rapid dose titration, (3) presence of other drugs with proconvulsant properties (4) presence of central nervous system pathology, (5) abnormal electroencephalogram, and (6) personal and family history of epilepsy.

Sensible guidance would be to (1) be alert for seizure worsening, (2) use newer medications such as selective serotonin reuptake inhibitors (SSRIs) or novel antipsychotics, and (3) always perform a thorough risk assessment and clearly identify potential seizure exacerbation as a potential danger.

In clinical practice this issue is rarely a problem, and in all likelihood more patients remain unexposed to potentially useful treatment, particularly for depression and anxiety, than have seizure deterioration as a side effect.

CONCLUSION

The ever-increasing treatment options available to people with epilepsy offer considerable hope for PWMD, but psychologic and behavioral difficulties pose considerable obstacles to realization of this hope. Clinical assessment and management in a multiprofessional manner can overcome most of these obstacles.

*R*eferences

1. Lhatoo SD, Sander JWAS. The epidemiology of epilepsy and learning disability. *Epilepsia* 2001; 42(Suppl 1):6–9.
2. Sillanpää M. Epilepsy in the mentally retarded. In: Wallace S, ed. *Epilepsy in Children.* London: Chapman and Hall, 1996:417–427.
3. Sillanpää M. Learning disability: occurrence and long-term consequences in childhood-onset epilepsy. *Epilepsy Behav* 2004; 5:937–944.
4. Lund J. Epilepsy and psychiatric disorder in the mentally retarded adult. *Acta Psychiatr Scand* 1985; 71:557–562.
5. Corbett JA. Epilepsy and mental handicap. In: Laidlaw J, Richens A, Oxley J, eds. *A Textbook of Epilepsy.* Edinburgh: Churchill Livingstone, 1988:533–538.
6. Corbett JA. Epilepsy and mental retardation. In: Trimble MR, Reynolds EH, eds. *Epilepsy and Psychiatry.* Edinburgh: Churchill Livingstone, 1981:138–146.
7. Deb S, Hunter D. Psychopathology of people with mental handicap and epilepsy. I: Maladaptive behaviour. *Br J Psychiatry* 1991; 159:822–826
8. Deb S, Hunter D. Psychopathology of people with mental handicap and epilepsy. II: Psychiatric illness. *Br J Psychiatry* 1991; 159:826–830.
9. Espie CA, Pashley ES, Bonham KG, Sourindhrin J, et al. The mentally handicapped person with epilepsy: a comparative study investigating psychosocial functioning. *J Ment Defic Res* 1989; 33:123–135.
10. Lewis JN, Tonge BJ, Mowat DR, et al. Epilepsy and associated psychopathology in young people with intellectual disability. *J Paediatr Child Health* 2000; 36:172–175.
11. Motte J, Trevathan E, Arvidsson JFV, Barrera MN, et al. Lamotrigine for generalized seizures associated with the Lennox-Gastaut syndrome. The Lamictal Lennox-Gastaut Study Group. *N Engl J Med* 1997; 337:1807–1812.
12. Sachdeo RC, Glauser TA, Ritter F, et al. A double-blind randomized trial of topiramate in Lennox-Gastaut syndrome. Topiramate YL Study Group. *Neurology* 1999; 52: 1882–1887.
13. Kerr MP, Baker GA, Brodie MJ. A randomized, double-blind, placebo-controlled trial of topiramate in adults with epilepsy and intellectual disability: impact on seizures, severity, and quality of life. *Epilepsy Behav* 2005; 7:472–480.
14. Morgan CL, Baxter H, Kerr MP. Prevalence of epilepsy and associated health service utilization and mortality among patients with intellectual disability. *Am J Ment Retard* 2003; 108:293–300.
15. Brown EC, Aman MG, Lecavalier L. Empirical classification of behavioral and psychiatric problems in children and adolescents with mental retardation. *Am J Ment Retard* 2004; 109:445–455.
16. Reid AH. Psychiatry of mental handicap: a review. *J R Soc Med* 1983; 76:587–592.

17. Rutter M, Graham P, Yule W. A neuropsychiatric study in childhood. London: Heinemann Medical, 1970.
18. Eyman RK, Moore BC, Capes L, Zachofsky T. Maladaptive behavior of institutionalized retardates with seizures. *Am J Ment Defic* 1970; 74:651–659.
19. Capes L, Moore BC. Behavior differences between seizure and non-seizure retardates. *Ariz Med* 1970; 27:74–76.
20. Steffenberg S, Gillberg C, Steffenberg U. Psychiatric disorders in children and adolescents with mental retardation and active epilepsy. *Arch Neurol* 1996; 53:904–912.
21. Ross EM, Peckham CS. School children with epilepsy. In: Parsonage M, Grant RHE, Craig AG, eds. *Advances in Epileptology; XIV Epilepsy International Symposium.* New York: Raven Press, 1983; 213–220.
22. Fryers T, Russell O. Applied epidemiology. In: Fraser W, Kerr M, eds. *Seminar Series in the Psychiatry of Learning Disabilities.* London: Gaskell, 2003:43.
23. Forsgren L. Prevalence of epilepsy in adults in northern Sweden. *Epilepsia* 1992; 33: 450–458.
24. Goulden KJ, Shinnar S, Koller H, et al. Epilepsy in children with mental retardation: a cohort study. *Epilepsia* 1991; 32:690–697.
25. Appleton R. Aetiology of epilepsy and learning disorders: specific epilepsy syndromes; genetic, chromosomal and sporadic syndromes. In: Trimble M, ed. *Learning Disability and Epilepsy.* Guildford, UK: Clarius Press, 2003:47–63.
26. Tatsuno M, Hayashi M, Iwamoto H, et al. Epilepsy in childhood Down syndrome. *Brain Dev* 1984; 6:37–44.
27. Veall RM. The prevalence of epilepsy among Mongols related to age. *J Ment Defic Res* 2000; 14:99–106.
28. Wisniewski KE, Segan SM, Miezejesji EA, et al. The Fra(X) syndrome: neurological, electro-physiological and neuropathological abnormalities. *Am J Med Genet* 1991; 38:476–480.
29. Hunt A. Development, behavior and seizures in 300 cases of tuberous sclerosis. *J Intellect Disabil Res* 1993; 37:41–51.
30. Sillanpää M, Lähdetie J. The genetics of learning disorders. In: Trimble M, ed. *Learning Disability and Epilepsy.* Guildford, UK: Clarius Press, 2003:27–46.
31. Bebin E, Gomez R. Prognosis in Sturge-Weber syndrome: comparison of unihemispheric and bihemispheric involvement. *J Child Neurol* 1988; 3:181–184.
32. Aicardi J. Epileptic syndromes in childhood. *Epilepsia* 1988; 29(Suppl 3):551–555.
33. Melville C, Cameron J. Autism. In: Fraser W, Kerr M, eds. Seminar series in the psychiatry of learning disabilities. London: Gaskell, 2003:115–134.
34. Expert Consensus Guideline Series: Treatment of psychiatric and behavioral problems in mental retardation. *Am J Ment Retard* 2000; 105:159–207.

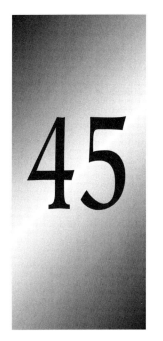

45

Family Factors and Psychopathology in Children with Epilepsy

Audrey Ho
Kevin Farrell

ehavioral problems occur more commonly in children with epilepsy than in children with other chronic diseases such as diabetes, asthma, or rheumatoid arthritis (1). Anxiety is common, particularly in adolescents, and depression is often not recognized and is left untreated. Although underlying brain dysfunction may play a role in behavioral abnormalities, family factors are also important and are more likely to be amenable to treatment. The observation that stress is associated with an increase in interictal spikes in a primate model of epilepsy (2), together with studies suggesting that management of stress may improve seizure control in children, emphasize further the importance of examining the psychosocial impact of epilepsy on the child and family (3, 4).

The diagnosis of epilepsy in a child can have a significant impact on the cognitive processing, affect, and behavior of the parents. Feelings experienced by the parents can include (1) loss of a perfect child, (2) realization that the child may always be different, and (3) a sense of stigma and fear that stigmatization may extend to other family members. Such feelings alter the dynamics of the family and influence parental behavior toward both the child with epilepsy and the siblings. Thus, the impact of the diagnosis of epilepsy in a child is not limited to the child but can extend to all family members (5).

Despite the high prevalence of psychopathology, there have been few studies on the treatment of behavioral abnormalities in children with epilepsy (6). The small number of studies resembles clinical practice, in which behavioral comorbidity is often not recognized in children with epilepsy or is considered to be an essential part of epilepsy and not treated specifically. This chapter addresses some of the family factors that may contribute to behavioral difficulties and suggests that management of psychologic comorbidity in the child and family adjustment should play an integral role in caring for the child with epilepsy (6).

THE CHILD

Children with epilepsy may exhibit a wide range of behavioral problems including depression, distractibility, inattention, hyperactivity, anxiety, and aggression (1, 6). The higher incidence of conduct disorders, attention deficit disorder, and pervasive developmental disorder in children with epilepsy complicated by other neurologic abnormalities suggests that organic brain dysfunction can play an important role (6). Disorders of attention are common in children with epilepsy but differ in some ways from those in the general childhood population. In children with attention deficit disorder attending psychiatry outpatient clinics, the male/female ratio has varied from 3:1 to 9:1, whereas a male/female ratio of 1:1 has been reported in children attending an epilepsy clinic (7). Furthermore, children with epilepsy are likely to have the inattentive type of attention deficit disorder, whereas most children attending a psychiatry clinic have the combined type (7). This may have implications for drug selection in those children in whom methylphenidate has not been effective. Although concerns have been raised that methylphenidate lowers the seizure threshold, this drug was effective in children with temporal lobe epilepsy and was not associated with an increased seizure frequency (7). A systematic study of antiepileptic drugs failed to demonstrate an effect of the drugs on behavior (8). However, certain antiepileptic drugs are associated with behavioral side effects, and the physician must remain alert to the possibility that the treatment may be contributing to behavioral difficulties.

Social factors also play an important role in behavioral difficulties in these children. Children with epilepsy may experience stigmatization, teasing, and bullying from peers and different expectations from their caregivers. Children in lower socioeconomic status appear to be at particular risk of behavioral difficulties (9). Adolescents with epilepsy are more likely to have psychiatric problems than their peers. Even the adolescents with epilepsy who scored within normal limits on a self-report questionnaire reported a higher impact of their perceived difficulties on daily life than adolescents without epilepsy (10). Perception of social stigma and a negative attitude to their disorder are factors that increase the risk of emotional difficulties. Children who have a negative attitude to their illness develop more problems related to self-concept and are more likely to develop depression, possibly as a consequence of "learned helplessness" (9).

It is also important to consider factors that influence the resilience of children in adverse situations. Good seizure control is one of the strongest predictors of improved behavior. In a longitudinal study of children with new-onset seizures, there was a trend for behavioral difficulties to improve in children who had no further seizures and to remain unchanged in those with recurrence of seizures (1). Studies have failed to demonstrate a clear association between the age of the child and the behavioral difficulties. This may reflect their use of chronological age as the variable studied. The psychologic maturation of the child at the onset of the epilepsy may be a more important predictor of coping and resilience. Thus, resilience and coping may be influenced by psychologic factors such as (1) the child's stage of premorbid organization of personality, (2) the child's resourcefulness and vulnerabilities, and (3) the child's cognitive capacity for understanding the complex nature of epilepsy and the implications of the diagnosis (11). Stresses within the family also influence the ability of the child to cope and increase the risk of behavioral problems. Similarly, how the family perceives epilepsy and interacts with the child may play an important role, and these are discussed in the following section. Whereas many studies have examined factors that increase the risk of behavioral problems, there are fewer studies that have examined resilience and how children with epilepsy cope successfully.

THE FAMILY

Parental Coping and Psychopathology

People who feel that they have some control over the events of their lives are better able to cope with stress than those who feel that their lives are determined by external forces. Parents usually experience a degree of shock at the time of the seizure and at the time of the diagnosis. This is often followed by a fear of the stigma associated with epilepsy. In parents who perceive that epilepsy has eroded their personal control, the fear of a further seizure may be a constant reminder of their initial traumatic experience. Thus, in one study, 31% of parents of children with epilepsy met the criteria for posttraumatic stress disorder, a prevalence similar to that in parents of children with potentially life-threatening illness (12). Furthermore, 32–37% of mothers of children with epilepsy score above the clinical cutoffs for depression (1, 13, 14).

Parental uncertainty as to what extent the child's behavior is influenced by either seizures or medications may also compromise the ability of the parent to have a set of expectations for the child and to establish reasonable rules for the management of certain behaviors. This may have an impact on children with epilepsy, who have been demonstrated to have a lower self-concept and higher level of depressive symptoms when the parents differ in their perception of the child's ability to cope (15). Studies on other chronic health conditions have also demonstrated that families are more likely to be overwhelmed when the parents have different approaches to parenting (15). When role ambiguity was less, mothers of children with epilepsy were better able to cope and had more self-esteem and better psychologic well-being (16). Similarly, uncertainty in the father compromises his ability to cope and is predictive of paternal depression (17). The lack of clarity in the child's role within the family makes it more difficult to determine new and appropriate roles and tasks within the family and is positively correlated with difficulty in parenting and maternal depression. It is therefore not surprising that parents often perceive that they lack competence in their parenting (18).

The parents' psychologic well-being and their sense of control over events have a significant impact on psychopathology in the child with epilepsy. Depression occurs in approximately one-third of parents of children with epilepsy, and there is a significant correlation between maternal depression and psychopathology in the child (13, 19–21). Similarly, lack of parental confidence in child discipline is a strong predictor of behavior problems in children with epilepsy (22). Lack of information on epilepsy is an important and potentially preventable family stressor that may contribute to family stress and maladjustment (5, 23). Although most studies have involved mainly mothers, studies examining paternal attitudes suggest that they also have considerable problems (17). This emphasizes the importance of epilepsy education, which ideally should include the entire family.

Parent–Child Relationship

The parent–child relationship can have a significant impact on the behavior of children with epilepsy. Maternal warmth correlates significantly with lower levels of antisocial behavior and somatic complaints. Similarly, positive remarks by the mother are associated with lower levels of neuroticism, somatic problems, and depression (13). In contrast, maternal criticism is associated with higher levels of overall psychiatric disturbances and antisocial behavior (13). Furthermore, the child's rating of parental overcontrol correlates directly with higher levels of depression, impulsiveness, and home and school behavior problems (24). Several studies support this observation, and children do less well in families that are overcontrolling (9, 22).

In a literature review of 35 studies between 1970 and 2004 that examined family factors and psychopathology in children with epilepsy, interactions between parent and child were considered to exert the greatest influence on child psychopathology (25). Parents of children with epilepsy tended to be less supportive than parents of healthy children. Fathers were less affectionate and less performance oriented, and both fathers and mothers were less stimulating. In addition, the parents tended to favor the child with epilepsy, had problems limit setting, and demonstrated more inconsistency in parenting that child.

Family Cohesiveness

The help and support that the family provide for one another plays an important role in the child's behavior. Measures of conflict and cohesion within the family were considered a major predictor of negative outcome in one study (26). Similarly, children with high scores in inattention, hyperactivity, social dysfunction, and thought disturbance were more likely to be from a family that scored high on the conflict dimension and low on the cohesion dimension of the Family Relations Index (26). This is significant in that families of children with epilepsy tend to be more rigid and less close than control families and

seem to have more problems with family functioning and family stress than control families (25). Family cohesiveness shows a negative correlation with seizure frequency and seizure duration (26). A causal relationship has not been demonstrated, but it has been speculated that the emotional climate of the family might have an impact on seizure frequency. Animal studies have demonstrated that psychosocial stress may correlate with interictal discharges. Thus, Lockard (2) observed that monkeys low in the social hierarchy had more epileptic discharges when exposed to dominant monkeys in the group.

Parental Perception, Parenting Differences, and Marital Conflict. Family members of children with epilepsy report high levels of depression, anger, guilt, helplessness, and frustration (5). More than 20% of mothers who had children with epilepsy had histories of nervous breakdowns (27). Thus, epilepsy in a young family member places the entire family at risk for problems involving family communication, cohesion, and integration (28).

Mothers have been the main caregivers in most studies (29), and there have been relatively few studies of fathers. Emotional overinvolvement by the mother with the child who has epilepsy is relatively common. This may result in overprotectiveness and lead to emotional immaturity, poor social skills, and difficulty in the child's ability to make normal peer relationships (5). Fathers of children with epilepsy, but not mothers, report a lack of competence in parenting when compared with parents of healthy children. In addition, fathers of children with epilepsy have expectations of the child that exceed their child's actual abilities to a much greater extent than fathers of unaffected children (30). This emphasizes the importance of including the father in the epilepsy education.

The parents' belief system and personalities can influence their interpretation of epilepsy and their reactions (31). When parents have different perceptions of epilepsy, this can have an impact on their expectations and their approaches to parenting. These can result in interparental conflict on how the child's behavior should be managed, which leads to increased stress on the family and child. For example, differences in how each parent perceives the child's ability to cope can lead to delays in obtaining support for the child or may result in a parent not being willing to participate in family or marital therapy (15). Sheeran et al. (32) also observed that the husbands of mothers who had difficulties dealing with the stress engendered at the time of the diagnosis perceived less cohesion and affection in their marriage. When parents differ in their perceptions and expectations of the child, there is a risk that a parent–child coalition might develop instead of the more ideal parental coalition. In such a situation, the child's relationship with one parent may be very different from his or her relationship with the other parent. This may not be ideal in that family system theory suggests that strong cross-generational coalitions may be detrimental to the well-being of family members and to the family unit as a whole. The most damaging aspect of such coalitions is that the parental behavior in parent–child interactions is likely to be in response to the parent's needs rather than the needs of the child (15, 33). Thus, children with epilepsy and behavior problems are more likely than other children with epilepsy to live in families characterized by marital conflict, divorce, or psychopathology in other family members (34). Despite the acceptance that problems with family functioning are more common when a child has epilepsy, there have been very few studies of marital conflict, one of the most important contextual variables related to child psychopathology, in families of children with epilepsy (25).

Effect on Siblings.   The diagnosis of epilepsy often has an underrecognized impact on siblings, who may observe the seizures and the reaction of their parents to the seizures. The siblings will also be affected by the parental adjustment to the diagnosis of epilepsy and, if they attend the same school, may experience the reactions of the school staff and of other students at the school. In a study of children between 8 and 12 years of age, the siblings reported concerns about their brother or sister getting hurt or dying as a result of a seizure, and the younger siblings more often reported feeling left out (35). Friends, school teachers, and even relatives may see the family as a unit and "parenticize" the siblings, looking to them for information or support. Even siblings of children with infrequent seizures report concern that people might make fun of them because of their brother's or sister's seizures. They also express concerns that they did not know what to do if their sibling has a seizure. One might expect that siblings would have less time and stimulation from their mothers especially at the time of the initial diagnosis and if the child has complicated epilepsy. However, although the nurturance and support received by siblings is usually less, parental expectations in terms of school performance and socialization often remain high (28, 36). Thus, siblings face the additional challenge of less care and nurturance and the elevated expectations of the parents. This may explain the increased incidence of externalizing behaviors in siblings of children with frequent seizures (35). In our experience, siblings often feel that the time spent with them by the parents is much more limited. Furthermore, they often perceive that their sporting and social activities are curtailed because of the time demands of the child with epilepsy. Finally, siblings often indicate that the parents are not sensitive to their needs. We encourage parents to set aside one-to-one time with the other children and to be aware that all family members are often affected by the diagnosis. It is also important that the siblings receive some appropriate information on the child's epilepsy. In our experience,

siblings exhibiting behavioral difficulties often demonstrate a substantial improvement when a professional explains to them some of the basic facts about epilepsy and how it might affect the child with epilepsy.

SUPPORT SYSTEMS

The resourcefulness of the parent may play an important role in overcoming the demands of parenting a child with epilepsy (5). Mothers with college education had a lower level of depression compared to mothers with high school or lower education (16). Similarly, mothers who were optimistic dealt more effectively with the negative social stigma of epilepsy, helped their child more to accept the diagnosis, and also established more appropriate goals for the child's development and growth (16). Families who are able to deal with the child's epilepsy and feel confident that they can manage their child's problems transfer this confidence to the child and improve the quality of life of the child and family. Lack of information or education about epilepsy and an unclear expectation of the child's functioning can lead mothers to experience significant mental distress and become overinvolved (16).

Lack of support in the family or extended family can undermine parents and create distress for mothers. Families of children with epilepsy have significantly less family resources, such as extended family social support, than families of children with asthma (37). Low-income families and single-parent families are particularly vulnerable (10). In contrast, the mental health of the mother is enhanced by family members who have adequate emotional boundaries and whose roles and functions are clear to each other (38, 39).

A supportive attitude by the school can have a significant impact on the psychologic well-being of the child and family. Children older than 4 years are in school for 6 hours on a school day, and parents have fewer concerns if they perceive the school to be a safe and supportive environment. Furthermore, the attitude of the school staff may influence positively the development of social skills and academic achievement. Education of teachers and students in the classroom can influence their attitude to the child with epilepsy and limit stigma. A more positive attitude taken by the school staff toward a child with epilepsy is likely to lessen the teasing and bullying that can occur. School staffs that are afraid of handling seizures are more likely to develop rigid rules and regulations and call parents after the slightest change in the child's condition. This can have a major impact on the daily routine of parents, who feel they have to be always on call to the school. Despite the obvious importance of school support for children with epilepsy, there are limited data on its impact on school attendance, academic and social development, and adjustment in children with epilepsy. For the school to address the needs of the child with epilepsy, the teachers must have a clear understanding of the diagnosis and its implications. Thus, the process of epilepsy education should include the school staff as well as the child and family members. Children with learning difficulties should have a psychoeducational assessment to guide the development of an individual educational plan.

CONCLUSION

The diagnosis of epilepsy can have a profound psychologic effect on the child and family. Family dynamics can be markedly disrupted, and family members often experience psychologic distress. Professionals dealing with children with epilepsy often fail to recognize the extent of psychopathology in the child and family, and active management of these issues occurs infrequently. This is likely to compromise the emotional development of the child and family and may even have an impact on seizure control. Education of the child, family, and school staff should be an integral part of the care for children with epilepsy. In addition, the psychologic well-being of the child and other family members should be monitored and treatment instituted when required. In our experience, involvement of a psychologist in the management of families with psychologic symptoms can have a profound effect on the behavior of the child with epilepsy and on the family.

References

1. Dunn DW. Neuropsychiatric aspects of epilepsy in children. *Epilepsy Behav* 2003; 4:101–106.
2. Lockard JS. Social primate model of epilepsy. In: Lockard JS, Ward AA, eds. *Epilepsy: A Window To Brain Mechanisms*. New York: Raven Press, 1980:165–190.
3. Schmid-Schonbein C. Improvement of seizure control by psychological methods in patients with intractable epilepsies. *Seizure* 1998; 7:261–270.
4. McCusker CG, Hicks EM. Psychological management of intractable seizures in an adolescent with a learning disability. *Seizure* 1999; 8:358–360.
5. Ellis N, Upton D, Thompson P. Epilepsy and the family: a review of current literature. *Seizure* 2000; 9:22–30.
6. Davies S, Heyman I, Goodman R. A population survey of mental health problems in children with epilepsy. *Dev Med Child Neurol* 2003; 45:292–295.
7. Dunn DW, Austin JK, Harezlak J, Ambrosius WT. ADHD and epilepsy in childhood. *Dev Med Child Neurol* 2003; 45:50–54.
8. Bourgeois BF. Antiepileptic drugs, learning, and behavior in childhood epilepsy. *Epilepsia* 1998; 39:913–921.
9. Dunn DW, Austin JK. Differential diagnosis and treatment of psychiatric disorders in children and adolescents with epilepsy. *Epilepsy Behav* 2004; 5(Suppl 3):S10–S17.
10. Lossius MI, Clench-Aas J, van Roy B, Mowinckel P, et al. Psychiatric symptoms in adolescents with epilepsy in junior high school in Norway: a population survey. *Epilepsy Behav* 2006; 9:286–292.
11. Noeker M, Haverkamp-Krois A, Haverkamp F. Development of mental health dysfunction in childhood epilepsy. *Brain Dev* 2005; 27:5–16.
12. Iseri PK, Ozten E, Aker AT. Posttraumatic stress disorder and major depressive disorder is common in parents of children with epilepsy. *Epilepsy Behav* 2006; 8:250–255.
13. Hodes M, Garralda ME, Rose G, Schwartz R. Maternal expressed emotion and adjustment in children with epilepsy. *J Child Psychol Psychiatry* 1999; 40:1083–1093.
14. Shore CP, Austin JK, Huster GA, Dunn DW. Identifying risk factors for maternal depression in families of adolescents with epilepsy. *J Spec Pediatr Nurs* 2002; 7: 71–80.
15. Haber LC, Austin JK, Huster GR, Lane KA, et al. Relationships between differences in mother-father perceptions and self-concept and depression in children with epilepsy. *J Fam Nurs* 2003; 9:59–78.
16. Mu PF, Kuo HC, Chang KP. Boundary ambiguity, coping patterns and depression in mothers caring for children with epilepsy in Taiwan. *Int J Nurs Stud* 2005; 42:273–282.
17. Mu PF. Paternal reactions to a child with epilepsy: uncertainty, coping strategies, and depression. *J Adv Nurs* 2005; 49:367–376.
18. Pulsifer MB, Gordon JM, Brandt J, Vining EP, et al. Effects of ketogenic diet on development and behavior: preliminary report of a prospective study. *Dev Med Child Neurol* 2001; 43:301–306.
19. Hoare P. Psychiatric disturbance in the families of epileptic children. *Dev Med Child Neurol* 1984; 26:14–19.
20. Hoare P, Kerley S. Psychosocial adjustment of children with chronic epilepsy and their families. *Dev Med Child Neurol* 1991; 33:201–215.
21. Shore CP, Austin JK, Dunn DW. Maternal adaptation to a child's epilepsy. *Epilepsy Behav* 2004; 5:557–568.
22. Austin JK, Dunn DW, Johnson CS, Perkins SM. Behavioral issues involving children and adolescents with epilepsy and the impact of their families: recent research data. *Epilepsy Behav* 2004; 5(Suppl 3):S33–S41.
23. Beech L. Knowledge of epilepsy among relatives of the epilepsy sufferer. *Seizure* 1992; 1:133–135.
24. Carlton-Ford S, Miller R, Nealeigh N, Sanchez N. The effects of perceived stigma and psychological over-control on the behavioural problems of children with epilepsy. *Seizure* 1997; 6:383–391.
25. Rodenburg R, Meijer AM, Dekovic M, Aldenkamp AP. Family factors and psychopathology in children with epilepsy: a literature review. *Epilepsy Behav* 2005; 6:488–503.
26. McCusker CG, Kennedy PJ, Anderson J, Hicks EM, et al. Adjustment in children with intractable epilepsy: importance of seizure duration and family factors. *Dev Med Child Neurol* 2002; 44:681–687.
27. Rutter M, Graham P, Yule WA. A neuropsychiatric study in childhood. Philadelphia: JB Lippincott, 1970.
28. Ferrari M, Matthews WS, Barabas G. The family and the child with epilepsy. *Fam Process* 1983; 22:53–59.
29. Levin R, Banks S, Berg B. Psychosocial dimensions of epilepsy: a review of the literature. *Epilepsia* 1988; 29:805–816.
30. Kitamoto I, Kurokawa T, Tomita S, Maeda Y, et al. Child-parent relationships in the care of epileptic children. *Brain Dev* 1988; 10:36–40.
31. Miller L. The epilepsy patient: personality, psychodynamics, and psychotherapy. *Psychotherapy* 1994; 31:735–743.
32. Sheeran T, Marvin RS, Pianta RC. Mothers' resolution of their child's diagnosis and self-reported measures of parenting stress, marital relations, and social support. *J Pediatr Psychol* 1997; 22:197–212.
33. Christensen A, Margolin G. Conflict and alliance in distressed and non-distressed families. In: Hinde RA, Stevenson-Hide J, eds. *Relationships within Families: Mutual Influences*. New York: Oxford University Press, 1988:263–283.
34. Oostrom KJ, Schouten A, Kruitwagen CL, Peters AC, et al., Dutch Study Group of Epilepsy in Childhood. Behavioral problems in children with newly diagnosed idiopathic or cryptogenic epilepsy attending normal schools are in majority not persistent. *Epilepsia* 2003; 44:97–106.
35. Mims J. Self-esteem, behavior, and concerns surrounding epilepsy in siblings of children with epilepsy. *J Child Neurol* 1997; 12:187–192.
36. Long CG, Moore JR. Parental expectations for their epileptic children. *J Child Psychol Psychiatry* 1979; 20:299–312.
37. Austin JK, McDermott N. Parental attitude and coping behaviors in families of children with epilepsy. *J Neurosci Nurs* 1988; 20:174–179.
38. Burr WR, Klein SR. Reexamining family stress: new theory and research. Thousand Oaks, CA: Sage, 1994.
39. McCubbin WR, Dahl B. Marriage and family: individuals and life cycle. New York: Wiley, 1985.

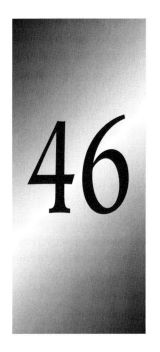

46 Learning and Behavior: Neurocognitive Functions in Children

Pirkko Nieminen
Kai Juhani Eriksson

his chapter will focus on the cognitive and neuropsychologic functioning in children and adolescents up to the age of 16 years with "epilepsy only," which is defined usually as a condition without any other neurologic signs or symptoms than seizures and without evident cognitive disabilities. We include all seizure, epilepsy, and syndrome types other than those with known association of severe cognitive or psychiatric disorders (e.g., Lennox-Gastaut and Landau-Kleffner syndromes) or major risk for significant developmental problems (e.g., West syndrome).

Epilepsy is one of the most common chronic neurologic conditions in childhood with a prevalence ranging from 3 to 6 per 1,000 (1) and an incidence of 25–100 per 100,000 per year, highest in children under the age of 3 years. Children with epilepsy are at an increased risk for developing cognitive and neuropsychologic problems, but they cannot be considered as a single group with a single disorder. Epilepsy in this age range is a heterogeneous condition, with evident additional neurodeficits such as mental retardation or cerebral palsy in up to 30% of all cases in population-based studies (2). However, more specific neuropsychologic problems have been described also in children with benign and idiopathic epilepsies and syndromes (e.g., rolandic epilepsy), and they have practical implications. These must be addressed in the clinical management of childhood epilepsy, which has goals such as seizure freedom and support of the motor, social, and neurocognitive development of the child.

DEVELOPING FUNCTIONS, DEVELOPING BRAIN, AND DEVELOPING CHILD

The effects of epilepsy on child development, learning, and behavior constitute a complex subject because all developing systems change over time. The development of the brain, the development of neurocognitive functions connected to brain development, and the development of social interactions between a growing child and her parents, siblings, and other meaningful people and even physical environment are greatly connected in the process of development. Thus it is scientifically a very difficult task to identify the meaningful factors during development. One way to approach the problem is to try to control some of these factors. Because epilepsy is often connected with various other diseases and dysfunctions, it is not surprising that the results of the studies about epilepsy and cognitive functions are contradictory and vary greatly. From clinical practice we know that there are children who are doing quite well in spite of epilepsy and there are children with many difficulties. Our focus to the problem is looking at the children with "epilepsy only."

The brain and brain functions are developing most rapidly in the first years and decades of life. Seizures and their treatment may interfere with the essential skills emerging at the age of epilepsy onset and thereafter. The immature brain has the capacity of reorganizing around insulted areas, thus rendering the damage less impairing, but this diminishes during maturation. Seizures and their treatment interfere with brain functions by overactivation, interruption, inhibition, and restructuring of vital functional pathways. Long and frequent seizures may alter neural circuits and neurotransmitter balances. This is seen especially in limbic systems (3).

Factors related to epilepsy may distort developmental processes in the developing brain, yet the developing brain may be able to overcome such distortions by alternative development processes. The developed brain is essentially matured and thus not apt to experience developmental disorders. However, any damage done at this age is a loss, because mature brain is limited in its ability to recover functions (3).

The brain is especially sensitive to insults in the earliest years of life. Recovery may be gained with age, but in part this may be more of compensation and rewiring of the developing nervous system. Children with severe seizure disorders in infancy are often more functionally handicapped than those with seizures of onset later in childhood, who again may be more handicapped than those with adolescent age at seizure onset.

From the brain development aspect the effects of epilepsy are connected to factors such as timing at onset of epilepsy; for example, what neuropsychologic functions are most actively developing at the time? The frequency of seizures is also important, of course, because frequent seizures do not allow time for the brain to recover.

When considering the cognitive, learning, and behavioral outcomes of childhood epilepsy, one way of approaching the problem is to study the psychologic and neuropsychologic development of the child and try to find out which functions are most vulnerable to the effects of epilepsy at different ages. We know the development of motor and language functions quite well, and we have good normative data and methods to assess the development. Our knowledge of the development of attention, executive functions, memory, and even visuospatial functions is not at all that precise. So it is much more difficult, from the developmental point of view, to consider the possible difficulties epilepsy brings to development.

The demands of environment and the challenges that family and social environment offer are also important when considering how children with "epilepsy only" in early childhood, school age, and adolescence solve their developmental tasks and gain social competency to manage later on in their life in society. So there is a complex interdependence of several neurologic, psychologic, and social factors influencing one another at the same time, and it is extremely difficult to isolate their individual impacts during development (4).

GENERAL COGNITIVE FUNCTIONS

Factors Contributing to Neurocognitive Functioning

The factors contributing to neurocognitive impairment in children with epilepsy are multifactorial, including, for example, the underlying etiology and neuropathology, electroencephalographic (EEG) discharges and seizures, antiepileptic drugs, and various psychosocial factors. Poor cognitive outcome is generally associated with early onset, long duration of the disease, and poor seizure control. There is evidence that cognitive functions may be impaired already at the onset of the disease, and that the maturation of cognitive functions in children is susceptible to the adverse influence of epilepsy (5).

Early age at onset of epilepsy can be regarded as one of the major risk factors for later impaired neurocognitive development. This might be due to the fact that this age is an era of rapid motor, social, and cognitive development, and early onset of seizures is likely to be associated with longer duration of the epilepsy. Also, seizure or epilepsy syndrome types at an early age are more often severe and symptomatic. Childhood is also a sensitive time period in the development of the central nervous system (CNS); that is, synaptogenesis and myelogenesis are active processes related to CNS maturation that can be disrupted by seizures, even by discharges. In clinical studies, early onset of temporal lobe epilepsy (6) has been associated with adverse neurodevelopmental impact on brain structure (white matter tissue volume loss) and cognition (full-scale IQ and verbal and nonverbal memory).

General Intelligence

The prevalence of cognitive, psychiatric, and behavioral disorders in children with epilepsy, as a group, is increased, and some of these difficulties have been described also in children with "epilepsy only." However, not all follow-up studies have observed clear differences between children with "epilepsy only" and age-matched controls in cognitive and behavioral performance over time; nonetheless, the results of a study with prospective, population-based methodology (7) imply that children even with idiopathic epilepsy are at risk for learning problems, regardless of normal IQ. Even though the intelligence scores have been found to be slightly lower in children with epilepsy compared to their siblings and children with migraine in follow-up studies, this difference has been shown to be quite stable (8).

Prognosis of Cognitive Functioning

A review of longitudinal cognitive studies in children and adolescents (9) on the neuropsychologic effects of seizures and epilepsies, having formal psychologic testing both at the beginning and at the end of the study, concludes that there is a mild but definite relationship between seizures and mental decline, but that future studies should include better assessment of the types and frequencies of seizures experienced. The cognitive effects of single seizures would need extensive study periods (more than 25 years). Cognitive studies should also include matched control groups for age and education, because developmental and aging changes should be considered in longitudinal investigations.

Long-term prognoses in idiopathic generalized and nonsymptomatic focal epilepsies and syndromes (5) include the following:

- Mild frontal lobe deficits with largely unknown but presumably favorable long-term outcome in juvenile myoclonic epilepsy
- Mild attentional problems with largely unknown outcome in generalized epilepsies with absence or generalized tonic-clonic seizures
- Mild heterogeneous deficits, with presumably favorable outcome, in idiopathic focal syndromes such as benign epilepsy with centrotemporal spikes (rolandic epilepsy) and occipital-lobe epilepsies
- Impaired executive and attentional functions with largely unknown outcome in nonsymptomatic frontal lobe epilepsies
- Material-specific episodic memory impairment with very slow deterioration in temporal lobe epilepsies
- Largely unknown and variable with unknown or heterogeneous outcome in parieto-occipital epilepsies

The general neurocognitive functioning of school-aged children with "epilepsy only" does not seem to differ significantly from age norms in formal neuropsychologic testing, but because of the heterogeneous nature of epilepsy and many confounding factors, future studies should focus on larger cohorts of children from different age groups and different epilepsy and syndrome types using matched control groups to determine those factors that can have impact on the neurocognitive performance at the individual level.

To predict the risk for neurocognitive problems in children with "epilepsy only" based on medical factors remains very difficult. Therefore, careful monitoring of educational progress and individual neuropsychologic tests when necessary should be included in the follow-up of children with epilepsy—especially of those children with learning problems at school—because the support for neurologic and cognitive development is an essential part of treating epilepsy in childhood.

SPECIFIC NEUROPSYCHOLOGIC FUNCTIONS

Neuropsychologic dysfunctions are not rare in children with idiopathic epilepsy who have normal IQs (10); the most common findings are deficits in memory and attention, mental slowing, slow reaction times, and problems in alertness; see for example, Aldenkamp et al. (11); Gulgönen et al. (12); and Aldenkamp and Arends (13). Difficulties have also been found in language functions (14) and visuomotor coordination (15). There are also studies, however, in which no dysfunctions have been found. Intact verbal memory and language functions were reported by Pavone et al. (16) and Boelen et al. (17), who found no differences between overall psychomotor development compared to controls. The findings are still controversial. We next take a more detailed look at the studies concerning problems in attention, memory, and language functions among children with "epilepsy only."

Attention

Attention is a construct of many subfunctions rather than a single special neurocognitive function. It is closely related to memory and executive functions (18). Attention refers to a general state of arousal, vigilance, and alertness—selective, focused, and sustained attention. Up to 60% of children attending an epilepsy clinic may have attentional problems (19). Alertness may be impaired unrelated to the seizure type or EEG activity. Studies that try to avoid the selection bias toward the more severe end of spectrum of childhood epilepsy show that epilepsy may be associated with specific deficits in attention unrelated to factors such as IQ or treatment (20). Also, in studies in which results indicate that neurocognitive functions in general are within expectations, the tasks that make use of verbal and visual attention skills are performed relatively more poorly, suggesting a special attentional impairment (14).

Studies of children with benign rolandic epilepsy (21) and children with other new-onset idiopathic epilepsies before formal diagnosis and without therapy (22) have shown that these children have more problems in attention tasks, but the differences were minor and were not seen in all domains of attention tested.

As Deonna et al. (23) point out, however, some children with focal epilepsies and a significant cognitive deficit may have fully preserved attentional capacities, indicating that epilepsy in general does not necessarily impinge on attentional mechanisms. In focal epilepsies of frontal origin, attentional deficits are a major problem—sometimes initially the only problem before other deficits become evident. Inattentiveness may be seen in "functional" focal epilepsies as in rolandic epilepsies.

Cognition and attention are closely related. In a critical review Sanchez-Carpintero and Neville (24) sum

factors are early onset, poor seizure control, high frequency and long duration of seizures, ineffective medication, and little support from the family. The findings concerning individual seizure-related factors of epilepsy and neurocognitive functioning are inconsistent (38), and one cannot find a single neuropsychologic profile among children with "epilepsy only." The picture is still quite diffuse, and more research work is needed.

The psychologic consequences of the epileptic disease for the child and the family are sometimes more important in children with mainly cognitive-behavioral manifestations of epilepsy, in whom seizures may be rare and not the main concern. In these situations,

psychologic reactions to the disease must be differentiated from quite similar symptoms that can be understood and explained as a direct effect of epilepsy (23). As Aicardi (39) writes:

... harmful effects are not entirely, or even mainly, the result of the cause of the epilepsy condition, or of the psychological consequences, but mostly the result of interference of chronic epileptic activity with neuronal function, with maturation, with post-synaptic structure and organization that may be sufficient, at the behavioral level, to preclude, transiently or permanently, a child's ability to normally interact with his/her environment and with learning.

References

1. Eriksson KJ, Koivikko MJ. Prevalence, classification, and severity of epilepsy and epileptic syndromes in children. *Epilepsia* 1997; 38:1275–1282.
2. Sillanpää M. Epilepsy in children: prevalence, disability, and handicap. *Epilepsia* 1992; 33:444–449.
3. Svoboda WB. Childhood epilepsy, language, learning and behavioral complications. Cambridge, UK: Cambridge University Press, 2004.
4. Andersson V, Northam E, Hendy J, Wrennall J. Developmental neuropsychology: a clinical approach. Hove, UK: Psychology Press, 2001.
5. Elger CE, Helmstaedter C, Kurthen M. Chronic epilepsy and cognition. *Lancet Neurol* 2004; 3:663–672.
6. Hermann B, Seidenberg M, Bell B, Rutecki P, et al. The neurodevelopmental impact of childhood-onset temporal lobe epilepsy on brain structure and function. *Epilepsia* 2002; 43:1062–1071.
7. Bailet LL, Turk WR. The impact of childhood epilepsy on neurocognitive and behavioral performance: A prospective longitudinal study. *Epilepsia* 2000; 41:426–431.
8. Deonna T, Zesiger P, Davidoff V, Maeder M, et al. Benign partial epilepsy of childhood. A longitudinal neuropsychological and EEG study of cognitive function. *Dev Med Child Neurol* 2000; 42:595–603.
9. Dodrill CB. Neuropsychological effects of seizures. *Epilepsy Behav* 2004; 5:21–24.
10. Sturniolo MG, Galletti F. Idiopathic epilepsy and school achievement. *Arch Dis Child* 1994; 70:424–428.
11. Aldenkamp AP, Overweg-Plandsoen WCG, Diepman LAM. Factors involved in learning problems and educational delay in children with epilepsy. *Child Neuropsychol* 1999; 5:130–136.
12. Gulgönen S, Demirbilek V, Korkmaz B, Dervent A, et al. Neuropsychological functions in idiopathic occipital lobe epilepsy. *Epilepsia* 2000; 41:405–411.
13. Aldenkamp AP, Arends J. Effects of epileptiform EEG discharges on cognitive function: Is the concept of "transient cognitive impairment" still valid? *Epilepsy Behav* 2004;5;25–35.
14. Williams J, Griebel ML, Dykman RA. Neuropsychological patterns in pediatric epilepsy. *Seizure* 1998; 7:223–228.
15. Hiementz JR, Hynd GW, Jimenez M. Seizure disorders. In: Brown RT, ed. *Cognitive Aspects of Chronic Illness in Children.* New York: The Guilford Press, 1999:238–261.
16. Pavone P, Bianchini R, Trifiletti RR, Incorpora G, et al. Neuropsychological assessment in children with absence epilepsy. *Neurology* 2001; 5:1047–1051.
17. Boelen S, Nieuenhuis S, Steenbeek L, Veldwijk H, et al. Effect of epilepsy on psychomotor function in children with uncomplicated epilepsy. *Dev Med Child Neurol* 2005:47; 546–550.
18. Mirsky AF. Disorders of attention, a neurological perspective. In: Lyon GR, Knasnegor NA, eds. *Attention, Memory and Executive Function.* Baltimore, MD: Paul H. Bookers, 1996:71–95.
19. Williams JP, Sharp GB, Griebel MI. Neuropsychological functioning in clinically referred children with epilepsy. *Epilepsia* 1992; 33(Suppl 3):17 (abstract).
20. Mitchell WG, Zhou Y, Chavez JM, Guzman BL. Reaction time, attention and impulsivity in epilepsy. *Pediatr Neurol* 1992:8;19–24.
21. Chevalier H, Metz-Lutz MN, Segalowitz SJ. Impulsivity and control of inhibition in benign focal childhood epilepsy. *Brain Cogn* 2000; 43:86–90.
22. Schouten A, Oostrom KJ, Pestman WR, Peters ACB. School career of children with epilepsy, who are otherwise healthy, is at risk before diagnosis of "epilepsy only." *Dev Med Child Neurol* 2001; 43:575–576.
23. Deonna T, Roulet-Perez E, Mayor-Dubois C. Childhood neuropsychology (developmental cognitive neuropsychology) in the context of epilepsy. In: Deonna T, Roulet-Perez E, eds. *Cognitive and Behavioral Disorders of Epileptic Origin in Children.* Cambridge, UK: Mac Keith Press/Cambridge University Press, 2005.
24. Sanchez-Carpintero R, Neville BGR. Attentional ability in children with epilepsy. *Epilepsia* 2003; 10:1340–1349.
25. Kadis DS, Stollstorff M, Elliott I, Lach L, et al. Cognitive and psychological predictors of everyday memory in children with intractable epilepsy. *Epilepsy Behav* 2004; 5:37–43.
26. Nolan MA, Redoblado MA, Lah S, Sabaz M, et al. Memory function in childhood epilepsy syndromes. *J Pediatr Child Health* 2004; 40:20–27.
27. Oostrom KJ, Teeseling VH, Smeets-Shouten A, Peters ACB, et al. Three to four years after diagnosis: cognition and behaviours in children with "epilepsy only"—a prospective, longitudinal, controlled study. *Brain* 2005; 128:1546–1555.
28. Henkin Y, Sadeh M, Kivity S, Shabati E., et al. Cognitive function in idiopathic generalized epilepsy of childhood. *Dev Med Child Neurol* 2005; 47:126–132.
29. Northcott E, Connolly AM, Berroya A, Sabaz M, et al. The neuropsychological and language profile of children with benign rolandic epilepsy. *Epilepsia* 2005; 46:924–930.
30. Cohen H, Le Normand M-TRS. Language development in children with simple partial left hemisphere epilepsy. *Brain Lang* 1998; 64:409–422.
31. Breier JI, Flechter JM, Wheless JW, Clark A, et al. Profiles of cognitive performance associated with reading disability in temporal lobe epilepsy. *J Clin Exp Neuropsychol* 2000; 22:804–816.
32. Leonard EL, George MRM. Psychosocial and neuropsychological function in children with epilepsy. *Pediatr Rehabil* 1999; 3:73–80.
33. Williams J, Sharp GB. Epilepsy. In: Keth Yeats M, Ris D, Taylor HG, eds. *Pediatric Neuropsychology. Research, Theory and Practice.* New York: Guilford Press, 2000:47–73.
34. Aldenkamp AP, Weber B, Overweg-Plandsoen WCG, Reijs R, et al. Educational underachievement in children with epilepsy: a model to predict the effects of epilepsy on educational achievement. *J Child Neurol* 2005; 20:175–180.
35. Fastenau PS, Shen J, Dunn DW, Perkins SM, et al. Neuropsychological predictors of academic underachievement in pediatric epilepsy: moderating roles of demographic, seizure, and psychosocial variables. *Epilepsia* 2004; 45:1261–1272.
36. Wakamoto H, Nagao H, Hyashi M, Morimoto T. Long-term medical, educational, and social prognoses of childhood-onset epilepsy; population based study in a rural district of Japan. *Brain Dev* 2000; 22:246–255.
37. Jalava M, Sillanpää M, Camfield C, Camfield P. Social adjustment and competence 35 years after onset of childhood epilepsy: a prospective study. *Epilepsia* 1997; 38:708–715.
38. Germanó E, Gagliano A, Magazú A, Sferro C, et al. Benign childhood epilepsy with occipital paroxysms: neuropsychological findings. *Epilepsy Res* 2005; 64:137–150.
39. Aicardi J. Foreword. In: Deonna T, Roulet-Perez E. *Cognitive and behavioral disorders of epileptic origin in children.* Cambridge, UK: Mac Keith Press/Cambridge University Press, 2005:xi–xiv.

47

The Landau-Kleffner Syndrome and Epilepsy with Continuous Spike-Waves During Sleep

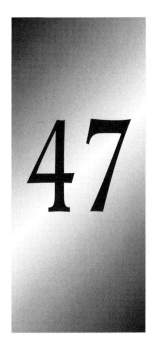

James J. Riviello, Jr.
Stavros Hadjiloizou

An epileptic seizure is a clinical event in which an observable alteration in neurologic function is associated with hypersynchronous neuronal discharges. Patients with epilepsy may also have associated cognitive and behavioral dysfunction. Cognitive and behavioral dysfunction may occur during the actual seizure or as a postictal phenomenon. Cognitive and behavioral dysfunction may also result from the underlying etiology of the epilepsy, the frequency of the actual seizures, side effects of antiepileptic drugs (AEDs), or comorbid psychologic or psychiatric disorders, such as or depression (1). Also, there are certain epileptic syndromes in which prominent neurologic, behavioral, and psychiatric manifestations are related to the abundance of epileptiform electroencephalographic (EEG) activity, usually occurring during sleep. These are called epileptic encephalopathies, disorders in which epileptiform abnormalities contribute to progressive dysfunction (2, 3).

The Landau-Kleffner Syndrome (LKS) and epilepsy with continuous spike-waves during slow sleep (CSWS) are specific epilepsy syndromes recognized by the International League Against Epilepsy (ILAE) (2–6) as epilepsies and syndromes undetermined as to whether they are focal or generalized (5). These two syndromes are now classified as epileptic encephalopathies (2). The other

defined epileptic encephalopathies are early myoclonic encephalopathy, Ohtahara syndrome, West syndrome, Dravet syndrome, myoclonic status in nonprogressive encephalopathies, and the Lennox-Gastaut syndrome (2). LKS and CSWS are also considered special syndromes of status epilepticus (SE) (7).

Patry and coworkers defined the term *electrical status epilepticus of sleep* (ESES) (8), prior to the definition of CSWS by the ILAE. However, ESES and CSWS are synonymous terms; status epilepticus during sleep (SES) is also used (9). The strict definition of ESES requires sleep-activated epileptiform activity in greater than 85% of slow wave sleep (6, 8). Veggiotti and colleagues emphasized the difference between the EEG pattern of CSWS and the epileptic syndrome of CSWS (10). Not all patients with sleep-activated EEG epileptiform activity consistent with ESES have the epileptic syndrome of CSWS. We use *ESES* to describe the EEG and *CSWS* to describe the epileptic syndrome, and we emphasize that these two epileptic syndromes are diagnosed by both the clinical manifestations and ESES, but not ESES alone.

Regression in intellectual or cognitive abilities is the hallmark of LKS and CSWS (3, 4). In fact, regression may be the presenting manifestation in some children, with language regression the hallmark of LKS and a more global neuropsychiatric regression in CSWS. Overt clinical seizures may not occur in all children with either syndrome, but behavioral and psychiatric disorders are very common. In general, cognitive regression should always raise the suspicion of a sleep-activated epileptic encephalopathy, especially in a child with an underlying developmental or neurologic disorder. Children require antiepileptic therapy for the seizures and epileptiform EEG activity and may require counseling or psychopharmacologic therapy for the associated behavioral disorders.

LKS and CSWS are rare pediatric epilepsy syndromes (11). In a recent 20-year epidemiologic study of childhood epilepsy, Kramer and colleagues reported LKS and CSWS in 0.2% each, compared with West syndrome in 9%, myoclonic seizures in 2.2%, and Lennox-Gastaut syndrome in 1.5% (12). Ohtahara syndrome and myoclonic astatic epilepsy also occurred in 0.2% each.

CLINICAL MANIFESTATIONS AND EVALUATION

LKS usually develops in children older than four years (13), with a range of 3 to 10 years (14), presenting with an apparent word deafness, or a "verbal auditory agnosia." Seizures and behavior disturbances, particularly attention deficits and hyperactivity, each occur in approximately two-thirds of children with LKS (3). The majority of cases are classified as "idiopathic," although any pathologic process affecting auditory cortex may cause LKS. Symptomatic cases have been described (see the section on Differential Diagnosis), and we have seen "symptomatic LKS" caused by a left temporal oligodendroglioma, with clinical improvement noted after resection.

The classical features of LKS are a verbal auditory agnosia (word deafness) followed by language regression, seizures, or both in a previously normal child who has an epileptiform EEG. The peripheral hearing must be normal, since a central disorder cannot be diagnosed with peripheral dysfunction. Children with sleep-activated epileptiform activity without the classic features of LKS may be referred to as "LKS variants" (15). LKS variants include EEG involvement of the more anterior language areas, with dysfunction characterized by oral-motor apraxia, sialorrhea, seizures, and an abnormal EEG (16) (anterior LKS); epileptiform EEGs in children with pervasive developmental delay (PDD; autism) with language regression (17–19); and epileptiform EEGs in children with congenital aphasias (20), also called developmental language disorders, with or without clinical regression (developmental LKS).

The evaluation includes a baseline history, physical examination, sleep-deprived EEG, a formal neuropsychologic evaluation, neuroimaging, with magnetic resonance imaging (MRI) preferred, long-term video-EEG monitoring (LTM), and, if needed, dipole analysis, functional neuroimaging with single-photon emission computed tomography (SPECT), positron emission tomography (PET), or magnetoencephalography (MEG) and the frequency-modulated auditory evoked response (FM-AER). The FM-AER is an evoked response that tests receptive language function and may be absent with a verbal auditory agnosia (21).

EEG Findings

An epileptiform EEG, especially with sleep activation, is the neurophysiologic hallmark of these disorders. ESES may occur in both syndromes, but not all children with ESES have these specific syndromes. Veggiotti et al. emphasized the difference between the EEG pattern of CSWS and the epileptic syndrome of CSWS (10). In 32 patients with CSWS, only 10 (34%) had features of the CSWS syndrome, whereas four had LKS, three had the acquired opercular syndrome, and 15 had symptomatic epilepsy. Van Hirtum-Das and colleagues identified 102 children with ESES, using a spike-wave index greater than 25% (22). In this group, only 18% had LKS. Although CSWS was named for sleep activation during slow wave sleep, this term is misleading, since EEG activation occurs in nonrapid-eye-movement (NREM) sleep, typically starting in drowsiness (9). This is our experience as well (23). The spike-waves become fragmented during rapid-eye-movement (REM) sleep, when focality may be seen, and the spike-wave-index usually decreases below 25% (9). Upon awakening, the spike-wave frequency dramatically decreases again.

The EEG in LKS shows bilateral, multifocal spikes and spike and wave discharges, occurring usually in the posterior regions, especially the more posterior regions, with a marked activation during NREM sleep. However, discharges occur in many locations and may be generalized. The strict definition of ESES (spike-wave index greater than 85%) is not required to diagnose LKS, since the spike-wave-index may only reach 50% (11). The EEG may improve over time, either spontaneously or with treatment (24, 25).

The language regression in LKS versus a more global neurobehavioral disorder in CSWS may be explained by the EEG findings (26, 27). Guilhoto and Morrell reported that a more focal ESES pattern was seen in LKS, whereas with a more generalized ESES pattern the CSWS syndrome with generalized neurobehavioral dysfunction was more likely (26). Guilhoto and colleagues subsequently reported 17 children with ESES. Five had LKS, and the EEG showed diffuse activity with accentuation in the centrotemporal region, whereas the others had widespread epileptiform discharges (27). Therefore, LKS and CSWS may have EEG patterns with different focality.

Pathophysiology

The underlying mechanisms of LKS and CSWS are not yet specifically identified; especially what generates the significant, interictal sleep-activated epileptiform activity and causes the intellectual regression. However, the neuropsychologic deficits presumably, at least partially, result from the epileptiform activity. Landau and Kleffner (4) suggested that "persistent convulsive discharges in brain tissue largely concerned with language communication result in the functional ablation of these areas." Hirsch and colleagues agree with this hypothesis (14). Poor daytime alertness due to sleep fragmentation may contribute to the neuropsychologic deficits (28). However, a causal relation between abnormal interictal discharges and neuropsychologic deficits is still controversial (29, 30). A valid argument is that the dysfunction may represent different manifestations of the same unknown, possibly genetically determined, underlying pathogenic mechanism. An argument against this hypothesis is that the suppression of discharges with medical or surgical therapy may, at least partly, reverse these cognitive deficits (31, 32).

Although a genetic predisposition was questioned, there is no strong evidence to support such predilection (33). The EEG response to corticosteroids raises the possibility of an autoimmune pathogenesis at least in a subset of patients, including CNS vasculitis or demyelination. IgG and IgM antibodies to brain endothelial cells have been identified in these disorders (15, 34), with higher levels in the patients than in controls. Brain derived neurotrophic factor (BDNF), BDNF autoantibodies, and IgM and IgG antibodies were elevated in some children with autism and childhood disintegrative disorder (CDD). The authors concluded that these findings suggest a previously unrecognized interaction between the immune system and BDNF (34). Autoantibodies to rat brain auditory cortex, brainstem, and cerebellum have been identified in children with LKS (35).

Interictal EEG abnormalities can clearly produce transient cognitive impairment (36–42). Furthermore, benign rolandic epilepsy may be not so "benign," since the interictal discharges may have a substantial effect on cognitive function (43, 44), at least for a subset of patients. Continuously abnormal discharges during sleep may disrupt hippocampal function and interfere with memory consolidation (45–47). More specifically, the occurrence of epileptiform discharges during a critical time of brain development may result in defective synaptogenesis and thalamocortical circuit formation. Secondary bilateral synchrony, facilitated by the corpus callosum with involvement of thalamocortical connections, was hypothesized as a possible mechanism for the generation of the epileptiform discharges (48–51). Hence, the potential impact of the persistent interictal discharges on brain plasticity is proposed as a mechanism for the resulting neuropsychologic impairment in these children.

Diagnostic Evaluation and Differential Diagnosis

Diagnosing these disorders starts by demonstrating an epileptic disturbance in the child with regression, usually first with a routine EEG. All pediatric epilepsy syndromes are classified as symptomatic, cryptogenic, or idiopathic. Symptomatic cases exist for both LKS and CSWS, although symptomatic cases are more frequent with CSWS. We have seen only one case of a "symptomatic LKS," in a child with a left temporal oligodendroglioma. However, other categories reported include infectious disorders, such as neurocysticercosis (52); inflammatory disorders, such as CNS vasculitis (53); demyelinating disease (54), and acute disseminated encephalomyelitis (ADEM) (55); congenital brain malformations, such as polymicrogyria (56); tumors, including temporal lobe astrocytomas and dysembryoplastic neuroepithelial tumors (DNET) (57–59); and, possibly, toxoplasmosis infection (60). ESES has been reported as occurring frequently in shunted hydrocephalus (61). Therefore, neuroimaging is warranted.

Typically, in the idiopathic cases, no structural abnormalities are seen with routine neuroimaging, although bilateral volume reduction in the superior temporal gyrus has been reported using an MRI cortical parcellation technique (62), and perisylvian polymicrogyria has been reported in a single case (56). Functional neuroimaging has demonstrated temporal dysfunction, with SPECT (63, 64), PET (65, 66), or MEG scans (67). These studies are usually done when epilepsy surgery is considered.

Sleep-activated epileptiform activity occurs in many epileptic disorders. However, sleep-activated EEGs are seen in LKS, CSWS, and PDD with regression, congenital aphasia or developmental language disorders, or the epilepsy syndromes benign focal epilepsy with centrotemporal discharges, benign focal epilepsy with occipital discharges, atypical benign partial epilepsy of childhood, Lennox-Gastaut syndrome, and myoclonic-astatic epilepsy (Doose syndrome) (2). Language or intellectual regression associated with behavioral problems may make the differential diagnosis difficult, and not all epilepsy syndromes are readily classified. In our experience, children with PDD with regression and an epileptiform EEG constitute the largest group of children referred for evaluation.

Clinical symptoms other than language regression have been reported with ESES. Hirsch and colleagues suggested that the term LKS should be expanded to include the acquired deterioration of any higher cortical function in association with sleep-activated paroxysmal features (68) and not only to language regression. Clinical manifestations include epileptic dysgraphia (69), visual agnosia (70), and an acquired frontal syndrome (71). We have seen one child with blindness and another child with a prosopagnosia, both demonstrating a more posterior ESES on EEG.

TREATMENT

All children with LKS and CSWS should have a formal neuropsychologic evaluation to guide their educational program and track developmental changes. Children with LKS will especially require intensive speech and language therapy. These two syndromes are associated with significant neuropsychiatric comorbidities, and treatment for hyperactivity, attention deficit disorder, mood instability, behavior problems, and even autistic symptoms may require psychopharmacologic agents or referral to a psychopharmacologist and psychologist. Despite control of seizures and EEG abnormalities, these children may have significant residual neurologic, psychologic, and psychiatric dysfunction.

LKS and ESES have similar treatment, but the specifics are debated. Smith and Hoeppner recommend that the treatment goal is the complete elimination of epileptiform activity within 2 years (11). Treatment options include standard AEDs, corticosteroids (adrenocorticotropic hormone [ACTH] or prednisone), high-dose benzodiazepines, intravenous immunoglobulins, or multiple subpial transections (MST). Although AEDs may control seizures, the language dysfunction may not improve, whereas corticosteroid treatment may control seizures and decrease the epileptiform activity and improve language (72–74). Early corticosteroid treatment has been considered the treatment of choice for LKS (74). Since relapse may occur, LKS often requires long-term corticosteroid treatment, which increases the risk of side effects (75). Despite either AED or corticosteroid treatment, many children continue with language dysfunction. Regardless of treatment, 50–80% of children have long-term language or neurobehavioral abnormalities (76–78). De Negri and colleagues used high-dose diazepam (DZP) for electrical status epilepticus (ESE) (79).

Tassinari et al. recommend trials with several different drugs and reported a long-lasting effect with valproic acid (VPA) along with clobazam, lorazepam, and clonazepam (9). Smith and Hoeppner recommended initial treatment with high-dose valproate, with or without a benzodiazepine and, if there was no response, then several months of corticosteroid therapy (11). Inutsuka and colleagues (80) reported treatment results in 15 children,

---

TABLE 47-1
Six-Month Dosing Schedule for Oral Prednisone

2 mg/kg/day for 1 month (maximum dose: 60 mg)
1.5 mg/kg/day for 1 month
1 mg/kg/day for 1 month
1 mg/kg every other day for 1 month
0.75 mg/kg every other day for 1 month
0.5 mg/kg/day every other day for 1 month

Note well: Immunizations should be up to date before the elective use of corticosteroids.

---

using the following protocol: (1) VPA at levels greater than 100 mg/L, (2) combination of VPA plus ethosuximide, (3) short cycles of high-dose DZP, (4) or intramuscular (IM) ACTH. Treatment with short cycles of ACTH (duration 11 to 43 days) or DZP (duration for 6 to 7 days) did not achieve long-term remission, whereas either high-dose VPA alone ($n = 7$) or in combination with ethosuximide ($n = 3$) achieved remission in 10 children (67%). We retrospectively analyzed our experience with ESES treatment in 12 children (81). Only 1/12 responded to initial short-term therapy with valproic acid. We used prednisone, for six months, in six children, with the dose schedule outlined in Table 47-1 (82); 5/6 had a positive response, but 4/5 (80%) relapsed, and required another course. Before the elective use of corticosteroids, immunizations should be up to date.

De Negri and colleagues introduced a high-dose diazepam protocol for ESE (79). A rectal dose of 1 mg/kg was given during EEG monitoring, and if there was a positive response, diazepam was then given orally at 0.5 mg/kg for several weeks. Children on chronic benzodiazepine treatment did not respond as well to this treatment. If a clinical relapse occurred, the diazepam was given again rectally. In De Negri's group with ESE, only 1 child had LKS and 1 had ESES. We modified this high-dose diazepam protocol, using 1 mg/kg, either orally or rectally, under EEG guidance, but then treated all children with a dose of 0.5 mg/kg, orally, for 3 to 4 weeks (83). If EEG showed no improvement, we rapidly tapered the DZP. If EEG showed an improvement, we tapered then by 2.5 mg/month. In our series, every child who initially responded and then had a rapid diazepam taper had either a clinical or electrographic regression. We now continue a maintenance diazepam dose, usually at a daily dose of 2.5 to 5 mg, for 2 years. The best responders to high-dose diazepam have been children with idiopathic LKS.

Immunoglobulins and the ketogenic diet have been tried, with case reports documenting efficacy, but long-term follow-up data are limited (84–88). MST has been done in selected children who failed medical therapy and may provide benefit (49, 89).

PROGNOSIS AND OUTCOME

In general, the outcome of epilepsy is favorable in both LKS and CSWS (90), whereas cognitive dysfunction occurs in the majority (11). LKS and ESES have been referred to as "benign" epileptic syndromes, referring to the resolution of seizures and EEG abnormalities, but given the devastating neuropsychologic deficits, we consider these as "malignant" epileptic syndromes.

The prognosis for LKS has varied. Mantovani and Landau conducted a long-term follow-up of the original children reported by Landau and Kleffner (91). In nine patients, with follow-up that varied from 10 to 28 years, four patients had full recovery, one had a mild language disability, and four had moderate disability. Later papers have not reported as positive an outcome. Bishop did a literature review of 45 children with LKS. The age of onset was related to the outcome, which was less favorable if onset occurred before four years of age (13). Shinnar and colleagues reported residual language dysfunction in 88% of children who had language regression, and most had autism or autistic features (76). Deonna et al. reported that only one of seven adult patients had normal language, with the six others demonstrating varying degrees of language deficits, some with complete absence of language (71). In a neuropsychologic follow-up study of 12 patients, Soprano et al. reported that 9/12 had a variable degree of persistent language deficit (78). Only 50% have been able to lead a normal life (49, 65).

The prognosis is poor in CSWS (92). In an adult follow-up study of seven patients, only one had active epilepsy, but only two had been educated in a normal school setting (93). The two patients with LKS had language deficits with a normal IQ, whereas the five with ESES had global mental deficiency. Scholtes et al. (94) did a long-term follow-up of ten children with ESES; a good recovery occurred in only one child, and a partial recovery in only four. Since CSWS is more likely symptomatic, the prognosis is not as good as for LKS, which is more likely to be idiopathic.

References

1. Bourgeois BFD. Determining the effects of antiepileptic drugs on cognitive function in pediatric patients with epilepsy. *J Child Neurol* 2004; 19(S1):S15–S24.
2. Engel J Jr. A proposed diagnostic scheme for people with epileptic seizures and with epilepsy: report of the ILAE Task Force on Classification and Terminology. *Epilepsia* 2001; 42:796–803.
3. Hadjiloizou S, Riviello JJ. Epileptic and epileptiform encephalopathies. Neurology, Emedicine, Boston, 2006. http://www.emedicine.com/neuro/topic547.htm.
4. Landau W, Kleffner FR. Syndrome of acquired aphasia with convulsive disorder in children. *Neurology* 1957; 7:523–530.
5. Commission on Classification and Terminology of the International League Against Epilepsy. Proposal for revised classification of epilepsies and epileptic syndromes. *Epilepsia* 1989; 30:389–399.
6. Tassinari CA, Bureau M, Dravet C, Dalla Bernardina B, et al. Epilepsy with continuous spikes and waves during slow sleep-otherwise described as ESES (epilepsy with electrical status epilepticus during slow sleep. In: Roger J, Bureau M, Dravet Ch, Dreifuss FE, et al, eds. *Epileptic Syndromes in Infancy, Childhood, and Adolescence*, 2nd ed. London: John Libbey, 1992:245–256.
7. Riviello JJ. Status epilepticus in children. In: Drislane F, ed. *Status Epilepticus: A Clinical Perspective*, Totowa, NJ: Humana Press, 2005: 313–338.
8. Patry G, Lyagoubi S, Tassinari A. Subclinical "electrical status epilepticus" induced by sleep in children: a clinical and electroencephalographic study of six cases. *Arch Neurol* 1971; 24:242–252.
9. Tassinari CA, Rubboli G, Volpi L, Meletti S, et al. Encephalopathy with electrical status epilepticus during slow sleep or ESES syndrome including the acquired aphasia. *Clin Neurophysiol* 2000:111(Suppl 2):S94–S102.
10. Veggiotti P, Beccaria F, Guerrini R, Capovilla G, et al. Continuous spike-and-wave activity during slow-wave sleep: syndrome or EEG pattern? *Epilepsia* 1999; 40:1593–1601.
11. Smith MC, Hoeppner TJ. Epileptic encephalopathy of late childhood: Landau-Kleffner syndrome and the syndrome of continuous spikes and waves during slow sleep. *J Clin Neurophysiol* 2003; 20:462–472.
12. Kramer U, Nevo Y, Neufeld MY, Fatal A, et al. Epidemiology of epilepsy in childhood: a cohort of 440 consecutive patients. *Pediatr Neurol* 1998; 18:46–50.
13. Bishop DVM. Age of onset and outcome in acquired aphasia with convulsive disorder (Landau-Kleffner syndrome). *Dev Med Child Neurol* 1985; 27:705–712.
14. Hirsch E, Valenti MP, Rudolf G, Seegmuller C, et al. Landau-Kleffner syndrome is not an eponymic badge of ignorance. *Epilepsy Res* 2006; 70(Suppl 1):S239–247.
15. Connolly AM, Chez MG, Pestronk A, Arnold ST, et al. Serum autoantibodies to brain in Landau-Kleffner variant, autism, and other neurologic disorders. *J Pediatr* 1999; 134:607–613.
16. Shafrir Y, Prensky AL. Acquired epileptiform opercular syndrome: a second case report, review of the literature, and comparison to the Landau-Kleffner syndrome. *Epilepsia* 1995; 36:1050–1057.
17. Tuchman RF, Rapin I. Regression in pervasive developmental disorders: seizures and epileptiform electroencephalogram correlates. *Pediatrics* 1997; 99:560–566.
18. Tuchman RF, Rapin I, Shinnar S. Autistic and dysphasic children. I: Clinical characteristics. *Pediatrics* 1991; 88:1211–1218.
19. Tuchman RF, Rapin I, Shinnar S. Autistic and dysphasic children. II: Epilepsy. *Pediatrics* 1991; 88:1219–1225.
20. Echenne B, Cheminal R, Rivier F, Negre C, et al. Epileptic electroencephalographic abnormalities and developmental dysphasias: a study of 32 patients. *Brain Dev* 1992; 14:216–225.
21. Stefanatos GA, Foley C, Grover W, Doherty B. Steady-state auditory evoked responses to pulsed frequency modulations in children. *Electroencephalogr Clin Neurophysiol* 1997; 104:31–42.
22. Van Hirtum-Das M, Licht EA, Koh S, Wu JY, et al. Children with ESES: variability in the syndrome. *Epilepsy Res* 2006; 7S;S248–S258.
23. Hadjiloizou S, Rotenberg A, Riviello J. Short-term sleep-onset EEG monitoring predicts electrical status epilepticus of sleep (ESES). *Epilepsia* 2006; 47(S4):31.
24. Bolanos A, Mikati M, Holmes G, Helmers S, et al. Landau-Kleffner syndrome: clinical and EEG features. *Neurology* 1995; 45(Suppl4):A180.
25. Bolanos A, Urion DK, Helmers SL, Lombroso CT, et al. Serial electroencephalographic changes in children with Landau-Kleffner Syndrome. *Epilepsia* 1997; 38(Suppl. 3):27. pl4:A180.
26. Guilhoto LMFF, Morrell F. Electrophysiological differences between Landau-Kleffner syndrome and other conditions showing the CSWS electrical pattern. *Epilepsia* 1994; 35(Suppl. 8):126.
27. Guilhoto LM, Machado-Haertel I.R, Manreza ML, Diament AJ. Continuous spike wave activity during sleep. Electroencephalographic and clinical features. *Arq Neuropsiquiatr* 1997; 55:762–770.
28. Kohrman MH, Carney PR. Sleep-related disorders in neurologic disease during childhood. *Pediatr Neurol* 2000; 23:107–113.
29. Holmes GL, McKeever M, Saunders Z. Epileptiform activity in aphasia of childhood: an epiphenomenon? *Epilepsia* 1981; 22:631–639.
30. Ben-Ari Y, Holmes GL. Effects of seizures on developmental processes in the immature brain. *Lancet Neurol* 2006; 5:1055–1063.
31. Matsuzaka T, Baba H, Matsuo A, Tsuru A, et al. Developmental assessment-based surgical intervention for intractable epilepsies in infants and young children. *Epilepsia* 42;2001 (Suppl. 6);9–12.
32. Holmes GL, Lenck-Santini PP. Role of interictal epileptiform abnormalities in cognitive impairment. *Epilepsy Behav* 2006; 8:504–515.
33. Landau WM. Landau-Kleffner syndrome: an eponymic badge of ignorance. *Arch Neurol* 1992; 49:353.
34. Connolly AM, Chez M, Streif EM, Keeling RM, et al. Brain-derived neurotrophic factor and autoantibodies to neural antigens in sera of children with autistic spectrum disorders, Landau-Kleffner Syndrome, and epilepsy. *Biol Psychiatry* 2006; 59:354–363.
35. Boscolo S, Baldas V, Gobbi G, Giordano L, et al. Anti-brain but not celiac disease antibodies in Landau-Kleffner syndrome and related epilepsies. *J Neuroimmunol* 2005; 160:228–32. Epub 2004.
36. Shewmon DA, Erwin RJ. The effect of focal interictal spikes on perception and reaction time. II. Neuroanatomic specificity. *Electroencephalogr Clin Neurophysiol* 1988; 69:338–352.
37. Shewmon DA, Erwin RJ. Transient impairment of visual perception induced by single interictal occipital spikes. *J Clin Exp Neuropsychol* 1989; 11:675–691.

38. Kasteleijn-Nolst Trenite DG, Bakker DJ, Binnie CD. Psychological effects of subclinical epileptiform EEG discharges. I. Scholastic skills. *Epilepsy Res* 1988; 2:111–116.

39. Aarts JH, Binnie CD, Smit AM, Wilkins AJ. Selective cognitive impairment during focal and generalized epileptiform EEG activity. *Brain* 1984; 107(Pt 1):293–308.

40. Binnie CD, Kasteleijn-Nolst Trenite DG, Smit AM, et al. Interactions of epileptiform EEG discharges and cognition. *Epilepsy Res* 1987; 1:239–245.

41. Binnie CD. Significance and management of transitory cognitive impairment due to subclinical EEG discharges in children. *Brain Dev* 1993; 15:23–30.

42. Binnie CD. Cognitive impairment during epileptiform discharges: is it ever justifiable to treat the EEG? *Lancet Neurol* 2003; 2:725–730.

43. Massa R, de Saint-Martin A, Carcangiu R, Rudolf G, et al. EEG criteria predictive of complicated evolution in idiopathic rolandic epilepsy. *Neurology* 2001; 57: 1071–1079.

44. Nolan MA, Redoblado MA, Lah S, Sabaz M, et al. Memory function in childhood epilepsy syndromes. *J Paediatr Child Health* 2004; 40:20–27.

45. Moruzzi G, Magoun HW. Brain stem reticular formation and activation of the EEG. *J Neuropsychiatry Clin Neurosci* 1995; 7:251–267.

46. Lorincz A, Buzsaki G. Two-phase computational model training long-term memories in the entorhinal-hippocampal region. *Ann N Y Acad Sci* 2000; 911:83–111.

47. Louie K, Wilson MA. Temporally structured replay of awake hippocampal ensemble activity during rapid eye movement sleep. *Neuron* 2001; 29:145–156.

48. Morrell F. Secondary epileptogenesis in man. *Arch Neurol* 1985; 42:318–335.

49. Morrell F, Whisler WW, Smith MC, Hoeppner TJ, et al. Landau-Kleffner syndrome: treatment with subpial intracortical transection. *Brain* 1995; 118:1529–1546.

50. Kobayashi K, Murakami N, Yoshinaga H, Enoki H, et al. Nonconvulsive status epilepticus with continuous diffuse spike-and-wave discharges during sleep in childhood. *Jpn J Psychiatry Neurol* 1988; 42:509–514.

51. Monteiro JP, Roulet-Perez E, Davidoff V, Deonna T. Primary neonatal thalamic haemorrhage and epilepsy with continuous spike-wave during sleep: a longitudinal follow-up of a possible significant relation. *Eur J Paediatr Neurol* 2001; 5(1):41–47.

52. Otero E, Cordova S, Diaz F, Garcia-Teruel I, et al. Acquired epileptic aphasia (the Landau Kleffner syndrome) due to neurocysticercosis. *Epilepsia* 1989; 30:569–572.

53. Pascual-Castroviejo I, Lopex Martin V, Martinez Bermejo A, Perez Higueras A. Is cerebral arteritis the cause of the Landau-Kleffner syndrome? Four cases in childhood with angiographic study. *Can J Neurol Sci* 1992; 19:46–52.

54. Perniola T, Margari L, Buttiglione M, Andreula C, et al. A case of Landau-Kleffner syndrome secondary to inflammatory demyelinating disease. *Epilepsia* 1993; 39:551–556.

55. Yoshikawa H, Oda Y. Acquired aphasia in acute disseminated encephalomyelitis. *Brain Dev* 1999; 21:341–344.

56. Huppke P, Kallenberg K, Gartner J. Perisylvian polymicrogyria in Landau-Kleffner syndrome. *Neurology* 2005; 64:1660.

57. Solomon GE, Carson D, Pavlakis S, Fraser R, et al. Intracranial EEG monitoring in Landau-Kleffner syndrome associated with left temporal lobe astrocytoma. *Epilepsia* 1993; 34:557–560.

58. Nass R, Heier L, Walker R. Landau-Kleffner syndrome: temporal lobe tumor resection results in good outcome. *Pediatr Neurol* 1993; 9:303–305.

59. Raymond AA, Halpin SFS, Alsanjari N, Cook MJ, et al. Dysembryoplastic neuroepithelial tumor: features in 16 patients. *Brain* 1994; 117:461–475.

60. Michaoowicz R, Jozwiak S, Ignatowicz R, Szwabowska-Orzesko E. Landau-Kleffner syndrome—epileptic aphasia in children-possible role of *Toxoplasma gondii* infection. *Acta Paediatr Hung* 1988–1989; 29:337–342.

61. Veggiotti P, Beccaria F, Papalia G, Termine C, et al. Continuous spikes and waves during sleep in children with shunted hydrocephalus. *Childs Nerv Syst* 1998; 14:188–194.

62. Takeoka M, Riviello JJ Jr, Duffy FH, Kim F, et al. Bilateral volume reduction of the superior temporal areas in Landau-Kleffner syndrome. *Neurology* 2004; 63:1289–1292.

63. O'Tuama LA, Urion DK, Janicek MJ, Treves ST, et al. Regional cerebral perfusion in Landau-Kleffner syndrome and related childhood aphasias. *J Nucl Med* 1992; 33: 1758–1765.

64. Guerreiro MM, Camargo EE, Kato M, Menezes Netto JR, et al. Brain single photon emission computed tomography imaging in Landau-Kleffner syndrome. *Epilepsia* 1996; 37:60–67.

65. Maquet P, Hirsch E, Dive D, Salmon E, et al. Cerebral glucose utilization during sleep in Landau-Kleffner syndrome: a PET study. *Epilepsia* 1990; 31:778–783.

66. da Silva EA, Chugani DC, Muzik O, Chugani HT. Landau-Kleffner syndrome: metabolic abnormalities in temporal lobe are a common feature. *J Child Neurol* 1997; 12: 489–495.

67. Paetau R, Granstrom M-L, Blomstedt G, Jousmaki V, et al. Magnetoencephalography in presurgical evaluation of Landau-Kleffner syndrome. *Epilepsia* 1999; 40:326–335.

68. Hirsch E, Maquet P, Metz-Lutz M-N, Motte J, et al. The eponym "Landau-Kleffner Syndrome" should not be restricted to childhood-acquired aphasia with epilepsy. In: Beaumanoir A, Bureau M, Deonna T, Mira L, et al, eds. *Continuous Spikes and Slow Waves During Slow Sleep/Electrical Status Epilepticus During Slow Sleep: Acquired Epileptic Aphasia and Related Conditions.* Mariani Foundation Paediatric Neurology 3. London: John Libbey, 1995:57–62.

69. DuBois CM, Zesiger P, Perez ER, Ingvar MM, et al. Acquired epileptic dysgraphia: a longitudinal study. *Dev Med Child Neurol* 2003; 45:807–812.

70. Eriksson K, Kylliainen A, Hirvonen K, Nieminen P, et al. Visual agnosia in a child with non-lesional occipito-temporal CSWS. *Brain Dev* 2003; 25:262–267.

71. Deonna T, Davidoff V, Maeder-Ingvar M, Zesiger P, et al. The spectrum of acquired cognitive disturbances in children with partial epilepsy and continuous spike-waves during sleep: a 4-year follow-up case study with prolonged reversible learning arrest and dysfluency. *Eur J Paediatr Neurol* 1997; 1:19–29.

72. McKinney W, McGreal DA. An aphasic syndrome in children. *Can Med J* 1974; 110: 637–639.

73. Marescaux C, Finck S, Maquet P, Schlumberger E, et al. Landau-Kleffner syndrome: a pharmacologic study of five cases. *Epilepsia* 1990; 31:768–777.

74. Lerman P, Lerman-Sagie T, Kivity S. Effect of early corticosteroid therapy for Landau-Kleffner syndrome. *Dev Med Child Neurology* 1991; 33:257–260.

75. Verhelst H, Boon P, Buyse G, Ceulemans B, et al. Steroids in intractable childhood epilepsy: clinical experience and review of the literature. *Seizure* 2005; 14:412–421.

76. Shinnar S, Rapin I, Arnold S, Tuchman RF, et al. Language regression in childhood. *Pediatr Neurol* 2001; 24:183–189.

77. Mantovani JF. Autistic regression and Landau-Kleffner syndrome: progress or confusion? *Dev Med Child Neurol* 2000; 42:349–353.

78. Soprano AM, Garcia EF, Caraballo R, Fejerman N. Acquired epileptic aphasia: neuropsychologic follow-up of 12 patients. *Pediatr Neurol* 1994; 11:230–235.

79. De Negri M, Baglietto MG, Battaglia FM. Treatment of electrical status epilepticus by short diazepam (DZP) cycles after DZP rectal bolus test. *Brain Dev* 1995; 17:330–333.

80. Inutsuka M, Kobayashi K, Oka M, Hattori J, et al. Treatment of epilepsy with electrical status epilepticus of sleep and its related disorders. *Epilepsy Behav* 2006; 28:281–286.

81. Albaradie RS, Bourgeois BFD, Thiele E, Duffy FH, et al. Treatment of continuous spike and wave during slow wave sleep. *Epilepsia* 2001; 42(Suppl 7):46–47.

82. Stefanatos GA, Grover W, Geller E. Case study: corticosteroid treatment of language regression in pervasive developmental disorder. *J Am Acad Child Adolesc Psychiatry* 1995; 34:1107–1111.

83. Riviello JJ, Holder DL, Thiele E, Bourgeois BFD, et al. Treatment of continuous spikes and waves during slow wave sleep with high dose diazepam. *Epilepsia* 2001; 42(Suppl 7):56.

84. Fayad MN, Choueiri R, Mikati M. Landau-Kleffner syndrome: consistent response to repeated intravenous gamma-globulin doses: a case report. *Epilepsia* 1997; 38:489–494.

85. Mikati MA, Saab R. Successful use of intravenous immunoglobulin as initial monotherapy in Landau-Kleffner syndrome. *Epilepsia* 2000; 41:880–886.

86. Mikati MA, Saab R, Fayad MN, Choueiri RN. Efficacy of intravenous immunoglobulin in Landau-Kleffner syndrome. *Pediatr Neurol* 2002; 26:298–300.

87. Lagae LG, Silberstein J, Gillis PL, Casaer PJ. Successful use of intravenous immunoglobulins in Landau-Kleffner syndrome. *Pediatr Neurol* 1998; 18:165–168.

88. Prasad AN, Stafstrom CF, Holmes GL. Alternative epilepsy therapies: the ketogenic diet, immunoglobulins, and steroids. *Epilepsia* 1996; 37 Suppl 1:S81–S95.

89. Irwin K, Birch V, Lees J, Polkey C, et al. Multiple subpial transection in Landau-Kleffner syndrome. *Dev Med Child Neurol* 2001; 43:248–252.

90. Bureau M. Outstanding cases of CSWS and LKS: analysis of the data sheets provided by the participants. In: Beaumanoir A, Bureau M, Deonna T, Mira L, et al, eds. *Continuous Spikes and Slow Waves During Slow Sleep/Electrical Status Epilepticus During Slow Sleep: Acquired Epileptic Aphasia and Related Conditions.* Mariani Foundation Paediatric Neurology 3. London: John Libbey, 1995:213–216.

91. Mantovani JF, Landau WM. Acquired aphasia with convulsive disorder: course and prognosis. *Neurology* 1980; 30:524–529.

92. Morikawa T, Seino M, Watanabe M. Long-term outcome of CSWS syndrome. In: Beaumanoir A, Bureau M, Deonna T, Mira L, et al., eds. *Continuous Spikes and Slow Waves During Slow Sleep/Electrical Status Epilepticus During Slow Sleep: Acquired epileptic aphasia and related conditions.* Mariani Foundation Paediatric Neurology 3. London: John Libbey, 1995:27–36.

93. Praline J, Hommet C, Barthez M-A, Brault F, et al. Outcome at adulthood of continuous spike waves of slow sleep and Landau-Kleffner Syndrome. *Epilepsia* 2003; 44:1434–1440.

94. Scholtes FB, Hendriks MP, Renier WO. Cognitive deterioration and electrical status epilepticus during slow sleep. *Brain Dev* 2005; 6:167–173.

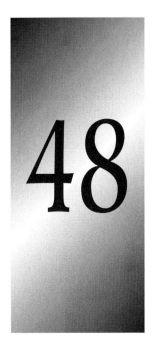

48

Effects of Antiepileptic Drugs on Psychiatric and Behavioral Comorbidities in Children and Adolescents

Ann M. Bergin

ll anticonvulsant drugs have their effect in the central nervous system. They affect neurotransmitter systems that are not only involved in generation and propagation of seizure activity, but also implicated in the pathogenesis of psychiatric disorders. As such, it is not surprising that there are interactions between anticonvulsant drugs and behavioral and psychiatric status in patients with epilepsy. At this time, many of the effects of anticonvulsant drugs on brain neurochemistry are known. However, in many instances the effect(s) responsible for the drugs' anticonvulsant effect is not clear. Similarly, although knowledge is increasing with respect to the neurochemical basis for psychiatric and behavioral disorders, precise understanding of pathophysiology is unknown. In this setting, it is not surprising that the interactions between these drugs and psychiatric and behavioral status appear complex.

There is relatively little good-quality clinical evidence regarding the impact of anticonvulsants on psychiatric and behavioral disorders in persons with epilepsy. This is particularly true of the older anticonvulsants. With respect to the newer agents, introduced over the last 10–15 years, there is a little more information from preclinical and subsequent studies. Unfortunately, until recently, separate studies in children were not required by the U.S. Food and Drug Administration (FDA), so

information remains relatively poor for effects in children. Recent federal laws requiring more detailed study of anticonvulsant drugs in children will be helpful in time.

The importance of comorbid disorders in epilepsy is increasingly recognized. Quality of life for patients with epilepsy is related to seizure frequency. However, in refractory epilepsy, depressed mood has been shown to be a powerful predictor of quality of life—indeed, the only variable predicting quality of life in this group (1). Depression is underdiagnosed and untreated in the majority of patients with epilepsy. Caplan et al. have described similar findings in pediatric epilepsy, with 33% of children with epilepsy having affective and anxiety disorders, compared to 6% in the normal control group (2). As with adults with epilepsy, only a minority had received mental health services. Disorders of behavior and attention are also more common in children with epilepsy than in the general pediatric population (3). Given the burden of behavioral and psychiatric disorders in childhood epilepsy, it is imperative to have an understanding of the impact of prescribed anticonvulsant medications on these disorders, in order both to avoid exacerbation of pre-existing conditions and, where possible, to improve symptoms.

This chapter will explore the effects of anticonvulsant drugs on the behavioral and psychiatric comorbidities affecting children and adolescents with epilepsy as far as it is known. References cited in the following sections are mainly to articles relevant to pediatric epilepsy patients, or work not cited by other authors. Two excellent recent reviews on this topic that provide the basis for otherwise unreferenced information in this chapter may be of interest to some readers (4, 5). Limitations in available data on this subject, particularly in children, signify plentiful opportunities for future well-designed studies.

POTENTIAL MECHANISMS OF EFFECTS

Effects of anticonvulsant drugs on behavioral and psychiatric comorbidities in epilepsy may be positive or negative. The mechanisms by which effects occur may be drug-related, often dose-dependent, or idiosyncratic, depending at least in part on the individual's underlying neuropsychiatric state. In general, anticonvulsant drugs that have predominantly gamma-aminobutyric acid (GABA) mechanisms of action have been considered to have sedating effects and perhaps to benefit individuals with anxiety or mania. On the other hand, those drugs with predominantly antiglutamatergic effects are considered activating, likely to be anxiogenic, and possibly antidepressant (6, 7). It is likely that other neurochemical pathways will also be shown to have an impact in mediating these effects.

Positive psychotropic effects may be induced by a number of different mechanisms, including the following:

1. Specific therapeutic actions for psychiatric disorders, as is considered to occur in mania and bipolar disease with treatment with valproic acid
2. A prophylactic effect of successful anticonvulsant treatment in those children and adolescents who experience peri- or postictal aggression or psychosis
3. Improvement due to reduced frequency of interictal epileptiform activity

Whether decreased interictal epileptiform activity can improve cognitive and behavioral disorders in epilepsy remains controversial. Pressler et al. report improvement in behavior problems in children who achieved reduction in interictal discharges during treatment with lamotrigine (8). This important question requires further study.

Negative psychotropic effects of anticonvulsant drugs may similarly be due to a direct action of the drug, whether inducing, unmasking, or exacerbating a disorder in a vulnerable individual. The occurrence of depression among children treated with phenobarbital provides an example (9). The relative contribution of individual susceptibility versus dose-related toxicity of the drug is difficult to discriminate. The phrase "forced normalization" describes the association of drug-induced rapid

improvement of epileptiform activity on the electroencephalogram (EEG) and the emergence of psychotic symptoms. The classical description is in children successfully treated for absence seizures with ethosuximide, in 2% of whom psychosis may occur. A higher rate, 8%, has been reported in adolescents and adults in similar circumstances. There are reports of treatment-emergent psychosis with a number of anticonvulsant drugs. Whether these represent forced normalization is unclear, and effect on EEG is not reported in most instances.

MEDICATIONS

The following discussion will summarize available information regarding effects of the anticonvulsant drugs on psychiatric and behavioral disorders. Where possible, studies of these effects in patients with epilepsy will be highlighted. Similarly, where available, information specific to children and adolescents being treated for epilepsy will be emphasized. Unfortunately, for many drugs, it is possible only to extrapolate from studies of the anticonvulsant drugs in nonepileptic persons. Two further considerations should be borne in mind. First, controlled studies designed to determine drug efficacy for refractory epilepsy for regulatory review may not accurately or completely identify behavioral and psychiatric effects of the drugs under study. Second, in many controlled studies as well as case series, the drug in question is part of a polytherapy regimen, limiting the ability to definitively attribute adverse effects solely to the drug under review.

Phenobarbital

Phenobarbital's anticonvulsant action is probably related to its ability to enhance GABA-mediated inhibition. In adults it has prominent sedating effects, to which tolerance usually develops. In contrast, children are more likely to experience behavioral effects, particularly aggression, hyperactivity, impulsivity, and sleep disturbance. These may occur at low serum levels. A double blind, placebo-controlled trial of phenobarbital in toddlers did not reveal significantly different behavioral problems between the treatment groups (10). Treatment with phenobarbital has been implicated in the occurrence of depression and suicidal ideation in children. Fifteen children with epilepsy aged 6–16 years treated with phenobarbital monotherapy were compared to 24 treated with carbamazepine monotherapy (9). Higher prevalences of depression (40% versus 4%) and suicidal ideation (47% versus 4%) were noted in those treated with phenobarbital. A family history of major affective disorder as well as stressful life events was also associated with depression in this study. These findings and concerns regarding cognitive function in the developing brain have resulted in decreased use of phenobarbital in childhood epilepsy.

Phenytoin

The anticonvulsant effect of phenytoin is related to sodium channel blockade. It is generally a well-tolerated drug whose clinical use is complicated by nonlinear kinetics, a high degree of protein binding, and, in infants, by high elimination rates. Behavioral adverse effects have been reported in children with epilepsy treated with phenytoin, just as with all anticonvulsants. However, a prospective, randomized, but not blinded, comparative study of monotherapy with phenobarbital, phenytoin, carbamazepine, and valproate in 167 children aged between 3 and 16 years with generalized tonic-clonic or partial seizures showed no significant difference in the rate of behavioral adverse effects between phenytoin (9%), carbamazepine (4%), and valproic acid (4%) (11). Cosmetic adverse effects have limited its use in children and adolescents, especially with the availability of newer drugs lacking these effects.

Carbamazepine and Oxcarbazepine

These related drugs probably exert their anticonvulsant effect by sodium channel blockade, though they have other sites of action also. In adults, studies in patients with bipolar disease suggest that carbamazepine is effective in mood stabilization compared to placebo. Only very limited data are available regarding mood stabilization effects of oxcarbazepine in adults. A randomized, multicenter, controlled trial of oxcarbazepine for bipolar disease in 116 children aged 7–18 years showed no benefit over placebo (12). Only one study suggested increased behavioral adverse effects in children treated with carbamazepine, but in general this is considered rare. This drug has been reported to improve alertness and attention in some children, though whether this is related to improved seizure control or to drug effect was unclear. Although carbamazepine is structurally related to tricyclic antidepressants, it is not considered to have significant antidepressant effect.

Valproic Acid

The mechanism of action of valproic acid is uncertain. Actions that may be responsible include potentiation of GABAergic function and inhibition of voltage-sensitive sodium channels. This drug is approved as a first-line agent in the treatment of acute mania in adults, and uncontrolled studies support efficacy for maintenance therapy for bipolar disease in childhood. There is no evidence to support a significant effect of valproic acid on behavioral status in childhood apart from bipolar disease.

Uncontrolled, open-label studies suggest a beneficial effect in children with aggressive behavior in bipolar and other psychiatric and behavioral disorders; however, there are no controlled studies in support of this effect. One small randomized, placebo-controlled study of 30 children and adolescents aged 6–20 years with pervasive developmental disorder and aggressive behavior revealed no difference between the treatment groups (13). A large placebo effect was noted in this study and complicates interpretation. There are no controlled studies of the effect of treatment with valproic acid in children with epilepsy and comorbid psychiatric disorders.

Gabapentin and Pregabalin

Despite their being analogs of GABA, the anticonvulsant actions of these two drugs are likely not related to effects on usual GABA binding sites. Mechanism of action remains unknown for both. In initial studies of efficacy in epilepsy patients, improvements in mood and symptoms of anxiety were noted. Controlled studies do not support an antidepressant effect for gabapentin, nor a mood stabilization effect, which had appeared promising in initial studies in bipolar disease. However, two placebo-controlled studies indicate efficacy in adults for social phobia and panic disorder. Five placebo-controlled studies of short-term treatment with pregabalin in generalized anxiety disorder showed significant benefit in adults, as did another placebo-controlled study of treatment of social anxiety. There are no controlled trials of pregabalin for anxiety in children, nor in epilepsy patients. There are three case reports describing 12 children with epilepsy who experienced increased aggressive and oppositional behaviors when treated adjunctively with gabapentin. All but two had developmental delay or mental retardation, and the behaviors represented an intensification of pre-existing difficulties in 8 of the 12.

Lamotrigine

Lamotrigine probably exerts its anticonvulsant effects via a combination of sodium channel inhibition and calcium channel effects. In early studies of efficacy in patients with epilepsy, effects on mood and quality of life were noted. Subsequent controlled studies in epilepsy and in nonepileptic populations have supported mood stabilization effects, and lamotrigine is approved for maintenance therapy of bipolar I disorder. In a recent placebo-controlled trial of lamotrigine for generalized tonic-clonic seizures in adults, there was a significant improvement in depressive symptoms in the group treated with lamotrigine versus the placebo-treated group. Lamotrigine is generally an activating rather than a sedating drug. Insomnia occurred in 6% of patients with newly diagnosed epilepsy on lamotrigine monotherapy, compared with 2% of those treated with carbamazepine. Use of lamotrigine for epilepsy in intellectually disabled patients has been associated with onset or exacerbation of aggressive or violent behaviors in a series of 19 adult patients. In another series of children and adults from a single center, four patients experienced improvement in behavioral disorders, while three others had deterioration with lamotrigine treatment. There are no reports of worsening of ADHD in children of normal intelligence treated with lamotrigine.

Topiramate

Topiramate has a wide range of potentially anticonvulsant actions, with antiglutamatergic action at kainate receptors, blockade of voltage gated sodium channels, and enhancement of GABAergic inhibition, and, as might be expected, topiramate has a broad spectrum of anticonvulsant activity. In polytherapy or with rapid introduction, treatment has been associated with a cognitive syndrome of psychomotor slowing and word-finding problems. Open-label trials have suggested efficacy for bipolar disease, but despite frequent use for this indication, there are no controlled studies confirming this effect. There are two controlled trials describing effect in treatment of aggression in borderline personality. However, topiramate may itself induce psychosis. This has been seen in children and adults and has included auditory and visual hallucinations, paranoid delusions, agitation, and aggression. Ten of 159 children or adolescents treated for epilepsy developed aggression or a psychotic syndrome, with a history of prior aggression recognized as a risk factor (14). Slow dose titration may reduce the risk of this side effect. There are small studies reporting small adverse effects on attention from topiramate treatment for epilepsy. Slow dose titration can ameliorate this effect. In a study of long-term treatment (24–61 months) in 277 children and adolescents, behavior disturbance or aggression occurred in 14 (5%), difficulty with concentration or attention in 11 (4%), and acute psychosis in 6 (2%) (15).

Levetiracetam

This drug has a specific CNS-limited binding site unique among the anticonvulsants. Its exact mechanism of anticonvulsant action is unknown. It is generally well tolerated. Initial studies reported up to 13% incidence of behavioral side effects, including agitation, hostility, anxiety, emotional lability, and symptoms of depression. Dose adjustment improved these symptoms, though in a case control study of long-term treatment with levetiracetam, 6.9% of 553 patients $\geq$ 16 years of age discontinued treatment because of behavioral symptoms (16). Psychiatric adverse effects seem to be more common in epilepsy patients than in those treated with levetiracetam for other reasons, such as cognitive disorders or anxiety,

and in some patients these effects may require emergency psychiatric treatment. In a recent double-blind, placebo-controlled study of levetiracetam treatment in refractory partial epilepsy in children, psychiatric adverse effects reported more frequently in the levetiractam-treated group were hostility (11.9% levetiracetam versus 6.2% placebo), nervousness (9.9% versus 2.1%), and agitation (5.9% versus 1%) (17). One child and four adolescents are reported in the literature who developed treatment-emergent psychotic symptoms, including visual and auditory hallucinations, paranoid delusions, and aggression. The majority had pre-existing cognitive impairment, and prior behavioral problems were common in the adolescents. All responded quickly to dose reduction or withdrawal of levetiracetam.

Zonisamide

This drug has a number of different effects in the brain which may be responsible for its anticonvulsant effects, including blockade of T-type calcium channels, inhibition of sodium channels, and possibly inhibition of glutamate release. There are very few reports regarding behavioral or psychiatric effects of zonisamide in those treated for epilepsy. An open-label study of adults for bipolar disorder showed mixed results, with improvements in measures of mood in some patients but a high rate of discontinuation due to worsening mood. Psychosis has been reported in patients with epilepsy treated with zonisamide. Fourteen of 74 patients treated with this drug and reviewed retrospectively had psychosis. The risk was greater in young patients, and obsessive-compulsive behavior was a feature in affected children. In this group zonisamide was part of a polytherapy regimen. One study of monotherapy with zonisamide in 27 children with idiopathic epilepsy for 2 years reported 2 children (7.4%) with behavioral disturbance. One 14-year-old child had selective mutism, violent behavior, and decreased concentration in the fourth year of treatment, and one 15-year-old child developed obsessive-compulsive disorder in the third year of treatment. This child responded to a decreased dose (18).

Tiagabine

Tiagabine inhibits neuronal and glial GABA reuptake, thereby enhancing GABA's inhibitory effect. In controlled trials of adjunctive use of tiagabine for refractory partial seizures, nervousness, abnormal thinking, and symptoms of depression were reported more commonly in the active treatment group than in the placebo group. The risk of psychosis does not appear to be increased by treatment with this agent. There are reports of nonconvulsive status epilepticus in both children and adults treated with tiagabine. Changes in behavior occurring while treated with this drug should therefore prompt EEG study.

Tiagabine's GABAergic action suggests it may be an effective anxiolytic agent. Open-label studies support such an effect, but controlled studies are needed for confirmation. To date, one double-blind, placebo-controlled study of tiagabine treatment of posttraumatic stress disorder in adults did not reveal a benefit over placebo (19).

Felbamate

Felbamate has a number of antiexcitatory effects, which account for its anticonvulant effects, including effects on N-methyl-D-aspartic acid (NMDA) and non-NMDA excitatory amino acid receptors as well as inhibition of voltage-gated sodium channels. It is relatively rarely used at present, because of serious hepatic and hematological adverse effects in some patients. Felbamate is an activating drug and may cause insomnia and irritability, particularly in children.

Vigabatrin

Vigabatrin exerts its anticonvulsant action by irreversibly binding to GABA transaminase, blocking degradation of GABA and increasing its concentration in the brain. It is not FDA-approved in the United States at this time and has been associated with irreversible peripheral visual field loss in a proportion of patients with chronic use, possibly upward of 30%, but it is otherwise available worldwide. Although drowsiness and sedation are common in adults, irritability, agitation, and aggression are more commonly seen in children.

CONCLUSION

Available information suggests that the anticonvulsant drugs in current use have, as expected, widespread effects on brain function. Even given the limited data available, it is evident that positive and negative psychotropic effects are common with use of these agents. Ideally, given the prevalence of behavioral and psychiatric disorders among children with epilepsy, physicians would be able to tailor choice of anticonvulsant drug with reference to the psychoactive profile of the drug. This would allow prescribers to avoid exacerbating pre-existing psychiatric disease, and possibly to improve symptoms and ultimately quality of life. Although current knowledge is insufficient to provide strong guidelines, the available information at least permits rational surveillance for adverse effects in children treated with these drugs.

Appropriate targets for future research in this area include greater understanding of the neurochemistry of psychiatric and behavioral disorders, as well as the mechanisms underlying anticonvulsant effects and psychotropic effects of these drugs. Epilepsy-specific vulnerabilities to these adverse effects, as well as the molecular basis of individual responses to these agents, also remain to be elucidated. In the clinical realm, controlled studies with greater numbers of patients are required to improve understanding of the effects and utility of these drugs in patients with epilepsy who also have psychiatric disorders. Consideration should also be given to examining both negative and potentially positive effects of polytherapy in this area.

References

1. Boylan LS, Flint LA, Labovitz DL, Jackson SC, et al. Depression but not seizure frequency predicts quality of life in treatment-resistant epilepsy. *Neurology* 2004; 62(2):258–261.
2. Caplan R, Siddarth P, Gurbani S, Hanson R, et al. Depression and anxiety disorders in pediatric epilepsy. *Epilepsia* 2005; 46(5):720–730.
3. Schubert R. Attention deficit disorder and epilepsy. *Pediatr Neurol* 2005; 32(1):1–10.
4. Ettinger AB. Psychotropic effects of antiepileptic drugs. *Neurology* 2006; 67(11):1916–1925.
5. Schmitz B. Effects of antiepileptic drugs on mood and behavior. *Epilepsia* 2006; 47 Suppl 2:28–33.
6. Ketter TA, Post RM, Theodore WH. Positive and negative psychiatric effects of antiepileptic drugs in patients with seizure disorders. *Neurology* 1999; 53(5 Suppl 2):S53–S67.
7. Glauser TA. Behavioral and psychiatric adverse events associated with antiepileptic drugs commonly used in pediatric patients. *J Child Neurol* 2004; 19 Suppl 1:S25–S38.
8. Pressler RM, Robinson RO, Wilson GA, Binnie CD. Treatment of interictal epileptiform discharges can improve behavior in children with behavioral problems and epilepsy. *J Pediatr* 2005; 146(1):112–117.
9. Brent DA, Crumrine PK, Varma RR, Allan M, et al. Phenobarbital treatment and major depressive disorder in children with epilepsy. *Pediatrics* 1987; 80(6):909–917.
10. Camfield CS, Chaplin S, Doyle AB, Shapiro SH, et al. Side effects of phenobarbital in toddlers; behavioral and cognitive aspects. *J Pediatr* 1979; 95(3):361–365.
11. de Silva M, MacArdle B, McGowan M, Hughes E, et al. Randomised comparative monotherapy trial of phenobarbitone, phenytoin, carbamazepine, or sodium valproate for newly diagnosed childhood epilepsy. *Lancet* 1996; 347(9003):709–713.
12. Wagner KD, Kowatch RA, Emslie GJ, Findling RL, et al. A double-blind, randomized, placebo-controlled trial of oxcarbazepine in the treatment of bipolar disorder in children and adolescents. *Am J Psychiatry* 2006; 163(7):1179–1186.
13. Hellings JA, Weckbaugh M, Nickel EJ, Cain SE, et al. A double-blind, placebo-controlled study of valproate for aggression in youth with pervasive developmental disorders. *J Child Adolesc Psychopharmacol* 2005; 15(4):682–692.
14. Reith D, Burke C, Appleton DB, Wallace G, et al. Tolerability of topiramate in children and adolescents. *J Paediatr Child Health* 2003; 39(6):416–419.
15. Grosso S, Franzoni E, Iannetti P, Incorpora G, et al. Efficacy and safety of topiramate in refractory epilepsy of childhood: long-term follow-up study. *J Child Neurol* 2005; 20(11):893–897.
16. White JR, Walczak TS, Leppik IE, Rarick J, et al. Discontinuation of levetiracetam because of behavioral side effects: a case-control study. *Neurology* 2003; 61(9):1218–1221.
17. Glauser TA, Ayala R, Elterman RD, Mitchell WG, et al. Double-blind placebo-controlled trial of adjunctive levetiracetam in pediatric partial seizures. *Neurology* 2006; 66(11):1654–1660.
18. Hirai K, Kimiya S, Tabata K, Seki T, et al. Selective mutism and obsessive compulsive disorders associated with zonisamide. *Seizure* 2002; 11(7):468–470.
19. Davidson JR, Brady K, Mellman TA, Stein MB, et al. The efficacy and tolerability of tiagabine in adult patients with post-traumatic stress disorder. *J Clin Psychopharmacol* 2007; 27(1):85–88.

49 Social Competence

Lesley C. Stahl
Rochelle Caplan

oncerted efforts have been made, in examining the social worlds of children, to distinguish children's social competence from their social skills. It has been suggested that the general domain of social competence is defined as the ability to identify and interpret social situations, as well as generate appropriate social responses (1). In contrast, others have defined social competence as the behavioral responses in any given social situation that prove effective or maximize the probability of producing positive effects for the individual (2, 3). Kavale and Forness have defined social skills as situation-specific actions exhibited in various social situations that require competent performance and result in interpersonal effectiveness (1). Thus, social competence might refer more to a trait, whereas social skills are more likely to represent the behavioral responses a child employs.

Understanding the nuances of children's social skills and competence are particularly important because social relationships are associated with the child's development of emotional regulation and sense of social self (4). In addition, relationships with peers enable young children to provide each other with emotional support in unfamiliar situations. They also enable children to acquire training in the wide range of social and cognitive skills necessary for facilitation of interpersonal relationships later in life (5).

A child's ability to negotiate positive social relationships varies with multiple factors, such as the child's psychosocial environment, cognitive skills, linguistic abilities, and behavior. Unfortunately, many children, including those with epilepsy (6–8), have difficulty establishing and maintaining social relationships, especially those with peers. Most importantly, the negative peer status of children with social skill deficiencies is a consistent predictor of poor long-term outcomes in a variety of domains (e.g., the interpersonal, psychiatric, employment, and legal realms) during adolescence and adulthood (9–16). Given the evidence for long-term poor social outcomes of children with epilepsy (17–19), clinicians should be aware of the need for early assessment and identification of social deficits and poor peer relationships in these children and, most importantly, effective intervention for these problems.

This chapter begins with a discussion of the predictive importance of poor peer relationships in children in general and current measurements used to assess children's social competence. The focus then shifts to the social cognitive mechanisms of children's social adjustment, with an emphasis on social information processing models that delineate the steps children go through cognitively and behaviorally when socializing with peers. Because of the high rate of cognitive and behavioral comorbidities in children with epilepsy (20), the chapter then provides a brief discussion on the social functioning of children with cognitive deficits and psychiatric disorders. Since epilepsy is a recurrent and chronic illness, the next section of this chapter describes the social competence of children with chronic illnesses. It then describes the social competence of children with epilepsy and the role stigma plays in peer relationships. The chapter concludes with recommendations for future directions, with an emphasis on a critical examination of the wide range of factors that might make children with epilepsy vulnerable to poor social competence and the need for intervention studies.

PREDICTIVE IMPORTANCE OF PEER RELATIONSHIP PROBLEMS

In comparison to popular children, children who are rejected by their peers show greater consistency in their negative peer status over time and report increased feelings of loneliness and social dissatisfaction (12). In addition, children with peer problems and peer rejection frequently have low academic achievement and poor school performance relative to other children (13, 14, 16, 21).

Peer rejection is also repeatedly noted to predict children's long-term adjustment. Specifically, Parker and Asher found that poor peer relationships contribute to 46–54% of male and 14–35% of female school dropout rates. Peer rejection is also considered a strong predictor of future criminal activity (15). Approximately 10–50% of children who have poor peer relationships are likely to engage in juvenile and adult criminal behaviors (15). The same study also found a significant relationship of peer rejection with increased frequencies of both poor occupational adjustment and adult suicide.

There is sufficient evidence to support the assertion that children who are rejected by their peers or who experience social difficulties are at risk for multiple maladaptive outcomes later in life (9–11, 14, 21–24). As previously reviewed, the maladaptive long-term outcomes for socially rejected children underscore the importance of understanding the social worlds of children with epilepsy in the hopes of providing effective interventions, since improvement of social functioning among peers is important for long-term adjustment in life (9–16).

SOCIAL COGNITIVE MECHANISMS IN CHILDREN'S SOCIAL ADJUSTMENT

The examination of the mechanisms underlying children's social cognitive processing reveals key variables that predict whether children are rejected or accepted by their peers. A child's response to social situations comprises a series of social information-processing steps, outside of the child's awareness, that reflect previous social interactions and experiences (25). Fraser noted that normal development of positive peer relationships in children requires the mastery of skills for assessing social situations, communication with peers, and the resolution of conflicts without aggression (25). For many children, the development and mastery of social cognitive skills is rather effortless. Children with deficient social skills may be more inclined to presume hostile intent of peers' behaviors or choose inappropriate responses to social situations and may exhibit difficulty in enacting appropriate social responses.

In many ways, social information processing is the way in which children interpret their social worlds and make sense of interpersonal interactions (12). Social information processing has been described as steps in a series of feedback loops in which each step may influence others during information processing of social situations and cues (25, 26). There has been an increased focus on the intricate process by which children perceive their interactions with peers and select a response and the method by which they behaviorally deliver their response. Thus, previous findings have emphasized the importance of understanding children's social cognitive processes, given that they may reflect specific cognitive styles and consequent behavioral styles that may eventually lead to social maladjustment (9). Of note, in addition to predicting social maladjustment, social cognitive processes contribute to the way a child perceives him- or herself in the social realm as well as the ways in which he or she chooses to perceive others (14).

Social Information-Processing Models

One model developed by Dodge et al. focuses on encoding of cues, interpretation of those cues, selection of a goal or response, and the behavioral enactment as domains of social information processing. In this particular model, children with skills deficits may also have knowledge deficits that contribute to their inability to interact appropriately with peers in social situations (27).

The social information-processing model developed by Dodge et al. provides a more detailed construct for the specific and complex steps children go through in perceiving and responding to social situations (27). The model includes six steps for social information processing that interact with one another in a series of continuous feedback loops. The steps are: (a) observation and encoding of social cues (e.g., attending to specific cues in the environment), (b) interpretation and attribution of the behavior and cues (e.g., assigning meaning to the cues), (c) selection of a goal or goals to be enacted (e.g., orientation to a particular set of outcomes), (d) construction of a response based on access (e.g., identification of various alternative responses to social situations), (e) response decision (e.g., selection of a response that can be enacted in the current situation), and (f) behavior enactment (e.g., executing the response selected) (1, 14, 25, 28).

However, for other children, such as those with cognitive impairments and psychopathology, the development of healthy social skills is limited by deficient social cognitive processing and impaired behavioral modulation. Socially inept children are less attentive to relevant social cues (e.g., decreased vigilance to peer behavior signaling conflict, or failure to notice behaviors or verbal responses indicating benign intent in interactions) (14). Children with deficient social skills may also be more inclined to presume hostile or negative intent of peers' behaviors, choose inappropriate responses to social situations, or exhibit difficulty in enacting appropriate social responses.

Measurement of Children's Social Competence and Social Functioning

The assessment of children's social competence and overall social functioning is somewhat challenging as there are relatively few measures that adequately assess children's social competence and social skills. Of the measures that do evaluate children's social skills and problematic behaviors, many use different methodologies and sources of information. Such methods include clinical interviews, direct behavioral observations (naturalistic or simulated observation), behavior-rating scales, peer reports (ratings or nominations), and self-report measures (e.g., perceptions about competence, acceptance, or status) (1, 29). In addition to the wide range of assessment methods, these measures employ multiple informants and sources of data (2, 29, 30).

Previous literature has strongly emphasized multimethods, multisources, and multisettings to be used in gathering data when examining children's social competence and skills, including peers, teachers, parents, and children's self-perceptions (2, 29, 30). The purpose behind this approach is to obtain a comprehensive and reliable evaluation of a child's social skills across a variety of settings including home, school, and community environments (29). With regard to a child's social competence and social skills, peer ratings appear to be the best measure, as they are less influenced by academic achievement than teacher ratings, less subject to social desirability than self-ratings, and more accessible than parent ratings (1).

Children's self reports provide valuable information regarding their own internal states. The Perceived Competence Scale for Children (PCSC) (31) is a child self-report measure that has been used in previous research studies and is designed to assess children's self-perceptions of competence across three domains: cognitive competence, reflected primarily in school or academic performance; social competence, reflected through popularity with one's peers; and physical competence, reflected through ability at sports and outdoor games. In addition to the PCSC, the Asher Loneliness Scale (ALS) (32) assesses

children's perceived relationships, social interaction, and loneliness including statements that tap into feelings of loneliness, peer status, and social adequacy (e.g., "I'm good at working with other teens").

The Matson Evaluation of Social Skills with Youngsters (MESSY) (33) evaluates how often a child engages in a range of verbal and nonverbal social behaviors. The MESSY also provides scales for both appropriate and inappropriate social skills so that users do not focus exclusively on the negative aspects of a child's behavior but also take into account positive aspects. Children are asked to report on their own perceptions of their social behaviors and on whether they feel the behaviors were appropriate or inappropriate. Although children may provide important information about their own internal emotional states, younger children may demonstrate limited self-awareness of their own thoughts and actions and, therefore, may not report information consistent with their actual behaviors (34).

In comparison to children's self-reports, parent-reported observations provide more objective information on a child's externalizing behaviors (35). One of the most frequently used parent-report measures assessing children's social functioning is the Achenbach Child Behavior Checklist (CBCL) (36). The CBCL includes broadband Externalizing and Internalizing scores in addition to reviews of children's friendships, weekly contacts with other children, and the quality of the child's relations with siblings and parents.

Similar to the child self-report forms, several studies have obtained parent's reports of children's social competence using the adult versions of the PCSC (31) and the MESSY (33). Both parent-report measures of the PCSC and MESSY include similar items to the child self-report measures and assess similar domains of functioning. Among the parent-report measures already noted, the Children's Assertive Behavior Scale (CABS) (37) is a parent-report measure that rates a child's social functioning with items placed on a continuum between socially passive behaviors to socially aggressive behaviors. Although parents are in a position to provide useful information about a child's externalizing behaviors, parents may be biased to the extent that they are often in a position of authority and may notice only children who consistently act in a disruptive or aggressive manner.

Much as with parent observations, teachers often provide valuable information on a child's externalizing behaviors and academic functioning (35). The CBCL Teacher Report Form (TRF) (36) is a measure often utilized to assess a child's academic, social, and emotional functioning based on teacher's observations. Similar to the CBCL parent form, the TRF provides broadband Externalizing and Internalizing scales and individual subscores reflecting problems with social withdrawal, unpopularity, immaturity, anxiety, and depression.

In addition to teacher reports, peers' inferences of a child's social competence have been obtained using peer nominations (e.g., "Who is your most favorite classmate?", "Who is your least favorite classmate?") or ratings (e.g., "How much would you like this child to be your friend?"). Peer sociometric measures are the most commonly used methods of identifying a child's social competence and determining a child's social status relative to his or her peers. The benefit of using this method rather than parent or teacher reports is that peer nominations or ratings can be used to identify "rejected" or "accepted" children, because peers are generally the ones who determine a child's social status.

VARIABLES ASSOCIATED WITH IMPAIRED SOCIAL FUNCTIONING IN CHILDREN

The Social Functioning of Children with Cognitive Disorders

Overall, children's social information processing is an intricate process including children's perceptions of their interactions with peers, their selection of a response, and the method by which they behaviorally enact the response (12, 14). Although children with poor peer relationships have been noted to exhibit deficiencies in their social information processing (14), the type and severity of deficiencies these children exhibit are variable depending on the presence of specific cognitive or psychiatric disorders. The high rates of cognitive and psychiatric comorbidities in pediatric epilepsy (20) underscore the importance of understanding how these variables are associated with social skills impairment in children.

Several previous studies have consistently demonstrated that students with learning disabilities (LD) have significant problems with social competence that are manifested in an assortment of social skill deficits (1, 38). One study in particular found that three out of four students with LD were evaluated as deficient in social skills on the basis of teacher and peer ratings (1). These authors also reported that eight out of ten students with LD were rejected by their non-LD peers, and 7 out of 10 students with LD were not considered as friends by their non-LD peers (1). Thus, social interaction for students with LD is defined most prominently by their peers through the dimension of rejection (1, 38, 39).

When considering potential factors that contribute to peer rejection, it has been suggested that peers perceive LD children as less competent in communication (verbal and nonverbal) and not as cooperative in social interactions (1). Interestingly, students with LD also perceive their social functioning to be negatively affected by a decreased competency in nonverbal communications and a deficiency in social problem-solving skills (1). These factors, considered collectively, could decrease interactions with peers and consequently lead to frequent rejection by peers. Of note, these studies all used peer nominations (38, 39) or teacher reports of social competence based on the Social Behavior at School Questionnaire (38).

The Social Functioning of Children with Psychopathology

Attention-Deficit/Hyperactivity Disorder (ADHD). Children with ADHD often have considerable difficulties in creating and maintaining relationships with their peers (40–43). Barkley estimates that more than 50% of ADHD children experience problems in their social relationships with peers (44). As a whole, boys with ADHD are more rejected and less popular with their peers than non-ADHD boys, and they appear to establish negative first impressions that put them at risk for further rejection in later interactions with peers (45).

These children are often perceived by their peers as annoying and aversive (42, 43). Studies have attributed this frequent rejection by peers to a multitude of variables including the ADHD child's lack of awareness to social cues, noncompliance, aggressive behaviors (22, 42, 43), distractibility from structured activities, hostile attribution of others' intentions, and inappropriate social agendas (43).

Additionally, ADHD children's behavior often elicits negative or hostile responses from peers (42). During social interaction, deficits in performance ("doing what you know") rather than knowledge ("knowing what to do") often contribute to the poor peer relationships of children with ADHD. In essence, although ADHD children typically want to develop positive peer relationships and know the appropriate responses or behaviors, they lack the behavioral repertoire and self-control to implement them. Wheeler and Carlson suggest that ADHD children may have frequent skill, performance, and self-control deficits when attempting to establish and maintain relationships with peers (16).

Anxiety Disorders. Children with anxiety disorders often exhibit significant difficulties in their relationships with peers. Several studies have demonstrated that children's anxiety and their maladaptive social functioning may be interrelated (46). In particular, anxiety in children has been associated with pervasive unpopularity among peers, decreased social interactions, and increased dependency on adults to facilitate social situations. These findings are consistent despite use of different measures both to identify anxiety and to assess social competence in these children (46). In general, anxious and depressed children are noted to have friendships of shorter duration, fewer visits with peers, and generally disturbed relationships compared to nonclinic children (47). Strauss et al. found that anxious children were liked significantly less than nonreferred children and were most likely to be socially neglected by peers (48).

Earlier studies noted several factors that may contribute to anxious children's poor peer relationships. In particular, anxious children frequently display a unique pattern of social deficits in that they exhibit shy and withdrawn social behaviors, whereas children with externalizing disorder are often perceived as aggressive, negative, and inappropriately assertive in their peer interactions (46). Thus, children with anxiety display increased levels of loneliness, poor social competence, and reduced rates of appropriate social skills compared to nonanxious children (46). The studies reviewed included the following measures in assessing social competence in anxious children: children's self-perceptions based on the ASL, PSCS, and MESSY (46), peer nominations (48), teacher reports of social competence based on the PSCS and MESSY (46), and parent reports using the PSCS and MESSY (46) or parent interviews (47).

Depression. As a whole, depressed mood in children is correlated with depressogenic beliefs, low self-esteem, self-control deficits, and impaired social skills (49). Blechman et al. found that children who are socially incompetent have the highest levels of peer-nominated and self-reported depression (2). Although studies have confirmed that depression and social skill deficits are correlated in children, they have not been able to conclusively determine the direction of causal influence (2, 49). While a child's level of depressive symptoms acts as a moderating variable in the relationship between social skills and subsequent depressive symptoms (49), others studies have implicated deficits in social competence as both a cause and consequence of depression in children (2, 50).

Children with depression are often described as exhibiting significantly more negative self-concepts and less social self-confidence than nondepressed children. Depressed children initiate interpersonal behavioral sequences that foster social strain and possible social isolation (50). In particular, they often seek personal assurances from others, but then tend to refuse or deny the reassurances they receive. Subsequently, these children experience significant interpersonal distress that can lead nondepressed children to withdraw from them and leave them socially isolated (50). The social competence of children with depression was assessed using peer nominations and ratings (2, 50), teacher reports based on the TRF (50), parent reports using the CBCL and MESSY (46) or parent interviews (47), and children's self-reports based on the MESSY (49) and PCSC (2, 50).

In summary, studies have consistently revealed that children and adolescents diagnosed with a wide range of psychopathology, ADHD (40–43), anxiety disorders (46, 47), and depression (2, 49, 50) are at an increased risk for peer rejection and poor social functioning.

The Social Functioning of Children with a Chronic Illness

The social functioning of chronically ill children and adolescents has received increased attention in research with the intent of better understanding the impact of chronic illness on children's daily lives (30, 51, 52). Reviews of the psychosocial literature reveal that children and adolescents with chronic illness are at a significantly greater risk of developing more psychosocial problems than their healthy peers (30, 51, 52). Often the daily demands and management of a chronic illness can disrupt or interfere with leisure activities and increase the likelihood that children and adolescents miss important time socializing with peers (53). In addition, children and adolescents with a chronic illness are twice as likely to report being unhappy compared to healthy children (51).

Examining the social functioning of children with cancer, La Greca found that teachers and peers perceived children with cancer to be less sociable and more socially isolated than their healthy peers (30). Chronic disease has been seen as affecting children's and adolescents' self-esteem, sense of identity, and overall sense of autonomy (54). Furthermore, children with chronic illness have fewer close friends and are less likely to date even when they are not physically prevented by their disability from participating in social activities (51).

Illness visibility might play a role in decreased social functioning in children with chronic illness (52, 53). Thus, children with a highly visible illness may experience greater levels of rejection, teasing, and invasive questioning than those with less illness visibility (52, 53). These experiences may perpetuate feelings of unattractiveness and undesirability in these children (53).

Yet there is evidence that children with a variety of chronic diseases who appear "normal" often have worse social functioning than ill children whose appearance was perceived as "abnormal" (53). It is possible that children with less-visible illnesses often struggle with the decisions to disclose their disease to peers and consequently struggle to appear "normal" and suppress symptoms that reveal their underlying disease.

However, studies examining the relationship between illness variables (e.g., age of onset, severity) and poor social functioning have found that physical restrictions and pain were associated with restricted social activities but not with limitations in social interactions (55). Some investigators have suggested that the poor social functioning that children with chronic illness experience may reflect associated psychopathology, such as anxiety and depression (56), rather than illness related variables.

The discrepancies found between various studies examining the social functioning in children with chronic illness may be related to the use of different types of measures or other methodological differences (e.g., sample size, type of disease). In addition, each of the studies reviewed employed various forms of measurement in assessing children's social competence, such as children's self-perceptions of their social competence based on the Social Self Efficacy Scale (51), Perceived Loneliness Scale (53), PSCS, or MESSY (55). Parents' reports were obtained using the CBCL (55), Children's Assertive Behavior Scale (55), and parent interviews (30), and peer reports were acquired using peer ratings of how much they liked a child (52). None of the studies reviewed obtained teachers' perceptions of social competence in children with chronic illness.

In summary, chronic illness is related to impaired social functioning in children. Inconsistent findings about the possible role of illness visibility in prior studies highlight the need to better understand how chronic disease interferes with normative social functioning in children and adolescents (53).

The Social Competence of Children with Epilepsy

As described throughout this part of the book, epilepsy is a chronic condition that impacts every aspect of development. Children with new-onset seizures and chronic epilepsy have been noted to exhibit impairment in their behavioral, emotional, cognitive, and linguistic functioning (7, 57–66).

Yet, despite the previously reviewed role played by these variables and chronic illness in children's social functioning, little research has been conducted on the social skills of children and adolescents with epilepsy (7, 8, 53, 61, 67–71). Of note, these studies all used parent or teacher reports of social competence based on the CBCL (36). None of the studies of social skills in children with epilepsy have used multiple informants, child self-reports, or peer reports.

Furthermore, only one study has examined for the possible effects of all these variables on social competence findings (7). Controlling for IQ, socioeconomic, and seizure variables, these authors found that subtle cognitive deficits along with externalizing behaviors (e.g., impulsivity, poor social judgment, and disruptive behaviors) were associated with decreased social involvement and low overall social competence (7). Austin et al. reported an association of social competence deficits with both internalizing and externalizing behaviors in a large sample of children with chronic epilepsy (57). Hermann et al. demonstrated an association of poor social competence with neuropsychologic deficits in children with epilepsy (61). The findings of these studies are consistent with the poor social competence found in the general population of children with learning disorders (1, 38), externalizing behaviors found in ADHD (23, 42, 43), as well as internalizing behaviors found in children with depression (50), and anxiety disorders (46).

Regarding linguistic and social communication deficits, children with epilepsy, particularly those with cryptogenic epilepsy with complex partial seizures (CPS), who have difficulty using language to formulate and organize their thoughts, are not competent social communicators (59). Their peers, perceiving them as "different," become reluctant to play or interact with them. Externalizing behaviors and disruptive disorder diagnoses, as well as poor peer interaction and academic achievement, in CPS children with more thought disorder might further contribute to this perception (59).

In terms of illness variables, findings are inconsistent across studies. Some studies demonstrate an association with seizure variables (8, 61, 70) while others do not (7). Variability in the findings of these studies might reflect sample differences in terms of size, associated mental retardation and educational difficulties, and demographic features as well as the inter-relationship between seizure variables, such as age of onset, duration of illness, seizure frequency, and antiepileptic drugs.

Similar to variables found for children with chronic illness (e.g., social restrictions, illness visibility, being unhappy), epilepsy might interfere with children's social interactions and time for socializing with peers (53). In addition, the degree to which a child's epilepsy is visible to peers may impact a child's overall social functioning (52, 53). Further studies are needed to determine whether, as found for children with chronic illness (52, 53), the visibility of a child's seizures and the decision to disclose this diagnosis to peers may have a greater impact on social functioning than seizure-related variables in these children (52, 53).

The Social Competence of Children with Epilepsy and the Impact of Stigma

Individuals are stigmatized because they have a feature that is considered undesirable (72) and may subsequently result in their disapproval and rejection by others (73). Studies examining the effects of stigma have emphasized the important dimension of visibility or concealability in relation to illness symptom presentation (72). As previously described for chronic illness, the more visible an illness is, the more a child is likely to be perceived as dissimilar and the less accepted by his or her peers (52, 53). Thus, the degree to which children with epilepsy experience social rejection could depend in part on the visibility of symptoms involved with the illness and its effects on their peers' perceptions of dissimilarity (52).

These findings suggest that peers' attitudes and beliefs may create a social atmosphere that contributes to feelings of stigma in the lives of children and adolescents with epilepsy, resulting in decreased social competence and acceptance by peers. Previous studies have revealed that children with epilepsy, fearful of experiencing stigmatization by their peers, choose to limit disclosure of their illness to others in an attempt to feel and appear less different from their peers (73). Children with epilepsy might, therefore, experience increased stress and decreased feelings of social competency as a result of how they manage their disorder and try to conceal their illness from others (72, 73).

In summary, additional information is clearly needed to understand the relationship of the stigma of epilepsy with the role of the previously reviewed cognitive, psychiatric, and social communication comorbidities in children on their social competence. More specifically, do children with epilepsy with poor social skills feel peer rejection because of the stigma of epilepsy rather than because of their comorbid cognitive, behavioral, and communication problems?

CONCLUSIONS AND FUTURE DIRECTIONS

Negative peer status of children with social skill deficiencies in childhood is a consistent predictor of poor long-term outcomes in adulthood. A child's response to social situations comprises a series of social information-processing steps that result from previous social interactions and experiences. Therefore, children with epilepsy with cognitive difficulties, including learning disorders and social communication deficits, as well as psychiatric disorders might experience difficulty in establishing positive peer relationships. Furthermore, children with a chronic illness often experience difficulty coping with illness-related frequent interruptions in their social activities, which result in the loss of important time socializing with peers and consequently poor peer relationships. All these variables increase the likelihood that children and adolescents with epilepsy are at risk for poor peer relationships as they cope with the daily demands of a chronic illness in addition to cognitive, linguistic, and psychiatric problems (Figure 49-1).

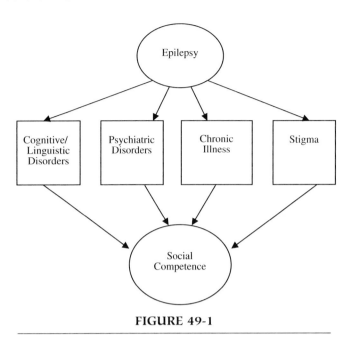

FIGURE 49-1

Social competence and contributing factors in poor peer relationships in children with epilepsy.

Future research should focus on examining the relationship among psychopathology, cognitive problems, linguistic deficits, and stigma in children with epilepsy, because poor social competence may reflect the interaction between these comorbid conditions. These studies should incorporate measures of how peers perceive the social skills of children with epilepsy and, in turn, whether their perception is related to cognitive, behavioral, and social communication problems of children with epilepsy.

The frequency of social impairment among children with epilepsy and its prognostic significance highlights that the social world may be an important point of intervention. Enabling the development of better peer relationships could improve the overall long-term outcomes in adult life. Finally, the findings of the previously reviewed studies emphasize the need to educate clinicians, parents, teachers, and children with epilepsy about the social skill deficits associated with epilepsy and, more importantly, the need for early assessment and intervention.

References

1. Kavale KA, Forness SR. Social skill deficits and learning disabilities: A meta-analysis. *J Learn Disabil* 1996; 29(3):226–237.
2. Blechman EA, McEnroe MJ, Carella ET, Audette DP. Childhood competence and depression. *J Abnorm Psychol* 1986; 95(3):223–227.
3. Foster SL, Ritchey WL. Issues in the assessment of social competence in children. *J Appl Behav Anal* 1979; 12(4):625–638.
4. Hartup W, Abecassis M. Friends and enemies. In: Smith P, Hart C, eds. *Blackwell Handbook of Childhood Social Development*. New York: Blackwell Publishers; 2002:285–305.
5. Asher S, Hymel S. Children's social competence in peer relations: sociometric and behavioral assessment. In: Wine J, Smye M, eds. *Social Competence*. New York: Guilford Press; 1981:125–156.
6. Austin JK, Smith MS, Risinger MW, McNelis AM. Childhood epilepsy and asthma: comparison of quality of life. *Epilepsia* 1994; 35(3):608–615.
7. Caplan R, Sagun J, Siddarth P, Gurbani S, et al. Social competence in pediatric epilepsy: insights into underlying mechanisms. *Epilepsy Behav* 2005; 6:218–228.
8. Williams J, Sharp G, Bates S, et al. Academic achievement and the behavioral ratings in children with absence and complex partial epilepsy. *Educ Treat Child* 1996; 19:143–152.
9. Crick N, Dodge K. A review and reformulation of social information-processing mechanisms in children's social adjustment. *Psychol Bull* 1994;115(1):74–101.
10. Dodge K. Behavioral antecedents of peer social status. *Child Dev* 1983; 54:1386–1399.
11. Dodge K, Coie J, Pettit G, Price J. Peer status and aggression in boys' groups: developmental and contextual analyses. *Child Dev* 1990; 61:1289–1309.

12. Henker B, Whalen C. The social worlds of hyperactive (ADDH) children. *Clin Psychol Rev* 1985; 5(5):447–478.

13. Hymel S, Vaillancourt T, McDougall P, Renshaw P. Peer acceptance and rejection in childhood. In: Smith P, Hart C, eds. *Blackwell Handbook of Childhood Social Development*. New York: Blackwell Publishers, 2002:265–284.

14. McFayden-Ketchum S, Dodge K. Problems in social relationships. In: Mash E, Barkley R, eds. *Treatment of Childhood Disorders*. New York: Guilford Press, 1998:338–360.

15. Parker J, Asher S. Peer relations and later personal adjustment: Are low-accepted children at risk? *Psychol Bull* 1987; 102(3):357–389.

16. Wheeler J, Carlson C. The social functioning of children with ADD and hyperactivity and ADD without hyperactivity: a comparison of their peer relations and social deficits. *J Emot Behav Disord* 1994; 2(1):2–12.

17. Wirrell EC, Camfield CS, Camfield PR, Dooley JM, et al. Long-term psychosocial outcome in typical absence epilepsy: sometimes a wolf in sheep's clothing. *Arch Pediatr Adolesc Med* 1997; 151(2):152–158.

18. Sillanpaa M. Long-term outcome of epilepsy. *Epileptic Disord* 2000; 2(2):79–88.

19. Sillanpaa M, Haataja L, Shinnar S. Perceived impact of childhood-onset epilepsy on quality of life as an adult. *Epilepsia* 2004; 45(8):971–977.

20. Austin J, Caplan R. Behavioral and psychiatric comorbidities in pediatric epilepsy: toward an integrative model. *Epilepsia*, in press.

21. Ollendick T, Weist M, Borden C, Green R. Sociometric status and academic, behavioral, and psychological adjustment: a five-year longitudinal study. *J Consult Clin Psychol* 1992; 60(1):80–87.

22. Coie JD, Dodge KA, Coppotelli H. Dimensions and types of social status: a cross-age perspective. *Dev Psychol* 1982; 18(4):557–570.

23. Coie J, Kupersmidt J. A behavioral analysis of emerging social status in boys' groups. *Child Dev* 1983; 54:1400–1416.

24. Johnston C, Pelham W, Murphy H. Peer relationships in ADDH and normal children: a developmental analysis of peer and teacher ratings. *J Abnorm Child Psychol* 1985; 13(1):89–100.

25. Fraser MW. Cognitive problem solving and aggressive behavior among children. *Fam Soc* 1996; 77(1):19–32.

26. Erdley C, Asher S. A social goals perspective on children's social competence. *J Emot Behav Disord* 1999; 7(3):156–168.

27. Dodge K, Pettit G, McClaskey C, Brown M. Social competence in children. *Monogr Soc Res Child Dev* 1986; 51(2):1–85.

28. Schippell P, Vasey M, Cravens-Brown L, Bretveld R. Suppressed attention to rejection, ridicule, and failure cues: a unique correlate of reactive but not proactive aggression in youth. *J Clin Child Adolesc Psychol* 2003; 32(1):40–55.

29. Merrell KW, Streeter AL, Boelter EW, Caldarella P, et al. Validity of the home and community social behaviors scales: comparisons with five behavior-rating scales. *Psychol Sch* 2001; 38(4):313–326.

30. LaGreca AM. Peer influences in pediatric chronic illness: an update. *J Pediatr Psychol* 1992; 17(6):775–784.

31. Harter S. Perceived Competence Scale for Children. Manual: Form O. Denver, CO: University of Denver.

32. Asher S, Hymel S, Renshaw P. Loneliness in children. *Child Dev* 1984; 55:1456–1464.

33. Matson, JL, Rotatori AF, Helsel WJ. Development of a rating scale to measure social skills in children: the Matson Evaluation of Social Skills with Youngsters (MESSY). *Behav Res Ther* 1983; 21:335–340.

34. Fergurgur MK. Childhood depression: relationships between parent, child, and clinician reports. Psy.D. diss., Alliant International University, 2002.

35. Dedmon AM. The availability, use, and participation of multiple informants in the assessment of child and adolescent psychopathology in research and practice. Ph.D. diss., Texas Tech University, 1999.

36. Achenbach T. Manual for the Child Behavior Checklist/4-18 and 1991 profile. Burlington, VT: University of Vermont Department of Psychiatry, 1991.

37. Michelson L, Wood R. Development and psychometric properties of the Children's Assertive Behavior Scale. *J Behav Assess* 1986; 4:3–13.

38. Nabuzoka D, Smith PK. Sociometric status and social behavior of children with and without learning difficulties. *J Child Psychol Psychiatry* 1993; 34(8):1435–1448.

39. Stone WL, La Greca AM. The social status of children with learning disabilities: a reexamination. *J Learn Disabil* 1990; 23(1):32–37.

40. Anastopoulos A, Klinger E, Temple E. Treating children and adolescents with attention-deficit/hyperactivity disorder. In: Hughes J, LaGreca A, Conoley J, eds. *Handbook of Psychological Services for Children and Adolescents*. Oxford: Oxford University Press, 2001:245–263.

41. Barkley RA. Attention-deficit/hyperactivity disorder. In: Mash E, Barkley R, eds. *Treatment of Childhood Disorders*. New York: Guilford Press, 1998:55–97.

42. Cunningham C, Cappelli M. Attention-deficit hyperactivity disorder. In: Bellack A, Hersen M, eds. *Handbook of Behavior Therapy in the Psychiatric Setting*. New York: Plenum Press, 1993:513–540.

43. Henker B, Whalen C. Hyperactivity and attention deficits. *Am Psychol* 1989; 44(2):216–223.

44. Barkley RA. Comorbid disorders, social relations, and subtyping. In: *Attention-Deficit Hyperactivity Disorder: A Handbook for Diagnosis and Treatment*. New York: Guilford Press, 1998:139–163.

45. Bickett L, Milich R. First impressions formed of boys with learning disabilities and attention deficit disorder. *J Learn Disabil* 1990; 23(4):253–259.

46. Strauss CC, Lease CA, Kazdin AE, Dulcan MK, et al. Multimethod assessment of the social competence of children with anxiety disorders. *J Clin Child Psychol* 1989; 18(2):184–189.

47. Puig-Antich J, Lukens E, Davies M, Goetz D, et al. Psychosocial functioning in prepubertal major depressive disorders: interpersonal relationships during the depressive episode. *Arch Gen Psychiatry* 1985; 42:500–507.

48. Strauss CC, Lahey BB, Frick P, Frame CL, et al. Peer social status of children with anxiety disorders. *J Consult Clin Psychol* 1988; 56:137–141.

49. Wierzbicki M, McCabe M. Social skills and subsequent depressive symptomatology in children. *J Clin Child Psychol* 1988; 17(3):203–208.

50. Cole DA, Martin JM, Powers B, Truglio R. Modeling causal relations between academic and social competence and depression: a multitrait-multimethod longitudinal study of children. *J Abnorm Psychol* 1996; 105(2):258–270.

51. Cappelli M, McGrath PJ, Heick CE, MacDonald NE, et al. Chronic disease and its impact: the adolescent's perspective. *J Adolesc Health Care* 1989; 10:283–288.

52. Potter PC, Roberts MC. Children's perceptions of chronic illness: the roles of disease symptoms, cognitive development, and information. *J Pediatr Psychol* 1984; 9(1):13–25.

53. Curtin LS, Siegel AW. Social functioning in adolescents with epilepsy. *Child Health Care* 2003; 32(2):103–114.

54. Kellerman J, Zeltzer L, Ellenberg L, Dash J, et al. Psychological effects of illness in adolescence: anxiety, self-esteem, and perception of control. *J Pediatr* 1980; 97(1):126–131.

55. Meijer S, Sinnema G, Bijstra J, Mellenbergh G, et al. Social functioning in children with a chronic illness. *J Child Psychol Psychiatry* 2000; 42:309–317.

56. Sandstrom MJ, Schanberg LE. Peer rejection, social behavior, and psychological adjustment in children with juvenile rheumatic disease. *J Pediatr Psychol* 2004; 29(1):29–34.

57. Austin JK, Dunn DW, Caffrey HM, Perkins SM, et al. Recurrent seizures and behavior problems in children with first recognized seizures: a prospective study. *Epilepsia* 2002; 43(12):1564–1573.

58. Caplan R, Siddarth P, Gurbani S, Ott D, et al. Psychopathology and pediatric complex partial seizures: seizure-related, cognitive, and linguistic variables. *Epilepsia* 2004; 45(10):1273–1281.

59. Caplan R, Siddarth P, Bailey C, Lanphier E, et al. Thought disorder: a developmental disability in pediatric epilepsy. *Epilepsy Behav* 2006; 8:726–735.

60. Davies S, Heyman I, Goodman R. A population survey of mental health problems in children with epilepsy. *Dev Med Child Neurol* 2003; 45(5):292–295.

61. Hermann BP, Whitman S, Hughes JR, Melyn MM, et al. Multietiological determinants of psychopathology and social competence in children with epilepsy. *Epilepsy Res* 1988; 2:51–60.

62. Hesdorffer DC, Ludvigsson P, Loafsson E, Gudmundsson G, et al. ADHD as a risk factor for incident unprovoked seizures and epilepsy in children. *Arch Gen Psychiatry* 2004; 61(7):731–736.

63. McDermott S, Mani S, Krishnaswami S. A population-based analysis of specific behavior problems associated with childhood seizures. *J Epilepsy* 1995; 8:110–118.

64. Rutter ML. Psycho-social disorders in childhood, and their outcome in life. *J R Coll Physicians Lond* 1970; 4(3):211–218.

65. Thome-Souza S, Kuczynski E, Assumpcao F Jr, Rzezak P, et al. Which factors may play a pivotal role on determining the type of psychiatric disorder in children and adolescents with epilepsy. *Epilepsy Behav* 2004; 5(6):988–994.

66. Wagner JL, Smith G. Psychological services in a pediatric epilepsy clinic: referral patterns and feasibility. *Epilepsy Behav* 2006; 8:39–49.

67. Apter A, Aviv A, Kaminer Y, Weizman A, et al. Behavioral profile and social competence in temporal lobe epilepsy of adolescence. *J Am Acad Child Adolesc Psychiatry* 1991; 30:887–892.

68. Austin J, Smith M, Risinger M, McNelis A. Childhood epilepsy and asthma: comparison of quality of life. *Epilepsia* 1994; 30:887–892.

69. Dorenbaum D, Cappelli M, Keene D, McGrath P. Use of a child behavior checklist in the psychosocial assessment of children with epilepsy. *Clin Pediatr (Phila)* 1985; 24:634–637.

70. McCusker C, Kennedy P, Anderson J, Hicks E, et al. Adjustment in children with intractable epilepsy: importance of seizure duration and family factors. *Dev Med Child Neurol* 2002; 44:681–687.

71. Schoenfeld J, Seidenberg M, Woodard A, Hecox K, et al. Neuropsychological and behavioral status of children with complex partial seizures. *Dev Med Child Neurol* 1999; 41:724–731.

72. Jacoby A, Snape D, Baker GA. Epilepsy and social identity: the stigma of a chronic neurological disorder. *Lancet Neurol* 2005; 4(3):171–178.

73. MacLeod JS, Austin JK. Stigma in the lives of adolescents with epilepsy: a review of the literature. *Epilepsy Behav* 2003; 4(2):112–117.

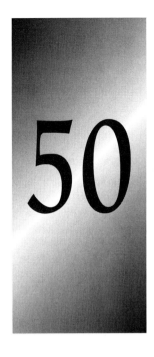

50 Academic Achievement

Joan K. Austin
David W. Dunn

cademic underachievement is common in children with epilepsy. In general, studies show children with epilepsy to be about one year behind academically, to have increased rates of school failure, and to use special education services at increased rates. Most of the research in this area has been cross-sectional in design and has investigated children who have had epilepsy for a number of years. In addition, because a number of seizure variables are interrelated (e.g., frequent seizures and polytherapy), it has been difficult to isolate specific factors that predict academic underachievement in this population. Nevertheless, some studies provide important information about risk and protective factors for academic underachievement in children with epilepsy. In this chapter we address three questions: When do academic problems begin? What are the risk factors for academic underachievement? What are the protective factors for academic achievement?

WHEN DO ACADEMIC ACHIEVEMENT PROBLEMS BEGIN?

Understanding when academic problems begin in this population is important because it both provides information about possible causes of problems and guides for treatment. Potential causes of academic achievement problems include underlying neurologic dysfunction, epilepsy syndrome, effects of seizures, and side effects of antiepileptic medications (AEDs). Academic achievement problems that are present before seizure onset or treatment with AEDs suggest underlying neurologic dysfunction as a cause of the problems rather than effects of seizures or side effects of AEDs. Moreover, academic problems that occur early suggest a need for clinicians to do early assessment and referral for these problems.

Only a few studies have investigated academic achievement in children with epilepsy early in the course of the disorder to determine when problems began. One research approach to identify when academic problems begin is to investigate the timing of use of special education services in the school. For example, in a prospective study of 542 children who had been diagnosed with epilepsy approximately 5 years earlier, Berg et al. studied the timing of use of special education services (1). In this study, 58% of the children had used such services at some point during this 5-year period. The finding of particular relevance to identifying when achievement problems begin was that 23% of the children had received special education services *before* the onset of their first unprovoked seizure. For 30% of the children, special education services were initiated after diagnosis, and for 5%, services were initiated between onset and diagnosis. The finding that at the time of the survey 47% were actively receiving special education services demonstrates that these academic achievement problems are enduring in a substantial percentage of children.

When Berg et al. explored which children were most at risk for service use, they found major differences based on etiology and epilepsy syndrome. Children were placed into two groups: (a) idiopathic and cryptogenic and (b) remote symptomatic and/or epileptic encephalopathy. Service use was lower in the former group, with 49% having received services at some point during the 5-year period and 15% having received services prior to the onset of epilepsy. In contrast, service use was substantially higher in the latter group, with 88% having ever received services and 54% having received services before onset of epilepsy. Although service use was lower in the idiopathic and cryptogenic group, it was still three times higher than the 13–14% rate of special service use in the general population of children during the same time period in the same geographical area.

Findings in a prospective study of 69 children with newly diagnosed epilepsy in the Dutch Study of Epilepsy in Childhood (2) also provide information on when academic achievement problems begin. Children in this study had normal intelligence and either idiopathic or cryptogenic epilepsy syndromes. Before diagnosis of epilepsy, 22% of the children had repeated one grade at school (compared to 11% in mainstream primary schools) and 54% of the children had required remedial assistance (compared to 23% of their healthy classmates). This study also provides empirical evidence that school performance problems begin before diagnosis of epilepsy in a large percentage of children who otherwise are normally developing.

In a study exploring academic achievement in children within the first year of seizure onset, data from teachers and academic achievement testing in the schools were used (3). The 106 children in the sample had normal intelligence and no other chronic conditions. Teachers' ratings at one year after the first seizure of the children's academic performance, and achievement testing carried out by the school, provided the data. Compared to national norms, the mean scores for the whole sample were in the normal range. However, approximately 25% of the children had total school performance scores at least one standard deviation below the norm based on the teacher's rating; 10% of the children had a total battery score on the achievement testing carried out by the school that was at least one standard deviation below the norm.

In summary, despite the few studies on academic achievement in children with new onset seizures and the variability in samples and methods, results are consistent. Findings provide strong evidence that problems in academic achievement occur very early in the course of epilepsy. Moreover, in almost one-fourth of children otherwise developing normally, achievement problems

occurred before the onset of seizures. In children with more severe epilepsy syndromes, over half of the children showed problems before seizure onset. These findings suggest that underlying neurologic dysfunction might be the cause of academic achievement problems in many children. Moreover, because problems were evident early in children otherwise developing normally, findings suggest that even subtle underlying neurologic problems can affect academic achievement in children with epilepsy.

Clinically, these findings suggest that families should be informed that some children with seizures, including those who appear to be developing normally, have academic achievement problems. At the time of seizure onset, and on a regular basis, the clinician should ask the parents how the child is doing at school. If problems are identified, a formal assessment of neuropsychologic functioning should be carried out, and if cognitive deficits are found, remedial help should be initiated. Because academic problems continue in a large number of children, it is important for the parents to be proactive in getting their children's educational needs met.

WHAT ARE THE RISK FACTORS FOR ACADEMIC UNDERACHIEVEMENT?

Understanding risk factors for academic underachievement should help to identify those children most at risk for problems. In addition, the identification of risk factors should guide the development of interventions to prevent or reduce achievement problems. Two groups of authors (4, 5) have proposed models that identify factors associated with academic achievement in children with epilepsy.

Fastenau Model

The model by Fastenau et al. describes how a variety of risk factors (neurologic dysfunction, seizure variables, neuropsychologic deficits, medication side effects, and child and family response) interact to predict academic achievement (6). Factors in the model that were proposed to be the most direct predictors of academic achievement were seizure variables, neuropsychologic deficits, and child and family response.

Relationships among seizure, neuropsychologic, and child and family variables were tested in a study of 173 children who had a diagnosis of at least 6 months duration (4). Children with another chronic condition or with diagnosed mental retardation were excluded. The study had two aims: (a) to investigate the relationship between neuropsychologic functioning and academic achievement and (b) to investigate the extent to which demographic, seizure, and psychosocial variables moderated the relationship between neuropsychologic functioning and academic achievement. Academic achievement was measured in three areas (reading, writing, and math) using standardized scales in an individual testing situation. Neuropsychologic functioning was measured using a comprehensive battery of cognitive tests. Three underlying constructs were identified using factor analysis on the battery: verbal/memory/executive functioning (VME), rapid naming/working memory (RN/WM), and psychomotor. Findings indicated that neuropsychologic functioning was strongly associated with academic achievement. VME had the strongest association, RN/WM had the next strongest association, and psychomotor had the weakest association with academic achievement.

Variables explored to determine whether they moderated the relationship between neuropsychologic function and academic achievement were demographic (child age, gender, and caregiver education), seizure (seizure type, seizure frequency, duration, and age at onset), child response (attitude toward having epilepsy, school self-concept, and attribution style), and family environment (family mastery). Of these variables only family mastery was found to have significant moderating effects. Specifically, the relationship between neuropsychologic functioning and academic achievement (writing and reading) was weaker when children's homes were more organized and supportive. When children lived in home environments that were less organized and unsupportive, their academic achievement was more influenced by neuropsychologic impairment.

Findings partially supported the model in that deficits in neuropsychologic functioning were strongly associated with academic underachievement. A major limitation of the study was that the epilepsy syndrome was not explored for relationships with academic achievement. On the other hand, a strength of the study was that it explored potential moderators, including some that were protective in nature. Those findings are further discussed in the section on protective factors.

Aldenkamp Model

The model proposed by Aldenkamp et al. describes how epilepsy factors (type of epilepsy/epilepsy syndrome, treatment [polytherapy], and frequency of epileptiform discharges) interact and lead to cognitive impairment [lower intelligence] and impaired vigilance (5). The direct predictors of academic underachievement in the model are cognitive impairment and impaired vigilance. The type of epilepsy or epilepsy syndrome is theorized to predict cognitive impairment and lower intelligence. Epileptiform electroencephalographic (EEG) discharges and polytherapy are proposed to predict impaired vigilance.

The Aldenkamp model is similar to the Fastenau model in that they both propose that neuropsychologic functioning predicts academic achievement. In the Aldenkamp model, however, epilepsy syndrome is the prominent variable that predicts neuropsychologic impairment, which in turn predicts academic achievement. In other words, neuropsychologic functioning is proposed to mediate (i.e., account for) the association between epilepsy syndrome and academic achievement. Compared to the Fastenau model, the Aldenkamp model is less comprehensive and does not include demographic or psychosocial variables as potential moderators.

Relationships proposed in the Aldenkamp model were investigated by Aldenkamp et al. in a study of 176 children with epilepsy ages 6–12 years and 113 control children similar in age and gender distribution (5). All of the children were in regular education classrooms. The four areas of educational achievement measured were reading, arithmetic, language, and visuospatial. Epilepsy variables studied were type of epilepsy/epilepsy syndrome (none, idiopathic generalized, localization-related, or symptomatic generalized), seizure type (none, partial, or generalized), epileptiform EEG discharges (none, sporadic, or frequent), and treatment (none, monotherapy, or polytherapy). Reaction time and memory function were tested to measure neuropsychologic function and vigilance.

Aldenkamp's findings supported relationships proposed in the model. The poorest academic achievement was found in children with localization-related and symptomatic generalized epilepsy. On average these children were approximately 14 months behind at school compared to controls. Those with symptomatic generalized epilepsy were 26 months delayed compared to controls. In contrast, children with idiopathic epilepsy did not show educational delay.

The dominant neuropsychologic factor associated with academic underachievement in Aldenkamp's study was lower intelligence. Children with localization-related epilepsy had a mean IQ that was 10 points below controls, and those with symptomatic epilepsies had a mean IQ that was 26 points lower. The other characteristics related to academic underachievement were frequent epileptiform discharges on the EEG and the use of polytherapy. Because these two factors were not independent of epilepsy syndrome, the predominant predictor of academic underachievement was epilepsy syndrome. Given that serious epilepsy syndromes are associated with brain dysfunction, the findings also suggest that underlying neurologic dysfunction predicts academic underachievement (5).

Based on these two models, there is substantial evidence that a major risk factor for academic underachievement is neuropsychologic impairment. It is also clear from studies by Berg et al. (1) and Aldenkamp et al. (5) that neuropsychologic functioning is not independent of epilepsy syndrome. In the McNelis et al. (3) study the authors did not measure epilepsy syndrome but did explore seizure severity. They placed the children into three groups based on seizure severity: 1 (only one seizure and no AED), 2 (only one seizure and treated with an AED), and 3 (more than one seizure and treated with an AED). Seizure severity was significantly associated with the teacher's rating of performance. Because the authors did not report on epilepsy syndrome, it is not known if those with higher seizure severity also had more severe syndromes. These findings suggest that, early in the course of epilepsy, assessment for neuropsychologic functioning should be carried out on children who have recurrent seizures and those with more severe epilepsy syndromes.

WHAT ARE PROTECTIVE FACTORS FOR ACADEMIC ACHIEVEMENT?

Identifying factors that might prevent the development of academic achievement problems or reduce them is of the highest clinical importance. Little research has been carried out to identify protective factors, especially psychosocial variables that are likely to be amenable to change in the clinical setting. In general, studies have been conducted (a) to investigate the association between academic achievement and psychosocial variables and (b) to identify psychosocial variables that moderate or weaken the relationship between neuropsychologic impairment and academic underachievement.

A few studies have investigated the relationship between psychosocial variables and academic underachievement. Demographic, seizure, and psychosocial variables have been explored for their relationships with academic achievement in cross-sectional studies. This approach was used by Austin et al. as part of a larger study of academic achievement in children with either epilepsy or asthma (7). Epilepsy subjects were 117 children who had been treated with an AED for at least one year. Children who were diagnosed with mental retardation or who had another chronic condition were excluded. Factors explored for relationships with academic achievement were child gender, seizure severity (combination of seizure type, frequency, and AED use), child attitude toward having epilepsy, child adaptive functioning at school, and school self-concept. Child attitude reflected beliefs and feelings about having epilepsy. Child adaptive functioning was measured by teachers' ratings of how hard the child was working at school, the appropriateness of the child's behavior at school, how well the child was learning at school, and the child's happiness at school. School self-concept measured the children's perceptions of their intellectual status and their school performance. In a multiple regression, these factors, along with child gender and seizure severity, were explored for relationships with academic achievement as measured by school-administered group tests given during the academic year.

Results from the multiple regression showed that, with the exception of self-concept, all of the variables were significantly associated with the total composite score on the achievement battery. Female gender, low seizure severity, more positive child attitudes, and more positive ratings of the child's adaptive functioning at school were significantly associated with higher academic achievement. This study points to two potential protective factors (attitudes and adaptive functioning at school) that should be amenable to change. Attitudes are based on beliefs, and feelings associated with beliefs, that are amenable to change. Adaptive functioning at school also should be amenable to change because it reflects the child's motivation and behavior at school. This study was limited by lack of information on neuropsychologic functioning and epilepsy syndrome, which might have affected the results. For example, children with poorer adaptive functioning might have had more cognitive impairments.

A more recent study also explored demographic, seizure, AED, psychosocial, and family variables for relationships with school performance in 73 adolescents (ages 12–18 years) in Nigeria (8). Demographic variables studied were child age, gender, and level of education. Seizure variables were age at onset, years of epilepsy, seizure frequency per month, and seizure type. AED variables were type, number, and presence of side effects. Psychosocial variables measured were adolescent perception of stigma, attitude toward having epilepsy, and psychopathology. Family variables were family functioning, socioeconomic status, caregiver perception of stigma, and caregiver psychopathology. Finally, to measure school performance, the mean scores on all subjects were obtained from school records for the prior three school terms. Data were analyzed using multiple regression.

Results indicated that six variables were significantly associated with school performance. Two family variables (caregiver psychopathology and family functioning), three adolescent psychosocial variables (attitude toward having epilepsy, perception of stigma, and externalizing behavior problems), and one seizure variable (years of epilepsy) were significant predictors of school performance. With the exception of the seizure variable, these variables are potentially amenable to change through behavioral interventions (8). This study (8) did not include information on epilepsy syndrome or neuropsychologic functioning.

Neuropsychologic functioning and psychosocial variables were measured in a study of a small sample ($n = 41$) of children with idiopathic epilepsy and explored for relationships with academic underachievement (9). Children were placed into three groups based on teacher rating of their school achievement: good, adequate, and poor. Psychosocial data collected from the teacher also included information on child behavior problems, maturity, attention, motivation, and social skills. Data were analyzed using one-way analysis of variance.

Results showed that 61% of the children had less academic progress than would have been expected given their IQ. No associations were found between school achievement and child gender, social background, and seizure variables (age of onset, seizure type, duration of the seizure disorder, EEG features, and AED treatment). Variables associated with poor academic achievement were visuomotor impairment, low IQ, and emotional maladjustment (e.g., poor self-esteem and low motivation). The finding that almost two-thirds of children with epilepsy who were otherwise normally developing were having problems academically suggests that psychosocial variables might play an important role in academic achievement (9). Because of the small sample, data analysis was limited to univariate analysis of variance. A strength of the study was that subjects were limited to those with idiopathic epilepsy.

Another approach to identifying protective factors is to identify variables that weaken the relationship between neuropsychologic impairment and academic underachievement. This approach was used in the previously described study by Fastenau et al. (4), which showed that family mastery moderated the relationship between cognitive deficits and achievement. Families with high mastery are able to accomplish tasks without difficulty; they plan ahead, have direction, and perceive that each family member contributes equally to family chores and activities. It might be that an organized family environment provides children with more neuropsychologic impairments with needed routine and structure that would facilitate their academic achievement. In addition, families who are high in mastery might also have regular study times and bedtimes for children, which in turn might lessen the academic risk associated with cognitive impairment. Based on this study, interventions should be considered that focus on improving the family environment. For example, interventions might focus on encouraging family members to emotionally support the child related to achievement problems and to help the child with activities and routines that would promote academic achievement in the children.

CONCLUSION

In summary, academic achievement problems are common in children with epilepsy. They appear to begin very early in the course of the disorder, and in some children they are present before the onset of seizures. Two variables that appear to be risk factors for achievement problems are neuropsychologic impairments and more serious epilepsy syndromes. Some psychosocial variables (e.g., child attitudes) that might serve as protective factors have been identified. However, these studies have not included neuropsychologic functioning or epilepsy syndrome. In addition, with few exceptions, studies have not tested these psychosocial variables to determine whether they moderate the relationship between neuropsychologic functioning and academic achievement.

References

1. Berg AT, Smith SN, Frobish D, Levy SR, et al. Special education needs of children with newly diagnosed epilepsy. *Dev Med Child Neurol* 2005; 47(11):749–753.
2. Schouten A, Oostrom K, Jennekens-Schinkel A, Peters ACB. School career of children is at risk before diagnosis of epilepsy only. *Dev Med Child Neurol* 2001; 43: 574–576.
3. McNelis AM, Johnson CS, Huberty TJ, Austin JK. Factors associated with academic achievement in children with recent-onset seizures. *Seizure* 2005; 14: 331–339.
4. Fastenau P, Shen J, Dunn D, Perkins S, et al. Neuropsychological predictors of academic underachievement in pediatric epilepsy: moderating roles of demographic, seizure, and psychosocial variables. *Epilepsia* 2004; 45(10):1261–1272.
5. Aldenkamp AP, Weber B, Overweg-Plandsoen WCG, Reijs R, et al. Educational underachievement in children with epilepsy: A model to predict the effects of epilepsy on educational achievement. *J Child Neurol* 2005; 20(3):175–180.
6. Fastenau P, Dunn D, Austin J. Pediatric epilepsy. In: Rizzo M, Eslinger P, eds. *Principles and Practice of Behavioral Neurology and Neuropsychology*. Philadelphia: W.B. Saunders, 2003:965–982.
7. Austin JK, Huberty TJ, Huster GA, Dunn DW. Academic achievement in children with epilepsy or asthma. *Devel Med Child Neurol* 1998; 40(4):248–255.
8. Adewuya AO, Oseni SBA, Okeniyi JAO. School performance of Nigerian adolescents with epilepsy. *Epilepsia* 2006; 47(2):415–420.
9. Sturniolo MG, Galletti F. Idiopathic epilepsy and school achievement. *Arch Dis Child* 1994; 70:424–428.

51

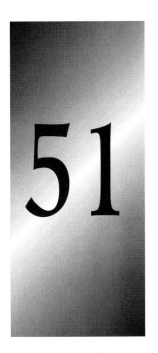

Psychosocial Intervention in Pediatric and Adolescent Epilepsy

Janelle L. Wagner
Gigi Smith

I t is well documented that youth with epilepsy are at increased risk for psychiatric symptoms and psychosocial maladjustment as a result of biological vulnerability, family, and individual (e.g., social, cognitive, self-efficacy, coping skills) variables (see Chapters 42–46, 49). One of the most difficult challenges posed to children with recurrent seizures and their families may be the noncontingency associated with epilepsy. Perceived control, self-esteem, and behavior management have been suggested as salient targets of intervention, for which psychopharmacological and medical interventions are not indicated (1). Thus, the current literature implies that interventions focused on changing youths' general perceptions and specific illness appraisals as well as enhancing coping skills may be an effective treatment for pediatric psychosocial maladjustment.

The importance of a mental health presence in pediatric epilepsy clinics has been underscored by the discrepancy between prevalence rates of psychiatric/psychosocial difficulties and access to adequate mental health services (2–4). Experts in the field of pediatric epilepsy have also highlighted the development of evidence-based standards of mental health care for children with epilepsy as a priority recommendation (5). Unfortunately, the extant literature, which is reviewed in the following paragraphs, is quite sparse.

PSYCHOLOGICAL INTERVENTIONS TARGETING PSYCHOSOCIAL ADJUSTMENT

Psychological interventions for children with epilepsy have primarily included educational (6), cognitive-behavioral (7–9), or family (10, 11) components, with most delivered in a group format (7–9, 12). Some interventions target caregivers or youth only (13); others include both caregivers and youth (7–9, 12). An example of an educational program for youth with epilepsy and their parents is the "Be Seizure Smart" program developed by Austin and colleagues (6). This program, delivered via telephone, targets family members' fears about epilepsy as well as seizure knowledge, management, information, and support needs. Results from ten families of children with newly diagnosed epilepsy revealed that children had significantly fewer epilepsy concerns and reduced need for information as well as higher general knowledge about seizures and better family functioning after this intervention. Parents also evidenced significantly greater knowledge about seizures and a reduced need for information and for supports.

Several studies have utilized cognitive-behavioral strategies with children and their families. For example, in a large international study, Lewis and colleagues (7) examined the efficacy of "The Children's Epilepsy Program," an intervention designed to provide knowledge about epilepsy as well as teach decision making and communication skills to youth aged 7 to 14 and their parents. Children and their parents were randomly assigned to the control (CO; $N = 126$) or the treatment condition (TX; $N = 126$). Parents and children in the CO group attended three two-hour joint didactic sessions. Four 90-minute TX sessions for youth covered understanding body messages, controlling seizures with medication, telling others about seizures, and coping skills/adaptation (bullying, teasing, and frustration; rehearsal and role-playing strategies to combat negative attitudes; anger management exercises; etc.). The four TX sessions for parents included education, decision making, working as a family system, and coping/adapting (9). Results revealed no significant pretreatment differences across youth groups. At the 5-month follow up, both groups of youth demonstrated significant improvement in seizure knowledge, but the TX group showed significantly greater knowledge than the CO group did. Additionally, at follow-up, after adjustment for covariates, results revealed that the TX group viewed themselves as being more competent than the CO group in social interactions and skills (7). Results also revealed that parents' knowledge improved significantly across both the TX and CO groups; however, parental anxiety was significantly more reduced in the TX group than in the CO group. In contrast to the initial hypotheses, data did not support the premise that, following intervention, parents in the TX group would be more supportive of their child's participation in activities (9).

In another study, Snead and colleagues (8) examined the effectiveness of a cognitive-behavioral/psychoeducational group intervention for adolescents and their parents. "Taking Charge of Epilepsy" was based in part on the work of DiIorio and colleagues (14) and focuses on medical aspects of epilepsy (adherence, education), healthy behaviors and attitudes (health habits, diet, exercise, sleep), stress management (anxiety, depression, emotions, cognitive-behavioral coping skills), social concerns (self-image and self-esteem, driving, dating), and interacting with family and peers (behavioral rehearsal of communication skills and negotiation with caregivers). An initial pilot study informed the development of a clinical trial in which six group sessions were presented to seven teens aged 13–18 and their families. T-tests revealed no significant pre–post intervention changes in quality of life reported by the teens on the Quality of Life in Epilepsy Inventory for Adolescents (QOLIE-AD-48) (15); however, nonparametric statistical analyses revealed a significant effect toward a positive change. No significant effects or trends were observed for depressive symptoms, reported through the Children's Depression Inventory (CDI) (16), or anxiety symptoms, reported on the Revised Children's Manifest

Anxiety Scale (RCMAS) (17). Finally, open-ended questions revealed family satisfaction with and perceived relevancy of the intervention.

Tieffenberg and colleagues (12) designed a group program to teach developmentally appropriate independence and illness self-management to children with epilepsy and asthma in Argentina. Participants were randomized to intervention (TX; 64 asthma and 54 epilepsy completers) or control (CO; 43 asthma and 45 epilepsy). Children and parents in the TX group received five two-hour sessions that included identification of bodily cues and personal triggers, recognition of the balance in life, understanding treatment, handling risk situations, and developing healthy decision-making strategies. Games, drawings, stories, videos, and role playing were utilized to illustrate key concepts of the program, and a booster session occurred 2 to 6 months after completion of the initial program. Results revealed that children in both the asthma and epilepsy TX groups showed a significant increase in internal health locus of control, which was maintained at one-year follow-up. Also, parents' knowledge improved, and fears and anxieties decreased in both TX groups. Finally, children with seizures in the TX group had significantly fewer seizures and visits to the physician's office as well as improved school attendance compared to children with seizures in the CO group.

In a series of family intervention studies, Hufford and colleagues examined the effectiveness of an interactive videoconferencing family therapy protocol for adolescents with epilepsy and their parents. In the first study (11), three teens and their mothers identified the most pertinent problems and completed between six and ten sessions. Outcomes were measured using self-report instruments developed by the researchers. Mothers reported a 40% reduction in problem severity and a 73% reduction in frequency of family problems. Similarly, teens reported 63% and 84% reductions in problem severity and family problems, respectively. Glueckauf and colleagues (10) expanded on the first study with 22 teens who were randomly assigned to one of three conditions: interactive videoconferencing-based family counseling (VFC), office-based family counseling (OFC), or waiting list (WL). For each participant, the therapist conducted a behavior-systems analysis of the primary problems and proposed strategies for interventions. Families were then taught how to set and track progress of goals, and discussion of weekly events, identification of and suggestions for removing barriers to goal accomplishment, praise for efforts, and review of assignments were also conducted. Nonparametric statistical analyses revealed significant reductions in parent- and child-reported problem severity and frequency across all treatment groups at 1 week post-intervention, and treatment gains regarding problem behaviors were maintained at 6 months. However, teachers reported an increase in behavior problems at the 6-month follow-up.

Three other studies, which were not specifically designed as clinical trials to examine the effectiveness of a psychological intervention but that provide descriptive information regarding psychological interventions in children with epilepsy, are outlined in the following paragraphs. In the first study the impact of epilepsy camp on attitudes towards epilepsy in children aged 8 to 16 was examined (13). Campers completed the initial assessment before arriving for camp and received a second questionnaire on the last day of camp to return in one month. Camp did not include educational programming on epilepsy. Results for 20 children revealed no pre–post-camp differences in attitudes toward epilepsy as reported on the Child Attitude Toward Illness Scale (18). Nonetheless, there was a trend for children with infrequent seizures (fewer than six seizures per year) to show improvement in attitudes over time; however, the sample size of 13 likely limited power in this analysis.

In the second study, Hoare and Kerley (19) designed a parents' group counseling program to reduce the psychological distress of children with epilepsy and their families and to identify the factors associated with psychosocial outcome. However, attendance for the program was abysmal, as only 12% of the 108 families who were initially approached participated. Moreover, of those 14 parents who attended the first meeting, attrition was high for subsequent sessions; therefore, the effectiveness of the intervention could not be examined. Descriptive statistics revealed that participants were more likely than nonparticipants to have marital problems, family stress, a child with more severe epilepsy, and greater concern over the effect of epilepsy on their child's development. Participating parents reported that individual sessions with a trained counselor would be more beneficial and indicated their preference for this counselor to be part of the clinic neurology team.

In the final study reviewed, Williams and colleagues (20) tracked psychological referral patterns in a university-based epilepsy clinic for 533 children aged 2 months to 27 years followed over two years. Of the 533 children seen, 101 were referred for psychological services. Specifically, 19% of all children were seen for brief psychological interventions, which focused on acceptance of the diagnosis and medical status, behavior management, clarification of myths about epilepsy, and concerns regarding medication side effects and adherence. Additionally, a significant number of children were referred for psychoeducational, neuropsychologic, speech, or behavioral evaluations. Outpatient psychotherapy for family, individual, or both was recommended for 14% of families, parent training for 4%, and state funded programs for severely disturbed

children for 2%. See Wagner and Smith (21) for a more detailed review of the articles presented.

STRENGTHS AND LIMITATIONS OF THE EXTANT LITERATURE

The studies just summarized make an important contribution to the literature by investigating the impact of psychological interventions on psychosocial adjustment in pediatric epilepsy. They are characterized by several strengths, including multiparticipant designs. To illustrate, several studies utilized parallel or combined parent and child interventions (6–8, 10, 12) and/or teacher report outcomes (7, 10). Study designs were also strengthened by the use of randomization in four of the nine studies (7, 8, 10, 12), and a comparison group of youth with asthma (12). Additionally, three studies utilized pilot data for streamlining their subsequent, more formalized intervention studies (7, 8, 10). Snead and colleagues (8) employed empirically supported information in the development of their intervention in addition to well-validated outcome measures. Select studies also attended to issues surrounding feasibility in dissemination of the intervention. For example, to minimize transportation difficulties, Glueckauf (10) utilized advanced technology in the form of videoconferencing. The Snead (8) and Lewis (7, 9) interventions were designed for a brief group format, and Williams (20) provided intervention at a medical center epilepsy clinic. Similarly, the Sawin study (13) was conducted in a naturalistic setting, though it was not intended to be a "true" psychological intervention.

These studies share familiar weaknesses, including lack of detailed information, poorly defined or validated outcome measures, small sample sizes, and design limitations. For example, details are absent regarding the intervention content (19) and sample characteristics such as pretreatment symptom severity (10, 20). As a result, readers of the literature are left unaware of how many participants evidenced clinical disorders (e.g., depression, anxiety) prior to the intervention. Exclusion of this data could significantly impact outcomes (e.g., regression to the mean if pretreatment scores are clinically elevated) and for whom the intervention is appropriate (e.g., those at risk, those with clinical symptoms, youth with epilepsy in general). Similarly, researchers have used outcome measures that are often ill defined or nonstandardized (6, 7). Traditionally, these measures have also not been readily accessible to clinicians for use or further validation. Accessibility to intervention protocols has also been limited.

With the exception of Lewis et al (7) and Tieffenberg (12), most studies are plagued by small sample sizes, potentially limiting the generalizability of findings and adequate power to detect significant findings.

Also, many of the studies have less than ideal study designs, including varying numbers of control and treatment sessions (7, 9). Other studies lack a control group to allow for stronger evidence that improvements were indeed attributal to the intervention and not extraneous factors (6, 8). It is also sometimes unclear in evidence-based psychosocial intervention what the level of training is for those who are providing the intervention (6, 7, 12). Additionally, although therapeutic relationship has a significant impact on treatment outcomes, it was assessed in only one study (10). Finally, studies (7, 12) frequently failed to control for potential psychological mediators that likely play a salient role in study findings. Notably, small sample sizes do limit the feasibility of advanced analyses required to examine these indirect relationships.

CONCLUSIONS AND FUTURE DIRECTIONS

In summary, the literature reviewed in this chapter (summarized in Table 51-1) provides support for the use of psychological interventions in youth with epilepsy; however, multisiteal comprehensive randomized clinical trials across sites are necessary before implications of effectiveness of psychosocial interventions for youth with epilepsy can be adequately surmised. Despite current limitations in the literature, several relevant points are highlighted. First, the nature of cognitive-behavioral interventions renders them amenable to epilepsy-specific psychosocial adjustment, and they should be promoted on that basis (22). Second, common pathogenic mechanisms for epilepsy and depression have been proposed, inferring that if depression is not treated, epilepsy may not be managed as effectively as possible (23). Similarly, behavioral interventions have been shown to reduce seizure severity and frequency as well as improve psychological adjustment (24). Thus, evidence-based psychological interventions for youth with epilepsy indeed seem relevant, and further steps should be taken to develop, research, and disseminate such interventions.

Historically, epilepsy research has focused on issues related to the basic science of seizures, medications, evaluation methods, and treatments such as vagus nerve stimulation, the ketogenic diet, and epilepsy surgery. Understanding the etiologies of seizures and effective management must continue to be examined; however, parallel endeavors to explore psychological interventions for youth with epilepsy must receive adequate attention, given the high comorbidity of psychosocial difficulties in these children. Unfortunately, physicians may often underestimate the impact of patients' stressors, environment, family, and fears. Consequently, behavioral approaches to epilepsy are neglected (25). Health care professionals are also challenged by "epilepsy-like dysthymia" instead of traditional presentations of depressive symptoms (26).

Indeed, Gilliam and colleagues (27) reported that 79% of neurologists who see epilepsy patients do not screen for depression in their clinic, but that they would if an evidence-based treatment improved compliance and quality of life.

Paralleling these critical points, the following clinical recommendations are offered. Brief cognitive-behavioral therapy and psychological consultation within epilepsy medical clinics are likely to benefit youth with epilepsy/ seizure disorders. Thus, the presence of a psychologist or psychiatrist in epilepsy clinics who could provide a variety of on-site psychologic services similar to those described by Williams et al. (20) would greatly benefit both epilepsy health care providers and families. Psychologists, social workers, and nurses with specialized training in epilepsy should be employed in the care of children with epilepsy (28) to provide interventions to youth and their families as well as provide consultation to medical professionals, school personnel, and state agencies providing resources for youth with epilepsy. These health care providers are encouraged to participate in school- and community-based programs to provide comprehensive education to parents, teachers, primary care health providers, peers, children with epilepsy, and the community.

With an emphasis on evidence-based medicine (5), the question becomes one of which intervention(s) to use. Until epilepsy-specific psychological assessment and intervention tools are readily available, those supported by research in the fields of psychology and psychiatry should be utilized. For example, evidence-based interventions focused on changing youths' perceptions and enhancing coping skills and self-efficacy (29) appear salient for use with youth with epilepsy. Alternatively, several of the interventions outlined in this chapter may also be applicable. Of course, factors such as group versus individual intervention, familial access to the clinic, and availability of trained mental health professionals will also inform decisions.

Finally, recommendations for the establishment of evidence-based psychological interventions for youth with epilepsy are offered. First, an efficient and standardized tool that assesses epilepsy-specific psychological adjustment must be validated in youth with epilepsy and sensitive to the measurement of clinical change. A recent study published promising findings for a similar measure for use in adults with epilepsy (30). Second, multisite randomized clinical trials should be designed to examine content and methods of delivery of cognitive-behavioral interventions adapted for youth with epilepsy and their families. Such studies would directly inform the practice of evidence-based medicine. For example, adaptation of an evidence-based cognitive-behavioral intervention focused on control enhancement, given the relevancy of learned helplessness and perceived control to epilepsy

TABLE 51-1

Characteristics of Studies Utilizing Psychological Interventions to Target Psychosocial Adjustment in Pediatric Epilepsy

STUDY	SAMPLE	TARGET OF INTERVENTION	STUDY DESIGN	INTERVENTION	RESULTS
Austin et al. 2002 (6)	10 families	Reduce concerns and fears, seizure management	Pre–post treatment group	Group family telephone conference, education by nurse, seizure management	Both parent and child knowledge about seizures improved, and informational needs were met.
Glueckauf et al. 2002 (10)	22 teens at risk and their parents	Reduce problem behaviors	Random assignment to video conference counseling [VC], office-based counseling [OB], or waiting list [WL]	Identification of problem, goal setting, barriers to goals	Parents and teens reported reductions in problem severity and frequency across VC and OB, discrepancy in parent and teacher report of prosocial behavior.
Hoare and Kerley 1992 (19)	14 parents	Reduce psychological distress	Descriptive	Nonspecific	Attrition was high. Participants more likely to have more family problems than nonparticipants.
Hufford et al 1999 (11)	3 adolescents and their mothers	Reduce problem behaviors	Pre–post treatment group	Emphasis on identifying problem, setting goals, and barriers to goals delivered via interactive videoconferencing	Mothers and teens reported reductions in problem severity and family problems.
Lewis et al. 1990 (7), 1991 (9)	252 families	Increase epilepsy knowledge and decision making skills	Random assignment to treatment [TG] or control [CG]	CG: didactic education TG: body cues, seizure management, coping skills, telling others	Children in TG showed greater knowledge compared to CG. TG children viewed themselves as more competent than CG. TG parents reported significant reduction in anxiety.
Sawin et al. 2001 (13)	20 children ages 8–16	Improve attitude towards epilepsy	Pre–post treatment group	Summer epilepsy camp. No formal epilepsy education. Interactions with other children with epilepsy.	No pre–post camp differences in attitudes towards epilepsy.
Snead et al. 2004 (8)	7 adolescents ages 13–18 and their parents [Pilot study of 4 families]	Improve epilepsy management, coping skills, communication	Pre–post treatment group	Cognitive-behavioral intervention focused on healthy behaviors, stress management, social concerns, communication	No significant pre–post changes in quality of life [QOL], depression, or anxiety. Significant effect toward positive change in QOL.
Tieffenberg et al. 2000 (12)	99 children and their parents	Improve independence and self-management of epilepsy	Random assignment to treatment [TG] and control [CG] group	Identify cues, recognize seizure triggers, understand treatment, handle risk, develop good decision making	Children showed significant increase in internal health locus of control. Parents' knowledge improved while fears/anxieties decreased. School attendance improved and visits to physician decreased for TG compared to CG.
Williams et al. 1995 (20)	101 children referred out of 533	Various targets	Descriptive information on referral patterns	Ranged from adjustment to epilepsy, discipline, epilepsy education, adherence	N/A

management (29), may be appropriate. Similarly, the relationship of self-efficacy to management of epilepsy–related depressive symptoms has been highlighted for the development of manualized interventions designed to enhance psychosocial adjustment to epilepsy (31). In addition, given the robust support for the impact of family adjustment on adherence, seizure control, and quality of life (32), a caregiver component should be included in the intervention. Specifically, caregiver guilt and struggles specific to parenting a child or teen with epilepsy (e.g., relaxed discipline, overprotectiveness) should be included because these issues may cause barriers to parenting and the enhancement of developmentally appropriate

independence (33). Interventions should also be age-specific and sensitive to challenges that may be specific to a particular age, such as adolescence. Within the design of the study, training for individuals who will be disseminating the treatment, as well as measures to ensure the fidelity of these interventions and adherence to treatment protocols, should be included. Reports of study findings should contain statistics such as effect size and clinical significance. Lastly, dissemination of the manualized treatments and training workshops for clinicians to promote the practical use of evidence-based medicine for youth with epilepsy should be a priority of researchers.

References

1. Dunn DW. Neuropsychiatric aspects of epilepsy in children. *Epilepsy Behav* 2003; 4(2):101–106.
2. Ott D, Siddarth P, Gurbani S, Koh S, et al. Behavioral disorders in pediatric epilepsy: unmet psychiatric need. *Epilepsia* 2003; 44(4):591–597.
3. Besag FM. Psychopathology in people with epilepsy and intellectual disability. *J Neurol Neurosurg Psychiatry* 2003; 74(11):1464.
4. McDermott S, Mani S, Krohn W. A population-based analysis of specific behavior problems associated with childhood seizures. *J Epilepsy* 2005; 8:110–118.
5. Living well with epilepsy II: report of the 2003 National Conference on Public Health and Epilepsy. Washington, DC: Epilepsy Foundation of America, 2003.
6. Austin JK, McNelis AM, Shore CP, Dunn DW, et al. A feasibility study of a family seizure management program: "Be Seizure Smart." *J Neurosci Nurs* 2002; 34:30–37.
7. Lewis MA, Salas I, de la Sota A, Chiofalo N, et al. Randomized trial of a program to enhance the competencies of children with epilepsy. *Epilepsia* 1990; 31(1):101–109.
8. Snead K, Ackerson J, Bailey K, Schmitt MM, et al. Taking charge of epilepsy: the development of a structured psychoeducational group intervention for adolescents with epilepsy and their parents. *Epilepsy Behav* 2004; 5:547–556.
9. Lewis MA, Hatton CL, Salas I, Leake B, et al. Impact of children's epilepsy program on parents. *Epilepsia* 1991; 32(3):365–374.
10. Glueckauf RL, Fritz SP, Ecklund-Johnson EP, Liss HJ, et al. Videoconferencing-based family counseling for rural teenagers with epilepsy: Phase 1 findings. *Rehabil Psychol* 2002; 47(1):49–72.
11. Hufford BJ, Glueckauf RL, Webb P. Home-based, interactive videoconferencing for adolescents with epilepsy and their families. *Rehab Psychol* 1999; 44(2):176–193.
12. Tieffenberg JA, Wood EI, Alonso A, Tossutti MS, et al. A randomized field trial of ACINDES: a child centered training model for children with chronic illnesses. *J Urban Health* 2000; 77(2):280–297.
13. Sawin KJ, Lannon SL, Austin JK. Camp experiences and attitudes toward epilepsy: a pilot study. *J Neurosci Nursing* 2001; 33(1):57–64.
14. DiIorio C, Faherty B, Manteuffel B. Epilepsy self-management: partial replication and extension. *Res Nursing Health* 1994; 17(3):167–174.
15. Cramer JA, Westbrook LE, Devinsky O, Perrine K, et al. Development of the Quality of Life in Epilepsy Inventory for Adolescents: the QOLIE-AD-48. *Epilepsia* 1999; 40(8):1114–1121.
16. Kovacs M. Children's depression inventory. North Tonawanda, NY: Multi-Health Systems, 1992.
17. Reynolds C, Richmond B. Revised Children's Manifest Anxiety Scale. Los Angeles: Western Psychological Services, 1985.
18. Austin JK, Huberty TJ. Development of the Child Attitude Toward Illness Scale. *J Pediatr Psychol* 1993; 18(4):467–480.
19. Hoare P, Kerley S. Helping parents and children with epilepsy cope successfully: The outcome of a group programme for parents. *J Psychosom Res* 1992; 36(8):759–767.
20. Williams J, Sharp GB, Griebel ML, Knabe MD, et al. Outcome findings from a multidisciplinary clinic for children with epilepsy. *Child Health Care* 1995; 24(4):235–244.
21. Wagner JL, Smith G. Psychosocial intervention in pediatric epilepsy: a critique of the literature. *Epilepsy Behav* 2006; 8:39–49.
22. Krishnamoorthy ES. Treatment of depression in patients with epilepsy: problems, pitfalls, and some solutions. *Epilepsy Behav* 2003; 4:S46–S54.
23. Kanner AM, Balabanov A. Depression and epilepsy: how closely related are they? *Neurology* 2002; 58(Suppl 5):S27–S39.
24. Williams DT, Gold AP, Shrout P, Shaffer D, et al. The impact of psychiatric intervention on patients with uncontrolled seizures. *J Nerv Ment Disord* 1979; 167(10):626–631.
25. Devinsky O. Therapy for neurobehavioral disorders in epilepsy. *Epilepsia* 2004; 45(Suppl 2):34–40.
26. Barry JJ, Jones JE. What is effective treatment of depression in people with epilepsy? *Epilepsy Behav* 2005; 6:520–528.
27. Gilliam FG, Santos J, Vahle V, Carter J, et al. Depression in epilepsy: ignoring clinical expression of neuronal network dysfunction? *Epilepsia* 2004; 45(Suppl 2):28–33.
28. National Association of Epilepsy Centers. Guidelines for essential services, personnel, and facilities in specialized epilepsy centers in the United States. *Epilepsia* 2001; 42(6):804–814.
29. Weisz J, Southam-Gerow M, Gordin E, Connor-Smith J. Primary and secondary control enhancement training for youth depression: Applying the deployment-focused model of treatment development and testing. In: Kazdin A, Weisz JR, eds. Evidence-based psychotherapies for children and adolescents. New York: Guilford Press; 2003: 165–186.
30. Gilliam FG, Barry JJ, Hermann BP, Meador KJ, et al. Rapid detection of major depression in epilepsy: a multicentre study. *Lancet Neurol* 2006; 5:399–405.
31. Caplin D, Austin JK, Dunn DW, Shen J, et al. Development of a self-efficacy scale for children and adolescents with epilepsy. *Child Health Care* 2002; 31(4):295–309.
32. Austin JK, Dunn DW, Johnson CS, Perkins SM. Behavioral issues involving children and adolescents with epilepsy and the impact of their families: recent research data. *Epilepsy Behav* 2004; 5 Suppl 3:S33–S41.
33. Shore CP, Austin JK, Dunn DW. Maternal adaptation to a child's epilepsy. *Epilepsy Behav* 2004; 5(4):557–568.

IX

OTHER DISORDERS ASSOCIATED WITH EPILEPSY THAT IMPACT BEHAVIOR, MOOD, AND COGNITION

52 Psychogenic Nonepileptic Seizures: An Overview

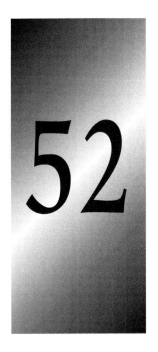

Markus Reuber
Christian E. Elger

sychogenic nonepileptic seizures (PNES) are episodes of altered movement, sensation, or experience resembling epileptic seizures, but not associated with ictal electrical discharges in the brain. Also, PNES cannot be explained by physiologic processes such as hypotension or bradycardia and do not fulfill the diagnostic criteria for pathophysiologically "explained" disorders such as migraine, sleep disorders, or paroxysmal dystonia.

PNES are one of the most important differential diagnoses in epilepsy clinics. What is more, they can occur in patients who also have epilepsy. PNES are often disabling and require a therapeutic approach that is very different from that appropriate for epileptic seizures. Failure to recognize PNES and treatment of PNES as epilepsy are associated with serious risks to patients. For these reasons, it is essential that doctors who see patients with epilepsy be able to recognize PNES and to communicate the diagnosis to their patients.

After a brief summary of the current knowledge about epidemiology and etiology of PNES, this chapter will focus on the aspect most important to neurologists: making the diagnosis and communicating it successfully

to patients. A final section will describe treatment options and outcome.

NOSOLOGY, EPIDEMIOLOGY, AND ETIOLOGY

Nosology

Although the fact that they are listed under the heading of dissociative disorders in the International Classification of Diseases (ICD-10), and under somatoform or conversion disorders in the *Diagnostic and Statistical Manual of Mental Disorders* (DSM-IV), suggests that PNES are an identifiable, separable, and separate disorder, we and others regard them as one manifestation of a range of interacting psychosocial conditions. It is likely that most PNES are an unintentional expression of psychologic distress, although there are currently no tests of intentionality and it is probable that at least some seizures are factitious or malingered. PNES are best understood as a manifestation of a range of different forms of psychopathology rather than a clearly delineated diagnostic entity. As such, they may be interpreted as a form of dissociation (in the sense that they disrupt the usually integrated functions of consciousness, memory, identity, or perception), although PNES not only are seen in dissociative disorders but also occur in other psychiatric disorders. Most commonly associated are other somatoform (22–84%), other dissociative (22–91%), posttraumatic stress (35–49%), depressive (57–85%), or anxiety disorders (11–50%). Twenty-five to 62% of patients with PNES fulfill the DSM-III or IV criteria for personality disorder (1). In a small minority of patients (perhaps one in 20), PNES seem to occur without any other psychiatric symptoms or in the absence of personal or social circumstances that could explain a dissociative or conversion process (2). It remains uncertain whether these patients have a pathophysiologically different disorder or whether they have not disclosed information that would have enabled a more comprehensive formulation of their symptoms.

Epidemiology

There is no reliable information on the incidence or prevalence of PNES in the general population. Studies based on patients referred to neurologic centers suggest an incidence of 1.5/100,000 per year (equivalent to about 4% that of epilepsy), or 3/100,000/year. However, given the setting of these studies in specialist centers and the fact that only video-encephalographically (EEG) proven cases were counted, these figures are likely to be an underestimate. One recent study that reportedly captured all patients first presenting to a neurologist, emergency room, or primary care physician with a blackout indicated that 57.4% had epilepsy, 22.3% had fainted, and 18.0% had PNES (3). PNES are diagnosed even more commonly in certain clinical settings. For instance, about 20% of patients referred for epilepsy surgery evaluation, and up to 50% of patients with refractory "status," have PNES rather than epilepsy (4).

Etiology

Like that of other functional ("medically unexplained") somatic syndromes, the etiology of PNES is perhaps best described by a multidimensional model that distinguishes between predisposing, precipitating, perpetuating, and (in the case of PNES also) triggering factors. Predisposing factors confer an increased vulnerability to PNES, precipitating factors determine the timing of the manifestation of seizures, perpetuating factors contribute to a chronically recurrent course, and triggering factors start off individual seizures. It is a particular advantage of this model that it can be used to produce an etiology-based formulation in an individual patient. The factors that need to be considered in such a formulation include biographical factors (e.g., childhood trauma, abuse, neglect, life events), relevant biological features (e.g., sex, presence of learning disability), psychologic features (e.g., coping styles, personality or "ego structure"), "psychiatric"

or "neurologic" comorbidity (e.g., depression, anxiety, epilepsy, or learning disability), and social factors (e.g., family environment, financial security) (2). Factors can interact with each other (a history of childhood neglect may become particularly relevant after a distressing life event in adult life), and one factor can act in different ways. Additional epileptic seizures, for instance, could act as a predisposing factor by reducing a patient's confidence to be able to remain in control in a moment of particular distress, an epileptic aura can precipitate or trigger a dissociative reaction, and certain environmental responses that patients experience when they have epileptic seizures could make a chronically recurrent course of PNES more likely.

MAKING AND COMMUNICATING THE DIAGNOSIS

Diagnostic Delay

Although PNES are not rare and much has been published about their semiology, it has been observed that the mean latency between manifestation and diagnosis remains unacceptably long at 7–16 years and that three-quarters of patients with PNES (and no additional epilepsy) are still treated with anticonvulsants initially. The rate of patients with PNES misdiagnosed as epilepsy has been found to be around 5% in seizure patients treated by family physicians, or 10% in patients with "refractory epilepsy" referred to a specialist epilepsy clinic.

Misdiagnosis

The early distinction of PNES from epileptic seizures is important because treatment with antiepileptic drugs (AEDs) is inappropriate for a psychologic problem and puts people at risk of drug toxicity, emergency interventions, and even death. As significantly, the failure to make the diagnosis means that clinically relevant psychopathology (including an increased risk of suicide) is likely to remain undetected and unaddressed. In addition, the misdiagnosis of PNES as epilepsy is very costly. The average annual medical mistreatment cost of PNES as epilepsy has recently been estimated as £316 ($626) in the UK (5). The indirect costs to society through loss of employment (of patients and carers) are likely to be even greater than the direct costs of inappropriately prescribed anticonvulsant drugs or professional time (although it has been shown that patients with undiagnosed PNES visit their doctors very frequently). It has been shown that 69% of PNES patients were working at the time of manifestation of seizures, but only 20% were still working at the time the diagnosis was made. An outcome study demonstrated that at a mean of 4.1 years after diagnosis, 41.4% of patients

TABLE 52-1
Differential Diagnosis of Paroxysmal Neurologic Disorders in Adults

Syncope
Reflex syncope (e.g., neurovasogenic synocpe, micturition syncope)
Cardiac syncope (e.g., with tachy- or bradycardia, long-QT syndrome, structural cardiac abnormalities, aortic stenosis, cardiomyopathies, arteriovenous shunts)
Perfusion failure (e.g., hypovolemia, autonomic failure)

Psychogenic attack
Psychogenic nonepileptic seizure
Depersonalization/derealization
Panic attack
Hyperventilation attack
Flashback

Transient ischemic attack

Migraine

Narcolepsy/cataplexy

Parasomnia

Paroxysmal dystonia

Hyperekplexia

Paroxysmal vertigo

Hypoglycemia

(with a mean age of 38.6 years) had retired on health grounds. Encouragingly, health care utilization costs are significantly reduced in the six months after diagnosis of PNES with video-EEG (4).

Differential Diagnosis

The differential diagnosis of paroxysmal neurologic disorders is wide (see Table 52-1). However, PNES can be distinguished from most of the conditions listed on the basis of the patient's history and a description of a typical event by a seizure witness alone. The commonest challenge is the differentiation of PNES from epileptic seizures and syncopal events. This differentiation cannot be based on any single observation, and no single semiologic feature is shared by all types of PNES.

History

One important reason why the diagnosis of PNES may not be made is that physicians fail to consider the differential diagnosis of nonepileptic seizures before diagnosing (and treating) presumed epilepsy. However, there are often many "red flags" in the patient's history that could alert clinicians to the possibility of a diagnosis of PNES (Table 52-2). A number of recent studies have demonstrated that the history given by patients with PNES does not only differ from the account given by patients with epilepsy in terms of facts relating to seizures (such

TABLE 52-2
Features in the History That Can Help to Determine the Likelihood of PNES, Epileptic Seizures, or Syncopal Events

FEATURE IN HISTORY	PSYCHOGENIC NONEPILEPTIC SEIZURES	EPILEPTIC SEIZURES	SYNCOPE
Manifestation <10 years of age	Unusual	Common	Occasional
Change of seizure semiology	Occasional (more dramatic with time)	Rare	Rare
High seizure frequency	Common	Occasional	Rare
Recurrent seizure status	Common	Rare	Never
Worsening with antiepileptic drugs	Occasional	Rare	Rare
Seizures in front of a doctor	Common	Unusual	Common (blood tests)
Multiple unexplained physical symptoms	Common	Rare	Rare
Multiple surgical procedures and investigations	Common	Rare	Rare
Psychiatric treatment	Common	Rare	Rare
Vascular risk factors, history of heart disease	Rare	Rare (except in elderly patients)	Not uncommon (common in patients with cardiogenic syncope)
Sexual and physical abuse	Common	Rare	Rare
Parasuicide	Common	Rare	Rare

TABLE 52-3

Overview of Linguistic Criteria Found Useful in the Differentiation of Interactions with Patients with Epileptic and Nonepileptic Seizures (6)

FEATURE	EPILEPTIC SEIZURES	NONEPILEPTIC SEIZURES
Subjective seizure symptoms	Typically volunteered, discussed in detail	Avoided, discussed sparingly
Formulation work related to seizures	Extensive, large amount of detail	Practically absent, very little detailing effort
Seizures as a topic	Self-initiated	Initiated by interviewer
Focus on seizure description	Self-initiated or readily maintained with prompting	Difficult or impossible ("focusing resistance")
Seizure description by negation	Rarely (negation usually explained and contextualized)	Common
Description of periods of reduced consciousness or self control ("gap")	Intensive formulation work Aiming at a precise, detailed description Attempts to fill "gap" Precise placement of period of lost consciousness in seizure context Display of willingness to know what happened during periods of unconsciousness Degree of unconsciousness can be interactively challenged	"Holistic" description of unconsciousness Naming of unconsciousness without further description Pointing out inability to remember anything No self-initiated detailed description Presentation of "gap" as most dominant or only element of attacks Completeness of unconsciousness cannot be challenged
Metaphors, conceptualization of seizures	Seizures as external independent agent Active fight against seizure threat	No coherent concept Seizures not definitely external No active struggle against seizure threat
Spontaneous reference to attempted seizure suppression	Often made	Rarely made

as the duration of attacks or a history of seizures in a doctor's office). There are also marked differences in how patients with epileptic and nonepileptic seizures interact with doctors when they talk about their seizure experiences. These features can be elicited if the doctor adopts a receptive stance, avoids early interruption, and opens the encounter with an open question (such as "How can I help you today?" or "What was your expectation when you came to see me?"), so that patients have an opportunity to stress those aspects of their experience that are subjectively most relevant (6). Some of the linguistic and interactional features that can help physicians to make the diagnosis of epilepsy or PNES when they give patients time to communicate their own agenda are summarized in Table 52-3. Doctors may also pick up other nonverbal or affective cues in their interaction with the patient or the interaction between patient and carer, such as signals of helplessness, submissiveness, delegation, inappropriate indifference, anger, or fear.

Semiology of PNES

Studies using cluster analysis suggest that several types of PNES can be differentiated. The commonest semiology

involves excessive movement of limbs, trunk, and head. Seizures with stiffening and tremor, or seizures with atonia, are less frequent in most series. A diagnosis of PNES is used most commonly in patients who describe impairment or loss of consciousness (LOC) during their attacks. However, if PNES are defined as paroxysmal events that resemble epileptic seizures, the diagnosis could also be applied to purely sensory or experiential attacks akin to simple partial seizures. Based on this understanding (and the fact that patients with PNES without LOC may have a similar profile and respond to similar treatments as those whose PNES involve LOC), patient series from epilepsy centers often also include individuals whose consciousness is unimpaired during attacks. However, it is likely that diagnostic categories are particularly ill-defined in this patient group. What is called "PNES" in an epilepsy center would probably (and justifiably) be labeled as "panic attacks," as "hyperventilation attacks," or as episodes of "derealization" or "depersonalization" elsewhere.

The clinical diagnosis of PNES is based on the description or observation of the semiologic details such as those listed in Table 52-4. As in the evaluation of other patients with paroxysmal disorders, it is crucial to interview a seizure witness as well as the patient himself. Perhaps

TABLE 52-4

Ictal Observations That Help in the Differentiation of PNES, Epileptic Seizures, and Syncope

OBSERVATION	PSYCHOGENIC NONEPILEPTIC SEIZURES	EPILEPTIC SEIZURES	SYNCOPE
Seizure provocation	Not uncommon (arguments, stress, doctor's office)	Rare (e.g., photosensitive epilepsy)	Common (from an upright position, not from a supine position)
Gradual onset	Not infrequent (often lasting several minutes)	Focal onset possible (aura, duration typically <30 seconds)	Common (presyncopal symptoms, duration often minutes)
Motor activity	Commonly undulating motor activity with sudden pauses but stable frequency	Typical seizure patterns (tonic, clonic, tonic-clonic)	Myoclonic jerks common (short duration, rapid recovery)
Asynchronous arm and leg movements	Common	Unusual	Not uncommon (multifocal myoclonus)
Purposeful movements	Occasional	Very rare	Rare
Rhythmic pelvic movements	Occasional	Rare	Never
Opisthotonus, "arc de cercle"	Occasional	Very rare	Occasional ("decerebrate" posturing)
Prolonged ictal atonia	Occasional	Very rare	Not >60 seconds
Skin	No cyanosis despite long seizure duration	Cyanosis common	Pallor, sweating
Ictal crying	Occasional	Very rare	Very rare
Closed eyes	Very common	Rare	Rare
Resistance to eye opening	Common	Very rare	Very rare
Maintained pupillary light reflex	Very common	Often abolished	Common
Ictal reactivity	Occasionally partially preserved	Rarely preserved	Rarely preserved
Ictal incontinence	Not uncommon	Not uncommon	Rare
Seizure duration >2 minutes	Common	Uncommon	Very uncommon (only if patient supported in upright posture)
Postictal reorientation	Often unexpectedly quick or slow	Mostly over minutes	<1 minute (exception: head injury caused by collapse/patient maintained in upright position)
Tongue biting	Occasional (tip)	Not infrequent (lateral)	Occasional (tip)
Injury	Common	Common (burns)	Rare
Seizures at night (from "sleep")	Not uncommon	Common	Rare

the most helpful pointers to a diagnosis of PNES are seizures that seem to be provoked by stressful situations or that occur in front of a doctor, seizures of long duration with motor activity that stops and starts, and closed eyes during tonic-clonic-like seizures. Patients with PNES are often very upset when they have a seizure, they may cry during or immediately after the event.

PNES can be particularly difficult to distinguish from epileptic seizures originating in the frontal lobes. Like the semiology of PNES, that of frontal lobe seizures may include emotionally charged screams, bilateral motor activity with retained consciousness, and ictal speech arrest with unimpaired postictal recollection of the event. A degree of ictal responsiveness may be preserved in focal frontal or temporal lobe seizures, although actions carried out during the seizure may later not be remembered. Semiologic factors that may help distinguish between frontal lobe seizures and PNES include the observations that frontal seizures very commonly arise from sleep, occur in clusters, and are very short. Although the semiology of frontal seizures may be dramatic and bizarre, it is more stereotyped than that of PNES (4).

Interictal Tests.   The role of interictal EEG, brain imaging, or neuropsychologic testing in the diagnostic categorization of seizures is limited. In line with an older study, we recently found that 22.3% of our patients with PNES (and no additional epilepsy seizures) had interictal epileptiform EEG abnormalities, lesions detected by magnetic resonance imaging (MRI), or neuropsychologic deficits. In view of the fact that not all patients had been fully investigated, the true proportion of the patients with such abnormalities would likely have been even higher (7). In a blinded comparative study, we found nonspecific EEG changes in 18% of patients with PNES (and no epilepsy) and 10% of age-matched healthy controls (8).

Abnormalities are therefore commoner in patients with PNES than in healthy individuals. This makes it harder to distinguish patients with PNES from those with epilepsy. Although abnormal findings are much commoner in patients with epilepsy as a group, individual patients with epilepsy can have normal investigations, whereas evidence of brain abnormality may well be found in patients with PNES (7).

Ictal EEG Recordings.   Even ictal EEG recordings can be misleading if the seizures do not involve loss of consciousness, because surface EEG shows ictal changes in only 10–20% of such focal epileptic seizures. Ambulatory EEG in particular, especially if undertaken with one of the older eight-channel EEG recorders, may miss ictal discharges or epileptiform interictal changes. When using such systems, the clearest indication of the seizure type is sometimes provided by the electrocardiographic (ECG) channel. It has been noted that the heart rate tends to increase suddenly in epileptic seizures, whereas the increase is more gradual in PNES (4).

Even in the absence of ictal epileptiform discharges or typical postictal EEG changes, the periodicity of ictal muscle artifacts can help in the distinction of epileptic and nonepileptic seizures: The frequency of muscle spasms in generalized tonic-clonic epileptic seizures shows a characteristic decrement, whereas the shaking seen in PNES tends to change during the course of a seizure only in terms of amplitude, not frequency (9).

Postictal Blood Tests.   The measurement of serum prolactin (or cortisol) 15 to 20 minutes after an ictal event can help in the differentiation of PNES and epileptic seizures. However, although a 3- to 5-fold prolactin rise above a baseline measurement taken at the same time of day provides reasonably reliable support for a diagnosis of epilepsy, the absence of an increase does not prove that the event was a PNES (especially if an epileptic seizure would have been classified as focal rather than generalized). It should be pointed out, though, that prolactin rises have been described after PNES and even after nonepileptic hypotensive syncope (4).

Seizure Observation.   The most important investigation in the diagnosis of PNES is the observation of a typical seizure. Occasionally, the recording of a seizure with a home video or even a still camera provides sufficient support to make the diagnosis. Footage from mobile phones or closed-circuit television cameras can be helpful. Sometimes physicians have the opportunity to observe a seizure directly and to examine a patient. In this case, the attempt to elicit the pupillary light reflex (forced lid closure, which is preserved in PNES but may be absent in epileptic seizures), the reaction to noxious stimuli (such as the corneal reflex or tickling the inside of the nose), the Babinski response, and the observation of purposeful movements (for instance, when the patient's hand is dropped over his head) can be helpful.

However, to date, the diagnostic reliability of diagnoses based on the patient's history and a video recording of an event or ictal examination by an expert has not been formally assessed. Occasionally, even epilepsy experts are uncertain about the etiology of a seizure happening in front of them. Given the implications and therapeutic consequences of the diagnosis, it is therefore much better if seizures are recorded simultaneously with EEG and video. About one-third of patients with PNES will have a seizure during a routine EEG recording. Otherwise PNES are often observed within the first 48 hours of monitoring. The likelihood of a seizure occurring rises to at least two-thirds if photo-stimulation and hyperventilation are combined with the suggestion that these provocation methods can cause seizures. It has been shown that use of the diagnostic "gold standard" in patients who were difficult to diagnose on the basis of history, witness account, and interictal investigations changes the clinical diagnosis in many cases (4).

Provocation Techniques. If no seizures occur during video-EEG monitoring, the monitoring time can be extended or provocation techniques may be used. Provocation with saline patches, vibration, and hypnosis has been described, but the most commonly used technique involves the suggestive intravenous injection of normal saline solution. This procedure can provoke typical seizures in over three-quarters of patients but provokes epileptic seizures exceptionally rarely. Although some authors have expressed ethical doubt about provocation techniques, we and others consider the use of placebo defensible, especially if the diagnosis of PNES is followed by an offer of treatment, because the failure to make a clear diagnosis can have devastating effects, especially if no diagnosis is made after referral to an epilepsy center.

In the final analysis, the diagnosis of PNES is based on the combination of history and seizure observation and the lack of a "physical" explanation for the seizures. The tools that may be used in the diagnostic process have been reviewed in great detail recently (10). However, in about one-third of patients seen in epilepsy centers, the situation is complicated by coexisting epileptic seizures—of course, the confirmation of PNES by video-EEG does not mean that patients do not have epilepsy as well (11).

Communicating the Diagnosis

Once the diagnosis of PNES has been made, clinicians are faced with the difficult task of telling patients that they do not have epilepsy (for which they may have been treated for years), but that their seizures are a manifestation of psychologic or social distress. The question of how the diagnosis should be communicated has attracted considerable interest. One reason why "good" communication is important at this point is that PNES resolve with an explanation of the problem, which is acceptable and comprehensible, in about 10% of patients. It has also been shown that longer-term outcome is better in PNES patients who accept that they have PNES than those who continue to think that they have epilepsy. At present, however, only three in five patients referred for a psychotherapy assessment interview turn up. Patients are often angry and confused about the communication of the diagnosis of PNES (12). Like other patients with somatoform illness, those who fail to accept their diagnosis are likely to remain heavy users of health care services. In the particular case of PNES, unsuccessful communication is also likely to increase the risk of continuing inappropriate treatment with anticonvulsants. We have previously shown that 41% of patients diagnosed with PNES (and no additional epileptic seizures) were taking AEDs four years

after the diagnosis of PNES had been communicated to them and their general practitioners (GPs) (13).

There are a number of reasons why the communication of the diagnosis of PNES can be a challenging task (14). Whereas patients with epilepsy quite readily accept "stress" as a trigger for seizures, it has been shown that patients with PNES (just like other patients with medically unexplained physical symptoms) are less likely to endorse stress or emotional factors as a possible cause of seizures (15). In fact, the majority of patients have difficulties with the recognition of emotions or the fact that emotions or traumatic experiences could be related to their seizures. This is reflected in the fact that over 90% of patients score as alexithymic using a validated self-report instrument (16).

Although a communication protocol has been put forward for this setting, its superiority to any other form of communication has not been established, and less than one-half of the patients diagnosed at a center where the protocol was in use engaged in psychotherapy (17). Physicians keen to improve their communication skills may benefit from using the "reattribution model," which has been widely used in other somatoform disorders (18). This model has been subjected to further scrutiny, and there is evidence for its acceptability and clinical effectiveness (14). Communication between doctors and patients in line with this model has been examined with the help of a linguistic content analysis. One study looking at the communication between family physicians and patients with medically unexplained problems identified different forms of normalization of the patients' illness experience that were harmful (basic reassurance, reporting negative test results, giving negative results and generic explanations) and some that had positive effects on psychosocial outcomes (giving explanations linking physical and psychologic factors based on the patients' experience) (19).

In the explanation of the disorder, physicians may want to consider using the term "functional seizures," which has been shown to be less offensive to patients than the term "PNES" (which is used here because it has become the most established term in recent publications on the subject) (20). Watching a video recording of a typical seizure with the patient may contribute to the shared understanding that seizures are real and disabling. The use of leaflets may help reduce feelings of loss (often of the diagnosis of epilepsy) and isolation.

TREATMENT AND OUTCOME

Neurologic Assessment

The diagnosis of PNES should be accompanied by a thorough neurologic assessment. Given the high prevalence of comorbid epilepsy, it is particularly important to determine whether patients require AED treatment.

In patients with additional epileptic seizures, particular effort is required to enable patients to understand that they have two different types of seizures and, ideally, to learn to differentiate between them. If a diagnosis of additional epilepsy is uncertain, AEDs should be avoided if at all possible. The risks associated with occasional epileptic seizures have to be weighed against those of anticonvulsant toxicity and inappropriate treatment of prolonged PNES as status epilepticus in emergency rooms and intensive care units (which is perhaps more likely if a patient takes AEDs prescribed by a neurologist).

Psychiatric Assessment

The neurologic assessment should be followed by a psychiatric examination. Axis-1 disorders such as depression, anxiety, or posttraumatic stress disorder may respond to psychologic or pharmaceutical treatments. In the many patients who show evidence of personality pathology, chronic somatization or dissociation tendencies treatment may more realistically aim at behavior modification rather than cure.

Psychotherapy

The current mainstay of treatment is psychologic in nature. In the great majority of patients a conflict, trauma, or "unspeakable dilemma" can be identified that can be used to engage patients in treatment, although they may initially see no connection between this and their attacks. It remains unclear whether a psychoanalytical, interpersonal psychodynamic, cognitive behavioral, or alternative approach (family therapy, hypnotherapy, eye movement desensitization and reprocessing, cognitive analytic therapy, biofeedback) is best. All have been used successfully in individual cases, but no meaningfully controlled studies have been completed (1). We currently offer a psychotherapeutic intervention based on a model of brief psychodynamic-interpersonal therapy. This approach was previously found to have equivalent effects to cognitive behavior therapy in the treatment of depression and was shown to be helpful and cost-effective in the treatment of functional bowel disorders. Key features of this model include (a) the assumption that the patient's problems arise from or are exacerbated by disturbances of significant personal relationships, with dysfunctional interpersonal patterns usually originating earlier in their lives, and the explicit linking of this to the patient's symptoms; (b) a tentative, encouraging, supportive approach from the therapist, using "understanding hypotheses" and metaphors to deepen insight into psychologic mechanisms, "linking hypotheses" to elucidate links and patterns in different aspects of the patient's life (e.g., between the somatic and the emotional, or between the patient's current or past relationship patterns and what is happening in the "here and now" of the therapy session), and "explanatory hypotheses" to move patients to a further level of understanding of themselves and their symptoms. Patients are encouraged to make changes in unhelpful patterns of interpersonal relationships and to express and process emotions more effectively, particularly in relation to unresolved issues. If appropriate, patients are also shown cognitive and behavioral strategies such as techniques for warding off threatened seizures, panic attacks, and flashbacks, and they are offered relaxation tapes (Reuber M, Burness C, Howlett S, Brazier J, et al., submitted). A cognitive behavioral approach has been described elsewhere (21).

Pharmacological Therapy

Psychologic treatment may be augmented by pharmaceutical therapy, even in the absence of axis-1 disorders such as depression. Studies in other patient groups have shown that selective inhibition of serotonin reuptake can be helpful in somatization and symptom syndromes (such as dissociation) and improve emotional dysregulation, which is one of the core problems in patients with PNES. The use of low-dose neuroleptics has also been described for quasi-psychotic states such as severe dissociation (4).

Outcome

On the whole, the seizure and social outcome in PNES patients seen in epilepsy centers is poor. We recently showed that after an average of 11 years after manifestation and 4 years after diagnosis, two-thirds of patients continued to have seizures, and over half were dependent on social security. Our results were in accord with those in other PNES patient groups. This means that outcome is considerably worse than in newly diagnosed epilepsy, although it is similar to that seen in other somatoform disorders (13).

Although a number of controlled treatment studies are finally under way, no form of treatment has so far been proven to improve the natural history in patients diagnosed with PNES. What is more, measuring outcome in patients with PNES is complex, and the reports of the (uncontrolled) studies that are available are difficult to compare (22). We have shown that our treatment program improves patient-centered outcome measures (SF-36, CORE outcome measure, somatic symptom count) by at least one standard deviation in about one-half of all patients and that this form of treatment appears cost-effective (Reuber et al., submitted). Others have demonstrated that seizures can stop with treatment and that illness perceptions can be influenced by cognitive behavioral therapy (21).

CONCLUSION

Patients with PNES show a tendency to seek medical attention, and they make up a considerable share of the workload of neurologists and epileptologists as well as emergency room and general physicians. The differentiation of PNES from other paroxysmal disorders is crucial if iatrogenic injury is to be avoided (Table 52-1). Apart from this, the correct diagnosis of PNES may lead patients and physicians to focus on relevant underlying or associated psychologic issues.

Although there is no single fact in the history that allows the physician to make the diagnosis of PNES, the history often contains "red flags" that make this diagnosis more likely. The general, social, and medical histories are often as helpful as the description of seizures by patients and witnesses. Especially, a history of recurrent emergency or intensive care admissions with "status epilepticus," other unexplained medical symptoms, many surgical procedures, or psychiatric disorders can provide hints (Table 52-2).

If they allow patients to develop their own communication agenda, physicians can also listen for a range of interactive and linguistic clues in the patient's communication behavior that suggest a diagnosis of epilepsy or PNES (Table 52-3). The diagnosis of PNES may not be hard to make once it has been considered. Especially in an emergency room setting, physicians often forget that not everything that shakes is epilepsy. The diagnosis is particularly easy when there is an opportunity for direct observation of a seizure and for ictal examination (see Table 52-4).

The distinction of PNES from epilepsy is only the first step to a full diagnostic formulation. A complete diagnosis should also characterize any underlying or associated psychopathology. Childhood trauma or neglect, stressful life events, a dysfunctional home and social environment, psychiatric comorbidity, personality pathology, epilepsy, learning disability, and other "organic" brain disorders and abnormalities can all play an etiological role. A better etiological understanding of the seizure disorder can help the physician to communicate the diagnosis more successfully to a patient who may consider the problem "purely physical" or may fail to recognize feelings or the relevance of emotional problems for the seizures.

In view of the diversity of etiological factors, treatment has to be adjusted to individual patients but can share common elements such as addressing unhelpful illness perceptions, improving insight into links between symptoms and emotions, and enhancing independence and coping skills.

Physicians should always consider the differential diagnosis of other paroxysmal disorders, including PNES, before diagnosing epilepsy. In all patients in whom the diagnosis of PNES is considered or in whom the diagnosis of epilepsy remains in doubt, in all patients admitted to hospital with "status epilepticus," and in patients who fail to respond to anticonvulsant treatment, a clear diagnostic categorization should be sought. This should involve the assessment of the patient by a physician versed in the diagnosis of seizure disorders and, if at all possible, the documentation of a typical seizure by video-EEG. At present, longer-term social and seizure outcome is often poor. In the absence of major new developments in the treatment of patients with PNES, outcome may be improved if the diagnosis is more actively sought, made earlier, and communicated more convincingly.

References

1. Reuber M, Howlett S, Kemp S. Psychologic treatment for patients with psychogenic nonepileptic seizures. *Expert Rev Neurother* 2005; 5:737–752.
2. Reuber M, Howlett S, Khan A, Grünewald R. Nonepileptic seizures and other functional neurological symptoms: predisposing, precipitating and perpetuating factors. *Psychosomatics*, 2007; May–Jun; 48(3):230–238.
3. Kotsopoulos IA, de Krom MC, Kessels FG, Lodder J, et al. The diagnosis of epileptic and non-epileptic seizures. *Epilepsy Res* 2003; 57:59–67.
4. Reuber M. Psychogenic nonepileptic seizures: diagnosis, aetiology, treatment, prognosis. *Schweiz Arch Neurol Psychiatr* 2005; 156:47–57.
5. Juarez-Garcia A, Stokes T, Shaw B, Camosso-Stefinovic J, et al. The costs of epilepsy misdiagnosis in England and Wales. *Seizure* 2006; 15:598–605.
6. Schwabe M, Howell SJ, Reuber M. Differential diagnosis of seizure disorders: a conversation analytic approach. *Soc Sci Med*, 2007; May 4; [Epub ahead of print].
7. Reuber M, Fernández G, Helmstaedter C, Qurishi A, et al. Evidence of brain abnormality in patients with psychogenic nonepileptic seizures. *Epilepsy Behav* 2002; 3:246–248.
8. Reuber M, Fernández G, Bauer J, Singh DD, et al. Interictal EEG abnormalities in patients with psychogenic non-epileptic seizures. *Epilepsia* 2002; 43:1013–1020.
9. Vinton A, Carino J, Vogrin S, Macgregor L, et al. "Convulsive" nonepileptic seizures have a characteristic pattern of rhythmic artifact distinguishing them from epileptic seizures. *Epilepsia* 2004; 45:1344–1350.
10. Cragar DE, Berry DTR, Fakhoury TA, Cibula JE, et al. A review of diagnostic techniques in the differential diagnosis of epileptic and nonepileptic seizures. *Neuropsychol Rev* 2002; 12:31–64.
11. Reuber M, Fernández G, Helmstaedter C, Bauer J, et al. Are there physical risk factors for psychogenic nonepileptic seizures in patients with epilepsy? *Seizure* 2003; 12:561–567.
12. Carton S, Thompson PJ, Duncan JS. Non-epileptic seizures: patients' understanding and reaction to the diagnosis and impact on outcome. *Seizure* 2003; 12:287–294.
13. Reuber M, Pukrop R, Bauer J, Helmstaedter C, et al. Outcome in psychogenic nonepileptic seizures: 1 to 10 year follow-up in 164 patients. *Ann Neurology* 2003; 53:305–311.
14. Reuber M, Mitchell AJ, Howlett S, Crimlisk CH, et al. Functional symptoms in neurology: questions and answers. *J Neurol Neurosurg Psychiatry* 2005; 76:307–314.
15. Binzer M, Stone J, Sharpe M. Recent onset pseudoseizures: clues to aetiology. *Seizure* 2004; 13:146–155.
16. Bewley J, Murphy PN, Mallows J, Baker GA. Does alexithymia differentiate between patients with nonepileptic seizures, patients with epilepsy and nonpatient controls? *Epilepsy Behav* 2005; 7:1165–1173.
17. Krahn LE, Reese MM, Rummans TA, Peterson GC, et al. Health care utilization of patients with psychogenic nonepileptic seizures. *Psychosomatics* 1997; 38:535–542.
18. Goldberg D, Gask L, O'Dowd T. The treatment of somatization: teaching techniques of reattribution. *J Psychosom Res* 1989; 33:689–95.
19. Dowrick CF, Ring A, Humphries GM, Salmon P. Normalisation of unexplained symptoms by general practitioners: a functional typology. *Br J Gen Pract* 2004; 54:165–170.
20. Stone J, Campbell K, Sharma N, Carson A, et al. What should we call pseudoseizures? The patient's perspective. *Seizure* 2003; 12:568–572.
21. Goldstein LH, Deale A, Mitchell-O'Malley S, Toone BK, et al. An evaluation of cognitive behavioral therapy as a treatment for dissociative seizures. *Cognitive Behavioral Neurology* 2004; 17:41–49.
22. Reuber M, Mitchell AJ, Elger CE. Measuring outcome in the treatment of psychogenic nonepileptic seizures: the limited relevance of seizure-freedom. *Epilepsia* 2005; 46:1788–1795.

53 Conducting Treatment Trials for Psychologic Nonepileptic Seizures

W. Curt LaFrance, Jr.

Patients with psychologic (psychogenic) nonepileptic seizures (NES) are often severely disabled, with episodes that are refractory to treatment, and are frequently encountered in neurology, psychiatry, and emergency departments. NES, also referred to as pseudoseizures, are paroxysmal behaviors resembling epileptic seizures that have psychologic comorbidities and are unresponsive to treatment with antiepileptic drugs (AEDs). The phenomenology of NES is well delineated, including a preliminary understanding of risk factors and prognostic features (1), and is discussed in Chapter 52. Numerous studies exist on the diagnosis of NES, ictal semiology, comorbid psychiatric diagnoses, and neurologic and neuropsychologic characteristics of patients with NES, but to date, no double-blind, randomized, placebo-controlled trial (RCT) has been completed for NES.

Given the paucity of systematic treatment trials for NES, much less is known about treatments for NES. A review of the NES treatment literature reveals that only class III and IV studies are available, and no effective treatments have been developed for NES (2, 3). Patients with NES present unique challenges given the overlap of neurologic and psychiatric presentations. The few studies in neurology and psychiatry journals addressing clinical trial methodology do not adequately address the compounded challenges encountered when combined neuropsychiatric issues are present in a single treatment trial.

Approaching the patient with NES from a biopsychosocial model yields a number of potential treatment targets (3) (Figure 53-1). In this chapter, the treatment targets, interventions to address the targets, and methodological issues in treatment trials are described to aid and inform future NES treatment trials.

APPROACHES TO DEVELOPING TREATMENT TRIALS FOR NES

Treatment strategies, in general, include prevention, risk factor reduction, and prophylactic and symptomatic interventions. Clinical observations in some patients reveal that as depression improves, NES frequency decreases. Because symptomatic treatment for NES does not yet exist, another approach is to treat the comorbid psychiatric conditions that frequently accompany NES (4). Research reveals that patients with NES often have comorbid psychiatric conditions such as major depressive disorder, anxiety disorders including posttraumatic stress disorder (PTSD), or symptoms of depression, anxiety, and impulsivity, in addition to their NES (5). Mood, anxiety, and impulsivity disorders are characterized by serotonin system dysregulation

TABLE 53-3

Example of Types of Assessment Ratings at Baseline and Completion (N = 6)

SCALE	CUTOFF	BASELINE (ENROLLMENT)		COMPLETION (WEEK 10)	
		MEDIAN	RANGE	MEDIAN	RANGE
Modified Hamilton Depression Scale (41)	[<7]	25	(13–28)	17	(7–35)
Beck Depression Inventory-II (42)	[<14]	26	(10–44)	11	(2.0–36)
Davidson Trauma Scale (43)	[<17]	26.0	(7–118)	22.5	(6–78)
Barrett Impulsivity Scale (44)	[<70]	80	(51–93)	68	(54–83)
Dissociative Experiences Scale (24)	[<5]	31.8	(11–44)	17.3	(8.6–63.5)
Symptom Checklist 90 (45)	[<120]	148	(42–201)	110	(11–176)
Global Assessment of Functioning* (46)	[>80]	49	(40–60)	55	(25–85)
Family Assessment Device:					
General Functioning Score (47)	[<2.00]	2.00	(1.33–2.58)	1.79	(1.00–2.83)
LIFE-RIFT (QoL measure) (48)	[<9]	20	(7–28)	15	(6–30)
Ways of Coping (49) (method most used) [seek social support/planful problem solving]		Escape/ avoidance		Seek social support	
NES frequency during trial (biweekly sum)		7.5	(1–34)	2	(0–64)

For all assessments except *, a higher score indicates a worse condition.
Cutoff scores in controls and healthy subjects are presented in brackets by the scale.
(p values were intentionally not analyzed in this feasibility open label trial, as it is not powered for such calculations).

average, these patients with NES had moderate to severe depression scores (Hamilton [<7] and Beck Depression Scales [<14]), symptoms related to trauma (Davidson Trauma Scale [<17]), moderate to severe impulsivity (Barrett Impulsivity Scale [<70]), dissociative experiences (Dissociative Experiences Scale [<5]), elevated somatic scores (Symptom Checklist 90 [<120]), impaired social functioning (Global Assessment of Functioning [>80] and LIFE-RIFT [<9, in recovery]), family dysfunction (Family Assessment Device [FAD General Functioning subscale <2.0]), and maladaptive coping patterns (Ways of Coping [seek social support, planful problem solving]).

DESIGNING NES TREATMENT TRIALS

The results of the open-label feasibility trial in patients with NES inform the conduct of future NES trials. The issues pertinent to NES treatment trials and to conducting research in a combined neuropsychiatric population are described in Table 53-4.

Monitoring Outcomes in NES Trials

The presence of pathologic scores on numerous scales reveals that these patients have a variety of psychosocial issues along with their events. These findings are similar to what van Merode and colleagues showed in their study on psychopathological symptoms in patients

with NES (23). Baseline scores were in the symptomatic range, indicating a need for looking at a broad set of measures for primary and secondary outcomes. Depression and anxiety scores were in the clinical range on scales, validating our focus on the commonly occurring comorbidities for treatment. Interestingly, the Dissociative Experiences Scale (DES) scores were consistent with a PTSD population, and not those with dissociative identity disorders (24). Patients with NES and comorbid psychiatric symptoms were able to complete the surveys and able to tolerate flexible-dose sertraline over the course of the trial.

TABLE 53-4

NES Treatment Trial Issues and Obstacles

- NES severity/frequency
- psychosocial symptom severity
- outcome differences in younger vs. older cohorts
- personal physical characteristics—hemiparesis and cognitive symptoms
- logistical restrictions—transportation/driving
- distinguishing mixed NES/epileptic seizures
- prior AED/antidepressant treatments
- choice of primary outcome measures

The Hawthorne Effect in NES Trials

Patients enrolling in a treatment trial receive more attention than they typically receive in routine medical encounters. This may be particularly true for patients diagnosed with NES. Giving focused attention to patients who are often seen in a limited fashion by several providers may impact the frequency of events. In statements with mixed relief and exasperation, several patients with NES reported appreciation that "at least now somebody is trying to help with this." The Hawthorne effect (the positive effect observed in patients from the attention received in a study) may come into play with trials enrolling these patients (25). We collected the retrospective 2-week seizure count at enrollment, and to address the potential Hawthorne effect, we compared it to the frequency in the 2-week treatment-free baseline period. Monitoring patients for seizures and symptoms before receiving the intervention may be essential to look for changes, either positive or negative, from enrollment to initiation of therapy. The Hawthorne effect may be due to the researcher's cumulative attention over time, so the baseline comparison may not truly assess the effect. The potential confound underscores the need for a placebo-controlled trial. A blinded baseline also may help to establish what effect trial enrollment may have on other symptoms.

Seizure Frequency and Severity in NES Trials

For statistical analysis, dichotomous groups based on symptom severity may need to be established. In our trial, patients with a baseline frequency of ten or more events every 2 weeks showed either worsening or no improvement in their seizure frequency. The cutoff of ten events every 2 weeks was an ad hoc finding; there was no preset cutoff for severity related to frequency. There is a large variance in the number of events that different patients with NES experience. This finding raises the possibility that a high baseline frequency may yield worse outcomes and may need to be addressed when designing treatment trials. Stratifying the subjects into high- and low-frequency groups may be helpful to better evaluate the impact of an intervention but may influence the statistical analysis. Analogously, patients with higher psychiatric symptom scores or psychosocial dysfunction may experience worse outcomes. The effect of stratification on sample size calculations would need to be explored in more detail for future randomized trials, and large numbers of patients may be needed to examine these potential stratification issues.

The Effect of Presenting the Diagnosis in NES Trials

It will be important to examine both the short-term and long-term outcomes in NES trials to monitor for a sustained treatment effect. After vEEG diagnosis of NES, patients may have an immediate reduction in the number of events (26); however, this effect is not long standing in the majority of patients (27). Because it is unclear why a temporary NES reduction occurs immediately following diagnosis, it will be important to follow patients after any intervention to assess its true benefit. The subjects in this open-label trial were followed with phone calls at 4, 8, and 12 months after enrollment to assess seizure status, medication usage, global functioning, and for treatment dropout rates. The analysis of the 12-month follow-up phase data of the study is not yet complete.

Children and Adults in NES trials

As noted previously, NES occurs across the lifespan, from children to the elderly. Outcomes in children, however, are better than in adults, and outcomes in the elderly are unknown. To limit age-effect bias, future trials may either focus on a population younger than 18 years old or may include patients older than age 65. The age restriction should not be overly limiting to recruitment. In general, clinical trials report retention rates of 10% to 15% from screen to completion (28). A 50% retention rate occurred in our open-label trial, arguing for the success of future NES trials.

Neurologic and Psychiatric Comorbidity in NES Patients

We encountered limitations in conducting treatment trials in NES with regard to the physical, social, logistical, and recruitment realms. The typical problems with recruitment and with retaining patients seen in neurologic clinical trials or in psychiatric clinical trials are compounded in a trial with combined neuropsychiatric issues present. For example, depression trials typically do not have to deal with driving restrictions, and epilepsy trials do not typically have to monitor for suicidality. Articles that address the complexities and patient challenges in a neuropsychiatric population together are lacking. Given this paucity of information, the methodologic issues that presented in the NES population are described in this chapter. These problems may arise in treatment trials with other neuropsychiatrically ill populations also, such as in traumatic brain injury.

Lability and Attrition in NES Patients

Crises, lability, and approach/avoidance patterns present significant challenges to recruitment and retention in this population. Several patients with NES present in crisis and with frequent events; however, when assistance is offered, they may reject the support. Two patients dropped out of the open-label trial the day after enrolling.

One patient who was admitted to the inpatient unit for an acute exacerbation of depression dropped out after reviewing the battery of questionnaires and did not want to switch from suboptimized paroxetine to sertraline. The other patient who dropped out was an inpatient in the epilepsy monitoring unit who experienced physical limitations that included developing dominant-handed hemiparesis following some of her NES.

Head Injury and Neurologic Conditions in NES

Cognitive and physical limitations in NES patients that may be neurologically based or that may be part of other somatoform symptoms may affect participation in trials. To obtain a comprehensive assessment, patients completed a large battery of self-report questionnaires measuring the frequency of NES, depression, anxiety, dissociative, somatoform, and trauma-associated symptoms, family functioning, quality of life, and other psychosocial variables. Patients with NES may have neurologic deficits (7) and a high frequency of nonseizure conversion disorders (5). If dominant hemiparesis, either of physiologic or of psychogenic etiology, exists, patients may be unable to fully participate in trials that document broad psychosocial factors via self-report batteries. Also, if patients are on numerous central nervous system active medications, cognitive slowing may be a limitation to timely completion of self-report batteries.

In this pilot trial, patients with focal findings and cognitive slowing were accepted and asked to complete all forms. This led to losing one participant and resulted in modifying the RCT. Researchers accept a certain attrition rate in trials. When designing studies, it is important to realize that not including patients with brain damage will potentially affect generalizabilty to other NES populations. If, on the other hand, these patients are to be excluded, an abbreviated battery or clinician ratings may be the "least common denominator" used in the final outcomes comparisons among all subjects in trials.

Driving in NES Trials

A logistic issue that may limit participation in NES trials not present in psychiatric trials is driving. Driving restrictions in patients with epilepsy vary by state (29). The issue of restricting the driving of patients with NES is less clear (30). A survey of neurologists revealed that many physicians recommend restricting driving privileges in patients with NES (31). In the same report, twenty patients with NES were found to have no difference in the number of accidents when compared to general population accident rates. Driving, and the often lengthy distance to a research center, may be a major limitation for patients. Patients with NES also expressed reservations about using mass transit, for fear of having an event on public transportation. Enlisting family or friends, or budgeting for taxis for patient transportation may be one way to address this potential problem in prospective trials for NES.

The Decision to Study Mixed NES/Epilepsy versus Lone NES

Given our current lack of knowledge in NES treatments, including mixed NES/ES patients may or may not be considered a limitation. Reports on comorbidity reveal that only 5 to 10% of patients diagnosed with NES have mixed NES/ES (32–34). To limit the possibility of inaccurate seizure frequency quantification, one could argue that the ideal treatment trial will select only patients with lone NES to use a more "pure" study population. Acknowledging the low prevalence of mixed ES/NES, for this feasibility trial, patients with mixed ES/NES who could readily distinguish between their events were enrolled. Trials with larger samples may opt for the "purist" approach of enrolling only lone NES patients, realizing that this may impact generalizability to the subset with mixed ES/NES.

Distinguishing Different Types of Seizures

One concern regarding the "ideal" NES population is the difficulty of diagnosing, enrolling, and then retaining this difficult-to-engage population. Including mixed NES/ES patients may shed light on similarities and differences between the NES and ES and mixed NES/ES populations. Many patients with mixed NES/ES are readily able to identify and distinguish their various events with a careful initial history. When asked about their seizure descriptions, patients with mixed NES/ES describe different physical characteristics of the different types. The following example illustrates a patient relaying his two different types of seizures.

> I have the seizures that occur at night, where I wake up, usually on the floor, and my whole body hurts. I have wet myself and I don't know what happened. . . . My other seizures occur during the day. I can be watching TV and there's a scene where a child is being abused, or I will have had an argument with someone, and then I'll have my other seizure. My arm shakes and I am out of it for a few seconds or minutes. I can't speak, but I can hear what is going on around me. I'm usually o.k. after a few minutes following that type of seizure.

These distinctions are documented with the absence of epileptiform activity on vEEG during the daytime NES, and the presence of epileptiform activity during the nocturnal generalized tonic-clonic seizures, which helps to validate the distinction of the two seizure types. When monitoring outcomes, training the patient and the family to record these different events separately will be essential.

Medication Issues: Drug-Naïve NES Patients (Do They Exist?) and Stopping the AED

When designing the treatment trial, based on our hypothesis testing the effect of an SSRI, we sought patients with NES who had not had prior treatment with psychotropic medications. Another population "purity" methodological issue in the NES population is finding psychotropic-naïve patients. Studies show that there is a 7-year diagnostic delay between onset of seizures and diagnosis of NES (35). In the ensuing time, patients are often treated with several AEDs and also with psychotropic medications (36). Most of the patients in the open-label study had prior exposure to antidepressants. However, the dosing, in many cases, may have been below optimal pharmacologic level. It is unclear if prior medication exposure limits potential response to an optimized drug. Also, from a clinical trials perspective, the effect of stopping a current medication may impact the outcome. Given that patients with NES have had AED and psychotropic exposures, the decision to discontinue all psychotropic medications, or AEDs, or to add the study medication to the current regimen, is one of considerable importance for future NES treatment trials. In our trial, patients stopped their antidepressants before enrolling.

Time Lag between Symptoms, Diagnosis, and Enrollment

The means and timing of establishing the NES diagnosis are linked to enrollment procedures. A 12-month delay occurred from vEEG diagnosis to obtaining treatment for NES in our study. Once referred for the study, patients who were eligible were enrolled within 1 month. This diagnostic delay deserves mention because the time lag may impact prognosis. Poorer prognosis is seen in patients with a long history of NES (37). One patient with NES for less than 12 months required fewer treatment sessions to reach cessation than those who had their events for more than a year (38). Several factors could account for delay in treatment after NES is diagnosed. Patients may not accept the diagnosis, moving from a "neurologic problem to a psychiatric one" (39). Referrals between neurologists and psychiatrists may be limited due to lack of interdisciplinary discussion (40). The diagnosis is most often made at tertiary care centers with vEEG monitoring, and communication of the diagnosis to the referring physician may not occur until a report is generated. The delay from vEEG diagnosis to treatment could be shortened by addressing the previously noted issues.

THE CHOICE OF OUTCOMES IN NES TRIALS

A common primary outcome in AED trials is number of seizures. In our trial, the patients scored at pathologic or symptomatic levels on several other measures of psychosocial functioning. Whether treating patients with nonepileptic or epileptic seizures, it is important for us to realize that preventing the ictus is not the only goal of therapeutic interventions for patients with seizures. Treatment trials that address various psychosocial issues in the lives of patients with NES may lead to improved treatment outcomes.

SUMMARY

In summary, prospective, controlled treatment trials in patients with NES are necessary to determine effective interventions. In demonstrating the feasibility of conducting an open-label trial, the methodological issues in conducting rigorous, randomized, controlled treatment trials in NES are addressed. From the feasibility trial, we learned relevant factors for trials in NES patients include the following: NES and psychosocial symptom severity, age differences, personal/physical characteristics, logistical restrictions, the presence of mixed NES/ES, prior AED/antidepressant treatments, and breadth of outcome measures. Being aware of these design and methodological issues may increase enrollment and retention, and inform appropriate outcomes, and facilitate future NES treatment trials.

Note: Portions of this chapter are taken from the following publication: LaFrance WC Jr, Blum AS, Miller IW, Ryan CE, Keitner GI. Conducting an open label pharmacologic trial in patients with psychologic nonepileptic seizures. *J Neuropsychiatry Clin Neurosci* 2007, in press.

References

1. Barry JJ. Nonepileptic seizures: an overview. *CNS Spectr* 2001; 6:956–962.
2. LaFrance WC Jr, Devinsky O. The treatment of nonepileptic seizures: Historical perspectives and future directions. *Epilepsia* 2004; 45(Suppl 2):15–21.
3. LaFrance WC Jr, Barry JJ. Update on treatments of psychological nonepileptic seizures. *Epilepsy Behav* 2005; 7:364–374.
4. LaFrance WC Jr, Devinsky O. Treatment of nonepileptic seizures. *Epilepsy Behav* 2002; 3(5 Suppl 1):S19–S23.
5. Bowman ES, Markand ON. Psychodynamics and psychiatric diagnoses of pseudoseizure subjects. *Am J Psychiatry* 1996; 153:57–63.
6. Vaswani M, Linda FK, Ramesh S. Role of selective serotonin reuptake inhibitors in psychiatric disorders: a comprehensive review. *Prog Neuropsychopharmacol Biol Psychiatry* 2003; 27:85–102.
7. Kanner AM, Parra J, Frey M, Stebbins G, et al. Psychiatric and neurologic predictors of psychogenic pseudoseizure outcome. *Neurology* 1999; 53:933–938.
8. Benbadis SR. A spell in the epilepsy clinic and a history of "chronic pain" or "fibromyalgia" independently predict a diagnosis of psychogenic seizures. *Epilepsy Behav* 2005; 6:264–265.
9. Burneo JG, Martin R, Powell T, Greenlee S, et al. Teddy bears: an observational finding in patients with non-epileptic events. *Neurology* 2003; 61:714–715.
10. Reuber M, House AO, Pukrop R, Bauer J, et al. Somatization, dissociation and general psychopathology in patients with psychogenic non-epileptic seizures. *Epilepsy Res* 2003; 57:159–167.
11. Murray C, Lopez A, eds. The World Health Report 2002. Reducing risks, promoting healthy life. Geneva, Switzerland: World Health Organization, 2002.

12. Fiszman A, Alves-Leon SV, Nunes RG, D'Andrea I, et al. Traumatic events and post-traumatic stress disorder in patients with psychogenic nonepileptic seizures: a critical review. *Epilepsy Behav* 2004; 5:818–825.

13. Freyd JJ, Putnam FW, Lyon TD, Becker-Blease KA, et al. Psychology. The science of child sexual abuse. *Science* 2005; 308:501.

14. Wyllie E, Friedman D, Luders H, Morris H, et al. Outcome of psychogenic seizures in children and adolescents compared with adults. *Neurology* 1991; 41:742–744.

15. Fakhoury T, Abou-Khalil B, Newman K. Psychogenic seizures in old age: a case report. *Epilepsia* 1993; 34:1049–1051.

16. Shulman KI, Silver IL. Hysterical seizures as a manifestation of "depression" in old age. *Can J Psychiatry* 1985; 30:278–280.

17. Lempert T, Dieterich M, Huppert D, Brandt T. Psychogenic disorders in neurology: frequency and clinical spectrum. *Acta Neurol Scand* 1990; 82:335–340.

18. Kellinghaus C, Loddenkemper T, Dinner DS, Lachhwani D, et al. Non-epileptic seizures of the elderly. *J Neurol* 2004; 251:704–709.

19. First MB, Spitzer RL, Gibbon M, Williams JBW. Structured clinical interview for DSM-IV axis I disorders clinician version (SCID-I). New York: Biometrics Research Department, New York State Psychiatric Institute, 1997.

20. Pfohl B, Blum N, Zimmerman M. Structured interview for DSM-IV personality. Washington DC: American Psychiatric Press, 1997.

21. Keller MB. Undertreatment of major depression. *Psychopharmacol Bull* 1988; 24:75–80.

22. Oquendo MA, Baca-Garcia E, Kartachov A, Khait V, et al. A computer algorithm for calculating the adequacy of antidepressant treatment in unipolar and bipolar depression. *J Clin Psychiatry* 2003; 64:825–833.

23. van Merode T, Twellaar M, Kotsopoulos IA, Kessels AG, et al. Psychological characteristics of patients with newly developed psychogenic seizures. *J Neurol Neurosurg Psychiatry* 2004; 75:1175–1177.

24. Bernstein EM, Putnam FW. Development, reliability, and validity of a dissociation scale. *J Nerv Ment Dis* 1986; 174:727–735.

25. West ED, Jackson A, Physentides A, Seenivasagan S, et al. Randomized comparative trial of a ward discussion group. *Br J Psychiatry* 1982; 141:76–80.

26. Farias ST, Thieman C, Alsaadi TM. Psychogenic nonepileptic seizures: acute change in event frequency after presentation of the diagnosis. *Epilepsy Behav* 2003; 4:424–429.

27. Wilder C, Marquez AV, Farias ST, Gorelik M, et al. Long-term follow-up study of patients with PNES [abstract 2.469]. *Epilepsia* 2004; 45(Suppl 7):349.

28. Keitner GI, Posternak MA, Ryan CE. How many subjects with major depressive disorder meet eligibility requirements of an antidepressant efficacy trial? *J Clin Psychiatry* 2003; 64:1091–1093.

29. Krauss GL, Ampaw L, Krumholz A. Individual state driving restrictions for people with epilepsy in the US. *Neurology* 2001; 57:1780–1785.

30. Iriarte J, Parra J, Urrestarazu E, Kuyk J. Controversies in the diagnosis and management of psychogenic pseudoseizures. *Epilepsy Behav* 2003; 4:354–359.

31. Benbadis SR, Blustein JN, Sunstad L. Should patients with psychogenic nonepileptic seizures be allowed to drive? *Epilepsia* 2000; 41:895–897.

32. Lesser RP, Lueders H, Dinner DS. Evidence for epilepsy is rare in patients with psychogenic seizures. *Neurology* 1983; 33:502–504.

33. Benbadis SR, Agrawal V, Tatum WO IV. How many patients with psychogenic nonepileptic seizures also have epilepsy? *Neurology* 2001; 57:915–917.

34. Martin R, Burneo JG, Prasad A, Powell T, et al. Frequency of epilepsy in patients with psychogenic seizures monitored by video-EEG. *Neurology* 2003; 61:1791–1792.

35. Reuber M, Fernandez G, Bauer J, Helmstaedter C, et al. Diagnostic delay in psychogenic nonepileptic seizures. *Neurology* 2002; 58:493–495.

36. de Timary P, Fouchet P, Sylin M, Indriets JP, et al. Non-epileptic seizures: delayed diagnosis in patients presenting with electroencephalographic (EEG) or clinical signs of epileptic seizures. *Seizure* 2002; 11:193–197.

37. Lempert T, Schmidt D. Natural history and outcome of psychogenic seizures: a clinical study in 50 patients. *J Neurol* 1990; 237:35–38.

38. Rusch MD, Morris GL, Allen L, Lathrop L. Psychological treatment of nonepileptic events. *Epilepsy Behav* 2001; 2:277–283.

39. LaFrance WC. How many patients with psychogenic nonepileptic seizures also have epilepsy? *Neurology* 2002; 58:990–991.

40. Kanner AM. More controversies on the treatment of psychogenic pseudoseizures: an addendum. *Epilepsy Behav* 2003; 4:360–364.

41. Miller IW, Bishop S, Norman WH, Maddever H. The Modified Hamilton Rating Scale for Depression: reliability and validity. *Psychiatry Res* 1985; 14:131–142.

42. Beck AT, Steer RA, Brown GK. Manual for The Beck Depression Inventory-second edition (BDI-II). San Antonio: Psychological Corporation, 1996.

43. Davidson J. Davidson Trauma Scale. New York: Multi-Health Systems, 1996.

44. Barratt ES, Patton JH. Impulsivity: cognitive, behavioral and psychophysiological correlates. In: Zuckerman M, ed. *Biological Basis of Sensation-Seeking. Impulsivity, and Anxiety.* Hillsdale, NJ: Lawrence Erlbaum, 1983:77–116.

45. Derogatis LR. Symptom Checklist 90-R: Administration, scoring, and procedures manual. 3rd ed. Minneapolis, MN: National Computer Systems, 1994.

46. Task Force on DSM-IVTR. Diagnostic and statistical manual of mental disorders: DSM-IV-TR. 4th, text revision ed. Washington, DC: American Psychiatric Association, 2000.

47. Epstein NB, Baldwin LM, Bishop DS. The McMaster Family Assessment Device. *J Marital Fam Ther* 1983; 9:171–180.

48. Leon AC, Solomon DA, Mueller TI, Turvey CL, et al. The Range of Impaired Functioning Tool (LIFE-RIFT): a brief measure of functional impairment. *Psychol Med* 1999; 29:869–878.

49. Folkman S. Ways of coping (revised). San Francisco: University of California, 1985. http://goodquestions.ucsf.edu/tools/surveys/pdf/Ways%20of%20coping.pdf.

54 Cortical Malformations

Megan Selvitelli
Bernard S. Chang

he study of malformations of cortical development can provide useful insights into epilepsy, behavior, and brain development. With improved detection via neuroimaging, cortical malformations are now the second most commonly recognized cause of medically refractory epilepsy in adults and account for nearly 40% of medically refractory seizures in children (1, 2). Most patients with cortical malformations also have some degree of developmental delay and may have focal neurologic deficits relating to the location of the malformation. Understanding of cortical malformations is crucial not only for epileptologists, but also for developmental neurobiologists, as recent research has helped elucidate some of the genetic causes of cortical malformations, thereby improving our understanding of brain formation.

Normal brain development begins in the second month of gestation with neuron and interneuron generation and proliferation within the ventricular epithelium and striatum (3). Neurons then migrate along radial and tangential glial tracts to the cortical surface (1). Subsequently, the cortex is laminated into six layers, with the later-arriving neurons forming the outermost cortical layer (1). Finally, cortical connections develop throughout gestation and infancy via synaptogenesis and are further modified by synapse pruning and cellular apoptosis (1).

Malformations of cortical development may result from alterations in any part of the sequence just described. If there is failure of neuronal proliferation, microcephaly may occur, whereas overabundant neuronogenesis may result in hemimegalencephaly. Abnormalities in neuronal migration may cause deposits of neurons along the glial migration tracts, resulting in periventricular nodular heterotopia, subcortical band heterotopia, or lissencephaly, depending on the site of neuronal migration arrest. Finally, abnormalities in neuronal organization may result in abnormally formed gyri, as in polymicrogyria, or in more restricted areas of cortical disorganization, as with focal cortical dysplasias.

This chapter provides information on the etiologies of these cortical malformations and gives details on the associated epilepsy and behavioral characteristics.

DISORDERS OF PROLIFERATION

Microcephaly

Microcephaly is defined by a significantly small head circumference, more than 2–3 standard deviations (SD) below the mean, which is used as a surrogate marker for brain size. It is associated with epilepsy in 40% and with mental retardation in most (4). Microcephaly may occur secondary to genetic factors (e.g., microcephaly vera), in association with various syndromes (e.g., inborn errors of metabolism), or as a result of environmental factors, such as maternal toxoplasmosis, syphilis, alcohol consumption, or hypoxic ischemic injuries (5–7).

Presumably, microcephaly represents a failure of neuronogenesis, resulting in decreased neuronal number and brain size (6). Microcephaly vera is an autosomal recessive disorder associated with microcephaly with preserved gyral patterns and brain architecture. Microcephaly vera may be due to mutations in several genes, including the ASPM (abnormal spindle-like microcephaly associated) gene or microcephalin gene. The ASPM gene encodes a protein believed to be important in mitotic spindle formation, and the microcephalin protein is involved in compressing DNA prior to DNA segregation during mitosis (6, 8). Thus, some inherited forms of microcephaly may be due to a failure of mitosis in generating sufficient neuronal numbers, resulting in a small brain. Furthermore, microcephaly associated with simplified gyral pattern is presumably due to abnormalities in both neuronogenesis and migration, resulting in a small brain with simplified gyri.

Forty percent of patients with microcephaly experience seizures (4). Classically, patients with microcephaly vera have been defined as not having seizures, although more recent studies suggest that seizures may occur in some patients (9). On the other hand, patients with microcephaly with simplified gyral pattern tend to have seizures that begin in infancy; these seizures are associated with generalized epileptiform discharges and variable control (3, 8, 10). Finally, patients with microcephaly associated with spasticity and severe developmental and motor delays may have a neonatal onset of myoclonic and tonic-clonic seizures associated with diffuse epileptiform discharges and perhaps hypsarrhythmia or burst suppression patterns (11). Interestingly, there is an increased risk of epilepsy in patients with lower cognitive function (4).

Thus, a failure of neuronal proliferation, from multiple etiologies, may result in microcephaly, mental retardation, and an increased incidence of epilepsy.

Hemimegalencephaly

On the other hand, in hemimegalencephaly, one hemisphere is abnormally large. On pathologic examination, there is a range of expression from mild lobar to entire hemisphere involvement with a thickened cortex, blurring of the gray–white junction, and an increased amount of white matter (12). There may also be associated neuronal heterotopia and abnormal cortical gyration patterns (12). Magnetic resonance imaging (MRI) reveals the unilateral hemisphere enlargement (Figure 54-1), with an increase in cortical thickness and white matter volume, and in some patients may also demonstrate macrocephaly, an asymmetrically enlarged skull, intracranial calcifications, and unilateral ventriculomegaly (13).

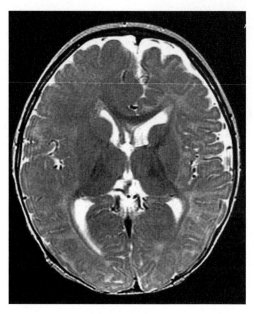

FIGURE 54-1

Hemimegalencephaly. This T2-weighted axial brain MRI of a patient with hemimegalencephaly demonstrates the enlargement of one cerebral hemisphere (in this case, right), with ipsilateral enlargement of white matter volume and a blurring of the gray–white junction.

Hemimegalencephaly may occur sporadically or in association with other syndromes, such as epidermal nevus syndrome, hypomelanosis of Ito, tuberous sclerosis, or Klippel-Trenaunay-Weber syndrome (14). Barkovich and Chuang have theorized that an insult during axonogenesis results in an increased release of nerve growth factors. These growth factors may cause an increased survival of neurons, which then migrate and create the enlarged and abnormal hemisphere (12).

Given the significant structural abnormality, it is no surprise that these patients are afflicted with medically refractory seizures and numerous neurologic deficits. Patients with hemimegalencephaly typically experience their first seizure within the first year of life, of which 62% are partial motor seizures, 11% are characterized as Ohtahara syndrome, 9% are infantile spasms, and 7% are generalized tonic seizures (14). As expected, the corresponding electroencephalographic (EEG) abnormalities include focal paroxysmal discharges from the affected hemisphere but may also include burst suppression patterns, hypsarrhythmia, and diffuse spike-wave complexes (14). These patients experience global developmental delay, including delayed and poorly developed language, hemiparesis, clumsiness, hypotonia, and possibly hemianopsia (13). Early hemispherectomy has been advocated as a means to control the seizures and improve speech, development, and quality of life in patients with early-onset, medically refractory seizures and hemiparesis (12–14). Therefore, patients with hemimegalencephaly have a significant brain malformation and are affected by severe seizures and neurologic deficits, which frequently require major surgery to arrest their progression.

DISORDERS OF MIGRATION

Disorders of migration result from arrest of neuronal migration along the radial glial tracts from the ventricular surface to cortex and are strongly associated with epilepsy.

Periventricular Nodular Heterotopia

Periventricular nodular heterotopia (PNH) are among the more common forms of cortical malformation (15–20%) and are seen in 2% of all epilepsy patients (15, 16). PNH are characterized by single or multiple rounded nodules of gray matter along the lateral ventricular walls. They may occur unilaterally or bilaterally and may be associated with other cortical malformations. Pathologically, they consist of normal-appearing neurons and glial cells, with bundles of myelinated fibers and a moderate degree of gliosis (15). The nodules may have reciprocal connections with the overlying cortex, which may show some degree of architectural dysplasia (15). The nodules are best visualized with MRI, on which the PNH show the same signal characteristics as the cortex on all imaging sequences (Figure 54-2).

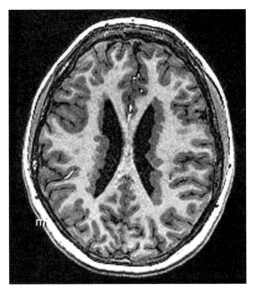

FIGURE 54-2

Periventricular nodular heterotopia. This T1-weighted axial brain MRI of a patient with periventricular nodular heterotopia demonstrates multiple confluent nodules of gray matter signal intensity lining the lateral walls of the ventricles bilaterally.

The nodules are presumed to be the result of a failure of neuronal migration. In female patients with bilateral PNH, a mutation at Xq28 in the filamin A (FLNA) gene may result in the bilateral failure of some neuronal migration. The FLNA gene encodes an actin-binding protein that may form the link between the plasma membrane and cytoskeleton, as well as participate in the formation of lamellipodia for neuron motility (8). The paucity of men with FLNA mutations is likely due to homozygous lethality in many cases, and its phenotype in women is assumed to be due to cellular mosaicism (8), although milder FLNA mutations have been described in males (17). Unilateral PNH may result from an insult during embryogenesis in the seventh through sixteenth weeks of gestation, when neuroblasts migrate along glia to the developing cortical plate (18). Given the high frequency of unilateral PNH occurring in watershed vascular distributions and the frequent association with prenatal vascular risk factors, Battaglia and coworkers (19) hypothesized that unilateral PNH are the result of ischemic events in utero that prohibit the migration of a local subset of neurons. Finally, the association of some cases of bilateral PNH with other cortical malformations, neurologic deficits, and mental retardation suggests a more global failure of migration due to an as-yet-undefined etiology.

PNH are associated with epilepsy in 80% of patients (18). The mean age of onset is in adolescence with a generalized tonic-clonic seizure (19). Nonetheless, the vast majority of patients more typically experience focal seizures that are often medically refractory (20). Patients with PNH in association with other cortical abnormalities often have multiple seizure types that are also medically refractory, including drop attacks, partial seizures, tonic seizures, and generalized tonic-clonic seizures (21).

EEG studies reveal interictal discharges either bilaterally in patients with bilateral disease or unilaterally over the affected hemisphere (20). The discharges are frequently temporal in localization, which may represent false localization. Seizures tend to originate in either hemisphere in bilateral patients or in the affected hemisphere in unilateral PNH (20). In studies using both depth and cortical electrodes, seizures originated from mesial temporal structures in 25%, from both mesial temporal regions and PNH simultaneously in 25%, and from PNH and widespread structures in 50% (18). Thus, the PNH may show intrinsic epileptogenicity in connection with the overlying cortex. Interestingly, patients with PNH have also exhibited photic driving on EEG over the affected hemisphere (19).

Li and coworkers (16) reported a poor response to surgery for patients with medically refractory seizures and PNH. In nine patients following variable degrees of temporal lobe resections, none were seizure-free at 12 months, and most had either Engel class III or IV outcomes. However, in two of ten patients in whom a temporal lobe resection also included removal of a portion of the PNH, the long-term seizure control was better maintained. More recently, Tassi and his fellow researchers (15) reported on ten patients who underwent corticectomy with partial removal of PNH. Seven of the ten patients had an Engel class Ia outcome at 1 year postoperatively. Given the presumed reciprocal connections between the PNH and overlying cortex and the frequent seizure onset from the PNH simultaneously with the overlying cortex, any surgical candidates would require extensive depth and cortical monitoring to determine the epileptogenic foci to remove.

Some patients with PNH show no deficits except their epilepsy. However, patients with associated cortical malformations or a more severe burden of PNH tend to have a lower intelligence and other neurologic deficits. More recently a study by Chang et al. (22) observed that many patients with PNH have a singular deficit in reading fluency out of proportion to their measured intelligence. They proposed that the PNH disrupt corticocortical connections, resulting in an impairment in processing rapidly presented stimuli.

In summary, PNH represent a failure of neuron migration beyond the periventricular region and are associated with medically refractory partial seizures and singular cognitive deficits.

Subcortical Band Heterotopia

Subcortical band heterotopia (SBH) are also due to a presumed failure of neuronal migration. SBH are symmetrical bands of subcortical heterotopic neurons separated from the cortex and ventricles by white matter. Pathologically, SBH consist of unlayered neurons interrupted by bundles of fibers (23). The overlying cortex may show a normal layering and thickness, whereas the intervening white matter may reveal scattered heterotopic neurons arranged in columns (23). On MRI (Figure 54-3), the SBH appear as a band of either symmetric or asymmetric gray matter of variable thickness, often with predominance in the frontocentral regions (24, 25). The overlying cortex may be normal or show a variable degree of simplified gyral patterns (24, 25).

SBH are presumably due to a failure of neuroblast migration along radial glial fibers during the third through fifth months of gestation. The "doublecortin" (DCX) gene on the X chromosome codes for a microtubule binding protein (26). A mutation in DCX may lead to a failure of microtubular bundling, resulting in abnormal neuronogenesis and migration (26). The DCX mutation is seen in 80% of sporadically affected women and in hereditary cases in which women express SBH and men develop lissencephaly (see the following subsection on lissencephaly for more details) (27).

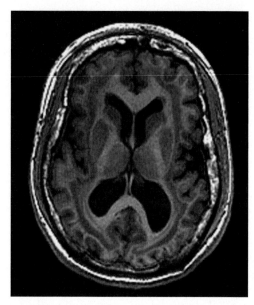

FIGURE 54-3

Subcortical band heterotopia. This T1-weighted axial brain MRI of a patient with subcortical band heterotopia demonstrates two bands of heterotopic gray matter that traverse the subcortical white matter and run the entire length of the cerebral hemispheres bilaterally.

The phenotypic expression of SBH is characterized by medically refractory seizures, developmental delay, and motor disability. Most patients experience multiple seizure types, including partial seizures (simple motor or complex partial seizures) and generalized seizures (atypical absence, drop attacks, or myoclonic seizures) (24, 25). Correspondingly, the EEGs reveal interictal and ictal SBH and cortical discharges focally, as well as generalized epileptiform discharges (23, 28). Consequently, very few patients benefit from epilepsy surgery, with only one patient in a series of eight who benefited from a resection (24).

The severity of developmental delays corresponds with the degree of SBH band thickness, younger age of onset of seizures, increased seizure frequency, type of seizures, and degree of ventricular enlargement (26). With formal neuropsychiatric testing, slowed processing speed, anxiety, depression, and poor social skills are detected (26, 29). These deficits may also reflect disruptions of the corticocortical connections by the SBH. Interestingly, these patients exhibit a relative preservation of verbal and visual episodic memory, which may reflect the typical lack of temporal involvement in SBH (29).

Classical Lissencephaly

Classical lissencephaly is described as a "smooth brain" and recognized by the absence of gyri or the presence of a few broad gyri separated by simple primary fissures and sulci. Microscopically, the cortex consists of only four layers: an outermost molecular layer, a thickened band of pyramidal neurons, a limited cellular myelinated layer III, and a broad band of disorganized small and medium-sized neurons in layer IV (30). The abnormal cortex is best seen posteriorly in the occipital areas, whereas a normal six-layered cortex is found in the temporal and inferior frontal lobes (30). On MRI, lissencephaly is identified by a thickened cortex of 10–20 mm, ventriculomegaly, decreased white matter volume with perhaps some neuronal heterotopia, and blurring of the gray–white junction (30).

Classical lissencephaly is also believed to result from abnormal neuronal migration. Interestingly, two genes have been found that account for 40% of patients with lissencephaly spectrum disorders (8). The LIS1 gene encodes a protein that may participate in cytoplasmic dynein-mediated nucleokinesis, somal translocation, cell motility, mitosis, and chromosome segregation. It produces posterior predominant lissencephaly and is found in 60% of patients with classical lissencephaly (a condition with no dysmorphic features) and 90% of patients with Miller-Dieker syndrome (a condition with micrognathia, ear abnormalities, anteverted nares, wrinkling of forehead, prominent superior lip, and bitemporal narrowing in addition to microcephaly, postnatal growth retardation, and profound mental retardation) (2, 31, 32). In contrast, the DCX gene, encoding the protein doublecortin, produces an anterior predominant lissencephaly in males and subcortical band heterotopia in females (31, 32). As stated previously, doublecortin is a microtubule-associated protein and may participate in regulation of cell adhesion and microtubular bundling, resulting in abnormal neuronogenesis and migration (8, 26). There are additional genes also associated with lissencephaly, most of which are presumed to function in neuronal migration. The ARX mutation and associated lissencephaly will be discussed separately in the following subsection.

More than 90% of patients with classical lissencephaly will experience seizures, typically before 6 months of age, including atypical absence and focal, tonic, and atonic seizures (2, 33). Most patients will suffer from infantile spasms, although they may not exhibit the classic hypsarrhythmic pattern on EEG (2, 33). Indeed, the EEG more commonly shows diffuse high-amplitude fast rhythms or extreme spindles, and sharp and slow-wave complexes with high amplitudes (2, 33). The seizures are often medically refractory, although one case report described significant reduction in seizures and resumption of development after a total corpus callosotomy (34). As might be expected from the global brain malformation and severe epilepsy, most patients with lissencephaly have profound mental retardation and spastic quadriparesis (2, 35).

Lissencephaly Associated with ARX Gene Mutations

Although most patients with classical lissencephaly are afflicted by global cortical malformation, severe epilepsy, and developmental delay, patients with lissencephaly associated with Aristaless-related homeobox (ARX) gene mutations display heterogeneous phenotypes. The ARX gene is expressed by the interneurons of the forebrain and the interstitium of the male gonad (31). ARX is involved in the differentiation of the embryonic forebrain and male testes; in particular, ARX is involved in the proliferation of neuronal precursors and tangential migration of GABAergic interneurons (31). Pathologically, the lissencephaly associated with the ARX mutation is characterized by a three-layered cortex, with a hypercellular molecular layer of small- and medium-sized neurons, a relative increase in pyramidal cell number in layer II, and a thick layer of small- and medium-sized neurons in layer III (30). As a result, the gray–white junction is relatively defined, in contrast to classical lissencephaly (30). On neuroimaging, a moderately thickened 5–10-mm cortex is observed, with gyral abnormalities more severe posteriorly, as well as abnormal white matter signal and cystic or fragmented basal ganglia (31, 36).

Patients with ARX mutations who have lissencephaly as described previously may suffer clinically from West syndrome, with infantile spasms, hypsarrhythmia, and mental retardation (37). Another syndrome of X-linked lissencephaly with abnormal genitalia (XLAG) is characterized by severe microcephaly, posterior predominant lissencephaly, agenesis of the corpus callosum, hypothalamic dysfunction (typically hypothermia), midbrain malformations, micropenis, cryptorchidism, and neonatal onset of intractable seizures (37). The ARX mutation is also associated with other syndromes, including XMESID (X-linked myoclonic epilepsy with spasticity and intellectual disability), Proud syndrome (X-linked mental retardation, agenesis of the corpus callosum, and abnormal genitalia), and Partington syndrome (X-linked mental retardation, dystonic hand movements, and myoclonic and tonic-clonic seizures) (36, 37). Thus, the ARX mutation, presumed to be involved in migration of interneurons and proliferation of neuronal precursors, may be expressed with widely different phenotypes that typically include epilepsy and mental retardation. One mechanistic explanation for the associated seizures centers on a disruption in GABAergic interneurons' inhibitory influence in the cortex, thus allowing for excessive cerebral synchronization.

DISORDERS OF ORGANIZATION

Polymicrogyria

Polymicrogyria is characterized by an irregular, excessively convoluted brain surface, which may be localized or diffuse. On microscopic examination, the cortex consists of four layers with evidence of tissue necrosis, likely fusing the gyri at the molecular layer (1). Another form of polymicrogyria exists that has no discernible cortical architecture (8).

Polymicrogyria may occur due to a postmigration disorder at approximately 20–24 weeks of gestation, which causes cortical necrosis and fusion (38). Environmental factors such as prenatal hypoxic-ischemic insults and congenital infections may account for this abnormality (39). However, in other patients, a genetic cause is implicated, which may be specific for different phenotypic expressions of polymicrogyria. For example, congenital bilateral perisylvian polymicrogyria (CBPP) is associated with X-linked inheritance, and bilateral frontoparietal polymicrogyria (BFPP) is due to autosomal recessive inheritance of mutations in the GPR56 gene, which may play a role in neuronal determination and cortical patterning (40–42).

Neuroimaging has been critical in the proper diagnosis of this cortical malformation. Polymicrogyria is typically seen as excessive cortical gyrations without true cortical thickening, thereby differentiating it from lissencephaly (Figure 54-4). There is also an irregular appearance to the gray–white junction (1).

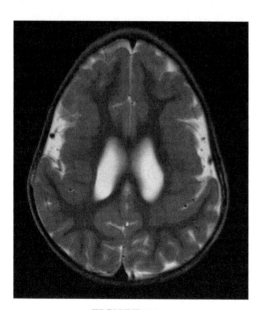

FIGURE 54-4

Congenital bilateral perisylvian polymicrogyria. This T2-weighted axial brain MRI of a patient with congenital bilateral perisylvian polymicrogyria demonstrates the irregular, excessive cortical convolutions characteristic of this malformation along the Sylvian fissures bilaterally. The polymicrogyric cortex appears abnormally thick, but close inspection reveals the irregular gray–white junction suggestive of polymicrogyria rather than true pachygyria.

The clinical expression of polymicrogyria is highly dependent on the location of the abnormal cortex, although most patients experience epilepsy. Patients with unilateral disease typically are affected by localization-related epilepsy or may have electrical status epilepticus of sleep (43). Patients with bilateral disease more often have multiple seizure types that are medically refractory and have an infantile onset (43). For example, patients with CBPP have seizures that are often generalized—either atonic, tonic, atypical absence, or generalized motor seizures—with neonatal onset and treatment resistance. The EEG abnormalities consist of generalized or multifocal epileptiform discharges, primarily involving the centrotemporal regions (40). Alternatively, CBPP patients may have seizures with a focal somatomotor onset (44). Similarly, patients with bilateral generalized polymicrogyria often experience generalized seizures (39), but patients with bilateral frontal polymicrogyria will more commonly experience partial and atypical absence seizures with onset in infancy or early childhood (2).

Patients with polymicrogyria demonstrate cognitive and behavioral deficits that correspond to the areas of greatest involvement. Therefore, patients with bilateral generalized polymicrogyria are often the most severely affected, with severe cognitive and motor delays (41), and patients with unilateral polymicrogyria may have a normal or borderline intelligence and contralateral hemiparesis permitting ambulation (38). Interestingly, patients with CBPP exhibit pseudobulbar palsy with dysarthria, dysphagia, drooling, and restricted tongue movements with spastic quadriparesis (40), findings that correlate with the bilateral perisylvian location of polymicrogyria in this group. On formal neuropsychologic testing, CBPP patients appear to have impaired language comprehension and expression, but intact frontal sorting abilities and borderline mental retardation, suggesting that they may benefit from alternative communication strategies such as sign language (44). Finally, patients with BFPP typically have dysconjugate gaze, pyramidal signs, cerebellar signs, and hypoplasia of the brainstem and cerebellum, as well as the more common developmental delay and spastic quadriparesis (39, 41). Nonetheless, despite deficits that seem to correspond to the areas of polymicrogyric cortex in many patients, functional MRI studies suggest that polymicrogyric cortex can be involved in normal cortical functioning in some patients (45).

Focal Cortical Dysplasia

Focal cortical dysplasias (FCD) encompass a heterogeneous disorder with presumably multiple causes, resulting in a focal area of cortical malformation. They are characterized by abnormal cortical lamination with or without dysplastic neurons, such as balloon cells (40, 46). They may be found throughout the cortex, often in frontal, temporal, or multiple locations (1, 47). FCD are best detected by MRI, which reveals gray matter thickening, blurring of the gray–white matter junction, and homogenous hyperintense signal in the subcortical white matter that tapers as it extends to the lateral ventricle (1, 40). Nonetheless, MRI may fail to detect up to 30% of FCD later identified by pathology, particularly in children with incomplete myelination, because the gray–white matter junction can be difficult to define in those cases (48).

FCDs are the cause of 5–10% of all focal epilepsies (46). The seizures begin in childhood or adolescence and are typically generalized tonic-clonic, tonic, hypomotor, or simple or complex partial seizures (47), whereas the more common chronic seizures consist of focal motor, complex partial, or secondarily generalized seizures (38). Furthermore, up to 30% of patients with FCD may experience either epilepsia partialis continua or generalized tonic-clonic status epilepticus (40, 46, 49) and some patients may experience continuous spike-waves during sleep (50). Similarly, the EEG may reveal either regional slowing or localized epileptiform discharges, although the discharges may be more extensive than the FCD location (1, 40). As seizures due to FCD are medically refractory in up to 76% of patients (47), surgical resections have been evaluated as potential cures. Seizure freedom may be achieved in 58–75% of patients with resection of FCD, particularly after complete resection of the FCD (1, 40).

Patients with FCD not only have medically refractory seizures but also experience motor and sensory deficits in 50–67%, lower intelligence, and possibly deficits related to the location of the FCD (40, 48, 50).

CONCLUSION

With the advent of improved neuroimaging techniques, malformations of cortical development are increasingly being recognized as an etiology of medically refractory epilepsy. Continued investigation into the causes of cortical malformations will improve our knowledge of normal brain development and may provide insights into epileptogenesis. Furthermore, this may translate into better treatments for epilepsy, including more advanced surgical techniques and targeted antiepileptic medications. Most of the malformations are characterized by varying degrees of cognitive impairments, which will also benefit from more refined descriptions and targeted therapies. Although malformations of cortical development comprise only a fraction of patients with epilepsy and developmental delay, they provide a useful framework for better understanding of seizures and mental retardation.

References

1. Sisodiya SM. Malformations of cortical development: burdens and insights from important causes of human epilepsy. *Lancet Neurol* 2004; 3:29–38.
2. Guerrini R. Genetic malformations of the cerebral cortex and epilepsy. *Epilepsia* 2005; 46(S1):32–37.
3. Pieffer A, Singh N, Leppert M, Dobyns WB, et al. Microcephaly with simplified gyral pattern in six related children. *Am J Med Genet* 1999; 84:137–144.
4. Abdel-Salam GM, Halasz AA, Czeizel AE. Association of epilepsy with different groups of microcephaly. *Dev Med Child Neurol* 2000; 42:760–767.
5. Woods CG, Bond J, Enard W. Autosomal recessive primary microcephaly (MCPH): a review of clinical, molecular, and evolutionary findings. *Am J Hum Genet* 2005; 76:717–728.
6. Woods CG. Human microcephaly. *Curr Opin Neurobiol* 2004; 14:112–117.
7. Mochida GH, Walsh CA. Molecular genetics of human microcephaly. *Curr Opin Neurol* 2001; 14:151–156.
8. Francis F, Meyer G, Fallet-Bianco C, et al. Human disorders of cortical development: From past to present. *Eur J Neurosci* 2006; 23:877–893.
9. Shen J, Eyaid W, Mochida GH, et al. ASPM mutations identified in patients with primary microcephaly and seizures. *J Med Genet* 2005; 42:725–729.
10. Mochida GH. Cortical malformation and pediatric epilepsy: a molecular genetic approach. *J Child Neurol* 2005; 20:300–303.
11. Straussberg R, Kornreich L, Harel L, Varsano I. Autosomal recessive microcephaly with neonatal myoclonic seizures: clinical and MRI findings. *Am J Med Genet* 1998; 80:136–139.
12. Jahan R, Mischel PS, Curran JG, Peacock WJ, et al. Bilateral neuropathologic changes in a child with hemimegalencephaly. *Pediatr Neurol* 1997; 17:344–349.
13. Flores-Sarnat L. Hemimegalencephaly: Part 1. Genetic, clinical, and imaging aspects. *J Child Neurol* 2002; 17:373–384.
14. Sasaki M, Hashimoto T, Furushima W, et al. Clinical aspects of hemimegalencephaly by means of a nationwide survey. *J Child Neurol* 2005; 20:337–341.
15. Tassi L, Colombo N, Cossu M, et al. Electroclinical, MRI, and neuropathological study of 10 patients with nodular heterotopia, with surgical outcomes. *Brain* 2005; 128: 321–337.
16. Li LM, Dubeau F, Andermann F, et al. Periventricular nodular heterotopia and intractable temporal lobe epilepsy: poor outcome after temporal lobe resection. *Ann Neurol* 1997; 41:662–668.
17. Sheen VL, Dixon PH, Fox JW, et al. Mutations in the X-linked filamin 1 gene cause periventricular nodular heterotopia in males as well as in females. *Hum Mol Genet* 2001; 10:1775–1783.
18. Aghakhani Y, Kinay D, Gotman J, et al. The role of periventricular nodular heterotopia in epileptogenesis. *Brain* 2005; 128:641–651.
19. Battaglia G, Granata T, Farina L, D'Incerti L, et al. Periventricular nodular heterotopia: epileptogenic findings. *Epilepsia* 1997; 38:1173–1182.
20. Battaglia G, Franceschetti S, Chiapparini L, et al. Electrographic recordings of focal seizures in patients affected by periventricular nodular heterotopia: role of heterotopic nodules in the genesis of epileptic discharges. *J Child Neurol* 2005; 20:369–377.
21. D'Orsi G, Tinuper P, Bisulli F, et al. Clinical features and long term outcome of epilepsy in periventricular nodular heterotopia. Simple compared with plus forms. *J Neurol Neurosurg Psychiatry* 2004; 75:873–878.
22. Chang BS, Ly J, Appignani B, et al. Reading impairment in the neuronal migration disorder of periventricular nodular heterotopia. *Neurology* 2005; 64:799–803.
23. Mai R, Tassi L, Cossu M, et al. A neuropathological, stereo-EEG, and MRI study of subcortical band heterotopia. *Neurology* 2003; 60:1834–1838.
24. Bernasconi A, Martinez V, Rosa-Neto P, et al. Surgical resection for intractable epilepsy in "double cortex" syndrome yields inadequate results. *Epilepsia* 2001; 42:1124–1129.
25. D'Agostino MD, Bernasconi A, Das S, et al. Subcortical band heterotopia in males: clinical, imaging and genetic findings in comparison with females. *Brain* 2002; 125:2507–2522.
26. Jacobs R, Anderson V, Harvey AS. Neuropsychological profile of a 9-year-old child with subcortical band heterotopia or "double cortex." *Dev Med Child Neurol* 2001; 43:628–633.
27. Leventer RJ. Genotype-phenotype correlation in lissencephaly and subcortical band heterotopia: the key questions answered. *J Child Neurol* 2005; 20:307–312.
28. Grant A, Rho J. Ictal EEG patterns in band heterotopia. *Epilepsia* 2002; 4:403–407.
29. Janzen L, Sherman E, Langfitt J, Berg M, et al. Preserved episodic memory in subcortical band heterotopia. *Epilepsia* 2004; 45:555–558.
30. Forman MS, Squier W, Dobyns WB, Golden JA. Genotypically defined lissencephalies show distinct pathologies. *J Neuropathol Exp Neurol* 2005; 64:847–857.
31. Kato M, Dobyns WB. Lissencephaly and the molecular basis of neuronal migration. *Hum Mol Genet* 2003; 12:R89–R96.
32. Gleeson JG. Classical lissencephaly and double cortex (subcortical band heterotopia): LIS1 and doublecortin. *Curr Opin Neurol* 2000; 13:121–125.
33. Kato M. A new paradigm for West syndrome based on molecular and cell biology. *Epilepsy Res* 2006; 70(S1):87–95.
34. Kamida T, Maruyama T, Fujiki M, Kobayashi H, et al. Total callosotomy for a case of lissencephaly presenting with West syndrome and generalized seizures. *Childs Nerv Syst* 2005; 21:1056–1060.

35. Pilz DT, Matsumoto N, Minnerath S, et al. LIS1 and XLIS (DCX) mutations cause most classical lissencephaly, but different patterns of malformation. *Hum Mol Genet* 1998; 7:2029–2037.

36. Sherr EH. The ARX story (epilepsy, mental retardation, autism, and cerebral malformations): one gene leads to many phenotypes. *Curr Opin Pediatr* 2003; 15:567–571.

37. Friocourt G, Poirier K, Rakic S, Parnavelas JG, et al. The role of ARX in cortical development. *Eur J Neurosci* 2006; 23:869–876.

38. Pascual-Castroviejo I, Pascual-Pascual SI, Viano J, Martinez V, et al. Unilateral polymicrogyria: a common cause of hemiplegia of prenatal origin. *Brain Dev* 2001; 23:216–222.

39. Chang BS, Piao X, Bodell A, et al. Bilateral frontoparietal polymicrogyria: clinical and radiological features in 10 families with linkage to chromosome 16. *Ann Neurol* 2003; 53:596–606.

40. Foldvary-Schaefer DO, Bautista J, Andermann F, Cascino G, et al. Focal malformations of cortical development. *Neurology* 2004; 62:S14–S19.

41. Chang BS, Piao X, Giannini C, et al. Bilateral generalized polymicrogyria: a distinct syndrome of cortical malformation. *Neurology* 2004; 62:1722–1728.

42. Piao X, Hill RS, Bodell A, et al. G protein-coupled receptor-dependent development of human frontal cortex. *Science* 2004; 303:2033–2036.

43. Ohtsuka Y, Tanaka A, Kobayashi K, et al. Childhood-onset epilepsy associated with polymicrogyria. *Brain Dev* 2002; 24:758–765.

44. Jansen AC, Leonard G, Bastos AC, et al. Cognitive functioning in bilateral perisylvian polymicrogyria (BPP): clinical and radiological correlations. *Epilepsy Behav* 2005; 6:393–404.

45. Araujo D, Araujo DB, Pontes-Neto OM, et al. Language and motor fMRI activation in polymicrogyric cortex. *Epilepsia* 2006; 47:589–592.

46. Bast T, Ramantani G, Seitz A, Rating D. Focal cortical dysplasia: prevalence, clinical presentation and epilepsy in children and adults. *Acta Neurol Scand* 2006; 113:72–81.

47. Fauser S, Huppertz H-J, Bast T, et al. Clinical characteristics in focal cortical dysplasia: a retrospective evaluation in a series of 120 patients. *Brain* 2006; 129:1907–1916.

48. Lortie A, Plouin P, Chiron C, Delalande O, et al. Characteristics of epilepsy in focal cortical dysplasia in infancy. *Epilepsy Res* 2002; 51:133–145.

49. Guerrini R, Filippi T. Neuronal migration disorders, genetics, and epileptogenesis. *J Child Neurol* 2005; 20:287–299.

50. Roulet Perez E, Seeck M, Mayer E, Despland P-A, et al. Childhood epilepsy with neuropsychological regression and continuous spike waves during sleep: epilepsy surgery in a young adult. *Eur J Paediatr Neurol* 1998; 2:303–311.

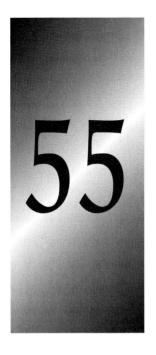

55 Chromosomal Abnormalities

Maurizio Elia

The prevalence of chromosome aberrations in live births, which can be ascertained using all the genetic techniques now available, is estimated at about 1:100 for balanced and unbalanced and at about 1:300 for unbalanced aberrations alone. However, considering the high number of deaths, especially in the early postnatal period, the prevalence at 1 year of age should be substantially lower than that in newborns. Furthermore, since epilepsy occurs in the first year of life in most cases of chromosome aberrations, but rarely during the first month of life, it is rather difficult to determine the prevalence of epilepsy with chromosome aberrations (1).

Approximately 6% of patients with learning disabilities and epilepsy have a chromosome abnormality. This figure rises to 50% in patients with major congenital malformations, although chromosome studies are often not included in the workup of children with learning disabilities and epilepsy, particularly if the child is not dysmorphic or if the child develops cognitive problems after the onset of epilepsy (2).

Obviously, there are many syndromes with epilepsy in which it is possible to find a chromosome abnormality. Singh et al. (3), analyzing the Oxford Medical Database and the PubMed database, identified 400 different chromosomal imbalances associated with seizures or electroencephalographic (EEG) abnormalities.

In the last few years, several syndromes has been described, caused by various chromosome abnormalities (i.e., monosomies, trisomies, deletions, duplications, translocations, inversions, etc.) or mutations, and associated with specific clinical and EEG features. However, clinical reports often resulted that were inadequate in describing the semiology of seizures or EEG characteristics.

In this review, some chromosome anomalies or mutations highly associated with epilepsy will be examined, and attention will be focused on the clinical features and course of epilepsy and EEG characteristics.

1p36 DELETION SYNDROME

1p36.3 deletions account for approximately 0.5–0.7% of cases with idiopathic mental retardation. The prevalence, originally estimated to be 1:10,000, is presently thought to be 1:5,000, because screening for terminal deletions is now available. So far, at least 100 cases of 1p36 deletion syndrome have been described. 1p36 deletion may be the result of a pure terminal deletion, or an interstitial deletion, or an unbalanced translocation, or a more complex rearrangement. The origin of the deletion can be paternal or maternal, and in the first instance the size of the deletion is larger (4).

The 1p36 deletion syndrome is primarily characterized by craniofacial dysmorphic features, brachydactyly or camptodactyly, short feet, and sensorineural hearing impairment. More rarely, epicanthal folds, highly arched or cleft palate, heart defects, hypothyroidism, and visual inattentiveness are reported. All patients have moderate to profound mental retardation. In more than 85% of cases muscle hypotonia is present.

Most subjects reach independent walking, which usually is characterized by broad-based gait and poor coordination. Behavioral disturbances have been reported, such as temper tantrums, aggressiveness, self-injuries, and autistic features (4).

Brain neuroimaging has shown cerebral atrophy, ventricular dilation or asymmetry, hydrocephalus, delay of myelination, focal cortical dysplasias, and leukodystrophy (4).

Seizures are present in more than half of the cases and are of different types: infantile spasms, simple or complex partial, generalized tonic-clonic, myoclonic, or absences. The onset is during infancy or childhood, and they are variably controlled by antiepileptic drugs (AEDs) (4).

Heilstedt et al. (5) reported 24 patients with 1p36 deletion, 11 of whom (46%) had seizures; these were divided in three subgroups: subjects with intractable seizures (3 of 11), subjects with infantile spasms (3 of 11), and patients with seizures well controlled by therapy (5 of 11). Another 3 patients (12.5%) had rare early seizures.

Of the 11 patients described by Kurosawa et al. in 2005 (6), 8 (about 73%) presented with epilepsy. The age at onset of seizures varied from 1 month to 7 years. The authors reported that most of the seizures were of the generalized tonic-clonic type; furthermore, in 6 cases epilepsy was drug resistant.

The EEG picture is variable and can show hypsarrhythmia, with focal or multifocal spikes or asymmetric slow-wave activity (4).

In 2001, Heilstedt et al. (5) proposed that haploinsufficiency for the voltage-gated K^+ channel beta-subunit gene (KCNAB2) is a significant risk factor for epilepsy. Eight patients (89%) in their series had deletions of the KCNAB2 gene and had epilepsy or EEG epileptiform abnormalities. On the other hand, of those not deleted, only 27% had seizures, and none presented with infantile spasms.

WOLF-HIRSCHHORN (4p⁻) SYNDROME

The Wolf-Hirschhorn or 4p⁻ syndrome (WHS) is a rare malformative condition that is caused by the distal deletion of the short arm of chromosome 4 (4p16). It is sporadic in about 85% of cases and originates from an unbalanced translocation in the remaining 15% of cases. Genetic molecular studies have shown that the deleted portion of the chromosome is usually of paternal origin but can be of maternal origin.

The prevalence of the WHS is estimated as 1:50,000; however it could be higher, considering the frequency of misdiagnosis due to lack of recognition or inadequate genetic analysis (7).

The shortest region of overlap of the different deletions found in patients with WHS (the "critical region") is approximately 165 kb long. The WHSC1 gene is a candidate gene for WHS and for Pitt-Rogers-Danks syndrome, which results from the absence of the same genetic segments as WHS but presents with minor clinical differences, likely due to allelic variation in the remaining homolog (8).

Zollino et al. (9) proposed a new critical region for WHS, referred to as WHSCR2, distally contiguous with the WHS critical region. Among the candidate genes in this region, the authors considered LETM1 likely to be pathogenetically involved in seizures. On the basis of an accurate genotype–phenotype analysis, a distinction in two different entities of WHS has been proposed: the "classical" and the "mild" form.

The WHS is characterized by low birth weight, severe growth retardation, severe mental retardation, microcephaly, "Greek helmet" profile, cleft lip or palate, coloboma of the eye, and cardiac septal defects. In approximately one-third of the cases death occurs in the first year of life because of severe systemic malformations, heart failure, or pulmonary infections (7, 8).

The following neuropathologic alterations have been reported: microcephaly, abnormal gyral pattern, gray matter heterotopia, dysplasia of the lateral geniculate bodies and dentate nuclei, and hypoplasia of the corpus callosum (7, 8).

Although the precise frequency of seizures in WHS is not known, they occur in 50–100% of subjects reported in the literature (7, 8). The clinical and EEG features of epilepsy in WHS have been reported only in some cases (7, 8, 10, 11).

Seizure onset usually occurs in the first 2 years of life. Different types of seizures have been described in association with WHS: simple or unilateral partial seizures, myoclonic seizures (often during status epilepticus), and generalized tonic-clonic seizures. More rarely, complex partial seizures or tonic spasms are present.

A peculiar clinical and EEG pattern has been found in nine Italian patients, described in two different studies (8). After the onset of unilateral or generalized tonic-clonic seizures, all of these patients presented with frequent atypical absences accompanied by myoclonic jerks induced by eye closure. These episodes were characterized by generalized slow spike-and-wave complexes on the EEG. Interictal EEG showed sequences of sharp waves localized over the central-parietal and occipital regions, unilaterally or bilaterally, atypical high-voltage spikes, and sharp waves often facilitated by the eye closure. This EEG pattern is very similar to that observed in Angelman syndrome. The same ictal or interictal EEG trait has been confirmed by other authors, and in at least in some cases, bursts of fast repetitive spikes over the posterior regions have been recorded (7).

The outcome of epilepsy in WHS is rather benign. Seizures are well controlled from 2 to 13 years of age in more than one-third of cases, and approximately 15% of patients can discontinue AED treatment (7). Most of the patients in the study by Kagitani-Shimono et al. (11) showed a gradual reduction of seizures and episodes of status epilepticus after 5 years of age. However, in the same study, one patient died during the first episode of status epilepticus.

Regarding antiepileptic drug treatment, the seizures observed in WHS can be usually controlled by valproic acid alone or in combination with ethosuximide. In some cases, benzodiazepines can be useful (7, 8 11). Sodium bromide for the treatment of status epilepticus has been proposed (11).

Similarities of the clinical picture and EEG pattern of WHS with that of Angelman syndrome, although disputable, have suggested an involvement of the gene coding for a subunit of the $GABA_A$ receptor (mapping on the short arm of the chromosome 4) in the pathogenesis of epilepsy in WHS. However, it is unlikely that the $GABA_A$ gene is involved because the $GABA_A$ gene maps proximally to the critical deletion region (WHSCR), specifically, 4p12–p13, far from the critical region of WHS. As previously discussed, LETM1, a gene possibly involved in calcium signaling or homeostasis, is a good candidate considering the seizures and neuromuscular problems in WHS (9).

6q TERMINAL DELETION SYNDROME

The 6q terminal deletion syndrome is a rare condition with mental retardation, facial dysmorphisms, genital hypoplasia, and structural anomalies of the CNS. Recently we reported five patients with 6q terminal deletion (ranging between 9 and 16 Mb) associated with a specific clinical and EEG pattern.

In all cases, seizures were characterized by vomiting, cyanosis, and head and eye deviation, with or without loss of consciousness. In four cases, the interictal EEG showed posterior spike-and-wave complexes, which were activated by sleep (Figure 55-1). No patient had status epilepticus or prolonged seizures. Brain magnetic resonance imaging (MRI) revealed colpocephaly and dysgenesis of the corpus callosum and brainstem in four patients; three of them also had hypertrophic massa intermedia. Seizure outcome was rather good in all patients (12).

TRISOMY 12p SYNDROME

This is a rare disorder, with an estimated prevalence of 1:50,000, which can be determined de novo (also in a mosaic fashion) or by an unbalanced translocation. The trisomy 12p syndrome is characterized by severe mental retardation, absent language, generalized muscle hypotonia, round

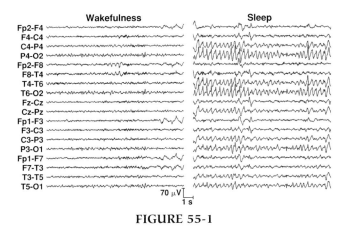

FIGURE 55-1

Awake EEG of a male subject with 6q terminal deletion syndrome. Note the presence of sharp waves over the posterior regions of the right hemisphere (a); during sleep, very long sequences of slow waves or spike-and-wave complexes are present over the posterior regions (b).

face, short neck, high and prominent forehead, flat occiput, hypertelorism, epicanthus, flat nasal bridge, long philtrum, prominent lower lip, low-set ears, and micrognathia.

Neuroimaging findings are various: basal ganglia calcifications, cortical and subcortical atrophy, dilatation of the cisterna magna, and signal alterations of the white matter (13, 14).

Seizures are present in about 30% of cases, and they are typically febrile or afebrile generalized tonic-clonic seizures or myoclonic seizures. In some patients atypical myoclonic absences occur after 3 years of age, and ictal and interictal EEG shows generalized spike- or polyspike-and-wave complexes at 3 Hz (13, 14) (Figure 55-2). The

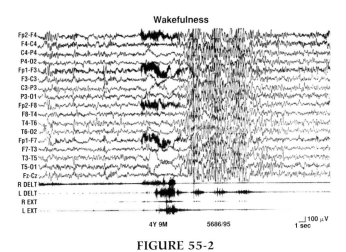

FIGURE 55-2

Awake EEG of a 4-year-9-month-old female with trisomy 12p syndrome, showing a myoclonic absence-like seizure. It is characterized by a discharge of high voltage, generalized spike-and-wave complexes, accompanied by rhythmical myoclonic jerks, prevalent over the left deltoid muscle (R = right, L = left, DELT = deltoid muscle, EXT = extensor muscle of the forearm).

seizures are usually controlled by valproate with or without ethosuximide.

It is interesting to note that in the region 12p13, included in the aberration, there is a cluster of three genes coding for voltage-gated K channels (13).

RING CHROMOSOME 14 SYNDROME

Ring chromosome 14 syndrome (r14S) is a rare disease mostly occurring as a mosaicism. The clinical phenotype is constituted by early-onset epilepsy, mental retardation (mostly severe or profound), language disturbance, microcephaly, and facial dysmorphisms. Ocular anomalies, such as cortical cataract, retinopathy, and refractive errors, can also be present (8).

Neuroimaging sporadically discloses corpus callosum hypoplasia, left temporal lobe hypodensity on computed tomographic (CT) scan, cortical atrophy, and ventricular dilation (8). In one patient, interictal single-photon emission computed tomography (SPECT) showed hypoperfusion over the frontal regions (15).

Epilepsy begins early, generally during the first year of life, with generalized seizures, but also with complex partial seizures. A frontal-temporal origin of seizures in some patients has also been reported. The interictal EEG is often focal, with spikes localized over the frontal-temporal, central, or temporal regions (15). Seizures are mostly drug resistant.

The pathogenesis of the seizures is not well understood. However, they are usually present in the cases with linear 14q terminal deletion, so epileptogenesis seems to be correlated with the ring. Two hypotheses have been proposed: (1) the mitotic instability induces the somatic mosaicism, with genetic variations among tissues; and (2) the telomere p reduces the expression of the genes on the adjacent region 14q (15)

ANGELMAN SYNDROME

Angelman syndrome (AS) is characterized by severe mental retardation, minimal expressive language, ataxia, myoclonic jerks, paroxysmal inappropriate laughter, and seizures (8, 14).

The prevalence of AS is approximately 1:62,000, but it could be an underestimated value, because some authors reported a higher prevalence rate (1:12,000). In more than 70% of cases of AS, a deletion of the long arm of chromosome 15 of maternal origin (15q11–13) is present; in approximately 2–3% of cases a paternal uniparental disomy (UPD) is recognizable; and in 3–5% of patients a defect of the imprinting center causes the absence of the typical maternal pattern of methylation of DNA. In addition, since 1997 numerous sporadic and familial cases of AS

have been reported (5–10%) with mutations of the UBE3A gene (ubiquitine protein ligase 3A), which is localized in the region 15q11–13. At least 50% of these mutations involve exons 8 and 9 of the UBE3A gene (16).

The genotypes just mentioned determine AS phenotypes of variable severity, more severe in the subgroup with 15q11–13 deletion, less severe in that with UBE3A mutations, and milder in those cases with paternal UPD and with a defect of the imprinting center (17).

Among the various transgenic animal models of AS available, those with absence of the GABRB3 gene present some clinical and EEG characteristics similar to those observed in humans (8, 14).

Presently, it is not clearly understood how inactivation of the UBE3A gene can result in AS. An interesting hypothesis recently proposed is that the UBE3A deficit could act directly through a defect of activation of the Plic-1 protein, which regulates the number of $GABA_A$ receptors containing the beta-3 subunit, thus reducing GABAergic strength (18).

Neuroimaging studies usually do not show a specific malformative pattern. Cerebral atrophy of various degrees and dilation of lateral ventricles are frequently present (8, 14).

The EEG picture in AS is very peculiar, common in the different genotypes, and is characterized by slow background activity and paroxysmal abnormalities, mostly spike-and-wave complexes, prevalent over the occipital or frontal regions. There is a diffuse discharge of spike-and-wave complexes, which are sometimes accompanied

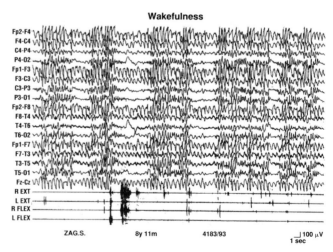

FIGURE 55-3

An 8-year-11-month-old female with AS. The awake EEG shows a slow background activity and quasi-continuous high voltage, diffuse spike-and-wave complexes, prevalent over the frontal regions. A surface EMG of extensor and flexor muscles of the forearms shows that myoclonic jerks are present, which are rarely correlated with the paroxysmal abnormalities (R = right, L = left, EXT = extensor muscle of the forearm, FLEX = flexor muscle of the forearm).

by myoclonic jerks. The myoclonic jerks, which are rhythmical and bilateral and sometimes quasi-continuous, do not correlate well with the EEG abnormalities. The typical pattern is a "myoclonic status epilepticus," clinically associated with marked ataxia, myoclonic jerks, and hyperactivity (Figure 55-3). In stages 1 and 2 of non-REM sleep, the spike-and-wave discharges become continuous, and spindles are not recognizable; in stages 2 and 3 of the subsequent sleep cycles, the activation of paroxysmal abnormalities is lower and spindles are better represented. In slow-wave sleep, myoclonic jerks tend to disappear; they appear again during awakening and, eventually, during REM sleep, when diffuse discharges are not evident and a theta activity appears over the vertex and the rolandic regions (19)

Back-averaging study of myoclonus in AS, during myoclonic status epilepticus or myoclonic absences, demonstrates a cortical origin, with a rostral-caudal pattern of activation. Furthermore, in some patients a fast focal or multifocal quasi-continuous rhythmical myoclonus, at approximately 11 Hz, of cortical origin and involving hands or face, has been described (14).

Seizures, present in about 90% of cases, usually begin in infancy, often during the first year of life, and they are rather polymorphous: spasms, myoclonic, myoclonic-atonic, tonic-clonic, simple partial, complex partial, atypical absences (Figure 55-4), myoclonic absences, and febrile convulsions (8, 14). Seizure onset is earlier and epilepsy is

more severe in patients with 15q11–13 deletion than in patients with another genotype (17).

Epilepsy in AS is relatively benign from later childhood on, and treatment is usually based on valproic acid, also in association with ethosuximide, or benzodiazepines. Topiramate was efficacious in a series of five patients with AS (8). Cortical myoclonus can be treated with high doses of piracetam (140 mg/kg/day) (14).

INV-DUP(15) SYNDROME

An inverted duplication of chromosome 15, or inv-dup(15) syndrome, is the most common genetic disorder in the group of the extrastructurally abnormal chromosomes. The prevalence at birth is estimated as 1:30,000 (1).

The phenotype can be quite variable, presenting with mental retardation, behavior disturbances, pervasive developmental disorders, and epilepsy. In most cases neuroimaging studies do not show significant alterations (20).

It has been suggested that the clinical severity of inv-dup(15) syndrome could be correlated directly with the extent of the duplicated segment, but some data contradict this statement (21). More probably, the clinical phenotype appears associated with the dosage of the 15q11–13 region, which is critical for Prader-Willi and Angelman syndromes (20). Among genes with a presumable role in the inv-dup(15) syndrome phenotype there are those coding for the alpha-5 and beta-3 subunits of the GABA receptor and the OCA2 gene (oculocutaneous albinism type II gene, formerly called the P gene), which is essential for normal pigmentation and is likely involved in the production of melanin.

Tetrasomy of these genes could alter the activity of the GABA receptor and cause some of the main clinical characteristics of the syndrome, such as seizures, hyperactivity, aggressiveness, and autistic behavior. Another gene, SLC12A6, which codes for a chloride cotransporter and is expressed in the brain, could be involved in the pathogenesis of seizures (20).

Epilepsy has a variable age of onset, between 6 months and 9 years of age, and it can present in the form of infantile spasms, symptomatic generalized epilepsy, or Lennox-Gastaut syndrome (Figure 55-5) (20). In this case, epilepsy has a severe prognosis, with tonic, atonic, tonic-clonic seizures and atypical absences with onset between 4 and 8 years. Myoclonic, complex partial seizures, and reflex myoclonic absences have been also reported (20, 22).

EEG features have been extensively reported only in a few studies: a slow background activity, multifocal paroxysmal abnormalities during wakefulness, and the typical pattern of Lennox-Gastaut syndrome during sleep have been noted (8, 20). Furthermore, a patient with central-temporal spikes in the interictal EEG has been described (8).

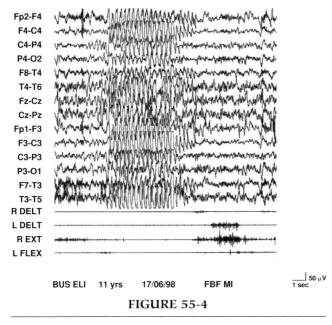

FIGURE 55-4

An 11-year-old female with AS. The EEG shows an atypical absence, which is correlated with the interruption of the motor activity, as evident from surface EMG of deltoid muscles and extensor muscles of the forearms (R = right, L = left, DELT= deltoid muscle, EXT = extensor muscle of the forearm, FLEX = flexor muscle of the forearm).

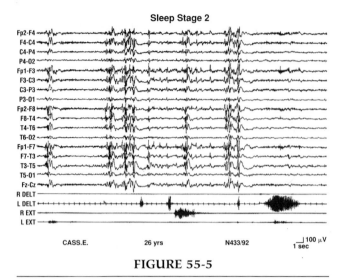

Sleep Stage 2

CASS.E.   26 yrs   N433/92   ⌐100 μV
                                            ⌐1 sec

FIGURE 55-5

A 26-year-old female with inv-dup(15) syndrome. The EEG during non-REM sleep shows numerous short runs of fast polyspikes, such as in typical Lennox-Gastaut syndrome (R = right, L = left, DELT = deltoid muscle, EXT = extensor muscle of the forearm).

CLASSICAL LISSENCEPHALY

Classical lissencephaly is distinguished into Miller-Dieker syndrome (MDS) and isolated lissencephaly sequence (ILS). Lissencephaly is a severe abnormality of neuronal migration occurring between the twelfth and the sixteenth week of gestation, consisting of a four-layered cortex instead of a normal six-layered cortex. MDS is characterized by profound mental retardation and, often, by absence of psychomotor achievements, typical facial anomalies with bitemporal narrowing, short nose, prominent superior lip, and small jaw; in ILS only the neurologic signs of lissencephaly but no gross dysmorphic features are present (23).

Classical lissencephaly is quite rare, with a prevalence of about 1:85,470 (23).

The LIS1 gene (PAFAH1B1), responsible for MDS, is located on chromosome 17p13.3 and codifies for the beta subunit of platelet-activating factor acetylhydrolase (PAFAH) isoform Ib, an inactivating enzyme for platelet-activating factor (PAF); the LIS1 gene has an important role in the stabilization of microtubules, which intervene during neuronal migration (23).

MDS is caused by large deletions of LIS1 gene and other contiguous genes (in about 92% of cases). Approximately 65% of subjects with ILS have a mutation involving the LIS1 gene; among these, 40% present with a deletion of the entire gene, while 25% have an intragenic mutation. Patients with missense mutations have a milder degree of lissencephaly than do those presenting

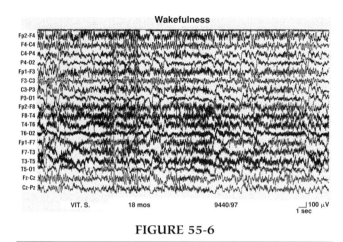

Wakefulness

VIT. S.   18 mos   9440/97   ⌐100 μV
                                            1 sec

FIGURE 55-6

An 18-month-old child with lissencephaly. Awake EEG showing a high-voltage diffuse theta activity, prevalent over the anterior regions of both hemispheres.

truncating or deletion mutations. Classic lissencephaly in males can also be due to mutations of the XLIS gene that, in females, instead determines a subcortical band heterotopia (SBH) or double cortex. Lissencephaly is mainly anterior in patients with mutations of the XLIS gene, posterior in those with mutations of the LIS1 gene (23).

Beginning in the first year of life, the EEG shows characteristic high-voltage fast rhythms that can be mixed with theta and delta activity, sometimes resembling a hypsarrhythmic-like picture (Figure 55-6). Subsequently, the slow activity disappears and is replaced by an alpha- or beta-like activity, prevalent over the rolandic or parietal regions, or by faster rhythms (15–25 Hz), more prominent over the posterior areas of the scalp (8).

Seizures, present in more than 90% of cases, invariably begin during the first 6 months of age and are of different types: spasms, myoclonic, simple or complex, tonic, atonic, subclinical seizures, and atypical absences (8, 23). Seizures in the lissencephalies are intractable, and lifespan is usually no longer than 20 years (23). Some improvement may be obtained with corticosteroids or benzodiazepines.

RING CHROMOSOME 20 SYNDROME

Ring chromosome 20 syndrome (r20S) is a rare condition. So far, more than 30 cases have been described, which were mostly sporadic or in mosaicism. The phenotype is characterized by mental retardation of variable degree, without relevant dysmorphic features; in 90% of cases drug-resistant seizures are present. In some patients, structural anomalies on MRI, such as cortical dysplasias, or functional abnormalities on positron emission tomography (PET), involving frontal lobe and basal ganglia, have been recognized (8, 24).

The telomeric regions p13 and q13 of chromosome 20, which are lost in r20S, contain genes involved in the pathogenesis of dominantly inherited epileptic syndromes, such as benign neonatal familial convulsions and autosomal dominant nocturnal frontal epilepsy, which differs from r20S. However, there is evidence supporting the view that r20S may also be a channelopathy (8).

Interictal EEG in r20S shows slow waves, spikes, or spike-and-wave complexes prevalently localized over the frontal regions. An apparently subclinical EEG pattern with multifocal theta waves at 5 Hz, mostly localized over the temporal regions, has been described (8).

Seizures are heterogeneous, but more frequently they are of the partial type (frontal) or secondarily generalized, with a variable age of onset, usually in infancy. Occurring concomitantly with the onset of seizures are frequent episodes of nonconvulsive status epilepticus. During these episodes, patients present with a disturbance of consciousness, bizarre behaviors, motor and verbal automatisms, and wandering and mimic of fear; myoclonic jerks involving eyelids and perioral region can be also present (8). Seizures can be triggered by video games or psychologic stress (8).

The ictal EEG is characterized by sequences of slow waves intermixed with spikes, and the frequency of spike-and-wave complexes can change during the discharge (Figure 55-7). The episodes of nonconvulsive status occur daily or weekly and can also have a duration of 1 hour (8, 24).

Epilepsy is intractable and persists in adulthood. Surgery was not effective in one subject with cortical dysplasia (8). In another case seizures were controlled by vagal nerve stimulation (25).

DOWN SYNDROME

Down syndrome (DS), or trisomy 21, is the most common chromosomal disorder in subjects with mental retardation. Its prevalence is approximately 1:700 live births. The phenotype is characteristic: mental retardation, microbrachycephaly, upward-slanted eyes, epicanthal folds, microtia, short neck, simian crease, and congenital heart malformations (26).

Trisomy 21, due to failure of disjunction of chromosome 21 during meiosis, is the cause of DS in 95% of cases; approximately 4% of patients present with an unbalanced translocation and about 1% of cases have mosaicism; in a minimal percentage of subjects a duplication of 21q22.3 region is evident.

From a neuropathologic point of view the pattern of cortical gyri appears simplified, and cytoarchitectonic changes, such as decreased GABAergic small granular cells, reduced neuronal density, delayed myelination, and dysgenesis of dendritic spines have been observed (8).

Seizures are present in about 10% of cases, although their prevalence is different in the various prospective and retrospective studies. They are rather heterogenous. In fact, approximately 35% of patients present with infantile spasms, with evolution sometimes to the Lennox-Gastaut syndrome, which in DS can have a later onset than in other conditions. In addition, subjects with benign myoclonic epilepsy or reflex epilepsy have been reported (14).

Age at onset of spontaneous and reflex seizures tends to coincide in DS (2–24 years). Reflex seizures are triggered by different unexpected stimuli; their frequency is usually high, with many per day. The same stimulus can evoke different types of seizures, such as atypical absences or tonic seizures.

Outcome of epilepsy in DS is generally rather benign, with a progressive reduction of seizures and the focalization of paroxysmal abnormalities.

Effectiveness of antiepileptic treatment is strictly correlated with the epileptic syndrome presented by the patient. Myoclonic seizures usually are well controlled by valproate, benzodiazepines, or vigabatrin. In some cases, with more resistant spasms, corticosteroids can be useful (8, 14).

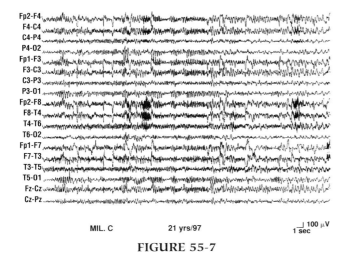

MIL. C   21 yrs/97   100 μV
                                          1 sec

FIGURE 55-7

A 21-year-old male with r20S. The EEG during nonconvulsive status epilepticus is characterized by sequences of slow waves intermixed with spikes; the frequency of the spike-and-wave complexes changes during the status.

FRAGILE-X SYNDROME

Fragile-X syndrome (FraXS) is one of the most common causes of inherited mental retardation, with a prevalence of 1:1,500 males. The physical phenotype is characterized

7. Battaglia A, Carey JC. Seizure and EEG patterns in Wolf-Hirschhorn (4p-) syndrome. *Brain Dev* 2005; 27:362–364.

8. Gobbi G, Genton P, Pini A, Gurrieri F, et al. Epilepsies and chromosomal disorders. In: Roger J, Bureau M, Dravet Ch, Genton P, et al.eds. *Epileptic Syndromes in Infancy, Childhood and Adolescence.* 3rd ed. London: John Libbey & Co, 2002:431–455.

9. Zollino M, Lecce R, Fischetto R, et al. Mapping the Wolf-Hirschhorn syndrome phenotype outside the currently accepted WHS critical region and defining a new critical region, WHSCR-2. *Am J Hum Genet* 2003; 72:590–597.

10. Battaglia D, Zampino G, Zollino M, et al. Electroclinical patterns and evolution of epilepsy in the 4p- syndrome. *Epilepsia* 2003; 44:1183–1190.

11. Kagitani-Shimono K, Imai K, Otani K, et al. Epilepsy in Wolf-Hirschhorn syndrome (4p⁻). *Epilepsia* 2005; 46:150–155.

12. Elia M, Striano P, Fichera M, et al. 6q terminal deletion syndrome is associated with a distinctive EEG and clinical pattern. A report of five cases. *Epilepsia* 2006; 47:830–838.

13. Elia M, Musumeci SA, Ferri R, Cammarata M. Trisomy 12p and epilepsy with myoclonic absences. *Brain Dev* 1998; 20:127–130.

14. Guerrini R, Gobbi G, Genton P, Bonanni P, et al. Chromosomal abnormalities. In: Engel J Jr, Pedley TA, eds. *Epilepsy: A Comprehensive Textbook.* Philadelphia: Lippincott-Raven, 1997:2533–2546.

15. Morimoto M, Usuku T, Tanaka M, et al. Ring chromosome 14 with localization-related epilepsy: three cases. *Epilepsia* 2003; 44:1245–1249.

16. Russo S, Cogliati F, Viri M, et al. Novel mutations of ubiquitin protein ligase 3A gene in Italian patients with Angelman syndrome. *Hum Mutat* 2000; 15:387.

17. Lossie AC, Whitney MM, Amidon D, et al. Distinct phenotypes distinguish the molecular classes of Angelman syndrome. *J Med Genet* 2001; 38:834–845.

18. Dan B, Boyd SG. Angelman syndrome reviewed from a neurophysiological perspective. The UBE3A-GABRB3 hypothesis. *Neuropediatrics* 2003; 34:169–176.

19. Dalla Bernardina B, Fontana E, Darra F. Myoclonic status in non-progressive encephalopathies. In: Roger J, Bureau M, Dravet Ch, Genton P, et al., eds. *Epileptic Syndromes in Infancy, Childhood and Adolescence.* 3rd ed. London: John Libbey, 2002:137–144.

20. Battaglia A. The inv dup(15) or idic(15) syndrome: a clinically recognisable neurogenetic disorder. *Brain Dev* 2005; 27:365–369.

21. Chifari R, Guerrini R, Pierluigi M, et al. Mild generalized epilepsy and developmental disorder associated with large inv dup(15). *Epilepsia* 2002; 43:1096–1100.

22. Elia M, Guerrini R, Musumeci SA, Bonanni P, et al. Myoclonic absence-like seizures and chromosome abnormality syndromes. *Epilepsia* 1998; 39:660–663.

23. Guerrini R, Sicca F, Parmeggiani L. Epilepsy and malformations of the cerebral cortex. *Epileptic Disord* 2003; 5(Suppl 2):S9–S26.

24. Elia M, Musumeci SA, Bottitta M, et al. Sindrome del cromosoma 20 ad anello ed epilessia: descrizione di un caso. *Bollettino Lega Italiana contro l'Epilessia* 1998; 101/103:265–266.

25. Chawla J, Sucholeiki R, Jones C, Silver K. Intractable epilepsy with ring chromosome 20 syndrome treated with vagal nerve stimulation: case report and review of the literature. *J Child Neurol* 2002; 17:778–780.

26. Romano C. La sindrome di Down. Linee guida per la diagnosi, l'assistenza ed il follow-up. In: Balestrazzi P, editore. *Linee guida assistenziali nel bambino con patologia malformativa.* Parma: Centro Studi Humana, 1994:91–101.

27. Neri G, Opitz JM, Mikkelsen M, Jacobs PA, et al. Conference Report: third international workshop on the fragile X and X-linked mental retardation. *Am J Med Genet* 1988; 30: 1–29.

28. Musumeci SA, Bosco P, Calabrese G, et al. Audiogenic seizures susceptibility in transgenic mice with fragile X syndrome. *Epilepsia* 2000; 41:19–23.

29. Ferri R, Musumeci SA, Elia M, Del Gracco S, et al. BIT-mapped somatosensory evoked potentials in the fragile X syndrome. *Neurophysiol Clin* 1994; 4:413–426.

30. Giuffrida R, Musumeci S, D'Antoni S, et al. A reduced number of metabotropic glutamate subtype 5 receptors are associated with constitutive homer proteins in a mouse model of fragile X syndrome. *J Neurosci* 2005; 25:8908–8916.

31. Musumeci SA, Ferri R, Elia M, Colognola RM, et al. Epilepsy and fragile X syndrome: a follow-up study. *Am J Med Genet* 1991; 38:511–513.

32. Musumeci SA, Hagerman RJ, Ferri R, et al. Epilepsy and EEG findings in males with fragile X syndrome. *Epilepsia* 1999; 40:1092–1099.

33. Tarani L, Raguso G, Lampariello S, Colloidi F, Bruni LA. Sindrome di Klinefelter: proposta di protocollo assistenziale. In: Balestrazzi P, editore. *Linee guida assistenziali nel bambino con patologia malformativa.* Parma: Centro Studi Humana, 1996:119–129.

34. Tatum WO 4th, Passaro EA, Elia M, Guerrini R, et al. Seizures in Klinefelter's syndrome. *Pediatr Neurol* 1998; 19: 275–278.

35. Elia M, Musumeci SA, Ferri R, Scuderi C, et al. Seizures in Klinefelter's syndrome: a clinical and EEG study of five patients. *Ital J Neurol Sci* 1995; 16:231–238.

36. Engel J Jr. A proposed diagnostic scheme for people with epileptic seizures and with epilepsy: report of the ILAE Task Force on Classification and Terminology. *Epilepsia* 2001; 42:796–803.

56 Autism

Susanna Danielsson

utism, particularly if combined with mental retardation (MR), may affect all major areas of functioning. When a measure such as the World Health Organization's International Classification of Functioning, Disability and Health (ICF) is used, the severe functional consequences of autism in daily life become obvious, as well as the difficulties in participation. The high occurrence of epilepsy in children with autism is one of the more evident signs that autism has a neurobiologic basis, in much the same way as MR. Epilepsy may influence functional skills, social participation abilities, morbidity, and mortality, both in individuals with and in those without autism, especially if pharmacoresistant. This chapter focuses on autism and its relationships to epilepsy.

DEFINING AUTISM

The definitions of autism include impairment and disability in three broad areas: social reciprocal interaction abilities, reciprocal communicative abilities, and behavioral problems, including a narrow range of stereotypic behaviors, activities, and interests. In the following sections, the term *autism* will be used when referring to this broad definition of the syndrome.

The term *autistic spectrum disorders* (ASD) is synonymous with the term *pervasive developmental disorders* (PDD) and includes—according to the *Diagnostic and Statistical Manual of Mental Disorders*, Fourth Edition (DSM-IV)—the diagnoses autistic disorder (AD), Rett syndrome, disintegrative disorder, Asperger syndrome, and PDD not otherwise specified, roughly equivalent to the terms *atypical autism* and *autistic-like conditions*.

Developmental abnormalities are present from the first years of life in the majority of cases, but about one-third of parents of children diagnosed with AD report that their child first seemed to develop quite normally but then had a loss of already acquired language and social relatedness skills in the second or third year of life—that is, an autistic regression. The regression is rarely documented except by parents' reports, so it may be disputed, and recent data suggest that most of these children also demonstrate previous, subtle developmental delays of social and communicative behaviors (1).

Autism is one of the developmental disorders, as are, for instance, attention deficit hyperactivity disorder (ADHD), developmental speech and language disorders, and developmental coordination disorder. Developmental disorders often occur together, an observation that supports the hypothesis of multiple primary neurologic deficits rather than a single localized lesion. The neurobiologic basis of social interaction abilities extends over multiple brain regions. On the more severe end of the autism spectrum (i.e., AD), 65–88% of cases have MR. There are specific conditions with a higher prevalence of autism than in the general population, for example, fragile X syndrome, tuberous sclerosis, and Rett syndrome. In many of the syndromes associated with ASD, mental retardation (MR) is also part of the clinical picture.

Etiology

Autism is a behaviorally defined syndrome with a multitude of different etiologies. In most cases specific causes are not detectable, but in 12–35% an underlying medical disorder can be identified (2). Associated medical conditions in autism are chromosomal abnormalities, neurocutaneous disorders (e.g., tuberous sclerosis), Rett syndrome, central nervous system (CNS) infections, and some metabolic disorders. Genetic factors are said to play a primary role, and the evidence for this comes from twin and family studies. Multiple genes are probably important for the manifestation of autism, because there is an absence of consistent significant findings in studies (3). The RELN gene, which codes for an extracellular protein guiding neuronal migration, has been implicated in autism, as have X-linked neuroligin genes, which are important in synaptogenesis during early brain development. Macrocephaly, acceleration followed by deceleration of brain growth, and increased neuronal packaging and decreased cell size in the limbic system, particularly in the amygdala, and a decreased number of Purkinje cells in the cerebellum, are but some of the neuropathologic findings that have been replicated in autism.

Epidemiology

Higher awareness and changed diagnostic criteria have altered the concept that autism is rare (4). The prevalence rate of AD is 0.1–0.2%, and the prevalence rate of ASD is considerably higher, 0.5–1%. AD is three to four times more common in males than in females. The sex ratio is lower among cases with severe MR (SMR; IQ < 50) and higher in those with normal IQ. Autism is much more common in individuals with MR: at least one of ten with mild mental retardation (MMR; IQ 50–70) and one of three with SMR have ASD (5).

Intervention

The assessment procedure leading to the diagnosis of autism will explain the individual's sometimes seemingly illogical or odd behavior and painful lack of social reciprocity. It will often be a turning point in the lives of these families. A diagnosis makes it possible to get access to the services for the disabled. The individual and his or her family can find information and learn from professionals, from other parents in support groups, and from the experiences of high-functioning individuals with autism. It will also be possible to strive for a more autism-friendly environment at home and at preschool, school, or at work. The medical workup will lead to the etiology in some cases. The risk for future siblings or children can be discussed on the basis of the knowledge evolving from the genetic studies on autism.

A recent review article (6) summarized the current treatment options in autism. The author concludes that there is not yet a single treatment that has been demonstrated to be efficacious in well-controlled studies. However, based on current knowledge, behavioral techniques and structured teaching based on visual cues are the most effective interventions. Examples of psychoeducational or behavioral approaches include TEACCH (The Treatment and Education of Autistic and Related Communication Handicapped Children), applied behavior analysis (Lovaas), alternative communication, PECS (Picture Exchange Communication System), and social skills training.

When behavioral problems fail to improve by appropriate behavioral and educational methods, medication can be used to facilitate management and to improve symptoms. Pharmacologic interventions are important in epilepsy, sleep disturbance, and coexisting neuropsychiatric disorders such as ADHD, depression, or obsessive-compulsive disorder.

Prognosis

Follow-up studies of children with AD show that outcome is variable, but that a majority of affected individuals have a low social functioning ability in adulthood, and few live independently or are capable of employment. Furthermore, the autistic symptoms most often persist throughout life (7, 8). Positive prognostic factors are the ability to use verbal communicative language in preschool years and a relatively higher IQ level. Conversely, coexisting conditions, such as SMR and epilepsy, are considered negative prognostic factors (9). Given that SMR is so often a comorbid feature in autism, and that epilepsy is so often a comorbid feature in SMR, it has been difficult to separate the prognostic effects of epilepsy and SMR. For the individual child diagnosed with autism, a cautious approach must be taken when discussing prognosis with the parents and the individual.

AUTISM IN EPILEPSY

There are few studies on the prevalence of ASD in individuals with epilepsy, but ASD and ADHD are probably the two most common neuropsychiatric disorders in children with epilepsy (10), especially if the epilepsy is therapy resistant. The results from more studies in the interface between neurology and psychiatry will shed more light on these issues, and there will be an increasing need for child psychiatrists and pediatric neurologists to work closer together concerning children with epilepsy, neurodevelopmental disorders, or both.

In one study of children with MR and active epilepsy, the prevalence of ASD was 38% (11). Severe behavioral problems had been undiagnosed despite parental concern in many of these cases. In a tertiary epilepsy clinic the prevalence of ASD was 32% in children, when screened with an Autism Screening Questionnaire (designed by Michael Rutter and Catherine Lord) (12).

Among children with therapy-resistant epilepsy being assessed before resective epilepsy surgery, the frequency of ASD varies between 19% and 38% (13, 14).

EPILEPSY IN AUTISM

There is a comorbidity of epilepsy, autism, and MR (9, 11, 15, 16). Literature reports on epilepsy in autism sometimes seem to be contradictory because of differences in sampling regarding cognitive level, etiology and age, diagnostic criteria for autism and epilepsy, and duration of follow-up. In the vast majority of cases, epilepsy is not the cause of the brain dysfunction causing autism, but epilepsy may aggravate the disability.

Epilepsy is more common in people with autism, with or without MR, than in the general population (16, 17). The reported rate has varied from 7% to 42% and is highest in studies including adolescents and young adults with moderate and severe MR and lowest in studies with children with ASD and no MR. Epilepsy is more common in females than in males with autism (9), which has been ascribed to a higher prevalence of cognitive and motor deficits in females with autism than in males or to the fact that females are less likely to exhibit autism if they do not have more severe brain dysfunction (16). In a population-based cohort of 120 individuals diagnosed with autism in childhood (84% with MR) and followed into adulthood (94% with MR), Danielsson et al. (9) showed that at least 38% (45 of 120) had epilepsy at some point in their lives and that the risk for epilepsy was highest in the first years of life and decreased from puberty and onward. In another study in which cases with acquired or congenital encephalophathy with AD were excluded (18), two-thirds of 18 cases with AD and MR had epilepsy onset after age 12. A bimodal distribution of epilepsy onset with a peak in both the toddler and adolescent periods has also been described (16), but not in an epidemiologically representative sample.

A majority of children and adults with autism have partial seizures with or without secondarily generalized seizures (9, 15).

According to Tuchman (19), it is reasonable to hypothesize that many autistic symptoms represent underlying dysfunction in overlapping structures in the CNS, as well as dysfunction in neurochemical systems, and that abnormalities in these systems may be responsible for the higher rates of epilepsy in this population. Tuberous sclerosis is one established cause of ASD and epilepsy, and it has been used as a model for testing theories of the brain basis of ASD (20). Individuals with tuberous sclerosis are at very high risk of developing ASD if the onset of seizures is within the first 3 years of life, and when temporal tubers are present and associated with temporal lobe epileptiform discharges.

Epileptiform EEG Abnormalities in Autism without Epilepsy

The reported rate of epileptiform abnormalities on electroencephalogram (EEG) in children with ASD without epilepsy has ranged from 6% to 61%, with lowest rates if only routine EEG is used and highest rates with 24-hour ambulatory EEG (21). Several studies have shown that a history of autistic regression without epilepsy is not correlated with epileptiform activity. There are studies showing normalization of EEGs in children with autism who receive valproic acid (21), but no studies showing whether future epilepsy can be prevented by treatment or whether there is a positive influence on the core symptoms and prognosis of autism. It has not been satisfactorily shown that treating subclinical epileptic spikes in this population improves behavior. Possible side effects from antiepileptic drugs (AEDs)—somatic, cognitive, and behavioral—must be considered, because there are few studies on treatment and long-term effects on groups with MR with or without autism. It is possible in this group that even modest cognitive AED side effects may have significant consequences. On the other hand, there are preliminary studies showing that some AEDs may have positive psychotropic effects in a subgroup of children with autism (22).

One must be aware that AD, Asperger syndrome, and autistic-like conditions are behaviorally defined diagnoses, in contrast to the epileptic encephalopathies, for example, Landau Kleffner syndrome or the syndrome of continuous spike wave of slow sleep (CSWS). These latter diagnoses are based on specific EEG findings together with specific clinical symptoms and signs. The functional deficits, including cognitive and/or language regression, seen in these children are potentially reversible and treatable as they are presumed to be caused by epileptiform activity. Some children have severe behavioral problems, and epilepsy is not always a prominent feature. These conditions remind us of the importance of not only neuropsychologic and educational, but also medical and neuropsychiatric, assessment of children with autistic symptoms. This assessment should include a detailed medical and psychiatric history, a general physical, neurodevelopmental and neurologic examination, and medical workup including EEG when indicated. A rapid or atypical onset of symptoms or fluctuating symptoms and recovery is not typical in autism.

In summary, it cannot be recommended to support widespread use of anticonvulsant medication in children with ASD without seizures, until more controlled studies support their use.

Prognosis

Abnormal mental or neurologic development, such as MR and autism, are negative prognostic factors for seizure remission. There are few studies addressing the long-term prognosis of seizure disorders in children with autism; but in a population-based follow-up study only 16% of childhood-onset epilepsy cases with autism were free of seizures and medication as adults (9). The majority of children with autism, MR, and epilepsy will be adults with the same diagnoses and have a low adaptive level in life. There is a need for regular medical checkups in this severely communication-disabled population. Collaboration across disciplines and specialist care are required for the adequate management not only in childhood, but in adulthood as well. The prognosis for seizure remission in children with autism without MR has not been described in a population-based sample.

TREATMENT AND INTERVENTION IN CASES WITH AUTISM AND EPILEPSY

The treatment options considered should be the same as in patients with only one of the two diagnoses. Treatment of epilepsy is not limited to the prescription of AEDs but also includes education and support to parents, teachers, and the person with epilepsy. Educational, learning, and behavioral problems must be addressed. There is a great challenge in meeting the needs of these persons. Because their communicative abilities are often very limited or very special, they need to have a spokesman. Side effects of AEDs must be considered carefully with regard to potential effects on cognition and behavior. It is important to respect the dignity of individuals with autism and not put them in stressful and frightening situations. On the other hand, such respect must never be an excuse for not investigating, diagnosing, and treating epilepsy in individuals with autism. It has been shown that children with autism can participate in prolonged EEG monitoring (21), and so can adults. Patients who do not achieve adequate seizure control with older AEDs deserve a trial with newer AEDs. For individuals with medically therapy-resistant epilepsy, the treatment approach must be multiprofessional, and the possibility of epilepsy surgery should be considered.

For those not suitable for resective surgery, ketogenic diet or vagus nerve stimulation could be an alternative.

A major issue is the need for education concerning epilepsy in the "autism-friendly" environment and for education about the needs of a person with ASD in the "epilepsy-friendly" environment.

EPILEPSY SURGERY AND AUTISM

Epilepsy surgery may be considered in adults, and at any age in the pediatric population, to control medically intractable epilepsy in patients with partial seizures and in those with generalized seizures that are caused by a localizable cortical abnormality. Most surgical procedures aim at seizure freedom, especially in patients with defined lesions. However, in children with catastrophic epilepsy, the aim may be to reduce seizures to prevent cognitive and behavioral decline. The catastrophic epilepsy disorders begin in children younger than 5 or 6 years, are difficult to control, and are strongly associated with MR and neuropsychiatric disorders such as ASD. Seizure outcome after epilepsy surgery is well documented, as are cognitive effects. Full-scale IQ remains stable in most cases. Better seizure outcome after surgery is reported in patients with vascular malformations and tumors, and worse outcome in patients with malformations of cortical development and gliosis. Not only the histopathologic diagnosis, but also the localization of the lesion and the surgical procedure have implications for outcome. Hemispherectomies carry the best prognosis (60–85% seizure-free) followed by temporal lobe resections (60% seizure-free). Most studies of psychiatric disorders and epilepsy have been performed in adult patients. It is known that partial seizures with an ictal focus in the temporal lobes are associated with a high rate of psychiatric disorders in children. Outcome, considering psychiatric and behavioral sequelae in the childhood population, has achieved more attention during the last 10 years. Reports of behavioral outcome after surgery have often relied on anecdotal information, often without neuropsychiatric assessment before surgical intervention. There are positive reports on postsurgical developmental and behavioral outcome in children with intractable epilepsy, but there are also less favorable reports. In the adult population it has until recently been assumed that patients with MR are poor candidates for epilepsy surgery. This has been challenged by Bjørnæs et al. (23), showing good seizure outcome after resective surgery in adult patients with focal epilepsy and IQ less than 70, provided that the operation was not done more than 12 years after the onset of epilepsy.

Until recently there have been very few prospective follow-up studies concerning the outcome of epilepsy surgery in cases with ASD in whom the effect on the core symptoms of autism is reported, and there are no reports with age-matched nonoperated controls. Partial recovery of social and language regression was reported in two children with focal epilepsy after surgical treatment (24), and there are additional case studies. Szabo et al. (25) reported neurologic, neuropsychologic, and psychiatric outcome after epilepsy surgery in five children with ASD. Four children had temporal lobe resections, and one had a temporo-parieto-occipital resection. Two years after surgery, all children still had ASD and developmental delay, but one child showed substantial improvement on all measures, despite persistent seizures. Four children were seizure free: two demonstrated mild improvement, one no improvement, and one decline. McLellan et al. (14) have followed-up the largest prospective cohort ($n = 60$), including children with ASD ($n = 23$), and therapy-resistant epilepsy, undergoing temporal lobe resection. Mean length at follow-up was 5 years 2 months (range 2–10 years). They found that ASD was significantly associated with younger age at seizure onset, right temporal lobe lesions, and MR. Among the sixteen children with ADHD, nine also had ASD. Among the twenty-three with ASD, twenty-one still had ASD at follow-up. They were described as improved ($n = 11$), no change ($n = 7$), or deteriorated ($n = 3$).

The results thus far suggest that families should be made aware that autistic symptoms in children with focal epileptogenic lesions may or may not improve after epilepsy surgery. To inform parents about this is an important part of the presurgical neuropsychiatric assessment. It makes it even more important to diagnose ASD before surgery; otherwise parents' expectations may be too high. There is also a risk that the autistic symptoms they did not conceptualize before surgery may be more obvious if seizures are improved after surgery.

Discussing epilepsy surgery and the effects on autistic symptoms is a completely different matter from surgical treatment of autistic regression in cases with epileptiform activity but without clinical seizures. In most countries surgery for autistic regression is not performed. There are published reports (26–28), but some are considered controversial, and ethical concerns have been raised (19, 29). In cases with autism without intractable epilepsy or specific epileptic encephalopathies, there are no data at the present time to support the use of surgical intervention.

References

1. Rogers S. Developmental regression in autism spectrum disorders. *Ment Retard Dev Disabil Res Rev* 2004; 10:139–143.
2. Gillberg C, Coleman M. Autism and medical disorders: a review of the literature. *Dev Med Child Neurol* 1996; 38:191–202.
3. Volkmar F, Pauls D. Autism. *Lancet* 2003; 362:1133–1141.
4. Wing L, Potter D. The epidemiology of autistic spectrum disorders: is the prevalence rising? *Ment Retard Dev Disabil Res Rev* 2002; 8:151–161.
5. Nordin V, Gillberg C. Autism spectrum disorders in children with physical or mental disability or both. Part I: clinical and epidemiological aspects. *Dev Med Child Neurol* 1996; 38:297–313.
6. Francis K. Autism interventions: a critical update. *Dev Med Child Neurol* 2005; 47: 493–499.
7. Howlin P, Goode S, Hutton J, Rutter M. Adult outcome for children with autism. *J Child Psychol Psychiatry* 2004; 45:212–229.
8. Billstedt E, Gillberg IC, Gillberg C. Autism after adolescence: population-based 13-22-year follow-up study of 120 individuals with autism diagnosed in childhood. *J Autism Dev Disord* 2005; 35:351–360.
9. Danielsson S, Gillberg IC, Billstedt E, Gillberg C, et al. Epilepsy in young adults with autism: a prospective population-based follow-up study of 120 individuals diagnosed in childhood. *Epilepsia* 2005; 46:918–923.
10. Besag F. Childhood epilepsy in relation to mental handicap and behavioural disorders. *J Child Psychol Psychiatry* 2002; 43:103–131.
11. Steffenburg S, Gillberg C, Steffenburg U. Psychiatric disorders in children and adolescents with active epilepsy and mental retardation. *Arch Neurol* 1996; 53:904–912.
12. Clarke D, Roberts W, Daraksan M, Dupuis A, et al. The prevalence of autistic spectrum disorder in children surveyed in a tertiary care epilepsy clinic. *Epilepsia* 2005; 46:1970–1977.
13. Taylor D, Neville B, Cross H. Autistic spectrum disorders in epilepsy surgery candidates. *Eur Child Adolesc Psychiatry* 1999; 8:189–192.
14. McLellan A, Davies S, Heyman I, et al. Psychopathology in children with epilepsy before and after temporal lobe resection. *Dev Med Child Neurol* 2005; 47:666–672.
15. Olsson I, Steffenburg S, Gillberg C. Epilepsy in autism and autistic-like conditions. *Arch Neurol* 1988; 45:666–668.
16. Volkmar FR, Nelson DS. Seizure disorders in autism. *J Am Acad Child Adolesc Psychiatry* 1990; 29:127–129.
17. Tuchman RF, Rapin I. Epilepsy in autism. *Lancet Neurol* 2002; 1:352–358.
18. Rossi PG, Posar A, Parmeggiani A. Epilepsy in adolescents and young adults with autistic disorder. *Brain Dev* 2000; 22:102–106.
19. Tuchman R. AEDs and psychotropic drugs in children with autism and epilepsy. *Ment Retard Dev Disabil Res Rev* 2004; 10:135–138.
20. Bolton P, Park R, Higgins N, Griffiths P, et al. Neuro-epileptic determinants of autism spectrum disorders in tuberous sclerosis complex. *Brain* 2002; 125:1247–1255.
21. Chez G, Chang M, Krasne V, Coughlan C, et al. Frequency of epileptiform EEG abnormalities in a sequential screening of autistic patients with no known clinical epilepsy from 1996 to 2005. *Epilepsy Behav* 2006; 8:267–271.
22. Martino A, Tuchman R. Antiepileptic drugs: affective use in autism spectrum disorders. *Pediatr Neurol* 2001; 25:199–207.
23. Bjørnæs H, Engberg Stabell K, Heminghyt E, Røste G, et al. Resective surgery for intractable focal epilepsy in patients with low IQ: predictors for seizure control and outcome with respect to seizures and neuropsychological and psychosocial functioning. *Epilepsia* 2004; 45:131–139.
24. Neville B, Harkness W, Cross H, et al. Surgical treatment of severe autistic regression in childhood epilepsy. *Pediatr Neurol* 1997; 16:137–140.
25. Szabo CA, Wyllie E, Dolske M, Stanford LD, et al. Epilepsy surgery in children with pervasive developmental disorder. *Pediatr Neurol* 1999; 20:349–353.
26. Patil A, Andrews R. Surgical treatment of autistic epileptiform regression. *J Epilepsy* 1998; 11:368–373.
27. Lewine JD, Andrews R, Chez M, et al. Magnetoencephalographic patterns of epileptiform activity in children with regressive autism spectrum disorders. *Pediatrics* 1999; 104:405–418.
28. Nass R, Gross A, Wisoff J, Devinsky O. Outcome of multiple subpial transections for autistic epileptiform regression. *Pediatr Neurol* 1999; 21:464–470.
29. Kanner A. Commentary: the treatment of seizure disorders and EEG abnormalities in children with autistic spectrum disorders: are we getting ahead of ourselves? *J Autism Dev Disord* 2000; 5:491–495.

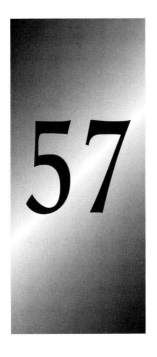

57 Attention Deficit Hyperactivity Disorder

Paul B. Augustijn

Attention deficit hyperactivity disorder (ADHD) is the most common behavioral disorder of childhood. It affects 3–5% of the school population, with a male-to-female ratio of 3 or 4:1. Symptoms seem to abate with age, although recent studies indicate that ADHD persists into adulthood in 30–70% of the cases. Symptoms include inattentiveness, distractibility, motoric overactivity, and impulsivity. Patients with ADHD appear to have a deficit in executive control, which is the ability to plan and implement a strategy to achieve a particular goal (1).

The *Diagnostic and Statistical Manual of Mental Disorders, Fourth Edition* (DSM-IV) discriminates three subtypes of ADHD: (1) predominantly inattentive type, (2) predominantly hyperactive type, and (3) combined type (for diagnostic criteria see Appendix 57-1) (2).

In children with ADHD the combined type is the most prevalent one: 87% of the affected boys and 65% of the affected girls in the age group 4–10 years have the combined type. During adolescence the type–ratio changes; in a study of young adolescents with ADHD (3), 52% had the combined type, 35% the inattentive type, and 13% the hyperactive-impulsive type (1).

Comorbidity is common, and ADHD is associated with several other psychiatric disorders such as anxiety, depression, conduct disorder, antisocial personality disorder, tics, oppositional defiant disorder, and substance abuse.

ADHD affects normal social and personal relationships; compared to normal control subjects it appears to be closely associated with educational problems in those with ADHD and has a negative influence in these patients on occupational pursuits compared to normal control subjects (4).

THE NEUROBIOLOGY OF ADHD

Children and adolescents with ADHD have difficulties in several attentional and neuropsychologic domains: problem solving, planning, orienting, alerting, cognitive flexibility, sustained attention, response inhibition, and visual working memory.

There is growing evidence from electrophysiologic studies that ADHD involves hypofunction of catecholaminergic circuits, particularly those that project to the prefrontal cortex. In particular, dopamine-mediated frontostriatal circuitry is thought to play a role in the pathophysiology of ADHD. Molecular genetic studies support these electrophysiologic markers. Researchers hypothesize that many different, probably interacting genes contribute to the ADHD phenotype. Several genes including dopamine receptor genes, dopamine transporter genes, and serotonin receptor genes have been associated with ADHD. Structural imaging studies supporting these insights found smaller total brain volumes, especially of the right frontal lobe, caudate nucleus, cerebellar hemispheres, and vermis. Anomalies in the frontal lobes and basal ganglia were confirmed by positron emission tomography (PET) and single-photon emission computed tomography (SPECT) studies. Functional magnetic resonance imaging (fMRI) studies revealed abnormal functioning of the dorsolateral prefrontal cortex and anterior cingulate cortex on tasks requiring inhibitory control. Functional neuroimaging studies also give insights in the underlying mechanisms by studying treatment response. An fMRI study related methylphenidate and enhanced performance on interference tasks to functional changes in the brain areas mentioned previously. In this study, event-related fMRI was used to study selective attention by using a paradigm that compared children with ADHD (on or off methylphenidate) and normal control subjects. Selective attention was abnormal in those with ADHD, but after treatment with methylphenidate results were equivalent to those of normal control children (5).

EPILEPSY AND ADHD

In epilepsy, comorbidity of ADHD is common and has a substantial impact on functioning, treatment, and prognosis. The relation between epilepsy and ADHD is complex. From the perspective of daily clinical practice, several issues with respect to this relationship should be addressed. These topics include the following:

1. The relationship between epilepsy and ADHD: Do epilepsy patients have an increased prevalence or risk of ADHD? Are certain epilepsy syndromes or seizure types associated with ADHD? Does ADHD in epilepsy patients have special features? Are ADHD symptoms in epilepsy patients caused by the epilepsy or do both share a common underlying cause? Should epilepsy be considered a contraindication to treat ADHD symptoms with stimulant drugs, for example, methylphenidate? Does a comorbid diagnosis of epilepsy and ADHD alter the prognosis of either condition? Can antiepileptic drugs (AEDs) provoke ADHD-like symptoms?
2. The association between ADHD, epileptiform electroencephalogram (EEG) features, and epilepsy: Do ADHD patients have an increased prevalence or risk of having a comorbid diagnosis of epilepsy, and if so, what kind of epilepsy? Do ADHD patients have an increased risk of having an abnormal EEG with epileptiform features and does this have implications for treatment? Are these EEG features a

contraindication to treat with stimulant drugs such as methylphenidate?

THE RELATIONSHIP BETWEEN EPILEPSY AND ADHD

Estimations of the prevalence of ADHD in children, adolescents, and adults with epilepsy vary widely depending on the sample studied and the measures used to establish the ADHD diagnosis. Many studies examining the relationship between ADHD and epilepsy are outdated. Diagnostic criteria have changed since these studies were conducted. Prevalence figures of individuals with symptoms of ADHD, whether they actually meet the full diagnostic criteria, have ranged from 8% to 77%.

Several studies have focused on only one or a limited number of ADHD symptoms, with controversial results (1). Semrud-Clikeman and Wical (6) evaluated attentional difficulties in children with complex partial seizures. They compared four groups of children: children with complex partial seizures with (7) and without ADHD (8), children with ADHD (9), and normal children (10). Children with partial seizures and ADHD performed the poorest on scales measuring attention. In general, children with partial seizures showed an attention deficit regardless of their ADHD status. A population study by McDermott et al. (11) showed that children (0–18 years) with seizures (prevalence 0.9%; $N = 121$) were 4.7 times (31.4%) more likely to have a behavior problem, whereas children with cardiac problems were 3 times (21.1%) more likely to have behavior problems, compared to normal control subjects (8.5%). Hyperactivity was found to be the most troublesome behavior for children with epilepsy in this study (11).

Poor seizure control was associated with increased behavioral problems, including hyperactivity, by Carlton-Ford and coworkers (12), who investigated the effects of epilepsy on social and psychological adjustment of children studied in the National Health Interview Survey. The odds of being among the most impulsive children (the top 10%) were more than 3 times greater for children with inactive epilepsy and more than 12 times greater for children with active epilepsy compared to children without epilepsy.

On the other hand, Oostrom et al. (13) did not find attention deficit to be characteristic of schoolchildren with newly diagnosed idiopathic/cryptogenic epilepsy. Fifty-one children with epilepsy were compared with 48 matched classmates and assessed within 48 hours after the diagnosis and before AED treatment, and later on at 3 and 12 months. Prior school and behavioral difficulties and maladaptive reaction to the onset of epilepsy, rather than the epilepsy variables, were found to be related to decreased attentional efficiency.

In studies using standardized measures such as behavioral checklists or parent and teacher questionnaires about ADHD symptoms in children with epilepsy, the prevalence ranged from 14% to 40% (1).

Dunn et al. (1) assessed a group of 175 children with normal intelligence (age 9–14 years) with chronic epilepsy for evidence of ADHD. Children were recruited from private practices of child neurologists and a child neurology clinic of a university hospital. Sufficient data on seizure type and epilepsy type were available in 151 children. Behavior was measured using the Child Behavior Checklist (CBCL) in combination with either the Child Symptom Inventory-4 (CSI) or the Adolescent Symptom Inventory-4 (ASI). The primary caregiver completed both scales: 58% of the children and 42% of the adolescents were in the at-risk range on the CBCL attention problems subscale, and 37% of the children and 25% of the adolescents scored as high as in the clinical range.

Based on CSI and ASI, the prevalence of possible ADHD combined type was 11.4%, 24% for the inattentive type, and 2.3% for the hyperactive-impulsive type. Overall, 38% of the children potentially qualified for a diagnosis of ADHD. Although the study of Dunn et al. (1) is not a population-based study, the prevalence of symptoms of ADHD was quite similar to that reported by Hempel et al. (14) (36%), McDermott et al. (11) (hyperactive impulsivity 34%), Carlton-Ford et al. (12) (28.1%), Hesdorffer et al. (15) (problems with attention 42.4%), and others.

Insight into the association between epilepsy type or seizure type classification and ADHD is limited. Hempel et al. (14) found that patients with intractable epilepsy and generalized ictal and interictal abnormalities (52%) were more likely to hold the ADHD diagnosis than patients with lateralized, independent bilateral, or indeterminate ictal onset (26%). Those with less frequent seizures (<12/yr) were more likely than those with more frequent seizures to have ADHD. No relation with IQ, age of seizure onset, seizure type, etiology, EEG, MRI, and number or type of AEDs was found. Dunn et al. (1) investigated the relationship between seizure classification (not the epilepsy syndrome classification) and ADHD. Children with tonic-clonic seizures had a prevalence rate of ADHD-combined type of more than 20%, whereas children with absence seizures or complex partial seizures with secondary generalization had rates below 15%. However, these differences were not statistically significant. A distinction between well-controlled generalized seizures and intractable seizures was not made in this study. The study did look at the relation between the focus of interictal activity and ADHD. They classified interictal activity as being of frontal, temporal, central, parietal/occipital, or generalized origin or independent multifocal. The prevalence of ADHD-

combined type in children with a frontal, temporal, or central focus was 6–12%, and the prevalence of the ADHD-primary inattentive type was 22–27%. Although the numbers of participants were too small to allow further subclassification, children with a frontal lobe focus appeared to have a similar prevalence of ADHD when compared to those with a temporal or central focus.

As stated previously, in the general population males have ADHD 3–4 times more often than females. In epilepsy patients, however, an even sex ratio was found. Dunn et al. (1) concluded that more females with epilepsy (44%) than males with epilepsy (32%) were diagnosed as having ADHD. This trend was not significant, neither in children in the 9–11-year-old group nor in the group of the 12- to 14-year-old adolescents.

This study on ADHD in children with epilepsy is unique because it used formal DSM-IV criteria to establish the diagnosis and then subdivided the subjects into the ADHD subclasses. In contrast to children with ADHD but without epilepsy, of whom the majority have the ADHD combined type (children 65–87%, adolescents 52%), they found that the minority of children with epilepsy (11.4%) had the combined type, whereas the inattentive type was found in 24% of the cases.

Based on these differences in sex ratio and ADHD type, it is postulated that the causes of ADHD in patients with epilepsy differ from those in nonepilepsy patients. "Epilepsy, including the CNS-lesion, repetitive electrical discharges and AEDs may cause dysfunction in multiple areas, thus causing inattention without hyperactivity seen in traditional ADHD" (1). However, causality could not be defined.

Other investigators found that children with new-onset seizures had significantly more attention problems than their siblings, measured by the CBCL, suggesting an underlying neurologic dysfunction causing both seizures and attention problems (16).

As a group, schoolchildren with newly diagnosed cryptogenic or idiopathic epilepsy have more behavioral problems than healthy classmates. However, behavioral problems, seen in 26% of the children, are perceived to occur already in the earliest stage of the disease. Preexisting adversity, such as family trouble and long-standing learning or behavior problems, and difficulty adapting to the upheaval and uncertainty around the diagnosis may be causative (7). These findings also suggest that it is not the epilepsy alone that causes behavioral problems.

Disruption of attention could also be attributed to subclinical epileptic discharges, producing so-called transient cognitive impairment, which could explain why the ADHD (especially the ADHD-inattentive type) is more common among children with epilepsy (17).

Studies comparing the prognosis of ADHD in children with or without epilepsy are lacking, although

APPENDIX

The following sections have been reproduced from the DSM-IV (2) by permission of the American Psychiatric Association.

Attention-Deficit Hyperactivity Disorder (ADHD)

When problems with attention, hyperactivity, and impulsiveness develop in childhood and persist, in some cases into adulthood, this mental disorder may be diagnosed.

Diagnostic Criteria for Attention-Deficit Hyperactivity Disorder

A. Either (1) or (2):

(1) Inattention: six (or more) of the following symptoms of inattention have persisted for at least 6 months to a degree that is maladaptive and inconsistent with developmental level:
   (a) Often fails to give close attention to details or makes careless mistakes in schoolwork, work, or other activities
   (b) Often has difficulty sustaining attention in tasks or play activities
   (c) Often does not seem to listen when spoken to directly
   (d) Often does not follow through on instructions and fails to finish school work, chores, or duties in the workplace (not due to oppositional behavior or failure to understand instructions)
   (e) Often has difficulty organizing tasks and activities
   (f) Often avoids, dislikes, or is reluctant to engage in tasks that require sustained mental effort (such as schoolwork or homework)
   (g) Often loses things necessary for tasks or activities (e.g., toys, school assignments, pencils, books, or tools)
   (h) Is often easily distracted by extraneous stimuli
   (i) Is often forgetful in daily activities

(2) Hyperactivity-impulsivity: six (or more) of the following symptoms of hyperactivity-impulsivity have persisted for at least 6 months to a degree that is maladaptive and inconsistent with developmental level:

   Hyperactivity.
   (a) Often fidgets with hands or feet or squirms in seat

   (b) Often leaves seat in classroom or in other situations in which remaining seated is expected
   (c) Often runs about or climbs excessively in situations in which it is inappropriate (in adolescents or adults, may be limited to subjective feelings of restlessness)
   (d) Often has difficulty playing or engaging in leisure activities quietly
   (e) Is often "on the go" or often acts as if "driven by a motor"
   (f) Often talks excessively

   Impulsivity.
   (g) Often blurts out answers before questions have been completed
   (h) Often has difficulty awaiting turn
   (i) Often interrupts or intrudes on others (e.g., butts into conversations or games)

B. Some hyperactive-impulsive or inattentive symptoms that caused impairment were present before age 7 years.
C. Some impairment from the symptoms is present in two or more settings (e.g., at school [or work] and at home).
D. There must be clear evidence of clinically significant impairment in social, academic, or occupational functioning.
E. The symptoms do not occur exclusively during the course of a pervasive developmental disorder, schizophrenia, or other psychotic disorder and are not better accounted for by another mental disorder (e.g. mood disorder, anxiety disorder, dissociative disorder, or a personality disorder).

Coding Based on Type

314.01 Attention-Deficit/Hyperactivity Disorder, Combined Type: if both criteria A1 and A2 are met for the past 6 months
314.00 Attention-Deficit Hyperactivity Disorder, Predominantly Inattentive Type: if criterion A1 is met but criterion A2 is not met for the past 6 months
314.01 Attention-Deficit Hyperactivity Disorder, Predominantly Hyperactive-Impulsive Type: if criterion A2 is met but criterion A1 is not met for the past 6 months

Coding note: For individuals (especially adolescents and adults) who currently have symptoms that no longer meet full criteria, "In Partial Remission" should be specified.

References

1. Dunn WD, Austin KA, Harezlak J, Ambrosius WT. ADHD and epilepsy in childhood. *Dev Med Child Neurol* 2003; 45:50–54.

2. American Psychiatric Association. Diagnostic and statistical manual of mental disorders, 4th ed. Washington, DC: American Psychiatric Association, 1994.

3. Rhode LA, Biederman J, Busnello EA, Zimmermann N, et al. ADHD in a school sample of Brazilian adolescents: a study of prevalence, comorbid conditions, and impairments. *J Am Acad Child Adolesc Psychiatry* 1999; 88:716–722.

4. Murphy P. McIntyre Burnham W. Behavioral comorbidities: attention deficit hyperactivity disorder—human and animal studies. In: Blume WT, ed. *Advances in Neurology. Volume 97: Intractable Epilepsies.* Philadelphia: Lippincott Williams & Wilkins, 2006:339–343.

5. The neurology of attention deficit/hyperactivity disorder [editorial]. *Brain Dev* 2005; 27:541–543.

6. Semrud-Clikeman M, Wical B. Components of attention in children with complex partial seizures with and without ADHD. *Epilepsia* 1999; 40:211–215.

7. Oostrom KJ, Schouten A, Kruitwagen CLJJ, Peters ACB, et al. Behavioral problems in children with newly diagnosed idiopathic or cryptogenic epilepsy attending normal schools are in a majority not persistent. *Epilepsia* 2003; 44:97–106.

8. Gonzalez Heydrich J, Pandina GJ, Fleisher CA, Hsin O, et al. No seizure exacerbation from risperidone in youth with comorbid epilepsy and psychiatric disorders: a case series. *J Child Adolesc Psychopharmacol* 2004; 2:295–310.

9. Bourgeois BFD. Antiepileptic drugs, learning, and behavior in childhood epilepsy. *Epilepsia* 1998; 39:913–921.

10. Gucuyener K, Erdemoglu AK, Senol S, Serdaroglu A, et al. Use of methylphenidate for attention-deficit hyperactivity disorder in patients with epilepsy or electroencephalographic abnormalities. *J Child Neurol* 2003; 18:109–112.

11. McDermott S, Mani A, Krishnaswami S. A population-based analysis of specific behaviour problems associated with childhood seizures. *J Epilepsy* 1995; 8:110–118.

12. Carlton-Ford S, Miller R, Brown M, Nealeigh N, et al. Epilepsy and children's social and psychological adjustment. *J Health Soc Behav* 1995; 36:285–301.

13. Oostrom KJ, Schouten A, Kruitwagen CLJJ, Peters ACB, et al. Attention deficits are not characteristic of schoolchildren with newly diagnosed idiopathic or cryptogenic epilepsy. *Epilepsia* 2002; 43:301–310.

14. Hempel AM, Frost MD, Ritter FJ, Farnham S. Factors influencing the incidence of ADHD in pediatric epilepsy patients [abstract]. *Epilepsia* 1995; 36(Suppl 4):122.

15. Hesdorffer DC, Ludvigsson P, Olafsson E, Gudmundsson G, et al. ADHD as a risk factor for incident unprovoked seizures and epilepsy in children. *Arch Gen Psychiatry* 2004; 61:731–736.

16. Austin JK, Harezlak J, Dunn DW, Huster GA, et al. Behavior problems in children before first recognized seizures. *Pediatrics* 2001; 107:115–122.

17. Marsden D, Besag F, Binnie CD, Fowler M. Effects of transitory cognitive impairment on psychosocial functioning of children with epilepsy: a therapeutic trial. *Dev Med Child Neurol* 1993; 35:574–581.

18. Steer CR. Managing attention deficit/hyperactivity disorder: unmet needs and future directions. *Arch Dis Child* 2005; 90(Suppl 1):119–125.

19. Gross-Tsur V, Manor O, van der Meere J, Joseph A, et al. Epilepsy and attention deficit hyperactivity disorder: is methylphenidate safe and effective? *J Pediatr* 1997; 130:670–674.

20. Tan M, Appleton R. Attention deficit and hyperactivity disorder, methylphenidate, and epilepsy. *Arch Dis Child* 2005; 90:57–59.

21. Nissen SE. ADHD drugs and cardiovascular risks. *N Engl J Med* 2006; 354:1445–1448.

22. Kratochvil CJ, Heiligenstein JH, Dittman R, Spencer TJ, et al. Atomoxetine and methylphenidate treatment in children with ADHD: a prospective randomized open label trial. *J Am Acad Child Adolesc Psychiatry* 2002; 41:776–784.

23. Schubert R. Attention deficit disorder and epilepsy. *Pediatric Neurol* 2005; 32:1–10.

58 Migraine in Children and Relation with Psychiatric and Sleep Disorders

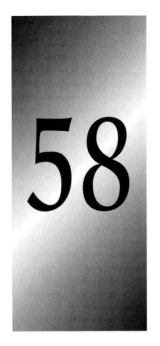

Vincenzo Guidetti
Federica Galli
Oliviero Bruni

Migraine is a disabling and common condition, affecting both adults and children or adolescents. Epidemiology, clinical characteristics, and comorbid disorders of migraine are related to age. Migraine occurs in 2% to 5% of preschool children, 10% of school-aged children, and 20% to 30% of adolescent girls (1, 2). No sex difference is apparent until age 11. Female preponderance begins at about age 12 during adolescence, with a female–male ratio of about 2 to 1 (3), maintaining this ratio in the adult population.

Migraine changes in clinical characteristics with age, even if differences exist from case to case. Gastrointestinal symptoms seem a more typical expression of childhood migraine than in adults. Preschool children frequently exhibit episodes involving vomiting and abdominal pain, with crying, irritability, and need to go to sleep. School-children may experience bilateral pain, with nausea, vomiting, photophobia, phonophobia, and change in mood; the child usually stops activities and sometimes goes to bed in the dark. Older children and adolescents tend to show unilateral location of pain. When young children show a stable unilateral location a diagnostic caution is imperative, because of a higher risk of secondary headache (4). The severity of childhood headache is usually milder than in adults. Furthermore, migraine attacks in children can be more brief and frequent than in adults.

An age effect on migraine characteristics must be stressed: younger children (less than 12 years old) show a shorter average duration of attacks, a lower proportion of throbbing headache, a higher proportion of frontal pain, and difficulties in describing pain (5).

At this moment, we do not have a specific system to classify headache in children, even though age-related clinical characteristics have been in part mentioned by the current system of classification of headache, the International Classification of Headache Disorders, 2nd edition (ICHD-II) (6), mainly for migraine without aura. The first edition of ICHD-I (7) evidenced limitations of applicability in childhood migraine, and some modifications of diagnostic parameters have been discussed (8–11). The changes outlined in ICHD-I criteria referred to shorter duration, not always unilateral localization, and photophobia and phonophobia not always present. The ICHD-II provides footnotes stressing differences from adults: attacks in children may last 1–72 hours (for adults the minimum is 4 hours); attacks are commonly bilateral in young children, and an adult pattern of unilateral pain usually emerges in late adolescence or early adult life; occipital headache in children, whether bilateral or unilateral, is rare and calls for diagnostic caution; in young children phonophobia and photophobia may be inferred from their behavior. In the ICHD, the criteria to define pain intensity in children are not specified. Studies found that the pain intensity, together with aggravation of headache by physical symptoms and vomiting, were the most important features for distinguishing migraine from tension-type headache (12). It is very important to bear in mind that the behavior of children (13) during headaches may yield elements to rate the "attack intensity."

Children may experience different types of migraine or headache. Migraine can be with or without aura. The former occurs in 10% to 20% of children with migraine. The aura usually precedes the headache by less than 30 minutes and lasts for 5 to 20 minutes, and may also be present without headache. The visual aura is the most common form as it happens in adults, even though the symptoms are likely difficult to describe for children and require insistent questioning. Visual disturbances are the most typical symptoms of aura (around 30–50%) in young migraine patients, but sensory or motor and speech disorders are also well recognized.

Chronic paroxysmal hemicrania was first described in 1973 (14), but very few cases have been reported in children (15). Many adult patients, however, report onset in childhood. Clinical features are characterized by cyclical and multiple attacks (range of 1 to 30) of excruciating unilateral pain in the ocular, frontal, and temporal areas, both day and night. Lacrimation, nasal stuffiness, and rhinorrhea, sometimes with ptosis, miosis, and upper lid edema, accompany headache. Nausea and vomiting are rare.

The clinical features are similar to cluster headache, but chronic paroxysmal hemicrania is totally relieved by indomethacin and is much more (80–90% of the cases) frequent among females.

Furthermore, the presence of migraine in the context of chronic daily headache (CDH) must be mentioned, differentiating it from chronic migraine (16). The diagnosis of CDH is a function of a quantitative parameter (an almost daily frequency of crises). We do not have clear qualitative parameters (a certain symptomatological characterization of the crises). The ICHD-II is an unquestionable advance for classifying CDH, in spite of the fact that no reference is given for pediatric CDH. However, evidence suggests differences compared to adults, even if findings on the clinical characterization of CDH in children and adolescents are unclear.

The application of Silberstein's model (17, 18) in the youngest age group does not give us an exhaustive diagnostic framework, leading to the hypothesis of specific symptomatologic expression of CDH in children and adolescents. By the application of Silberstein's criteria (17, 18), Gladstein and Holden (19) found that 35% of children and adolescents did not fit into these categories. However, the category that they called "comorbid pattern" (migraine crises in comorbid association with tension-type headache) helped the classification of almost all patients (19).

According to Abu-Arefeh's findings (20), the ICHD-I criteria for classifying chronic headache seem to apply even to the youngest, with all patients meeting the diagnostic parameters (70.6% with chronic tension-type headache [CTTH] and 30.4% with CTTH and migraine without aura). No data support the hypothesis of a probable transformation of migraine or episodic tension-type headache to CDH, as suggested for adults (17, 18). Hershey et al. (21) found that 27% of CDH patients could not be classified according to ICHD-I criteria. They underlined the predominance of migrainous characteristics of CDH in children and highlighted a temporal trend of the crises: frequent, daily intermittent and daily continuous headache. A recent population-based study confirmed the presence of migrainous features of CDH in adolescents (22). Migrainous characteristics of CDH in children have been evidenced and hypothesized to be related to the transformation of migraine over time, according to that suggested for adults (17, 18). However, according to our study (23), CDH with de novo onset prevails in the youngest, even if the clinical and differential characteristics must be clarified with respect to adults and different stages of patient development.

VARIANTS OF MIGRAINE

There are few epidemiological data concerning hemiplegic migraine (HM), basilar migraine (BM), and ophthalmoplegic migraine (OM) in childhood, even if case reports suggest that their onset and frequency are more common in children and adolescents than in adults (24). Conspicuous and persisting specific neurologic symptoms are associated with usual diagnostic criteria for migraine. HM is the first form of migraine to be linked to a genetic cause: a point mutation on chromosome 19, found in approximately 50% to 60% of families experiencing this clinical symptomatology. BM occurs most typically in adolescent and preadolescent females, but onset is in an early age. OM is the commonest in children.

Confusional migraine (25), Alice in Wonderland syndrome (26, 27), and transient global amnesia (28, 29) are other variants of migraine characterized by alteration in consciousness and disordered thought process. These aspects suggest a differential diagnosis with epilepsy.

Migraine and Epilepsy

Comorbidity of migraine and epilepsy has been described (30, 31) and in some cases differential diagnosis is required. The presence of visual phenomena and electroencephalographic (EEG) abnormalities in migraine and occipital lobe epilepsy, as the comorbidity of the two disorders, may make the differential diagnosis more difficult.

Visual symptoms are almost always present in occipital lobe epilepsy, but they are present in migraine too. The prevalence of visual disturbances in young migraine patients is around 32–56% (31), even though several elements markedly distinguish visual seizures from visual aura of migraine (32). A study (33) of electrophysiological and clinical factors distinguishing epilepsy and migraine with occipital EEG abnormalities showed that a family history of epilepsy, visual symptoms such as colored hallucinations and micro- or macropsias, unilateral EEG abnormalities, and irregular response to intermittent photic stimulation (IPS) characterized epilepsy, whereas a family history of migraine, visual symptoms such as amaurosis and scotomata, bilateral EEG abnormalities, and no changes during IPS were significantly related to migraine.

To date, the likely relationship between migraine and epilepsy in children is not clarified, as shown by several studies on this topic (34–37).

Equivalents or Precursors of Migraine

The ICHD-II (6) advances a new diagnostic category: "childhood periodic syndromes that are commonly precursors of migraine." A precursor of migraine is essentially migraine without headache: abdominal pain, bilious attacks, cyclical vomiting, motion sickness, benign paroxysmal torticollis of infancy, benign paroxysmal vertigo of childhood, and other periodic syndromes that have high incidence in the past of migraine subjects. Traditionally these disorders have been considered as equivalents or precursors of migraine in children. The new classification recognizes only cyclical vomiting, abdominal migraine, and benign paroxysmal vertigo as precursors of migraine. Benign paroxysmal torticollis and alternating hemiplegia of infancy have been relegated to the appendix of the ICHD-II, because the evidence of a link, either clinical or epidemiological, with migraine is unclear.

However, prudence is necessary: the possibility that abdominal symptoms are due to metabolic disorders (celiac disease, urea cycle disorder, or mitochondrial cytopathy) or epilepsy should be unconditionally tested.

Prognosis

The prognosis is generally thought to be good in the long term (38–41). Several studies record a high tendency to improve (around 50% at 5–10-year follow-up) or remit spontaneously (30–40%), at least for several years. The possibility of unchanging or worsening migraine is about 20%. For males the outcome is better than females. The reason is unknown.

The presence of modifications in the type of headache has been more frequently recorded (38–41). The changes in different subtypes occur mostly from migraine to tension type (about 25%), but the converse occurs as well (about 10%). The prognosis is affected by headache type at onset: migraine has a less favorable outcome, in comparison to episodic tension type.

The presence of comorbid psychiatric disorders is a negative prognostic factor for all headache subtypes (23, 42).

MIGRAINE AND PSYCHOLOGIC FACTORS

Several studies that outline the relationship between childhood psychologic factors and migraine suggest often conflicting interpretations. Vahlquist (43) recorded neurovegetative instability, ambition and perfectionism, and anxiety among migrainous children. Bille (44) described migrainous children as more anxious, sensitive, deliberate, cautious, fearful, vulnerable to frustration, tidy, and less physically enduring than control group children. Among females the differences were stronger. Coch and Melchior (45) found signs of nervousness, mental instability, and immaturity in migrainous and nonmigrainous patients. They suggested "a decreased resistance to psychological stress and conflict situations, rather than overt psychological disorder, or endogenous disease." Maratos and Wilkinson (46) found higher rates of anxiety and depression associated with conflicting parental relationships. They suggested a disturbed physiologic constitution and emotional upset as triggering factor. Millichap (47) found symptoms of depression, anxiety, and emotional and personality disorders in half of the children with recurrent headaches. Guidetti et al. (48, 49) found a feeling of being excluded from the family group and repressed hostility toward important figures.

It has been commented recently that some of the personality traits commonly associated with headache are more akin to psychopathologic disorders than psychologic features (50). The term *psychiatric comorbidity* has been used to indicate the possible, but unexplained and not casual, relationship between migraine and psychiatric disorders. Population-based studies in young adult samples (51–53) have supported the relationship between migraine and specific psychiatric disorders (major depression, anxiety disorder, and panic disorder), without a significant difference for subjects with tension-type headache compared to headache-free control subjects.

The hypothesis of a syndromic relationship between migraine and psychiatric disorders (major depression and anxiety disorder), with anxiety in childhood and adolescence, followed by migraine and then depression (50), or with a bidirectional influence in which one, migraine or depression, increases the first onset of the other (51–53), is an interesting recent finding to examine closely, with clinical, treatment, and pathophysiologic implications. The alternative putative explanations are two: (1) migraine causes psychopathology or is caused by it; and (2) underlying pathological (genetic or environmental) mechanisms are shared by migraine and anxiety or depression. An alteration of the same neurochemical systems is the presumed mechanism of both migraine and depression.

Psychiatric studies frequently refer to headaches as a complaint "related to" or "readable as" a psychosomatic or somatization disorder (54, 55). The American Academy of Child and Adolescent Psychiatry (AACAP) (56) classifies migraine as a disease to consider for a differential diagnosis with anxiety, because it is "a physical condition that may mimic anxiety disorders."

Often research in child and adolescence psychopathology refers to "somatic complaints" (such as "abdominal pain or headaches") as co-occurring symptoms in young psychiatric patients. Livingston et al. (57) found that between 25% and 30% of children admitted to a psychiatric hospital had physical symptoms, including headache, food intolerance, abdominal pain, nausea, and dizziness. Different interpretations have been suggested by other studies. Andrasik et al. (58) found a greater number of somatic complaints in migraineurs and higher ratings of depression and anxiety among migrainous adolescents, compared to matched headache-free subjects. The hypothesis suggested is that "frequent, unexplainable and intense head pain would likely lead to heightened levels of depression and anxiety." Cunningham et al. (59), comparing migraine and chronic nonheadache pain samples, found no difference in anxiety and depression levels between the two groups with chronic pain, with respect to pain-free controls. It is noteworthy that studies looking for differences between migraine and other headache subtypes did not find specific psychologic characteristics of migraine sufferers (60). From a psychologic point of view, no differences exist between headache sufferers and recurrent abdominal pain sufferers (61).

It has been shown that chronic illness, in general, explains variations in psychologic functioning between chronically ill and healthy children, and not a specific disorder (62). The burden of childhood adversities on CDH does not differ between subjects with chronic migraine and subjects with chronic tension-type headache (population study) (63). This emphasizes that psychiatric disorders are not specifically related to migraine, but probably to migraine as a kind of disabling and recurrent pain. It does not mean a cause-and-effect relationship, because the pathophysiologic mechanisms are unknown.

Clarifying the relationship between psychologic factors and headache could be a significant aid for psychosomatic research, which often considers the psychosomatic nature of headaches to be an established assumption (54, 55), even if, often, the established criteria to define the headache sufferers are not specified. The ICHD-II (6) advances an innovative categorization for headache related to psychologic factors. For the first time, the main body of the ICHD-II recognizes a "direction"

(headache attributed to psychiatric disorders) in this relationship, even though related only to somatization and psychotic disorders. The new classification is a first step toward a better systematization of the chapter on "headache and psychiatric disorders," even though, to date, there is a very limited evidence supporting psychiatric causes of headache, as outlined in the general comment introducing the section of the ICHD-II. In the main body of the classification, no direct reference is given to pediatric psychiatric disorders, even if in the appendix we can find disorders that may be attributed to headache in children and adolescents as well (e.g., "headache attributed to separation anxiety disorder," "headache attributed to social phobia"). In the appendix are novel entities that have not been sufficiently validated by research studies, but once sufficient scientific evidence is ascertained, they will be moved in the main classification.

This brief overview shows the consistency of psychologic disorders associated with headache, but the nature (genetic, biological, or environmental predisposition, and environmental/physical or psychologic/emotional stressors), direction (headache as a cause of psychologic disorders or vice versa), and reciprocal correlation of these factors remain unclear. The explanation might have a clarifying role in etiology and pathophysiology as well as consequences for the treatment of headache.

Distinguishing between biological predisposition (basic vulnerability) and triggering factors (precipitants) and determining the role and the different meaning of personality traits, specific psychologic factors (including attentional and cognitive elements, role of stress, and emotional disposition) and psychiatric comorbidity, should avoid a confounding overlap among these different elements.

MIGRAINE AND SLEEP

Relationship between Headache and Sleep

The reciprocal relationship between headache and sleep has been documented in medical literature for more than a century, and clinical texts allude to the importance of sleep as a headache precipitant. The precise nature and magnitude of the headache–sleep association and underlying mechanisms remain poorly understood (64).

Sleep represents the only well-documented behavioral state related to the occurrence of some headache syndromes. Sleep disorders are observed among all headache subgroups and headaches that occur during or after sleep are suggestive of sleep disorders.

In adults, the presence of a specific sleep disorder has been identified in 55% of subjects with onset of headache during the night (65), and treatment of the underlying sleep disorders improved the headache. More recently (66), a direct correlation between the increase in sleep disturbance and headache severity has been found.

On the other hand, headache may cause various degrees of sleep disruption and seems to be associated with several sleep disturbances either in adults or in children. Headaches are known to occur during sleep, after sleep, and in relationship with various sleep stages. Furthermore, sleep deprivation and sleep schedule changes are common headache triggers: an excess or lack of sleep or a bad quality or inadequate duration of sleep may cause headache. Many chronic headache patients, whatever the type of headache, may complain of insufficient sleep, lack of restoration in the morning, and severe snoring (67).

Different studies proposed a model of interaction between headache and sleep (65, 67). Lack of sleep triggers both migraine and tension-type headache, together with stress or tension, not eating on time, and fatigue (68). Even in children, one of the commonest self-perceived triggers of head pain was the lack of sleep (69).

Sleep, either spontaneous or induced by hypnotics, seems effective for relief of head pain or even to terminate the headache attacks (70, 71), even in the youngest sufferers.

Sleep is the most potent antimigraine treatment. Frequency of falling asleep during attacks is significantly more common in patients younger than 8 years of age than in older children, and in these children there is higher resolution of attacks with sleep (72). The intrinsic mechanism that leads to head pain relief is still unknown and understudied; the hypothesis that sleep could trigger an autonomic reset seems to be the most reasonable (73). However, the power of sleep in terminating the attack is counterbalanced by the ability to precipitate the attack. Although sleep was more commonly referenced as a relieving factor for migraine (70%), migraine attack was also precipitated by sleep deprivation in 24% and by sleep excess in 6% of cases (74). It is noteworthy that sleep deficiency may act differently according to headache subtype: one study (75) found a relationship between sleep disturbances and headache in 30.8% of subjects with migraine with aura, in 18.8% of subjects with migraine without aura, and in 3.8% of those with tension-type headache.

Sleep is a precipitating factor for either nocturnal headache (awakening during a usual sleep period with a headache) or morning arousal with headache (headache present at arousal at the end of a behaviorally defined sleep period). It has been hypothesized that depth of sleep could be responsible for the migraine attack, and the use of a technique named "sleep rationing," consisting of the reduction of total sleep time and of relaxed sleep and thereby leading to a reduction of REM sleep and slow-wave sleep, was successful in reducing both the intensity and the severity of the migraine attacks (76).

Another important point supporting this relationship is that treating headache improves sleep (5-HT, serotoninergic drugs) and, conversely, that treating sleep improves headache (continuous positive airway pressure [CPAP] treatment, sleep hygiene, dopaminergic agents for periodic limb movement/restless legs syndrome [PLM/RLS], stimulants for narcolepsy, and fibromyalgia treatment) (77).

Epidemiological Study in Children

Literature data show an association between headache and behavioral manifestations of sleep disorders. Parasomnias are the sleep disorders most commonly associated with headache: a history of sleepwalking has been reported in different groups of migraine patients with prevalence ranging from 21.9% to 30% (78).

A case control study in school age children confirmed a strong association between migraine or headache and different sleep disorders. Children with migraine and tension-type headache showed a higher prevalence of disorders of initiating and maintaining sleep (mainly shorter sleep duration, longer sleep latency, bedtime struggles, and night awakenings), of parasomnias (sleep talking, bruxism, nightmare but not sleepwalking, bedwetting, and sleep terrors), of restless sleep, and of daytime sleepiness. The group with migraine was the one with the more "disturbed sleep," with increased prevalence of nocturnal symptoms such as sleep breathing disorders and certain parasomnias, although no statistical differences between children with migraine and children with tension-type headache have been found (79). Further studies confirmed this first report showing that children with migraine headaches experienced more sleep disturbances compared to healthy controls and reported shorter sleep duration, bruxism, co-sleeping, and snoring; in this study the frequency of migraine predicted parasomnias and sleepwalking and duration predicted sleep anxiety and bedtime resistance (80).

A more recent report confirmed the presence of excessive daytime sleepiness, narcolepsy, and insomnia in children with headaches but failed to corroborate the higher prevalence of symptoms of sleep apnea, restlessness, and parasomnias, as reported in the previous studies (81).

From a different point of view, a recent study in children showed that migraine without aura was a sensitive risk factor for disorders of initiating and maintaining sleep, that chronic tension-type headache was a sensitive risk factor for sleep breathing disorders, and that headache disorder as a whole was a cumulative risk factor for disorders of excessive somnolence (82).

It is possible that the pathogenetic mechanism underlying headache or migraine and sleep could act since early life and that migraine variants are the presenting symptoms of a later developing headache. From this perspective an interesting association was reported between migraine and hyperreactivity syndrome during infancy (83), in which night awakenings and falling asleep difficulties are typical symptoms; and furthermore, in a retrospective evaluation of six children younger than 3 years of age, one of the early presenting signs of migraine was represented by sleep disorders (84). These early developmental disorders (e.g., feeding difficulties or sleep disorders) may also have a prognostic value because they were present in 78% of children with enduring headache (85).

Moreover, early sleep disorders have been also related to psychiatric comorbidity and involved in the endurance of headache in children and adolescence (23, 86).

Polysomnographic and Actigraphic Studies

Evaluation of the sleep–wake cycle in ten subjects with migraine on a long-term basis (2 weeks) using the actigraph showed that during the interictal period, sleep parameters of children suffering from migraine did not differ from those of control subjects; timing of the attack showed that it affected nocturnal motor activity, which presented the lowest values on the night before the attack, indicating a decrease in cortical activation during sleep preceding migraine attacks, supporting the hypothesis of a dopaminergic imbalance in children with migraine (87).

In children there is a real paucity of polysomnographic studies. In a preliminary study we demonstrated that the main feature of sleep organization in children with migraine was represented by a high degree of sleep instability as demonstrated by an increased number of stage shifts and increased movement time (88).

The description of changing diagnoses in several adults with headaches (65) after a polysomnographic study (periodic limb movements of sleep, fibromyalgia syndrome, and obstructive sleep apnea syndrome) suggested the possibility of similar conditions in pediatric patients.

Combined Treatment of Sleep and Headache

Indirect evidence for the role of sleep disorders in headache has been given by the improvement of migraine frequency and duration after the application of sleep hygiene guidelines (89).

Instructions to improve sleep hygiene include practices addressed to promote continuous and effective sleep, such as regularity of bedtime and rising time, restriction of beverage and foods that tend to disrupt sleep, and regular exercise. The application of sleep hygiene guidelines could represent an alternative approach to the treatment of migraine by correcting an inappropriate sleep behavior without resorting to pharmacological treatment.

On the other hand, sleep disorders may be an index of comorbid psychiatric disorders (e.g., shared symptom with anxiety, mood, adjustment, or posttraumatic stress disorders). This suggests the possibility of an approach to comorbid sleep disorders in headache sufferers that stresses the role of a systematic psychologic assessment.

Moreover, sleep disorders most implicated by headache include obstructive sleep apnea, primary insomnia, and circadian phase abnormalities, and their treatment improves headache. Patients suffering from chronic morning or nocturnal headache should be considered for the possible presence of a treatable sleep disturbance, such as obstructive sleep apnea or upper airway resistance syndrome, or a comorbidity with insomnia or circadian rhythm disorders (77, 90, 91).

Evidence for the association of headache and sleep disorder suggests the necessity to understand the reciprocal relationship, to make clear the direction, meaning, and implications in etiology, diagnosis, and therapy. The high prevalence, the wide diagnostic subtypes, the unclear pathophysiologic pathways for both disorders add complexities—even more so when we study the comorbid occurrence. However, ways toward a better understanding of such a relationship have been opened in pathophysiologic (actigraphic studies), diagnostic (polysomnographic and psychiatric studies), and therapeutic (e.g., sleep hygiene study) dimensions.

References

1. Abu-Arefeh I, Russell G. Prevalence of headache and migraine in schoolchildren. *BMJ* 1994; 309:765–769.
2. Aromaa M, Silanpää M, Rautava P. Childhood headache at school entry: a controlled clinical study. *Neurology* 1997; 17:488–491.
3. Sillanpää M, Aro H. Headache in teenagers: comorbidity and prognosis. *Funct Neurol* 2000; 15(Suppl):116–121.
4. Guidetti V, Fabrizi P, Galli F, et al. Unilateral headache in early and late childhood. *Int J Neurol Sci* 1999; 20:S56–S59.
5. Hershey AD, Winner P, Kabbouche MA, et al. Use of the ICHD-II criteria in the diagnosis of pediatric migraine. *Headache* 2005; 45:1288–1297.
6. Headache Classification Subcommittee of International Headache Society. The International Classification of Headache Disorders, 2nd edition. *Cephalalgia* 2004; 24(Suppl 1):1–151.
7. International Headache Society. Classification and diagnostic criteria for headache disorders, cranial neuralgias, and facial pain. *Cephalalgia* 1988;(Suppl 7):1–96.
8. Prensky AL, Sommer D. Diagnosis and treatment of migraine in children. *Neurology* 1979; 29:506–510.
9. Silberstein SD. Twenty questions about headaches in children and adolescents. *Headache* 1990; 30:716–724.
10. Rothner AD. Headache in children: a review. *Headache* 1979; 19:156–162.
11. Guidetti V, Bruni O, Cerutti R, et al. How and why childhood headache and migraine differ from that of the adults. In: Gallai V, Guidetti V, eds. *Juvenile Headache*. Amsterdam: Excerpta Medica, 1991:27.
12. Wöber-Bingol C, Wöber C, Wagner-Ennsgraber C, et al. IHS criteria for migraine and tension-type headache in children and adolescents. *Headache* 1996; 36:231–238.
13. Rossi LN, Cortinovis I, Menegazzo L, et al. Behavior during attacks and assessment of intensity in primary headaches in children and adolescents. *Cephalalgia* 2005; 26:107–112.
14. Neubauer D, Kuhar M, Ravnik I. Antihistamine responsive cluster headache in a teenaged girl. *Headache* 1997; 37:296–298.

15. Sjaastad O, Dale I. Evidence for a new (?) treatable headache entity. *Headache* 1976; 14:105–108.
16. Mack KJ. Episodic and chronic migraine in children. *Semin Neurol* 2006; 26:223–231.
17. Silberstein SD. Tension-type and chronic daily headache. *Neurology* 1993; 43: 1644–1649.
18. Silberstein SD, Lipton RB, Solomon S, et al. Classification of daily and near-daily headaches: proposed revisions to the IHS criteria. *Headache* 1994; 34:1–7.
19. Gladstein J, Holden EW. Chronic daily headache in children and adolescents: a 2 year prospective study. *Headache* 1996; 36:349–351.
20. Abu-Arafeh I. Chronic tension-type headache in children and adolescents. *Cephalalgia* 2001; 21:830–836.
21. Hershey AD, Powers SW, Bentti AL, et al. Characterization of chronic daily headaches in children in a multidisciplinary headache center. *Neurology* 2001; 56:1032–1037.
22. Wang SJ, Fuh JL, Lu SR, et al. Chronic daily headache in adolescents. Prevalence, impact, and medication overuse. *Neurology* 2006; 66:193–197.
23. Galli F, Patron L, Russo PM, Guidetti V. Chronic daily headache in childhood and adolescence: clinical aspects and a 4-year follow-up. *Cephalalgia* 2004; 10:850–859.
24. Hockaday JM. *Migraine in childhood and other non-epileptic paroxysmal disorders.* London: Butterworths, 1988:66.
25. Evans RW, Gladstein J. Confusional migraine or photoepilepsy? *Headache* 2003; 43: 506–508.
26. Evans RW, Rolak LA. The Alice in Wonderland syndrome. *Headache* 2004; 44: 624–625.
27. Gencoglu EA, Alehan F, Erol I, et al. Brain SPECT findings in a patient with Alice in Wonderland syndrome. *Clin Nucl Med* 2005; 30:758–759.
28. Rami A, Shapira Y, Flusser H, et al. Basilar migraine manifesting as transient global amnesia in a 9-year-old child. *Headache* 1986; 26:17–18.
29. Riggs SR, Bodensteiner JB. Acute confusional migraine: variant of transient global amnesia. *Pediatr Neurol* 1995; 12:129–131.
30. Ottman R, Lipton RB. Comorbidity of migraine and epilepsy. *Neurology* 1994; 44: 2105–2110.
31. Guidetti V, Fornara R, Marchini R, et al. Headache and epilepsy in childhood: analysis of a series of 620 children. *Funct Neurol* 1987; 2:323–341.
32. Panayiotopoulos CP. Visual phenomena and headache in occipital epilepsy: a review, a systematic study and differentiation from migraine. *Epileptic Disord* 1999; 1:205–216.
33. Brinciotti M, Di Sabato ML, Matricardi M, Guidetti V. Electroclinical features in children and adolescents with epilepsy and/or migraine, and occipital epileptiform EEG abnormalities. *Clin Electroencephalogr* 2000; 31:76–82.
34. Wirrell EC, Hamiwka LD. Do children with benign rolandic epilepsy have a higher prevalence of migraine than those with other partial epilepsies or nonepilepsy controls? *Epilepsia* 2006; 47:1674–1681.
35. Stevenson S, Sharon B. Epilepsy and migraine headache: is there a connection? *J Pediatr Health Care* 2006; 20:167–171.
36. Piccinelli P, Borgatti R, Nicoli F, et al. Relationship between migraine and epilepsy in pediatric age. *Headache* 2006; 46:413–421.
37. Ludvigsson P, Hesdorffer D, Olafsson E, et al. Migraine with aura is a risk factor for unprovoked seizures in children. *Ann Neurol* 2006; 59:210–213.
38. Bille B. Migraine in childhood and its prognosis. *Cephalalgia* 1981; 1:71–75.
39. Congdon PJ, Forsythe WI. Migraine in childhood: a study of 300 children. *Dev Med Child Neurol* 1979; 21:209–216.
40. Dooley J, Bagnell A. The prognosis and treatment of headaches in children—a ten year follow-up. *Can J Neurol Sci* 1995; 22:47–49.
41. Guidetti V, Galli F. Evolution of headache in childhood and adolescence: an 8-year follow-up. *Cephalalgia* 1998; 18:449–454.
42. Guidetti V, Galli F, Fabrizi P, et al. Headache and psychiatric comorbidity: clinical aspects and outcome in an 8-year follow-up study. *Cephalalgia* 1998; 18:455–462.
43. Vahlquist B. Migraine in children. *International Archives of Allergy* 1962; 7:348–352.
44. Bille B. Migraine in schoolchildren. *Acta Paediatr* 1962; 51(Suppl 136):1–151.
45. Coch C, Melchior JC. Headache in childhood—a five year material from a pediatric university clinic. *Dan Med Bull* 1969; 16:109–114.
46. Maratos J, Wilkinson M. Migraine in children: a medical and psychiatric study. *Cephalalgia* 1982; 2:179–187.
47. Millichap JG. Recurrent headaches in 100 children. *Child's Brain* 1978; 4:95–105.
48. Guidetti V, Ottaviano S, Pagliarini N, et al. Psychological peculiarities in children with recurrent primary headache. *Cephalalgia* 1983; 41(Suppl 1):215–217.
49. Guidetti V, Mazzei G, Ottaviano S, et al. The utilization of Rorschach test in childhood migraine: a case controlled study. *Cephalalgia* 1986; 6:87.
50. Merikangas KR, Angst J, Isler H. Migraine and psychopathology. Results of the Zurich cohort study of young adults. *Arch Gen Psychiatry* 1990; 47:849–853.
51. Merikangas KR, Merikangas JR, Angst J. Headache syndromes and psychiatric disorders: association and familial transmission. *J Psychiatry Res* 1993; 2:197–210.
52. Merikangas KR. Psychopathology and headache syndromes in the community. *Headache* 1994; 34:S17–S26.
53. Breslau N, Davis GC, Andreski P. Migraine, psychiatric disorders and suicide attempts: an epidemiological study of young adults. *Psychiatry Res* 1991; 37:11–23.
54. Campo JV, Fritsch SL. Somatization in children and adolescents. *J Am Acad Child Adolesc Psychiatry* 1994; 33:1223–1235.
55. Greene JD, Walker LS. Psychosomatic problems and stress in adolescence. *Pediatr Clin North Am* 1997; 44:1557–1572.
56. AACAP Official Action. Practice parameters for the assessment and treatment of anxiety disorders. *J Am Acad Child Adolesc Psychiatry* 1993; 32:1089–1098.
57. Livingston R, Taylor JL, Crawford SL. A study of somatic complaints and psychiatric diagnosis in children. *J Am Acad Child Adolesc Psychiatry* 1988; 27:185–187.
58. Andrasik F, Kabela E, Quinn S, et al. Psychological functioning of children who have recurrent migraine. *Pain* 1988; 34:43–52.
59. Cunningham SJ, McGrath PJ, Ferguson HB, et al. Personality and behavioral characteristics in pediatric migraine. *Headache* 1987; 27:16–20.
60. Karwautz A, Wöber C, Lang T, et al. Psychosocial factors in children and adolescents with migraine and tension-type headache: a controlled study and review of the literature. *Cephalalgia* 1999; 19:32–43.
61. Galli F, D'Antuono G, Tarantino S, Viviano F, et al. Headache and recurrent abdominal pain: a controlled study by the means of the Child Behavior Checklist (CBCL). *Cephalalgia*, 2007; 27:211–219.
62. Brown LK, Fritz GK, Herzog DB. Psychosomatic disorders. In: Wiener JM, ed. *Textbook of Child and Adolescent Psychiatry.* Washington, DC: American Psychiatric Press, 1997:621.
63. Juang KD, Wang SJ, Fuh SR, et al. Association between adolescent chronic daily headache and childhood adversity: a community-based study. *Cephalalgia* 2004; 24:54–59.
64. Kelman L, Rains JC. Headache and sleep: examination of sleep patterns and complaints in a large clinical sample of migraineurs. *Headache* 2005; 45:904–910.
65. Paiva T, Batista A, Martins P, Martins A. The relationship between headaches and sleep disturbances. *Headache* 1995; 35:590–596.
66. Boardman HF, Thomas E, Millson DS, Croft PR. The natural history of headache: predictors of onset and recovery. *Cephalalgia* 2006; 26:1080–1088.
67. Sahota PK, Dexter JD. Sleep and headache syndromes: a clinical review. *Headache* 1990; 30:80–84.
68. Spierings ELH, Ranke AH, Honkoop PC. Precipitating and aggravating factors of migraine versus tension-type headache. *Headache* 2001; 41:554–558.
69. Roth-Isigkeit A, Thyen U, Sto¨ven H, Schwarzenberger J, et al. Pain among children and adolescents: restrictions in daily living and triggering factors. *Pediatrics* 2005; 115: e152–e162.
70. Wilkinson M, Williams K, Leyton M. Observations on the treatment of an acute attack of migraine. *Research and Clinical Studies in Headache* 1978; 6:141–146.
71. Blau JN. Resolution of migraine attacks: sleep and the recovery phase. *J Neurol Neurosurg Psychiatry* 1982; 45:223–226.
72. Aaltonen K, Hämäläinen ML, Hoppu K. Migraine attacks and sleep in children. *Cephalalgia* 2000; 20:580–584.
73. Dexter JD. Relationship between sleep and headache syndromes. In: Thorpy MJ, ed. *Handbook of Sleep Disorders.* New York: Marcel Dekker, 1990:663–671.
74. Inamorato E, Minatti Hannuch SN, Zukerman E. The role of sleep in migraine attacks. *Arq Neuropsiquiatr* 1993; 51:429–432.
75. Rossi LN, Cortinovis I, Menegazzo L, et al. Classification criteria and distinction between migraine and tension-type headache in children. *Dev Med Child Neurol* 2001; 43: 45–51.
76. Gans M. Treating migraine by sleep rationing. *J Nerv Ment Dis* 1951; 113:405–429.
77. Dodick DW, Eross EJ, Parish JM. Clinical, anatomical, and physiologic relationship between sleep and headache. *Headache* 2003; 43:282–292.
78. Zucconi M, Bruni O. Sleep disorders in children with neurological diseases. *Semin Pediatric Neurol* 2001; 8:258–275.
79. Bruni O, Fabrizi P, Ottaviano S, et al. Prevalence of sleep disorders in childhood and adolescence headache: a case control study. *Cephalalgia* 1997; 17:492–498.
80. Miller VA, Palermo TM, Powers SW, Scher MS, et al. Migraine headaches and sleep disturbances in children. *Headache* 2003; 43:362–368.
81. Luc ME, Gupta A, Birnberg JM, Reddick D, et al. Characterization of symptoms of sleep disorders in children with headache. *Pediatr Neurol* 2006; 34:7–12.
82. Carotenuto M, Guidetti V, Ruju F, Galli F, et al. Headache disorders as risk factors for sleep disturbances in school aged children. *J Headache Pain* 2005; 6:268–270.
83. Guidetti V, Ottaviano S, Pagliarini M. Childhood headache risk: warning signs and symptoms present during the first six months of life. *Cephalalgia* 1984; 4:237–242.
84. Elser JM, Woody RC. Migraine headache in the infant and young child. *Headache* 1990; 30:366–368.
85. Balottin U, Termine C, Nicoli F, Quadrelli M, et al. Idiopathic headache in children under six years of age: a follow-up study. *Headache* 2005; 45:705–715.
86. Guidetti V, Galli F, Fabrizi P, Giannantoni A, et al. Headache and psychiatric comorbidity: clinical aspects and outcome in an 8-year follow-up study. *Cephalalgia* 1998; 18:455–462.
87. Guidetti V, Bruni O, Violani C, Casiello B, et al. Sleep wake cycle variations in migrainous children. *Cephalalgia* 1999; 19:278.
88. Guidetti V, Bruni O, Canitano R, Romoli M, et al. Migraine and headache in childhood: sleep disorders and sleep organization. *Cephalalgia* 1995; S16:10–12.
89. Bruni O, Galli F, Guidetti V. Sleep hygiene and migraine in children and adolescents. *Cephalalgia* 1999; 19(S25):58–60.
90. Loh NK, Dinner DS, Foldvary N, Skobieranda F, et al. Do patients with obstructive sleep apnea wake up with headaches? *Arch Intern Med* 1999; 159:1765–1768.
91. Neau JP, Paquereau J, Mailbe M, Meuroce JC, et al. Relationship between sleep apnoea syndrome, snoring and headache. *Cephalalgia* 2002; 22:333–339.

59 Migraine in Adults

Alexei E. Yankovsky
Frederick Andermann
Andrea Bernasconi

A link between migraine and epilepsy has been known for more than a century, since Sir William Richard Gowers's time, but the nature of this association is still unresolved. Migraine and epilepsy are in many respects similar brain disorders. Both are common. Epilepsy may be, and migraine is, by definition, a primary, presumably genetic disorder. In a small proportion of patients, genes have been found in different forms of epilepsy and in familial migraine. Both epilepsy and migraine-like headache (HA) may be secondary to other brain disorders. Etiology may at times be similar for epilepsy and migraine-like HAs (i.e., in arteriovenous malformation [AVM]). Both present as chronic conditions with episodic manifestations. Attacks may occur without any specific reason or may be triggered by stress, sleep deprivation, alcohol, menses, or fatigue. There are partially overlapping symptoms in some types of both these disorders. Finally, cortical hyperexcitability is the basic underlying mechanism in both.

On the other hand, there are important differences between epilepsy and migraine. Most epileptic seizures are not associated with HA or migraine. The classical migraine aura with cortical spreading depression (CSD) usually lasts many minutes, whereas epileptic propagation habitually lasts seconds. Occipital cortex is the primary generator for migraine aura, and the brainstem is possibly the generator for HA, based on positron emission tomography (PET) studies. Occipital epilepsy, however, is quite rare. An epileptic focus can be removed and the epilepsy remit, but in migraine no resective surgery is possible. Vagal nerve stimulation is widely used as a treatment of epilepsy, but in migraine only uncontrolled studies are reported. Specific electroencephalographic (EEG) discharge is an epilepsy marker, but migraine diagnosis is at present purely clinical. Both disorders are common, but the incidence and prevalence of migraine are much greater.

EPIDEMIOLOGY

The overall incidence of epilepsy in developed countries is estimated to be 25–50 per 100,000 persons per year. Different age-specific incidences for migraine and epilepsy have been reported. The age-specific incidence of epilepsy is highest in the extremes of life. The incidence of migraine with aura (MA) in women peaks between ages 12 and 17 years, depending on whether an aura is present. In men the incidence of migraine with aura peaks several years earlier. The substantial sex differences reported for migraine (affecting 18% of women and 6% of men) are much smaller for epilepsy. Prevalence of epilepsy in the United States was found to be 0.6%. Epilepsy may have a strong catamenial component; hormonal factors generally act as triggers for seizures. Hormonal factors are crucial for the onset of migraine at menarche, as well as for individual attacks in many women. Epilepsy is relatively constant across developed nations and geographic locations. The prevalence of migraine is highest in the Americas and Europe, intermediate in Africa, and lowest in Asia. No race differences have been established for epilepsy, although increased prevalence has been reported in young African Americans. In the United States, migraine is more common in the white population than in African Americans and least common in Asians.

Ottman and Lipton (1) reported a migraine prevalence of 24% among probands with epilepsy and 26% in the relatives of these probands. The median prevalence of epilepsy in people with migraine is 5.9%. The two disorders, therefore, are more than twice as likely to occur in the same person. Three alternative models were proposed to account for the comorbidity of migraine and epilepsy (2). One possibility is a simple, unidirectional causal explanation. In this case the incidence of either migraine or epilepsy should be raised before, but not after, onset of the second disorder. For example, epilepsy could cause migraine by activating the trigeminovascular system, in which case we would expect an excess risk of migraine after the onset of epilepsy. In fact, there is an excess risk of migraine both before and after epilepsy onset, and unidirectional causal models are not that simple (2). Nevertheless, in some patients this mechanism appears to operate, and onset of epilepsy is definitely before onset of migraine. Furthermore, resection of an epileptogenic focus may relieve both epilepsy and migraine in these patients, as has been shown in some of our patients with peri-ictal HA on postsurgical follow-up.

A second possibility is that shared environmental risk factors may explain this comorbidity. Because the risk of migraine is significantly increased in people with idiopathic or cryptogenic epilepsy, known environmental risk factors cannot account for all the comorbidity.

A third possibility is that shared genetic risk factors may account for comorbidity. However, migraine was not more likely in individuals with familial epilepsy than in others.

Finally, it has been proposed that an altered brain state (increased excitability) may increase the risk of both migraine and epilepsy and account for comorbidity (2). This hypothesis draws support from the similar therapeutic options and recent experimental studies on rats (3). The lesion in both can be considered as a functional network abnormality. Brainstem aminergic neurons (such as the noradrenergic neurons of the locus coeruleus) are part of a migraine network, supported by functional brain imaging showing activation of the dorsolateral pons.

MIGRAINE PATHOPHYSIOLOGY

Cortical hyperexcitability is the basic underlying mechanism of epilepsy and migraine. This has long been known for epilepsy, but in migraine this hypothesis has gained support only recently. Activation of brainstem and cortex is followed by activation of ascending and descending pathways and, finally, trigeminal meningeal vasodilation and neurogenic inflammation (4). Possible explanations suggested for migrainous hyperexcitability were low concentrations of magnesium and gamma-aminobutyric acid (GABA) and high concentration of glutamate, mitochondrial dysfunction, nitric oxide, and calcium channel abnormalities.

Considerable clinical and experimental evidence is available showing that CSD is an important pathophysiological correlate of the migraine aura. CSD can be induced experimentally by cortical trauma, applying high concentrations of potassium or glutamate, inhibition of Na^+/K^+-ATPase, and several other stimuli. There is also a PET study that showed silent CSD during migraine without aura, which was similar to what is observed in migraine with aura (5). This may explain the effectiveness of migraine prophylaxis in migraine both with and without aura through reduction of CSD.

ACUTE AND PROPHYLACTIC ASPECTS OF MIGRAINE TREATMENT

Prophylactic treatment with sodium valproate and topiramate (TPM) for migraine is currently used. Valproic acid (VPA) increases concentrations of GABA in the brain, increases the postsynaptic response to GABA and potassium channel flow, produces neuronal hyperpolarization; stops the firing of the 5-hydroxytryptamine (5-HT, serotonin) neurons of the dorsal raphe nucleus, which is thought to control head pain; and reduces central trigeminal activation, which is demonstrated by decreased C-Fos activation in the trigeminal nucleus caudalis. Valproic acid also reduces experimental neurogenic inflammation in the trigeminal vascular system, which is mediated by $GABA_A$ receptor agonism.

Topiramate has multiple mechanisms of action through voltage-activated sodium and calcium channels, $GABA_A$ receptors, and the alpha-amino-3-hydroxy-5-methylisoxazole-4-propionic acid (AMPA) or kainate subtype of glutamate receptors. It has been suggested that these effects are mediated by protein phosphorylation, which may be related to the combination of pharmacological properties of TPM. These and other antiepilepsy drugs (AEDs) may help for both migraine and seizures. Both medications may reduce the hyperexcitability phase of migraine and epilepsy, and it has been recently proven by Ayata et al. (3) that artificially induced CSD in rats was reduced after treatment with VPA or TPM for at least 6–8 weeks. A dose–response relationship for VPA and TPM was found in this study. However, propranolol, amitriptyline, and methysergide, which are not effective for epilepsy prophylaxis, were found to reduce CSD in this study as well. Furthermore, antiepileptic medications do not reduce the neurovascular inflammation phase of migraine, which typically follows neuroexcitation. Studies showed that not all antiepileptic medications are effective in migraine. More research is required because we do not know the precise mechanisms of action of these drugs nor the full picture of the pathogenesis of migraine and epilepsy. Other AEDs such as gabapentin, levetiracetam, tiagabine, and zonisamide showed some efficacy in small uncontrolled studies.

Treatment of the acute attack is substantially different in migraine and epilepsy. This is not surprising, because pathogenic mechanisms in migraine are mainly serotonergic and the use of triptans, which do not have antiseizure properties, is effective. On the contrary, prolonged seizures (status epilepticus) are responsive to benzodiazepines.

No systematic study has been conducted for the treatment of peri-ictal migraine attacks. Such a study is warranted, because this condition is frequent and, at times, may be more disabling than the seizures themselves. Usually patients are not treated with triptans or other antimigraine medications in peri-ictal migraine. They use over-the-counter medications for any type of HA, with variable effect. This is probably related to lack of both awareness and specific inquiry by the patients' physicians. It may also be related to the lack of specific seizure-related categories of HA in the previous HA classification. We have only limited information about the efficacy of sumatriptan in peri-ictal migraine based on anecdotal reports. This practical therapeutic question awaits resolution by a systematic trial.

Headache and Migraine in Intractable Partial Epilepsy

We were interested to characterize HA types and other head sensations (HSens) in large populations of patients with well-defined forms of epilepsy. There have been few previous studies in such defined populations (6–11). We will review briefly the systematic study of pathologically verified patients with intractable partial epilepsy (12). The aim of our study was to analyze the incidence of HA in such a group, compare HA and non-HA patients, and investigate possible correlations with HAs or migraine in the pathologically verified group.

We considered all reported peri-ictal HA as pre-ictal HA (PreHA), ictal HA (IHA), or postictal HA (PostHA). All types could represent migraine as defined by the second edition of the International Classification of Headache Disorders (ICHD-2) (13). We interviewed 100 consecutive patients (45 males; mean age 33 years) according to a standard form. They were undergoing presurgical evaluation for pharmacologically intractable partial epilepsy (9). The interview began with a verbatim description of the HA by the patient. For each HA type, questions inquired about lateralization, localization, quality of pain, and results of treatment. Interictal HA was defined as not temporally related to seizures. Severity was assessed using the visual analogue scale (VAS) of pain (0–10 cm; 0 = no pain, 10 = worst possible pain). Each section contained an open-ended question, with the answer recorded verbatim, followed by specific questions. Migrainous character of the HA was determined according to the diagnostic criteria of the ICHD-2, except that in some cases duration was shorter than 4 hours (13). Family history of recurrent HAs or migraine was also documented. Demographic and clinical data were obtained through interviews with patients and their relatives and by review of hospital charts. Diagnosis and lateralization of the seizure focus was based on a comprehensive evaluation including seizure history and semiology, neurological examination, video-EEG telemetry with scalp electrodes, and neuropsychologic evaluation in all. The seizure focus was determined by predominantly ipsilateral interictal epileptiform abnormalities and by unequivocal seizure onset. In all patients, magnetic resonance imaging (MRI) scans were acquired on a 1.5-T scanner using T1-fast field echo, proton-density, T2-weighted, and fluid attenuation inversion recovery images.

Fifty-nine patients (59%; 31 females) reported recurrent HAs. Mean age was 31.8 years (range 8–52). Interictal HA (InterHA) were reported by 31 patients. Peri-ictal HAs were reported by 47 patients. Of those, 11 had PreHA and 44 had PostHA. Eight patients had both PreHA and PostHA. Twenty-nine of these 47 patients (62%) had frontotemporal HAs. Twenty-five had migraine-like HA without aura according to the diagnostic criteria of the ICHD-2. Headache occurred in 18 of 30 (60%) patients with temporal lobe epilepsy (TLE) and in seven of 17 (41%) of those with extratemporal epilepsy (ETE), including four with frontal lobe epilepsy (FLE) and three with occipital lobe epilepsy (OLE). Twenty-nine patients reported a family history of recurrent HA or migraine (precise diagnosis was impossible because of the lack of direct confirmation). The characteristics of HA variables are presented in Table 59-1.

Preictal HA. Eleven patients (11%) had PreHA. All but one had TLE. Four of the eleven (36%) patients with PreHA had a pattern compatible with migraine without aura. In two the duration was less than 4 hours. Eight patients had PreHA continuing to PostHA. Intensity of PreHA was moderate. Four (36%) patients used over-the-counter analgesics. Follow-up data on patients in the

TABLE 59-1

Characteristics of PreHA, PostHA, and InterHA in Fifty-nine Patients with Intractable Epilepsy and Recurrent HAs

HA CHARACTERISTICS	PreHA N = 11	PostHA N = 44	InterHA N = 31
Occurrence with seizures	75%	20 pts = almost 100%, 12 = 75%, 7 = 50%, 5 = 25%	—
Side of HA	R = 6, L = 5	R = 12, L = 14, Bil = 18	R = 1, L = 2, Bil = 23, R or L = 13
Location	F-T in all, Middle = 2	F-T = 32, Middle = 16, Posterior = 3	F-T = 26, Middle = 9, Posterior = 5
Spread	Ipsi = 2 Contra = 1	Ipsi = 8 Contra = 4	Ipsi = 8 Contra = 1
Quality: Throbbing Pressure	7 4	19 28	24 14
Intensity (VAS)	7.1 cm	6.7 cm	6.2 cm
Use of analgesics	4 (27%)	36 (81%)	25 (80%)
Analgesics	One = 2	One = 29 Two = 4	One = 21 Two = 4
Positive effect	Always = 2, sometimes = 2	Always = 11, sometimes = 18, never = 4	Always = 8, sometimes = 17, never = 2
Duration	EarlyPreHA (5–30 min, n = 7) ProdPreHA (30 min–24 h, n = 4)	5–60 min = 13, 60 min–12 h = 19, longer or shorter = 12	5–60 min = 6, 60 min–12 h = 18, longer or shorter = 7
Frequency	Related to Sz	Related to Sz	Daily = 2, <1/w = 9, 1/w–1/m = 14, 1/m–6/m = 5

Cm = Centimeters, L = left, R = right, pts = patients, numbers refer to numbers of patients, F = frontal, T = temporal, PreHA = preictal HA, PostHA = postictal HA, InterHA = interictal HA, Sz = seizures, h = hours, min = minutes, w = weeks, m = months, ipsi = ipsilateral, contra = contralateral, Prod = prodromal, Bil = bilateral.

PreHA group after surgery are presented in Table 59-2. Two illustrative patients with PreHA are presented herein:

R.D. A 40-year-old man had HA in 75% of his seizures. Both conditions started at the same age. HAs were always located over the left frontotemporal region, remained localized, and had a throbbing and pressure character. They were accompanied by nausea and photo- and phonophobia, worsened on physical activity, and lasted 15 minutes. They were severe: VAS was 9.0 and he had to go to bed, but tried not to take medications. He had no family history of HA and no postictal or interictal pain. He had

bilateral temporal spikes and MRI showed left mesial temporal atrophy. He underwent left anterior temporal lobectomy. Hippocampal sclerosis was documented on pathology. Follow-up after 20 months showed Engel class one seizure outcome without any HA.

J.B. A 36-year-old woman had HAs in relation to most of her seizures. They started on the day before major or minor seizures, were right fronto-centro-temporal, remained in the same location, had a throbbing or pressure character, and got worse on physical activity. They lasted up to 12 hours and were accompanied by nausea, vomiting, and photo- and phonophobia. Both conditions started at the same age. HA were severe with a VAS of 9.6, and she always used one

TABLE 59-2
Surgery and Follow-up Data on Seizures and PreHA in Eleven Operated Patients

#	SURGERY	PATHOLOGY	FOLLOW-UP AFTER SURGERY (MO)	SEIZURE OUTCOME (ENGEL'S CLASS)	HA OUTCOME
1	R C resection	FCD	85	Class 2: Rare ictal dysarthria and L arm numbness, no GTCS	PreHA and PostHA with migraine-like features without aura (as before surgery)
2	R ATR	H atr+gliosis	93	1a	No HA
3	R ATR	H atr+gliosis	93	1a	No PreHA, Inter HA (as before surgery)
4	R SAH	H gliosis	96	1a	No PreHA, Inter HA
5	L ATR	H atr+gliosis	78	1a	N o HA
6	L SAH	H gliosis	85	1a for 74 months, 3 CPS over last year	No PreHA, Inter HA
7	L ATR	Normal H, neocortical gliosis	84	2 (1–2 "absences" per year)	No HA
8	R SAH	H atr+gliosis	96	1b	No PreHA, Inter HA
9	R SAH	H atr+gliosis	88	1a	No HA
10	VNS	—	48	4	No PreHA, PostHA and InterHA (as before surgery)
11	R SAH	H atr+gliosis	84	1a	No HA

C = Central, mo = months, L = left, R = right, H = hippocampus, atr = atrophy, ATR = anterior temporal resection, SAH = selective amygdalo-hippocampectomy, VNS = vagal nerve stimulation, HA = headache, PreHA = preictal HA, PostHA = postictal HA, InterHA = interictal HA, FCD = focal cortical dysplasia, CPS = complex partial seizures, GTCS = generalized tonic-clonic seizures.

tablet of acetaminophen, stopped her activities, and went to bed. She also had interictal migraine attacks with visual, sensory, and vestibular auras since age 11. Her sister had migraine. EEG showed right temporal spikes. Her imaging and pathological findings were consistent with ipsilateral hippocampal sclerosis. She underwent right selective amygdalo-hippocampectomy with Engel class one seizure outcome at 24 months' follow-up, without any HA.

Postictal HA. Forty-four patients (44%) had PostHA. Duration was 1 to 12 hours in 19 patients and from 5 to more than 24 hours. Intensity of PostHA was moderate. Thirty-six (81%) patients used over-the-counter analgesics.

Lateralization and Location of HAs. In 29 of the 47 patients (62%) with peri-ictal HAs these were frontotemporal. They were ipsilateral to the epileptic focus in 27 of 30 (90%) patients with TLE and in only 2 of 17 (12%) of those with ETE. Lateralization of PreHA was ipsilateral to the epileptic focus in nine patients with TLE, contralateral in one with TLE and in one with frontal seizure onset.

Migrainous Quality. Twenty-five patients had peri-ictal migraine-like HAs without aura according to the diagnostic criteria of the ICHD-2 (13), except that in some patients duration was less than 4 hours. Eighteen patients had TLE and seven had ETE, including four with FLE and three with OLE. Four of 11 (36%) patients with PreHA had migraine, as did 21 of 44 (48%) with PostHA. Another two patients reported migraine with aura only in the interictal period. None of the patients were treated with triptans or any other specific antimigraine medication.

Pathologically Verified Group. We found adequate pathological diagnosis available in 59 of 68 patients who underwent surgery, and we compared the HA with the non-HA groups (Table 59-3). Of 37 TLE patients, 36 had hippocampal sclerosis (HS), and one had a glioma. There was no correlation between HS and HA: 20 had HAs and 16 did not. Of 22 ETE patients, 8 had focal cortical dysplasia (FCD) (5 with and 3 without HA), 5 had focal atrophy (3 with and 2 without HA), 4 had AVMs (3 with and 1 without HA), and one had a calcification and HA. One patient with an occipital glioma had HA. Three patients (1 with and 2 without HA) had normal

TABLE 59-3

Comparison between HA and nonHA Groups in Fifty-nine Pathologically Confirmed Patients of Sixty-eight Operated

VARIABLES	HA GROUP	NONHA GROUP
Pathology (*n* = 59)	(*n* = 34)	(*n* = 25)
HS	20 (59%)	16 (64%)
FCD	5 (15%)	3 (12%)
Glioma	1 (3%)	1 (4%)
AVM	3 (8.5%)	1 (4%)
Focal atrophy	3 (8.5%)	2 (8%)
Calcification	1 (3%)	—
Normal	1 (3%)	2 (8%)
Sz onset lateralization (*n* = 68)	(*n* = 43)	(*n* = 25)
R	22 (51%)	13 (52%)
L	21 (49%)	12 (48%)

HS = hippocampal sclerosis, FCD = focal cortical dysplasia, AVM = arteriovenous malformation, R = right, L = left.

tissue. The analysis of 59 pathologically verified patients did not show any significant difference in HA occurrence in relation to the lobar epileptogenic area: 29 of 46 (63%) in TLE, 6 of 9 (66%) in FLE, 5 of 7 (71%) in OLE, and 1 of 4 (25%) in parietal lobe epilepsy (PLE).

Other Head Sensations. Eighteen patients had, in addition, poorly localized and ill described HSens other than HAs: 5 as a prodrome, 9 in the preictal, 3 in the postictal, and 4 in the interictal phase. Most of the patients described their HSens as having a constant pressure quality. Intensity was low and duration was short. No clear lateralization to the seizure focus was found in this group of patients.

DISCUSSION

In our study of 100 patients with medically intractable partial epilepsy we found that 59 (59%) had recurrent HAs. Periictal HAs were reported by 47: either PreHA or PostHA. InterHAs were described by 31 patients. Most previous studies discussed PostHAs only, with a range of incidence from 37% to 51%. These results are similar to our findings of 44%. PostHA is the most frequent HA type associated with seizures.

Preictal Headache and Migraine

PreHAs have rarely been reported, and their characteristics have not been thoroughly studied. We found that 11 patients (11%) had PreHA (14). Little attention has been paid to PreHA lasting minutes to hours. A recent study of cerebral blood flow (CBF) in patients with TLE detected an increase several minutes before seizure onset (15). This increase in CBF may be related to changes in neuronal activity long before the obvious EEG or clinical seizure onset and may provoke HA through the trigeminovascular system causing the release of vasoactive sensory neuropeptides that increase the pain response. PreHA was a lateralizing preictal clinical symptom in patients with TLE, because it was ipsilateral to the seizure focus in nine of ten TLE patients. One patient with TLE and one with ETE had contralateral HA. A larger number of patients should be studied prospectively to confirm the lateralizing value of PreHA. In eight patients, PreHA continued into the postictal period. This may point to a similarity in the pathogenesis of both forms. All seven seizure-free patients stopped having PreHA, which again implies their pathogenic relationship. Five of these patients also stopped having the other HA types (postictal and interictal HA) they had preoperatively. It is possible that seizure freedom has a positive influence on any form of HA. This supports the theory of a unidirectional causal explanation in this small population, although it cannot be generalized to all patients with epilepsy and HA. Reduction of seizures after surgery may also stop HA as in one of our patients, although another patient with rare residual seizures still continued to have PreHA. Milder disease can probably modify PreHA in some patients. Seizure freedom may have a lasting effect on PreHA because, even after seizure recurrence, patient 6 (Table 59-2) did not have a return of PreHA. The patient who had a vagal stimulator continued to have postictal and interictal HA, but his PreHA stopped. Whether this is an effect of vagal stimulation or not remains unclear; her typical seizures remained unchanged. In addition, this may point to a dissociated pathophysiology between PreHA compared to postictal and interictal HA. There may be a link between migraine and seizures, at least in four of our patients with PreHA who had migrainous features. Individual susceptibility for activation of this system could explain why only some patients with partial epilepsy have PIHA. Recognizing the significance of PIHA may be valuable in seizure interruption using sensory stimulation or biofeedback.

Interictal Headache

The rate of unclassifiable HA in the InterHA group was high: 29 of 31 patients (94%). In the majority it was mostly a sensation of pressure or throbbing (24 and 14 patients, respectively), either unilaterally or bilaterally and had insufficient features to fulfill the ICHD-2 criteria of migraine or tension HA. They were also not of any other primary HA type. Nevertheless, 80%

of patients with unclassifiable HA used medications and therefore these may be considered to be clinically significant.

Migraine-like Headache

Migrainous HAs occurred in 27% of our total population and in 46% of patients with recurrent HAs. Of our eleven patients with PreHA four had migrainous HA. In other studies the frequency of migrainous HAs in epilepsy patients was similar to the rate we found. Some studies reported lower or higher numbers and this may have been related to methodological issues.

Prevalence and Lateralization of HAs and Seizures

The frequency of occurrence of HAs in patients with seizures was typically high and predictable in both PreHA (75% of attacks) and PostHA, where it occurred in 75–100% of attacks in 32 of 44 patients. Most HAs were frontotemporal. The consistent lateralization in individual patients was striking. Only 18 of 44 who had PostHA had bilateral HAs; the others described them as strictly unilateral. It seems that seizure foci tended to induce consistently lateralized HAs. These were ipsilateral in 90% of patients with TLE and only in 12% of patients with ETE. Studying the exposed human cerebral cortex during epileptic seizures, Penfield and Jasper (16) observed widespread vasodilation and reactive hyperemia in the region of the discharging epileptic focus. As noted previously, studies of CBF in patients with TLE detected an increase several minutes before seizure onset (15) and during the seizure, potentially leading to release of vasoactive sensory neuropeptides that increase the pain response. Activation of dural trigeminovascular afferents and subsequent release of calcitonin gene–related peptide (CGRP) appear to be central to the development of migraine HA. This process induces an inflammatory reaction that triggers the production and secretion of additional agents such as substance P and neurokinin A that contribute to the "neurogenic inflammatory" environment. Increases in brain levels of CGRP, neurokinin A, and substance P were reported in rats after kainic acid–induced and electroconvulsive seizures in various areas including the hippocampus. Neuropeptides may increase during seizures associated with HA, although there have been no studies reporting a buildup of these inflammatory agents. This buildup continuing after seizures may explain the increased intensity of postictal HA compared to PreHA in our eight patients. No direct evidence exists in humans. It may be worthwhile to measure blood flow and neuropeptides in the peri-ictal state in patients with migraine versus other HA and nonHA groups.

Intensity and Treatment

The intensity of PostHA was comparable with that of PreHA (6.7 and 7.1 cm on the VAS), but more patients used analgesics postictally (81% vs. 27% of PreHA patients). These medications were over-the-counter and had not been specifically prescribed. Antimigraine preparations were not prescribed for patients with migrainous HAs. This is in agreement with other studies with a similar average intensity of the HAs. A third of the patients self-administered over-the-counter analgesics on a regular basis. Two-thirds reported taking medications occasionally. The higher number of patients taking analgesics for PostHA compared to PreHA probably reflects the longer duration of PostHAs and therefore their more disabling nature.

Effect of Epilepsy Syndrome and Pathology on Headache

We compared pathological findings in HA and non-HA groups. Hippocampal sclerosis, FCD, glioma, AVM, focal atrophy, and calcification were found in decreasing frequency in both groups without any significant differences in prevalence. Although the number of patients with AVM is small, the association between HAs and AVM is well known, and HA with or without migrainous features is a frequent presenting symptom of AVM. Epilepsy syndromes in HA and non-HA groups are shown in Table 59-4. Although 37 of 60 (62%) patients with TLE had HA, 23 of 60 (38%) did not. It appears that in patients with TLE both PreHA and PostHA may have lateralizing value. We are not aware of any other studies of epileptogenic pathology with correlation to headache.

Epileptic Syndromes Associated with Migraine in Adults

Andermann and Lugaresi (17) have emphasized several epileptic syndromes associated with migraine. Some of these are pediatric, such as rolandic epilepsy,

TABLE 59-4
Correlation of HA and Epileptic Localization

EPILEPSY TYPE (n = 100)	HA GROUP (n = 59)	NONHA GROUP (n = 41)
TLE	37 (63%)	23 (56%)
FCLE	14 (24%)	12 (29%)
OLE	6 (10%)	2 (5%)
PLE	2 (3%)	4 (10%)

TLE = temporal lobe epilepsy, FCLE = frontocentral lobe epilepsy, OLE = occipital lobe epilepsy, PLE = parietal lobe epilepsy.

which is associated with migraine in both patients and relatives (18). Further documentation of this association would be welcome.

Epileptic attacks may be induced by a migraine aura ("migralepsy"). The ICHD-2 mentions "migralepsy" in the comment, defining it as a seizure occurring immediately after a migrainous aura and followed by the headache phase (13). It is rare, given the high prevalence of both migraine and epilepsy, and only a few documented cases have been published (19). No specific subcategory has been assigned to "migralepsy". A migrainous aura may activate seizures in susceptible cortex, as do many other precipitating factors. Some of the cases may represent occipital seizures with visual auras and headache. "Migralepsy" is a condition different from PreHA, which starts with headache (at times with migrainous features) lasting minutes to hours and only later occurrence of seizures. Understanding of both conditions is still very limited.

Epilepsy with Seizures No Longer Triggered by Migrainous Aura

Patients who initially have a seizure following a migrainous aura may develop seizures independent of such a trigger. There is, in such rare cases, evidence for temporal foci, possibly due to secondary epileptogenesis (21).

Migraine and Brain Infarction

Epilepsy may also be due to gross cerebral lesions caused by migraine (brain infarction). Brain infarcts have long been known to be associated with migraine, particularly migraine with aura. Neuroimaging studies showed different locations and types of migrainous infarcts. Many patients had occipital infarcts, but single and multiple infarcts of any size and location have been reported. One recent study showed that most lesions were located in the cerebellum, often multiple, and were round or oval shaped, with a mean size of 7 mm. The majority (88%) of infratentorial infarct-like lesions had a vascular border zone in the cerebellum. Brain infarcts were detected far more often than expected in migraine patients, were most pronounced in migraine with aura, and in the majority were clinically silent. Cerebellar infarctions may not be directly associated with seizures, as compared with supratentorial lesions. This issue also requires further clarification.

Malignant Migraine Related to Mitochondrial Encephalomyopathies and CADASIL

Ischemic stroke and migraine with aura are major features of three syndromes characterized by chronic alterations of the vessel wall of small arteries (20): mitochondrial myopathy, encephalopathy, lactic acidosis, and stroke (MELAS), mitochondrial encephalomyopathy with ragged red fibers (MERRF), and cerebral autosomal dominant arteriopathy with subcortical infarcts and leucoencephalopathy (CADASIL). Symptoms of MELAS may significantly overlap with MERRF. Migraine as a part of MELAS syndrome, associated with mitochondrial DNA mutations, raises the possibility that mitochondrial dysfunction could play a role in migrainous headache and stroke. Impairment of mitochondrial function has recently been observed in the seizure focus of human and experimental epilepsy. The broad variety of mutations of mitochondrial DNA that lead to the inhibition of the mitochondrial respiratory chain or directly of mitochondrial adenosine triphosphate synthesis in epileptogenic areas of the human brain has been associated with epileptic phenotypes. Because mitochondrial oxidative phosphorylation provides the major source of adenosine triphosphate in neurons, and mitochondria participate in cellular Ca^{2+} homeostasis, they can modulate neuronal excitability and synaptic transmission, which are important in both migraine and seizures. Furthermore, mitochondria are intimately involved in pathways leading to the neuronal cell death characteristic of the areas of epileptogenesis.

CADASIL

CADASIL is an autosomal dominant disease of vascular and smooth muscle cells that is due to Notch-3 mutations and is mostly characterized by leukoencephalopathy, small deep infarcts, and subcortical dementia. Migraine with aura is present in one-third of patients, and it is typically the first symptom of the disease, presenting about 15 years before the first ischemic stroke. There is a high rate of atypical attacks, with prolonged aura or with acute-onset aura without HA. Ten percent of patients have a history of epileptic seizures. The MRIs of patients with CADASIL show striking white-matter abnormalities and, later in the disease, small subcortical infarctions. These abnormalities must not be interpreted as migraine-related white-matter abnormalities. The mechanisms underlying migraine in these chronic small-artery diseases affecting the brain are not yet defined. In patients with CADASIL, MA is not a consequence of the subcortical infarcts that occur 10–20 years after migraine onset. One hypothesis is that migraine directly relates to dysfunction of smooth muscle cells of meningeal and cortical vessels, triggering spreading depression. An alternative explanation suggests that mutation-induced cells signaling abnormalities might extend and reach neurons, and hyperexcitability may result, expressing as spreading depression or seizures. Presentation of CADASIL with migraine is typical, although onset with seizures may also occur.

TIME RELATION OF MIGRAINE AND SEIZURES

ICHD-2 recognizes ictal (hemicrania epileptica) and post-ictal HA, and both may have features of migraine (12). The diagnosis of "hemicrania epileptica" requires the onset of headache and epileptiform discharges on EEG to be synchronous. PostHA is a well-described recognized entity and occurs commonly after both partial and generalized seizures and apparently is the most frequent peri-ictal type of HA. It is common in patients with and without a family history of migraine.

CONCLUSION

There is a clear association between epilepsy and HA including migraine with and without aura. This is apparent for different types of epilepsy: localization related and generalized, TLE and ETE. HA is probably underrecognized and underreported and insufficient attention is paid to it by physicians. It adds significantly to the burden of epilepsy. PreHA and even prodromal HA may be related to the epileptic discharge and may provide valuable, although not absolute, lateralizing information in TLE. The mechanism of activation of migraine by seizures remains uncertain. Epilepsy and migraine are chronic disorders with increased hyperexcitability and are connected by their symptom profiles, comorbidity, and response to treatment. The presence of one disorder increases the probability that the other may also be present. Migraine in patients with epilepsy and epilepsy in migraine sufferers are expected to occur twice as commonly as in the general population. There has been significant progress in the classification, epidemiology, and identification of risk factors and triggers, pathophysiology, and treatment of both disorders. Each area benefits from research and improved understanding of the other. Shared mechanisms offer the potential for further therapeutic advances.

References

1. Ottman R, Lipton RB. Is the comorbidity of epilepsy and migraine due to a shared genetic susceptibility? *Neurology* 1996; 47:918–924.
2. Haut SR, Bigal ME, Lipton RB. Chronic disorders with episodic manifestations: focus on epilepsy and migraine. *Lancet Neurol* 2006; 5:148–157.
3. Ayata C, Jin H, Kudo C, Dalkara T, et al. Suppression of cortical spreading depression in migraine prophylaxis. *Ann Neurol* 2006; 59:652–661.
4. Bolay H, Reuter U, Dunn AK, Huang Z, et al. Intrinsic brain activity triggers trigeminal meningeal afferents in a migraine model. *Nat Med* 2002; 8:136–142.
5. Geraud G, Denuelle M, Fabre N, et al. Positron emission tomographic studies of migraine. *Rev Neurol (Paris)* 2005; 161:666–670.
6. Schon F, Blau JN. Post-epileptic headache and migraine. *J Neurol Neurosurg Psychiatry* 1987; 50:1148–1152.
7. Schachter SC, Richman K, Loder E, Beluk S. Self-reported characteristics of postictal headaches. *J Epilepsy* 1995; 8:41–43.
8. D'Alessandro R, Sacquegna T, Pazzaglia P, Lugaresi E. Headache after partial complex seizures. In: Andermann F, Lugaresi E, eds. *Migraine and Epilepsy.* Boston, MA: Butterworth-Heinemann, 1987:273–278.
9. Bernasconi A, Andermann F, Bernasconi N, Reutens DC, et al. Lateralizing value of peri-ictal headache: a study of 100 patients with partial epilepsy. *Neurology* 2001; 56:130–132.
10. Ito M, Adachi N, Nakamura F, et al. Characteristics of postictal headache in patients with partial epilepsy. *Cephalalgia* 2004; 24:23–28.
11. Leniger T, Isbruch K, von den Driesch S, Diener HC, et al. Seizure-associated headache in epilepsy. *Epilepsia* 2001; 42:1176–1179.
12. Yankovsky AE, Andermann F, Bernasconi A. Characteristics of headache associated with intractable partial epilepsy. *Epilepsia* 2005; 46:1241–1245.
13. Headache Classification Subcommittee of the International Headache Society. The International Classification of Headache Disorders, 2nd edition. *Cephalalgia* 2004; 24(Suppl):1–160.
14. Yankovsky AE, Andermann F, Mercho S, Dubeau F, et al. Preictal headache in partial epilepsy. *Neurology* 2005; 65:1979–1981.
15. Baumgartner C, Serles W, Leutmezer F, et al. Preictal SPECT in temporal lobe epilepsy: regional cerebral blood flow is increased prior to electroencephalography-seizure onset. *J Nucl Med* 1998; 39:978–982.
16. Penfield W, Jasper HH. Epilepsy and the functional anatomy of the human brain. Boston, MA: Little, Brown, 1954.
17. Andermann F, Lugaresi E., eds. *Migraine and epilepsy.* Boston, MA: Butterworth-Heinemann, 1987.
18. Bladin PF. The association of benign rolandic epilepsy with migraine. In: Andermann F, Lugaresi E, eds. *Migraine and Epilepsy.* Boston, MA: Butterworth-Heinemann, 1987:145–152.
19. Marks DA, Ehrenberg BL. Migraine-related seizures in adults with epilepsy, with EEG correlation. *Neurology* 1993; 43:2476–2483.
20. Andermann F. Clinical features of migraine-epilepsy syndromes. In: Andermann F, Lugaresi E, eds. *Migraine and Epilepsy.* Boston, MA: Butterworth-Heinemann, 1987:18–21.

60 Brain Tumors in Children

Maria Augusta Montenegro
Marilisa M. Guerreiro

Normal child behavior depends on the child's age, personality, family expectations, and health. Children confronted with a chronic, life-threatening illness tend to present with severe stress and have more behavioral and emotional problems.

Having a child with a brain tumor is probably one of the most frightening situations a family can experience. When a brain tumor is associated with seizures, the impact on the life of the child is even worse. The psychologic impact of this diagnosis can produce a series of behavior abnormalities. However, the behavioral disturbances presented by children with epilepsy due to brain tumors are also a consequence of the neoplastic lesion itself. Brain tumors are the most common solid neoplasm in children and the second most common category of pediatric tumors after leukemia. Supratentorial lesions are more common in the first 2 years of life, as opposed to infratentorial tumors, which are more common in children between 3 and 11 years old.

The clinical presentation of brain tumors in childhood varies according to the child's age. Small children present with macrocrania, and older children present with increased intracranial pressure and focal neurologic signs. Behavioral changes may occur but are not the most common feature of brain tumors in childhood. When a brain tumor is identified in a child with behavioral abnormalities, the possibility of a link between the two conditions should be considered (1).

Brain tumors should always be considered as a possible diagnosis in a child with seizures. The diagnosis of a brain tumor is performed by magnetic resonance imaging (MRI) or computed tomography (CT). Although MRI is usually the method of choice for the evaluation of most brain tumors, CT should also be performed in all patients. The CT images are an excellent tool to identify calcifications and bone remodeling or erosion. Moreover, the pattern of tumor density shown by CT can be used together with the signal intensity shown by MRI to establish a preliminary histological diagnosis (2).

BRAIN TUMORS AND BEHAVIOR

Epilepsy, especially temporal lobe epilepsy (TLE), is frequently associated with serious behavioral problems. Behavioral disorders such as hyperactivity and aggressiveness are more frequent in children with TLE (3). For the families of these children, behavioral improvement is as important as seizure control.

Abnormal behavior associated with brain tumors in childhood can be related to the patient's seizures or can appear after epilepsy surgery. Although uncommon, violent acts may also result directly from seizures, either as ictal or postictal behavior abnormalities.

Postictal violence is most commonly characterized by resistive behavior secondary to attempts at restraint (4). Postictal violence most often occurs because (due to the postictal confusion) patients usually misinterpret the caretaker's attempt to protect them and hence they become aggressive. However, postictal violent acts due to postictal psychosis may also occur.

Aggressive acts, rage, confusion, and spitting have been described in children with TLE due to ganglioglioma or meningioma. After resection, these events were controlled (1, 5, 6). Temporal lobe tumors may be a rare cause of severe behavioral abnormalities in children. For this subgroup of patients, neurosurgical intervention can be curative (1).

The pathophysiology of behavioral abnormalities associated with brain tumors and epilepsy remains unknown. It is hypothesized that dysfunction of the amygdala could be one of the causes responsible for the aggressive behavior; however, other structures—such as the periaqueductal gray matter, the hypothalamus, or the frontal lobes—are probably also involved. Lesions of both the right and the left hemispheres may be associated with abnormal behavior; however, it seems that left temporal lobe dysfunction is more commonly associated with abnormal behavior (7).

Although there are reports of behavior improvement after epilepsy surgery, the behavioral disturbances may persist. Moreover, it is possible that severe behavior abnormalities may appear only after epilepsy surgery. This is an issue that should always be explained to the child's family, because it is common for the family to expect that the epilepsy surgery will not only control the seizures but also improve behavior.

In our institution, two patients developed behavior abnormalities after epilepsy surgery and complete seizure control (8). Both patients had a temporal lobe ganglioglioma (Figure 60-1). This finding is in keeping with another series published by Andermann et al. (9),

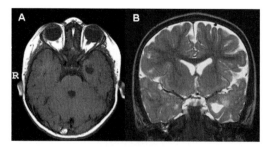

FIGURE 60-1

(A) Axial T1 and (B) coronal T1 images showing a left temporal lobe ganglioglioma.

in which delirium, depressive, paranoid, and schizophrenic symptoms occurred in children and adults after epilepsy surgery for ganglioglioma or dysembryoplastic neuroepithelial tumor (DNT) (Table 60-1). These psychiatric symptoms, presenting postoperatively in these patients, are difficult to classify within precise psychiatric categories.

Ganglioglioma is a benign tumor mainly located in the temporal lobe. Children with ganglioglioma often present with refractory seizures. Focal neurologic deficits and signs of increased intracranial pressure are unusual. Although the imaging appearance of this lesion is nonspecific, MRI usually shows a well-circumscribed lesion located peripherally, usually associated with cystic areas and calcification. Histologically these neoplasms are benign lesions with neuronal cells and astrocytic cells (Figure 60-2).

Dysembryoplastic neuroepithelial tumor is a benign tumor almost always associated with focal seizures. Histologically these neoplasms are benign, intracortical lesions composed of intermixed oligodendrocyte-like, astrocytic, and mature ganglion elements.

Both ganglioglioma and DNT can be associated with focal cortical dysplasia. Malignant changes in ganglioglioma and DNT are uncommon, and surgical prognosis is excellent. Szabó et al. (10) reported that behavioral disturbances in children might worsen after temporal lobectomy in patients with focal cortical dysplasia. The association between focal cortical dysplasia and developmental tumors is well established, and these tumors are classified as a type of malformation of cortical development (11).

One might speculate that the worsening of behavioral disturbances after epilepsy surgery and complete seizure control is due to so-called forced normalization (9, 12, 13). The daily epileptiform discharges and frequent seizures would make the patient more somnolent and calm, which could mask behavioral disturbances. Therefore, seizure control would enable the appearance of the behavioral abnormality.

Because only a few cases have been reported, we cannot conclude that patients with ganglioglioma are particularly prone to the development of behavioral abnormalities after epilepsy surgery. However, it is interesting to note that most patients were girls with left temporal lobe gangliogliomas. There is evidence that patients with a "foreign tissue" lesion that is surgically treated by temporal resection present with postoperative psychosis more often than patients who do not have these lesions (14).

Although there are organic explanations for behavioral worsening after epilepsy surgery, the psychologic aspects should not be neglected. Children with epilepsy have low self-esteem and increased psychiatric disturbances (15). It is possible that after epilepsy surgery and

TABLE 60-1

Patients with De Novo Behavioral Abnormalities after Epilepsy Surgery

AGE/GENDER	AGE AT FIRST SEIZURE	TYPE OF LESION	LOCALIZATION OF LESION
28/M#	10 yr	Ganglioglioma	Left temporal lobe
23/F#	3 yr	Ganglioglioma	Left temporal lobe
20/F#	14 mo	Ganglioglioma	Right temporal lobe
8/F#	2 yr	DNT	Right temporal lobe
18/F#	7	Ganglioglioma	Left sylvian area
27/F#	6 yr	Ganglioglioma	Left temporal lobe
2/F*	7 mo	Ganglioglioma	Left temporal lobe
6/F*	5 yr	Ganglioglioma	Left temporal lobe

#Andermann et al. (9); *Guimarães et al. (8).

seizure control, the family starts to pay more attention to behavior, which was not the most important concern before surgery.

There is not enough evidence to establish the relationship of ganglioglioma and postoperative psychosis; however, we recommend a careful preoperative psychiatric evaluation in patients with developmental lesions.

The management of behavioral disturbances associated with ganglioglioma resection may require antipsychotic drugs, such as risperidone. However, the prognosis is usually favorable, with behavioral improvement after a few months of treatment.

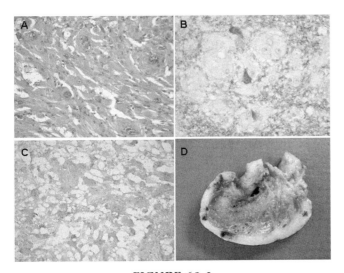

FIGURE 60-2

Ganglioglioma. (A) Hematoxylin-eosin; (B) immunohisto-chemistry: neuron-specific enolase; (C) immunohistochemistry: glial fibrillary acidic protein; (D) gross pathology. From the Department of Pathology, State University of Campinas (http://www.fcm.unicamp.br/departamentos/anatomia/neuro1.html). See color section following page 266.

BRAIN TUMORS AND COGNITION

In childhood, TLE is due to either hippocampal atrophy or lesions in the neocortical portion of the temporal lobe. Malformations of cortical development and tumors—such as DNT, astrocytoma, or ganglioglioma—are frequently associated with hippocampal atrophy (Figure 60-3).

Temporal lobe epilepsy in childhood has a wide range of clinical-electroencephalographic presentations. Children with TLE often have learning disabilities. A comprehensive neuropsychologic analysis (16) of children with TLE due to either hippocampal atrophy or neocortical lesions showed that although the IQs of these children were within normal limits, they had a lower cognitive performance. Moreover, they also presented with attention deficit; limited language performance with impairment in naming and verbal fluency; visuoperceptual and visuospatial deficits; and memory impairment in verbal learning, visual learning, verbal memory, and visual memory; delayed recall of verbal learning; and delayed recall for stories and recognition of stories. It is also interesting to note that these children had dysfunction of the frontal lobe characterized by abstract problem

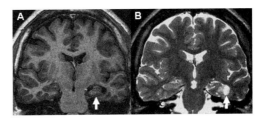

FIGURE 60-3

(A) Coronal T1 and (B) T2 images showing a ganglioglioma in the left temporal lobe associated with left hippocampal atrophy.

resolution impairment, planning deficit, perseveration, and lack of mental flexibility.

PROGNOSIS OF EPILEPSY ASSOCIATED WITH BRAIN TUMORS

The prognosis of epilepsy associated with brain tumors can be divided into two groups: children with malignant tumors and children with benign tumors. In the first group, the patient is often referred to an oncology center because of the severity of the disease. The child's clinical condition can deteriorate very quickly as a result of increased intracranial pressure. Therefore, treatment is aimed at the tumor itself, precluding a more detailed investigation of the epileptic manifestation. The prognosis of epilepsy has not been systematically evaluated because the emphasis is usually on the prognosis of the tumor itself.

However, when the child has a benign tumor, symptoms are usually slowly progressive. Moreover, children with low-grade tumors—gangliocytoma, ganglioglioma, DNT—will present with seizures as the only clinical manifestation associated with the neoplastic lesion. In this setting, seizures are frequently refractory to antiepileptic drug treatment. Epilepsy surgery is the treatment of choice, and the prognosis is related to the surgeon's ability to perform a complete resection of the tumor.

The most common causes of catastrophic epilepsy in children are focal malformations of cortical development and low-grade tumors. The chance of favorable seizure outcome after epilepsy surgery—that is, seizure freedom—is estimated at 60% to 65% for infants, 59% to 67% for children, and 69% for adolescents, compared

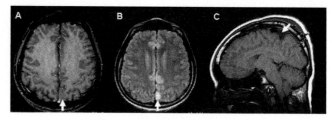

FIGURE 60-4

(A) Axial T1 and (B) FLAIR images showing a small gangliocytoma in the left parietal region. (C) After lesion resection the patient became seizure free (Engle 1). Follow-up, 3 years.

to 64% for adults. However, some subgroups of patients have higher percentages of seizure-free outcomes, especially those with hippocampal sclerosis or a low-grade tumor (17, 18).

In our experience, children with refractory epilepsy due to low-grade tumors have an excellent surgical outcome. As opposed to focal cortical dysplasia, the margin between the low-grade tumor and normal brain tissue is usually well demarcated, which enables a complete resection during surgery (Figure 60-4). Seizure freedom provides a fantastic improvement of the quality of life of these patients, which often is associated with improvement of the behavioral problems associated with refractory epilepsy, such as low self-esteem.

It is important to note that this dramatic improvement in behavior is much more frequently seen in children. Adults who become seizure free after epilepsy surgery may sometimes have difficulty adapting to "life without seizures."

References

1. Nakaji P, Meltzer HS, Singel SA, Alksne JF. Improvement of aggressive and antisocial behavior after resection of temporal lobe tumors. *Pediatrics* 2003; 112:e430–e433.
2. Tortori-Donati P, Rossi A, Biancheri R, Garrè L, et al. Brain tumors. In: Tortori-Donati P, ed. *Pediatric Neuroradiology: Brain.* Berlin: Springer-Verlag, 2005:329–436.
3. Franzon RC, Montenegro MA, Guimarães CA, Guerreiro CA, et al. Clinical, electroencephalographic, and behavioral features of temporal lobe epilepsy in childhood. *J Child Neurol* 2004; 19:418–423.
4. Delgado-Escueta AV, Mattson RH, King L, et al. The nature of aggression during epileptic seizures. *N Engl J Med* 1981; 305:711–716.
5. Kaplan PW, Kerr DA, Olivi A. Ictus expectoratus: a sign of complex partial seizures usually of non-dominant temporal lobe origin. *Seizure* 1999; 8:480–484.
6. Caplan R, Comair Y, Shewmon DA, Jackson L, et al. Intractable seizures, compulsions, and coprolalia: a pediatric case study. *J Neuropsychiatry Clin Neurosci* 1992; 4:315–319.
7. van Elst LT, Woermann FG, Lemieux L, Thompson PJ, et al. Affective aggression in patients with temporal lobe epilepsy: a quantitative MRI study of the amygdala. *Brain* 2000; 123:234–243.
8. Guimarães CA, Franzon RC, Souza EA, Schmutzler KM, et al. Abnormal behavior in children with temporal lobe epilepsy and ganglioglioma. *Epilepsy Behav* 2004; 5:788–791.
9. Andermann LF, Savard G, Meencke HJ, McLachlan R, et al. Psychosis after resection of ganglioglioma or DNET: evidence for an association. *Epilepsia* 1999; 4:83–87.
10. Szabo CA, Wyllie E, Dolske M, Stanford LD, et al. Epilepsy surgery in children with pervasive developmental disorder. *Pediatr Neurol* 1999; 20:349–353.
11. Barkovich AJ, Kuzniecky RI, Jackson GD, Guerrini R, et al. A developmental and genetic classification for malformations of cortical development. *Neurology* 2005; 65:1873–1887.
12. Taylor DC, Falconer MD. Clinical, socioeconomic, and psychological changes after temporal lobectomy for epilepsy. *Br J Psychiatry* 1968; 114:1247–1261.
13. Falconer MD, Taylor DC. Surgical treatment of drug-resistant epilepsy due to mesial temporal temporal sclerosis. *Arch Neurol* 1968; 19:353–361.
14. Taylor DC. Factors influencing the occurrence of schizophrenia-like psychosis in patients with temporal lobe epilepsy. *Psychol Med* 1975; 5:249–254.
15. Hermann BP, Austin J. Psycholgical status of children with epilepsy and the effects of epilepsy surgery. In: Wyllie E, ed. *The Treatment of Epilepsy: Principles and Practice.* Philadelphia: Lea & Febiger, 1993:1141–1148.
16. Guimarães CA, Li LM, Rzezak P, Fuentes D, et al. Temporal lobe epilepsy in childhood: comprehensive neuropsychological assessment. *J Child Neurol*, in press.
17. Saneto RP, Wyllie E. Epilepsy surgery in infancy. *Semin Pediatr Neurol* 2000; 7: 187–193.
18. Wyllie E. Surgical treatment of epilepsy in pediatric patients. *Can J Neurol Sci* 2000; 27:106–110.

61 Brain Tumors in Adults

Hermann Stefan

rain tumors in adults were discussed by Jackson in 1873 (1). In the early stages of the development of neurosurgery before imaging was available, seizures were a very important hint for the localization of an intracranial space-occupying process. Improved techniques for tumor and epilepsy therapy nowadays have led to long-term survival and treatment of many patients, often over 10–20 years. Progress in the diagnosis and treatment of brain tumors and epilepsy requires knowledge of special treatment options to improve quality of life during long-term treatment.

EPILEPTOGENESIS

Different mechanisms have been proposed to account for epileptogenesis in patients with brain tumors. Denervation hypersensitivity, caused by isolation of cortex from inhibitory subcortical influences, can result in epileptic activity (2). Disturbance of excitatory and inhibitory transmitter balance by changes of GABA and glutamate concentrations can be another factor (3–5). Brain tissue adjacent to a tumor often is alkaline, with increased expression of gap junction proteins. Consequently, hemosiderin and ischemic changes during disturbances of perfusion, as well as bleedings in the tumor or the neighborhood of the tumor, are another cause for the development of focal epilepsy. Hemosiderin can also promote epileptogenesis by perilesional gliosis but also by lipid peroxidase efficacy and neurotransmitter changes (6, 7). Finally, immunologic mechanisms and angiogenesis as well as invasion (8, 9) are other potential factors leading to the development of epilepsy.

EPIDEMIOLOGY

Brain tumors are recognized as the cause of seizures in 1–5% of patients with epilepsy. Whereas brain tumors in patients with seizures were found in a lower number by computed tomography (CT) investigations, nowadays approximately 35% or more are detected by magnetic resonance imaging (MRI). Most such tumors are supratentorial (22–68%) and only 6% are infratentorial. Concerning the different types of brain tumors, dysembryoplastic neuroepithelial tumors (DNET) are most often correlated with epilepsy (nearly 100%). Slowly growing tumors such as oligodendrogliomas (80%), astrocytomas (70%), and gangliogliomas (10–15%) are more frequently associated with epilepsy than are rapidly growing tumors such as glioblastomas (37%) and metastases (20%) (10).

DIAGNOSIS

Cerebral CT is not usually sufficient to detect small tumors, whereas MRI is nearly 100% sensitive but not predictive for the histologic type of tumor. The main problem is that nonexperts often reach conclusions on rather insufficient images. As a consequence, tumors are not recognized or tumors are wrongly diagnosed as nontumoral lesions. A comparison of MRI imaging recording and analysis by experts and nonexperts showed that nonexperts interpreted 61% of MRIs as normal, whereas experts interpreted only 22% as normal. Further, tumors were diagnosed by nonexperts using standard MRI recording techniques in approximately 8% of cases, whereas specific MRI recordings analyzed by experts showed tumors in more than 20% (11).

TREATMENT

The treatment of patients with tumors and epilepsy can be differentiated into the following categories:

1. Counseling of patients
2. Drug treatment
3. Surgery, radiation, or chemotherapy

Counseling is very important and should address life expectancy, seizure control, and psychologic and behavioral abnormalities. It is not within the scope of this chapter to discuss therapeutic strategies for different types of tumors with regard to radiation or chemotherapy, for example in patients with low-grade gliomas and seizures, because an individual consensus about the therapeutic strategy for each patient must be obtained. In each case one must decide whether to wait with treatment, to carry out radical tumor excision, to perform incomplete resections (for example, in elderly patients), to perform resections only, or to use radiation or chemotherapy.

Drug Treatment with Anticonvulsants

Seizure control most often is obtained by means of antiepileptic drug (AED) treatment. The most frequent routine strategy is to use phenytoin, carbamazepine, or even phenobarbital. This selection of AEDs is not without problems in tumor patients. Forty-five percent of patients with tumors suffer from epileptic seizures, and despite treatment with anticonvulsant drugs, nearly three-quarters have repeated seizures. In patients who are seizure free after tumor resection, long-term treatment is not recommended (12), whereas in patients with multiple or hemorrhagic tumors or increased intracranial pressure, long-term treatment can be worthwhile. In patients with tumoral epilepsy treated by phenytoin or carbamazepine,

25% exhibit exanthema (12). Other complications of drug treatments are encephalopathies or hematologic changes. The incidence of exanthema can be increased during steroid reduction after radiotherapy (13).

A major problem is the interaction of AEDs and chemotherapeutic drugs. The efficacy of AEDs can be decreased by chemotherapeutic drugs such as beta-chloro-nitrosourea (BCNU or carmustine), cisplatinum, carboplatinum, and taxol. This can be due to either a reduction of serum concentrations of AEDs or a decrease in absorption. Vincristine, for example, increases the clearance of carbamazepine and phenytoin by about 65% and shortens the half-life time by about 35% (14, 15).

Conversely, enzyme inducers such as phenytoin, carbamazepine, and phenobarbital decrease the bioavailability of dexamethasone and other chemotherapeutic drugs (16). In these instances, higher dosages of AEDs are often given because the serum concentration of the AED is lowered. However, this could lead to a further increase of the total serum concentration of the AED as well as its free fractions, and thus to intoxication and sometimes also, paradoxically, to an increase of seizure frequency. Thus, insufficient control of seizures and the emergence of psychologic symptoms may be wrongly interpreted as signs of tumor progression. Important interactions of the different AEDs and chemotherapeutic drugs are listed in the study by Vecht et al. (17). Another problem may arise because of the development of pharmacoresistance against AEDs. Carbamazepine, phenytoin, and other AEDs are substrates for multidrug-transporter (MDT) P-glycoprotein and multidrug-resistant–associated proteins (18, 19).

COGNITIVE DISTURBANCES AND DEPRESSION

In patients with epilepsy caused by low-grade gliomas, cognitive deficits are prevalent. These cognitive impairments may be due to the effects of the tumor itself, seizures, psychologic stress, chemotherapy, radiotherapy, and AEDs on brain function.

The lateralization and localization of the tumor, especially when situated in the temporal or frontal lobes, may cause specific and severe cognitive and emotional dysfunctions. Radiotherapy (RT) is often linked to cognitive impairment, but a recent study suggests that standard focal RT with fractional doses of less than 2 Gy is not generally associated with an increased risk of cognitive deficits, whereas higher fractional doses are likely to result in cognitive disability (20). The investigators found that the presence and severity of seizures or the use of AEDs was more strongly associated with cognitive deficits than was RT. Depression occurs frequently in patients with epilepsy and brain tumors, suggesting that it can be a specific sequela of both conditions as well as of therapeutic interventions.

In a simplified view, AEDs can be differentiated into GABAergic drugs (phenobarbital, primidone, benzodiazepines, valproate, vigabatrin, tiagabine, and gabapentin), which are more sedative, antimanic, and anxiolytic, and antiglutamatergic drugs (lamotrigine), which are antidepressant (21). AEDs are often used in high dosages in patients with tumoral epilepsy. Phenobarbital is not only sedating but also depressogenic. Sedation from benzodiazepines can also increase cognitive disturbances. Other negative effects on cognitive function can be caused by high dosages of carbamazepine, phenytoin, or topiramate. In tumoral epilepsy, high dosages of AEDs are used frequently in polytherapy with psychotropic medications. Not infrequently this practice leads to cognitive impairments, though cognitive adverse events are seen less frequently with lamotrigine than with carbamazepine (22).

Depressive symptoms are observed in 28% of patients with tumoral epilepsy who are treated with AEDs (23). Cognitive impairment and affective disorders may reduce the patient's capacity for compliance. Therefore a once daily or twice daily application of AEDs is recommended. An ideal AED for treatment of tumor patients should be effective in focal and secondary generalized seizures, should be simple to use (once or twice daily dose), should have no interactions, should be mood stabilizing, and ideally should also have an anticarcinogenic mechanism of action. Because of the rather high comorbidity of brain tumors, depression, and cognitive disturbance, newer anticonvulsants that are mood stabilizing or even antidepressant should be used in preference to first-generation AEDs. However, prospective studies using newer AEDs in tumoral epilepsy are rare. Wagner et al. (24) reported the use of levetiracetam in 26 patients who were not seizure-free during treatment with other AEDs, and 50% or greater seizure reduction control could be obtained by levetiracetam in 65% of the patients. Tiredness or dizziness was observed in 35%.

The influence of AEDs on seizure control, cognitive function, and quality of life in patients with low-grade glioma and epilepsy was investigated by Klein et al. (25). A total of 156 patients without clinical or radiological signs for recurrent tumor were compared with a control group; 50% of those patients taking AEDs were seizure-free. The patients with glioma had significantly worse information–processing speed and psychomotor and attentional functions, as well as verbal and visual memory and quality of life. These reductions in cognitive function were primarily related to AED therapy, whereas the decrease of quality of life was related most often to lack of seizure control.

Patients with low-grade gliomas are often impaired by neuropsychologic problems related to the severity of the epilepsy, the intensity of the drug treatment or other treatments such as chemotherapy or radiation. Therefore,

in patients with tumoral epilepsies, AEDs should be selected that not only control seizures but also do not cause or exacerbate cognitive, emotional, and other behavioral problems.

SURGERY

A complete tumor resection including the epileptogenic cortex leads to complete seizure control in up to 90% of the patients (26–29). However, a complete resection is not always possible because of localizations or extent of tumors. Seizure control can nonetheless be obtained if a critical tumor mass can be resected and, in addition, no multifocal secondary epileptogenic areas exist. Therefore, in patients with tumors and epilepsy, in addition to the localization of the tumor, the localization of uni- or multifocal epileptogenic areas is important. The spatial relation of the lesions to epileptogenic seizure generators, in our experience, is close in the case of oligodendrogliomas or gangliogliomas. DNET cavernomas and tuberogliosis show more variable conditions. Long-term outcome studies in patients with tumoral epilepsies showed that an early surgery is recommended. Follow-up studies with a mean of 8 years demonstrated good seizure control (Engel I in 82%, Engel II in 3%, Engel III in 13%, Engel IV in 5%); 41% of the patients were seizure-free without AEDs (some patients had recurrent seizures after 4 years). Predictors for a good prognosis were focal electroencephalographic (EEG) activity, no dual pathology, and no astrocytoma. With regard to the prognosis of astrocytoma it could be shown that a subtype, isomorphic long-time epilepsy-associated astrocytoma (LEA) exists, which has a more favorable survival time (30). The differentiation is possible by histochemical investigation (31).

New diagnostic devices permit a better differentiation of epileptogenic zones and the border of the tumor as well as control of the resection volume (4). A functionality-preserving neuronavigation guide technique also offers new possibilities for more precise excision (32). In addition to conventional electrophysiological techniques such as EEG and intraoperative electrocorticography, magnetoencephalography (MEG) also plays an increasing role in the functional presurgical exploration of tumor epilepsy. Noninvasively and preoperatively, localization of epileptic foci and their spatial relation to functionally important areas that must be preserved during surgery can thereby be delineated. These new investigational techniques offer the chance to avoid functional deficits and to increase the number of patients with tumors and epilepsy who can safely undergo surgery. The resulting increase in survival time of patients with tumoral epilepsy leads to a new challenge in treatment: the recognition and avoidance and treatment of behavioral problems in patients with tumors and epilepsies.

References

1. Jackson JH. On the anatomical, physiological, and pathological investigation of the epilepsies. *West Riding Lunatic Asylum Medical Reports* 1873; 3:315–339.

2. Echlin F. The supersensitivity of chronically isolated cerebral cortex as a mechanism in focal epilepsy. *Electroencephalogr Clin Neurophysiol* 1959; 11:697–722.

3. Bateman DE, Hardy JA, McDermott JR, Parker DS, et al. Amino acid neurotransmitter levels in gliomas and their relationship to the incidence of epilepsy. *Neurol Res* 1988; 10:112–114.

4. Buchfelder M. Fahlbusch R, Ganslandt O, Stefan H, et al. Use of intraoperative magnetic resonance imaging in tailored temporal lobe surgeries for epilepsy. *Epilepsia* 2002; 43:864–873.

5. Raymond A, Halpin S, Alsynjari N. Dysembryoplastic neuroepithelial tumor. Features in 16 patients. *Brain* 1994; 117:461–475.

6. Bakay RAE, Harris AB. Neurotransmitter, receptor and biochemical changes in monkey cortical epileptic foci. *Brain Res* 1981; 206:387–404.

7. Kraemer DL, Awad IA. Vascular malformations and basic mechanisms. *Epilepsia* 1994; 35:30–43.

8. Proescholdt A, Brawanski A. Behandlungsstrategien in der Warteschleife. *NeuroTransmitter* 2004; 3:62–67.

9. Wiendl H, Mitsdoerffer M, Weller M. Hide-and-seek in the brain: a role for HLA-G mediating immune privilege for glioma cells. *Semin Cancer Biol* 2003; 13: 343–351.

10. White JC, Liu CT, Mixter WJ. Focal epilepsy: a statistical study of its causes and the results of surgical treatment. I. Epilepsy secondary to intracranial tumors. *N Engl J Med* 1984; 438:891–899.

11. Oertzen von J, Urbach H, Jungbluth S, Kurthen M, et al. Standard magnetic resonance imaging is inadequate for patients with refractory focal epilepsy. *J Neurol Neurosurg Psychiatry* 2002; 73:643–647.

12. Moots PL, Maciunas RJ, Eisert DR, Parker RA, et al. The course of seizure disorders in patients with malignant gliomas. *Arch Neurol* 1995; 52:717–724.

13. Delattre JY, Krol G, Thaler HT, Posner JB. Distribution of brain metastases. *Arch Neurol* 1988; 45:741–744.

14. Gilbar P, Brodribb T. Phenytoin and fluorouracil interaction. *Ann Pharmacother* 2001; 35:1367–1370.

15. Villikka K, Kivistö K, Mäenpää H, Loensuu H, et al. Cytochrome P450-inducing antiepileptics increase the clearance of vincristine in patients with brain tumors. *Clin Pharmacol Ther* 1999; 66:589–593.

16. Gattis W, May D. Possible interaction involving phenytoin, dexamethasone and antineoplastic agents. *Ann Pharmacother* 1996; 30:520–526.

17. Vecht C, Wagner G, Wilms E. Interactions between antiepileptic and chemotherapeutic drugs. *Lancet* 2003; 2:404–408.

18. Löscher W. Current status and future directions in the pharmacotherapy of epilepsy. *Trends Pharmacol Sci* 2002; 23:113–118.

19. Wang Y, Zhou D, Wang B, Li H, et al. A kindling model of pharmacoresistant temporal lobe epilepsy in Sprague-Fawley rats induced by coriaria lactone and its possible mechanism. *Epilepsia* 2003; 44:475–488.

20. Taphoorn M. Neurocognitive sequelae in the treatment of low-grade gliomas. *Semin Oncol* 2003; 30(6 Suppl 19):45–49.

21. Ketter T, Post R, Theodore W. Positive and negative psychiatric effects of antiepileptic drugs in patients with seizure disorders. *Neurology* 1999; 53(Suppl 2):53–67.

22. Gillham R, Kane K, Bryant-Comstock L. A double-blind comparison of lamotrigine and carbamazepine in newly diagnosed epilepsy with health-related quality of life as an outcome measure. *Seizure* 1996; 9:375–379.

23. Trimble M, Schmitz B. The neuropsychiatry of epilepsy. Cambridge, UK: Cambridge University Press, 2002.

24. Wagner GL, Wilms EB, van Donselaar CA, Vecht ChJ. Levetiracetam: preliminary experience in patients with primary brain tumors. *Seizure* 2003; 12:585–596.

25. Klein M, Engelberts NH, van der Ploeg HM, Kasteleijn-Nolst Trinite DG, et al. Epilepsy in low-grade gliomas: the impact on cognitive function and quality of life. *Ann Neurol* 2003; 54:514–520.

26. Blume WT, Girvin JP, Kaufmann JCE. Childhood brain tumors presenting as chronic, uncontrolled focal seizure disorders. *Ann Neurol* 1982; 12:538–541.

27. Boon PA, Williamson PD, Fried I, Spencer DD, et al. Intracranial, intraaxial, space-occupying lesions in patients with intractable partial seizures: an anatomoclinical, neurophysiological and surgical correlation. *Epilepsia* 1991; 32:467–476.

28. Britton JW, Cascino GD, Sharbrough FW, Kelly PJ. Low-grade glial neoplasms and intractable partial epilepsy: efficacy of surgical treatment. *Epilepsia* 1994; 35:1130–1135.

29. Wyllie E, Lüders H, Morris HH. Clinical outcome after complete or partial resection for intractable epilepsy. *Neurology* 1987; 37:1634–1641.

30. Schramm J, Luyken C, Urbach H, Fimmers R, et al. Evidence for a clinically distinct new subtype of grade II astrocytomas in patients with long-term epilepsy. *Neurosurgery* 2004; 55:340–348.

31. Blümcke I, Luyken C, Urbach H, Schramm J, et al. An isomorphic subtype of long-term epilepsy-associated astrocytomas associated with benign prognosis. *Acta Neuropathol (Berl)* 2004; 107:381–388.

32. Nimsky C, Ganslandt O, Fahlbusch R. Functional neuronavigation and intraoperative MRI. *Adv Tech Stand Neurosurg* 2004; 29:229–263.

62 Sleep

Carl W. Bazil

Sleep is of vital importance to general health and optimal cognitive functioning; however, the busy modern world leads many people to minimize sleep or overlook sleep problems. Even so, everyone is aware of the drowsiness, inattention, and sluggish memory associated with acute sleep deprivation. It is becoming increasingly apparent, however, that chronic sleep deprivation, even by only an hour or two per night, can result in significant cognitive impairments.

Optimal memory and attention are important to all, but persons with epilepsy are more at risk for sleep-related problems because of additional factors that can worsen cognitive function, including seizures, underlying conditions causing epilepsy, and medication effects. Depression and anxiety are also common in persons with epilepsy, with additional risk of sleep disruption. This chapter begins with a discussion of the ways sleep and epilepsy interact. In the following section, the influence of sleep and sleep disorders on mood and cognition are discussed, with an emphasis on epilepsy patients. Finally, practical issues regarding attention to sleep in patients with epilepsy are highlighted.

INTERACTIONS BETWEEN SLEEP AND EPILEPSY

Sleep and epilepsy interact on several levels. First, sleep influences the frequency of interictal epileptiform discharges, with partial discharges occurring most commonly in deep, non-REM sleep (1). For this reason, sleep electroencephalograms (EEGs) can be important diagnostically. Whether interictal discharges have definite effects on cognition is an interesting question but will not be discussed here. Second, sleep influences the occurrence and secondary generalization of seizures. Third, seizures can disrupt sleep. Fourth, many sleep disorders are more common in patients with epilepsy than in the general population. Finally, anti-epileptic drugs (AEDs) have the potential to either worsen or improve sleep overall, and many affect specific sleep disorders. These last four interactions between sleep and epilepsy have potential influences not only on seizure occurrence but also on mood and cognition, and are discussed in depth in the remainder of this chapter.

Influences of Sleep on Seizures

Two large studies in an epilepsy monitoring unit looked at sleep and sleep stage in relation to onset and propagation of seizures, particularly those of partial onset (2, 3). Both studies found that sleep influences seizure onset, and this differs depending on the lobe involved. Temporal lobe seizures were more likely to begin during wakefulness, whereas frontal onset seizures more commonly began during sleep. Perhaps more interestingly, the pattern of spread differed. A frontal lobe seizure was more likely to secondarily generalize if beginning with the patient awake, but with temporal lobe seizures the reverse was true.

One of the implications for epilepsy patients has to do with the potential for sleep disruption. Because frontal lobe seizures are more likely to occur during sleep, and generalized seizures result in more profound sleep disruption, it is likely that frontal lobe seizures have a greater likelihood to disrupt sleep. This has not, however, been systematically studied. Anecdotally, there are many patients with frontal lobe seizures who nonetheless have profound difficulties in daytime cognition even though their seizures generally do not occur during wakefulness.

Influence of Seizures on Sleep

Intuitively, nocturnal seizures will disrupt sleep structure. Most will cause at least a brief awakening, and normal sleep is unlikely during a postictal state. It may seem that such disruption could be relatively minor, but actually even brief seizures can result in prolonged alterations in sleep structure. Treatment of nocturnal seizures has been shown to improve sleep (4, 5). Importantly, patients with partial seizures have been shown to have relatively normal sleep on seizure-free nights except for slightly decreased sleep efficiency with temporal lobe epilepsy (6).

The effects of individual temporal lobe seizures on sleep structure have been studied in patients in an epilepsy monitoring unit, who were recorded with polysomnography under baseline conditions (seizure-free), and following complex partial or secondarily generalized seizures (7). With daytime seizures, there was a significant decrease in REM the following night (12% vs. 18% for baseline) without significant changes in other sleep stages or in sleep efficiency. When seizures occurred at night, this decrease in REM was more pronounced (7% vs. 16%) and there were increases in stage 1 and decreases in sleep efficiency. These effects were amplified further when seizures occurred early in the night (Figure 62-1).

Therefore, seizures can have a profound, disruptive effect on sleep lasting much longer than the apparent postictal period, particularly when they occur early during sleep.

Prevalence of Sleep Disorders in Epilepsy Patients

Before specific sleep disorders are discussed, it must first be noted that two aspects of sleep are critical: obtaining

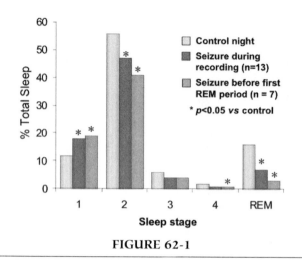

FIGURE 62-1

Effects of seizures on sleep structure in patients with temporal lobe epilepsy. Adapted from Bazil et al. (7). See color section following page 266.

sufficient sleep and adequate sleep hygiene. One of the more common reasons for inadequate sleep is perhaps the most obvious: failing to spend enough time in bed. This is common in the general population and is largely a cultural phenomenon. The demands of modern society, including work, family, and leisure time, often cause people to limit their sleep. Although most believe this to be benign, chronic sleep deprivation can clearly result in neurocognitive deficits (8). Epilepsy patients are certainly not immune from this; in fact, multiple studies suggest that epilepsy patients with sleep disruption suffer more than do healthy subjects without epilepsy (9, 10). This may be the most difficult of sleep disorders to treat; it requires convincing patients that sleep is more important than other activities.

Sleep hygiene is a fairly straightforward concept, but it is one with which many patients are unfamiliar. Review of sleep hygiene can also be time consuming, and in a busy office practice it is easy to overlook.

The basic principle of sleep hygiene is optimization of the conditions for sleep. Contrary to many people's beliefs and to the accepted norms of American society, humans do not have full voluntary control over sleep, as with (at least to a greater extent) eating and voiding. Many would like to believe that sleeping and waking are like a switch, on and off, but this is simply not true. Although sleep cannot be fully controlled, it can be encouraged, and this is the principle of sleep hygiene. Problems with sleep hygiene are prominent in patients with insomnia (11) and in patients with epilepsy (12). Principles of sleep hygiene are summarized in Table 62-1.

Specific sleep disorders most common in the general population, and in epilepsy patients, include obstructive sleep apnea (OSA), insomnia, periodic limb movements of sleep (PLMS), and restless legs syndrome (RLS). One prospective study of 100 epilepsy patients showed that sleep complaints were far more common than in

---

TABLE 62-1

Principles of Sleep Hygiene

General

1. Go to sleep at about the same time each night, and awaken at the same time each morning. Wide fluctuations between workdays and days off can further impair your sleep.
2. Try not to nap. If you do, restrict this to about an hour per day, and do it relatively early (before about 4 in the afternoon).
3. If you are not sleepy, either don't go to bed or arise from bed. Do quiet, relaxing activities until you feel sleepy, then return to bed.
4. Avoid doing stimulating, frustrating, or anxiety-provoking activities in bed or in the bedroom (watching television, studying, balancing the checkbook, etc.). Try to reserve the bedroom, and especially the bed, for sleep and sexual activity.

Use of drugs

1. Avoid coffee, tea, cola, or other caffeinated beverages after about noon. Also avoid chocolate late in the day.
2. If you smoke, avoid this in the hour or two before bedtime.
3. If you drink alcohol, limit this to 1–2 drinks per day and do not drink immediately before bedtime. Although you may find this relaxing, alcohol actually can interfere with sleep later in the night.
4. If you take prescription drugs or over-the-counter drugs that can be stimulating, discuss dosing times with your doctor.

Exercise

1. Exercise, particularly aerobic exercise, is good for both sleep and overall health and should be encouraged.
2. Avoid stimulating exercise in the evening (ideally at least 5 hours before bedtime).

Bedtime ritual

1. Perform relaxing activities in the hour before bedtime.
2. Make sure your sleeping environment is as comfortable as possible, paying attention to temperature, noise, and light.
3. Do not eat a heavy meal just before bedtime, although a light snack might help induce drowsiness.
4. It is sometimes helpful to place paper and pen by the bedside. If you find yourself worrying about completing or remembering a task the next day, write it down and let it go.

During the night

1. If you awaken and find you can't get back to sleep, arise from bed and do quiet, relaxing activities until you are drowsy. Then return to bed.
2. Place clocks so that the time is not visible from the bed.

---

90 normal control subjects; insomnia, excessive daytime sleepiness, OSA, and RLS were also more common although these did not reach statistical significance (13). Several other studies confirm that sleepiness and sleep disorders are common in epilepsy. De Weerd et al. (10) showed that patients with partial epilepsy have twice the incidence of drowsiness as control subjects, and this significantly worsens quality of life. Malow et al. (14) used the Epworth Sleepiness Scale to demonstrate that patients with epilepsy had increased drowsiness compared to control patients. Epilepsy was not a predictor of a high score when a sleep apnea scale was included, suggesting that this treatable condition may be responsible for much of the problem. Based on a survey given to parents of 89 children with idiopathic epilepsy (15), children with epilepsy showed more sleep problems than did control subjects, and these were associated with seizure frequency, age, paroxysmal activity on EEG, duration of illness, and behavioral problems.

OSA occurs in at least 3% of the general population (16). Evidence from subjective scales suggests that this disorder may be disproportionately responsible for excessive sleepiness seen in epilepsy patients (14). In selected epilepsy patients referred for polysomnography, up to 70% are found to have OSA (17, 18). Small series of epilepsy patients have shown that diagnosis and treatment of OSA can improve seizures in patients with epilepsy (18, 19).

While these studies show that OSA is common in a highly selected epilepsy population referred for polysomnography; the overall prevalence of the disorder and impact on quality of life in patients with epilepsy is less clear. There has been one prospective study of thirty-nine unselected patients with highly refractory epilepsy undergoing evaluation for epilepsy surgery, none of which had a previous diagnosis of sleep disorders (20). These patients were studied with overnight polysomnography during their evaluation. One-third were found to have

OSA as defined by respiratory disturbance index (RDI) > 5, and 13% had moderate to severe OSA. This study, although small, suggests that OSA may be more common in patients with refractory epilepsy than in the general population. Although these authors also did not evaluate the relationship between apneas and seizures, oxygen desaturation could result in cerebral irritation, or chronic sleep deprivation could worsen seizures. OSA is known to increase the risk of stroke and death (21); however, it is not known whether this condition contributes to death in patients with epilepsy or to sudden unexplained death in patients with epilepsy.

Insomnia occurs in more than 10% of the general population (22) and is more frequent in patients with epilepsy (10, 12). Sleep disturbance occurs in 39% of patients with intractable epilepsy, and most of the additional disturbance compared with controls is due to insomnia (10). According to the National Health Interview Study, adults with seizures are more than twice as likely to report insomnia and more than three times as likely to report excessive sleepiness as adults without epilepsy (23). Because depression and anxiety are known to be common in epilepsy patients (24), these are likely to be important contributors to insomnia in this population. No studies have looked specifically at this diagnosis in an epilepsy population using objective testing.

PLMS and RLS are both relatively common conditions. The incidence of RLS is about 10% and increases with age (25). PLMS occurs in about 5% of young adults; however, the prevalence may be as high as 44% in patients over age 64 (26–28). These conditions often occur together and have many characteristics in common; the main known effect of both is daytime somnolence. The study of epilepsy patients by de Weerd et al. (10) also suggested that RLS was more common in patients with epilepsy than in control subjects.

All of these studies underscore the increased prevalence of sleep disorders (particularly OSA) in the epilepsy population and the underutilization of polysomnography in these patients.

Effects of Anticonvulsant Medications

Early studies of AEDs showed an increase in sleep stability with all agents. In retrospect, much of this effect was likely due to a reduction in seizure activity, rather than an independent effect of the drug. More recently, the effects of AEDs have been studied independently of seizures, showing different effects (both detrimental and beneficial) of various AEDs on both sleep and specific sleep disorders.

Benzodiazepines and barbiturates are used less commonly for chronic treatment of seizure disorders, but they have the most convincing evidence for detrimental effects on sleep. Although both classes of medications reduce sleep latency, they also decrease the amount of REM sleep, and benzodiazepines reduce slow-wave sleep (29, 30). The effects of other AEDs are somewhat variable between studies, but some conclusions can be made. Phenytoin increases light sleep and decreases sleep efficiency, and most studies show decreased REM sleep (29, 31, 32). Findings for carbamazepine are more variable, but there also seems to be a reduction in REM sleep (31), particularly with acute treatment (33, 34). Valproate may increase stage 1 sleep (32) and (at least theoretically) could worsen OSA through weight gain.

Studies of newer agents in general suggest fewer detrimental effects on sleep. Lamotrigine has been shown to have no effect on sleep in one study (33), but another showed decreases in slow-wave sleep (35). Gabapentin, pregabalin, and tiagabine enhance slow-wave sleep and sleep continuity in patients with epilepsy (32, 33) and in normal volunteers (30, 36–40). Furthermore, gabapentin is effective in the treatment of one common sleep disorder, RLS (41), although carbamazepine and lamotrigine have also been used. A study of levetiracetam in epilepsy patients showed little effect on sleep (42); studies in normal volunteers have shown either little effect (42) or an increase in sleep continuity and slow-wave sleep (43). The effects of zonisamide, oxcarbazepine, and topiramate on sleep and sleep disorders are not known. Patients taking AEDs known to disrupt sleep (phenobarbital, phenytoin, carbamazepine, or valproic acid) have increased drowsiness compared to epilepsy patients who are not taking AEDs (44).

While the effects of AEDs on sleep have been known, and sleep changes were known to affect memory and performance, the most important aspect of this relationship is whether sleep changes due to AEDs actually affect performance. A study of tiagabine used during sleep deprivation addressed just that question (40). Thirty-eight healthy adults were restricted to 5 hours of sleep for four consecutive nights, and randomized to tiagabine 8 mg at bedtime or placebo. In a measure of attention (psychomotor vigilance task), subjects on placebo deteriorated during sleep restriction, but subjects receiving tiagabine did not (Figure 62-2). Subjects taking tiagabine also showed improved performance on the Wisconsin Card Sorting Task and reported more restorative sleep, but did not show improved wakefulness on the Multiple Sleep Latency Test and did not differ on several other measures of memory and alertness. However, it is intriguing that taking this sleep-enhancing drug resulted in modest improvement in subjects who were sleep-deprived. It is not known whether these changes would correlate to improved performance in epilepsy patients, or whether the findings would generalize to other AEDs that improve slow-wave sleep.

Effects of AEDs on various aspects of sleep and sleep disorders are summarized in Table 62-2.

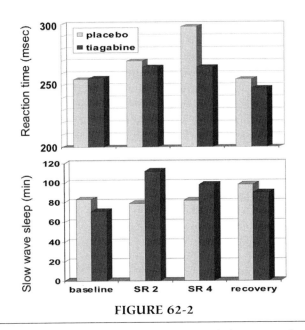

FIGURE 62-2

Effects of tiagabine on reaction time and slow-wave sleep in sleep deprivation. (Top) Effects on reaction time with the psychomotor vigilance task. (Bottom) Effects on total slow-wave sleep (p < 0.001). SR2, second night of sleep restriction. SR 4 (p = 0.24), fourth night of sleep restriction. Adapted from Walsh et al. (40).

EFFECTS OF SLEEP AND SLEEP DISORDERS ON MOOD AND COGNITION

Patients with epilepsy are probably more susceptible to the cognitive and functional consequences of sleep disruption than the general population. The most obvious aspect of this is drowsiness. Not a trivial problem, drowsiness contributes to increases in accidents and, particularly in the case of motor vehicles, to fatality. Patients with uncontrolled seizures are most susceptible to the drowsiness caused by seizures and medications. They should not be driving, but nearly one-third of patients with refractory epilepsy do drive (45). Additionally, patients with fully controlled seizures can still have disrupted sleep as a result of coincident sleep disorders or medications. Many patients with exclusively nocturnal events drive with the permission of their physicians and the state, but the impact of daytime drowsiness must be recognized.

Sleep disruption can affect many aspects of cognitive functioning. Although the exact function of sleep remains unclear, there is growing evidence that sleep in general, and REM and slow-wave sleep in particular, are required for optimal performance. Sleep loss has been clearly documented to affect both cognitive and procedural skills. This has been extensively studied in health care workers (46–48).

TABLE 62-2
Summary of AED Effects on Sleep

| AED | EFFECTS ON SLEEP | | EFFECTS ON SLEEP DISORDERS | |
	POSITIVE	NEGATIVE	IMPROVES/TREATS	WORSENS
Barbiturates	Decreased latency	Decreased REM	Sleep onset insomnia	OSA
Benzodiazepines	Decreased latency	Decreased REM, SWS	Sleep onset insomnia	OSA
Carbamazepine		Decreased REM?	RLS	RLS
Phenytoin	Decreased latency	Increased arousals and stage 1; decreased REM	None known	NE
Valproic acid		Increased stage 1	None known	OSA*
Felbamate	?	?	OSA*	Insomnia
Gabapentin	Increased SWS, decreased arousals	None	RLS	None known
Lamotrigine		Decreased SWS?	None known	None known
Levetiracetam	Increased SWS	None	None known	None known
Pregabalin	Increased SWS, decreased arousals	None	None known	None known
Tiagabine	Increased SWS	None	Insomnia	None known
Topiramate	?	?	OSA*	None known
Zonisamide	?	?	None known	None known

AED, Antiepileptic drug; REM, REM sleep; RLS, restless legs syndrome; SWS, slow-wave sleep; ?, unknown; note that some of these results represent small studies, and the effect may not occur in all patients. * Due to potential weight change.

There is also growing evidence that chronic sleep restriction by as little as 2 hours per night can severely impair neurobehavioral functions in normal individuals (8).

Both REM and slow-wave sleep are considered to be "essential sleep," and subjects who are deprived of sleep (at least in the short term) will "rebound" or make up most of the REM and slow-wave sleep that are lost. Very little stage 1 or 2 sleep is regained (25). Although the function of REM sleep remains speculative, there is considerable information suggesting that increased REM is correlated with enhanced learning of certain tasks (49–51). In addition, enhancement of REM sleep occurs with drugs useful in Alzheimer's disease (52, 53), and REM enhancement due to donepezil correlates with improved memory in normal individuals (54). Increased slow-wave sleep has also been correlated with certain types of learning in one human study (49).

OPTIMAL CARE OF THE EPILEPSY PATIENT WITH REGARD TO SLEEP

The most important aspect of sleep for the epilepsy patient is awareness of its importance. Too often, drowsiness and inattention are considered unavoidable effects of medication or seizures, but it is clear that sleep disruption is very common and can contribute to dysfunction. Seizures, sleep disorders, and mood disorders can easily form a cycle of dysfunction, with each independent problem contributing and worsening the others. Without attention to all aspects of the patient's care, optimal quality of life cannot be obtained.

In patients with persistent drowsiness, inattention, or cognitive problems a systematic approach is best. If the pattern is consistent with seizure occurrence, seizure control should clearly remain the major focus. But if seizures are controlled or at least minimized, attention to other disorders is warranted. Asking about sleep habits will help to ascertain whether the patient is receiving sufficient sleep or has problems with sleep hygiene. Any patient who shows persistent drowsiness and inattention without adequate explanation could have a coincident sleep disorder. A good subjective screen is the Epworth Sleepiness Test; and a patient with a score of 10 or more on this simple test should be considered for further workup. Medications taken by the patient should be considered, including anticonvulsant drugs, for possible adverse effects on sleep. A careful history may also show signs of specific sleep disorders. Even without demonstrable drowsiness, patients with snoring, subjective insomnia or hypersomnia, limb movements in sleep, or lack of other explanations for cognitive problems may have sleep disorders. When in doubt, referral to a sleep specialist for evaluation and possible testing should be considered.

CONCLUSIONS

Attention to sleep in patients with epilepsy has important implications for diagnosis, seizure control, memory and attention, and quality of life. Effects on mood have not directly been studied; however, poor sleep almost certainly contributes to the increased depression and anxiety seen in epilepsy patients. It is clear that independent sleep disorders frequently coexist with epilepsy and that seizures themselves cause sleep disturbance. The common complaint of drowsiness can no longer be dismissed in patients with refractory epilepsy, for whom sleep studies, diagnosis, and targeted therapy can clearly improve both seizure control and sleep. Any patient with persistent drowsiness should therefore be considered for study by polysomnography or video-EEG polysomnography.

Whether sleep disruption is caused by seizures, AEDs, or a coexisting sleep disorder, an adverse impact on daily functioning is likely. Decreased sleep efficiency and increased arousals result in daytime drowsiness, and are seen with seizures and with some AEDs. Chronic sleep deprivation, such as could occur with any of these, clearly has adverse consequences for neurocognitive performance. In any case, it is clear that the quality of sleep plays an important role in both seizure control and quality of life. Attention to seizures that may disrupt sleep, to possible concurrent sleep disorders, and to choice of anticonvulsant is therefore critical in the total care of the patient with epilepsy.

References

1. Sammaritano M, Gigli GL, Gotman J. Interictal spiking during wakefulness and sleep and the localization of foci in temporal lobe epilepsy. *Neurology* 1991; 41(2 Pt 1): 290–297.
2. Bazil CW, Walczak TS. Effects of sleep and sleep stage on epileptic and nonepileptic seizures. *Epilepsia* 1997; 38:56–62.
3. Herman ST, Walczak TS, Bazil CW. Distribution of partial seizures during the sleep–wake cycle: differences by seizure onset site. *Neurology* 2001; 56:1453–1459.
4. Touchon J, Baldy-Moulinier M, Billiard M, Besset A, et al. [Organization of sleep in recent temporal lobe epilepsy before and after treatment with carbamazepine]. *Rev Neurol (Paris)* 1987; 143:462–467.
5. Tachibana N, Shinde A, Ikeda A, Akiguchi, I,et al. Supplementary motor area seizure resembling sleep disorder. *Sleep* 1996; 19:811–816.
6. Crespel A, Baldy-Moulinier M, Coubes P. The relationship between sleep and epilepsy in frontal and temporal lobe epilepsies: practical and physiopathologic considerations. *Epilepsia* 1998; 39:150–157.
7. Bazil CW, Castro LH, Walczak TS. Reduction of rapid eye movement sleep by diurnal and nocturnal seizures in temporal lobe epilepsy. *Arch Neurol* 2000; 57:363–368.
8. Van Dongen HP, Maislin G, Mullington JM, Dinges DF. The cumulative cost of additional wakefulness: dose-response effects on neurobehavioral functions and sleep physiology from chronic sleep restriction and total sleep deprivation. *Sleep* 2003; 26:117–126.

9. Xu X, Brandenburg NA, McDermott AM, Bazil CW. Sleep disturbances reported by refractory partial-onset epilepsy patients receiving polytherapy. *Epilepsia* 2006; 47: 1176–1183.

10. de Weerd A, de Haas S, Otte A, Trenite DK, et al. Subjective sleep disturbance in patients with partial epilepsy: a questionnaire-based study on prevalence and impact on quality of life. *Epilepsia* 2004; 45:1397–1404.

11. Jefferson CD, Drake CL, Scofield HM, Myers E, et al. Sleep hygiene practices in a population-based sample of insomniacs. *Sleep* 2005; 28:611–615.

12. Bazil CW, DaGiau T, Salerni EA. Sleep disturbance in patients with epilepsy. *Epilepsia* 2006; 47 (Suppl 4): 276.

13. Khatami R, Zutter D, Siegel A, Mathis J, et al. Sleep-wake habits and disorders in a series of 100 adult epilepsy patients—a prospective study. *Seizure* 2006; 15:299–306.

14. Malow BA, Bowes RJ, Lin X. Predictors of sleepiness in epilepsy patients. *Sleep* 1997; 20:1105–1110.

15. Cortesi F, Giannotti F, Ottaviano S. Sleep problems and daytime behavior in childhood idiopathic epilepsy. *Epilepsia* 1999; 40:1557–1565.

16. Chervin RD, Guilleminault C. Obstructive sleep apnea and related disorders. *Neurol Clin* 1996; 14:583–609.

17. Malow BA, Fromes GA, Aldrich MS. Usefulness of polysomnography in epilepsy patients. *Neurology* 1997; 48:1389–1394.

18. Beran RG, Plunkett MJ, Holland GJ. Interface of epilepsy and sleep disorders. *Seizure* 1999; 8:97–102.

19. Devinsky O, Ehrenberg B, Barthlen GM, Abramson HS, et al. Epilepsy and sleep apnea syndrome. *Neurology* 1994; 44:2060–2064.

20. Malow BA, Levy K, Maturen K, Bowes R. Obstructive sleep apnea is common in medically refractory epilepsy patients. *Neurology* 2000; 55:1002–1007.

21. Yaggi HK, Concato J, Kernan WN, Lichtman JH, et al. Obstructive sleep apnea as a risk factor for stroke and death. *N Engl J Med* 2005; 353:2034–2041.

22. Chesson AL Jr, Anderson WM, Littner M, Davila D, et al. Practice parameters for the non-pharmacologic treatment of chronic insomnia. An American Academy of Sleep Medicine report. Standards of Practice Committee of the American Academy of Sleep Medicine. *Sleep* 1999; 22:1128–1133.

23. Strine TW, Kobau R, Chapman DP, Thurman DJ, et al. Psychological distress, comorbidities, and health behaviors among U.S. adults with seizures: results from the 2002 National Health Interview Survey. *Epilepsia* 2005; 46:1133–1139.

24. Jones JE, Hermann BP, Barry JJ, Gilliam F, et al. Clinical assessment of axis I psychiatric morbidity in chronic epilepsy: a multicenter investigation. *J Neuropsychiatry Clin Neurosci* 2005; 17:172–179.

25. Lavigne GJ, Montplaisir JY. Restless legs syndrome and sleep bruxism: prevalence and association among Canadians. *Sleep* 1994; 17:739–743.

26. Bixler EO, Kales A, Vela-Bueno A, Jacoby JA, et al. Nocturnal myoclonus and nocturnal myoclonic activity in the normal population. *Res Commun Chem Pathol Pharmacol* 1982; 36:129–140.

27. Ancoli-Israel S, Kripke DF, Mason W, Kaplan OJ. Sleep apnea and periodic movements in an aging sample. *J Gerontol* 1985; 40:419–425.

28. Mosko SS, Dickel, MJ, Paul T, LaTour T, et al. Sleep apnea and sleep-related periodic leg movements in community resident seniors. *J Am Geriatr Soc* 1988; 36:502–508.

29. Wolf P, Roder-Wanner UU, Brede M. Influence of therapeutic phenobarbital and phenytoin medication on the polygraphic sleep of patients with epilepsy. *Epilepsia* 1984; 25: 467–475.

30. Hindmarch I, Dawson J, Stanley N. A double-blind study in healthy volunteers to assess the effects on sleep of pregabalin compared with alprazolam and placebo. *Sleep* 2005; 28:187–193.

31. Drake ME Jr, Pakalnis A, Bogner JE, Andrews JM. Outpatient sleep recording during antiepileptic drug monotherapy. *Clin Electroencephalogy* 1990; 21:170–173.

32. Legros B, Bazil CW. Effects of antiepileptic drugs on sleep architecture: a pilot study. *Sleep Med* 2003; 4:51–55.

33. Placidi F, Diomedi M, Scalise A, Marciani MG, et al. Effect of anticonvulsants on nocturnal sleep in epilepsy. *Neurology* 2000; 54(5 Suppl 1):S25–S32.

34. Yang JD, Elphick M, Sharpley AL, Cowen PJ, et al. Effects of carbamazepine on sleep in healthy volunteers. *Biol Psychiatry* 1989; 26:324–328.

35. Foldvary N, Perry M, Lee J, Dinner D, et al. The effects of lamotrigine on sleep in patients with epilepsy. *Epilepsia* 2001; 42:1569–1573.

36. Foldvary-Schaefer N, De Leon Sanchez I, Karafa M, Mascha E, et al. Gabapentin increases slow-wave sleep in normal adults. *Epilepsia* 2002; 43:1493–1497.

37. Bazil C, Battista J, Basner R. Gabapentin improves sleep in the presence of alcohol. *J Clin Sleep Med* 2005; 1:284–287.

38. Mathias S, Wetter TC, Steiger A, Lancel M. The GABA uptake inhibitor tiagabine promotes slow wave sleep in normal elderly subjects. *Neurobiol Aging* 2001; 22:247–253.

39. Walsh JK, Randazzo AC, Frankowski S, Shannon K, et al. Dose-response effects of tiagabine on the sleep of older adults. *Sleep* 2005; 28:673–676.

40. Walsh JK, Randazzo AC, Stone K, Eisenstein R, et al. Tiagabine is associated with sustained attention during sleep restriction: evidence for the value of slow-wave sleep enhancement? *Sleep* 2006; 29:433–443.

41. Garcia-Borreguero D, Larrosa O, de la Llave Y, Verger K, et al. Treatment of restless legs syndrome with gabapentin: a double-blind, cross-over study. *Neurology* 2002; 59:1573–1579.

42. Bell C, Vanderlinden H, Hiersemenzel R, Otoul C, et al. The effects of levetiracetam on objective and subjective sleep parameters in healthy volunteers and patients with partial epilepsy. *J Sleep Res* 2002; 11:255–263.

43. Cicolin A, Magliola U, Giordano A, Terreni A, et al. Effects of levetiracetam on nocturnal sleep and daytime vigilance in healthy volunteers. *Epilepsia* 2006; 47:82–85.

44. Salinsky MC, Oken BS, Binder LM. Assessment of drowsiness in epilepsy patients receiving chronic antiepileptic drug therapy. *Epilepsia* 1996; 37:181–187.

45. Berg AT, Vickrey BG, Sperling MR, Langfitt JT, et al. Driving in adults with refractory localization-related epilepsy. Multi-center study of epilepsy surgery. *Neurology* 2000; 54:625–630.

46. Weinger MB, Ancoli-Israel S. Sleep deprivation and clinical performance. *J Am Med Assoc* 2002; 287:955–957.

47. Grantcharov TP, Bardram L, Funch-Jensen P, Rosenberg J. Laparoscopic performance after one night on call in a surgical department: prospective study. *Br Med J* 2001; 323:1222–1223.

48. Veasey S, Rosen R, Barzansky B, Rosen I, et al. Sleep loss and fatigue in residency training: a reappraisal. *J Am Med Assoc* 2002; 288:1116–1124.

49. Stickgold R, Whidbee D, Schirmer B, Patel V, et al. Visual discrimination task improvement: a multi-step process occurring during sleep. *J Cogn Neurosci* 2000; 12:246–254.

50. Stickgold R, Hobson JA, Fosse R, Fosse M. et al. Sleep, learning, and dreams: off-line memory reprocessing. *Science* 2001; 294:1052–1057.

51. Maquet P. The role of sleep in learning and memory. *Science* 2001; 294:1048–1052.

52. Holsboer-Trachsler E, Hatzinger M, Stohler R, Hemmeter U, et al. Effects of the novel acetylcholinesterase inhibitor SDZ ENA 713 on sleep in man. *Neuropsychopharmacology* 1993; 8:87–92.

53. Schredl M, Weber B, Braus D, Gattaz WF, et al. The effect of rivastigmine on sleep in elderly healthy subjects. *Exp Gerontol* 2000; 35:243–249.

54. Schredl M, Weber B, Leins ML, Heuser I. Donepezil-induced REM sleep augmentation enhances memory performance in elderly, healthy persons. *Exp Gerontol* 2001; 36:353–361.

X

CONCLUSION

63

Historical Perspectives and Future Opportunities

Giuliano Avanzini

T he behavioral aspects of epilepsy have been a matter of interest since the earliest available descriptions. Adopting a historical approach to a given discipline offers a unique perspective on its founding concepts and their evolution. This chapter will discuss some of the historical antecedents to current views on epilepsy-related behavioral changes and their relevance to future developments. Particular attention will be given to the history of epilepsy in the nineteenth century, when biased interpretations of clinical observations led to the construction of a general theory of the nature of epilepsy that can still teach us a valuable lesson about the risks underlying the misuse of scientific (or rather pseudoscientific) methods.

SEIZURE-RELATED BEHAVIORAL DISORDERS

Behavioral manifestations can occur acutely as an aspect of seizure phenomena or during the postictal phase. Typical examples are the more or less complex automatisms that express the involvement of high-level integration areas of the brain and may be associated with cognitive and psychic symptoms. Correlating observed symptoms with the putative origin and propagation of underlying epileptic discharges has made it possible to draw some interesting inferences concerning the roles of the cerebral regions responsible for the seizures, and these

have been complemented by the results of brain stimulations in epilepsy patients before or during surgery.

It is noteworthy that transient periictal symptoms are usually observed and analyzed by the members of multidisciplinary teams participating in the workup of patients with epilepsies. However, such teams do not normally include specialists in psychiatry, so, although the analysis of seizure phenomenology has significantly advanced our understanding of neuropsychologic functions and dysfunctions, its potential contribution to our knowledge of the neurobiology of psychiatric symptoms has so far been underexploited. This is regretable inasmuch as the rapidly evolving character of ictal symptoms could provide a privileged opportunity for analyzing the dissolution and reconstitution of psychic functions in a uniquely dynamic dimension. The situation now seems to be improving, as demonstrated by several excellent chapters concerning seizure-related behavioral disorders to be found in this book. Nevertheless, there are still many more contributions to be made concerning epilepsy-related neuropsychologic disorders.

THE NEUROPSYCHOLOGIC APPROACH TO EPILEPSY-RELATED BEHAVIORAL DISORDERS

The value of the neuropsychologic approach in characterizing the changes in memory and learning, attention and concentration, language, sensory–motor integration, and fluency that are associated with the epilepsies has become gradually clearer with the emergence of the concept of epileptic syndrome. According to the definition of the International League Against Epilepsy (ILAE), "epilepsy is a chronic condition of the brain characterized by an enduring propensity to generate epileptic seizures, and by the neurobiological, cognitive, psychologic, and social consequences of this condition" (1). An epileptic syndrome (i.e., a complex of signs and symptoms that defines a unique epilepsy condition) is not characterized only by the types of seizures and their natural history, but also by its particular cognitive profile.

The neuropsychologic assessment of patients undergoing surgery for intractable epilepsies plays a special role in confirming the lateralization and localization of epileptogenic areas, and defining the risk to memory and other cognitive functions. The combination of neuropsychologic tests, functional imaging, and neurophysiologic techniques has opened up very promising prospects for the analysis of cognitive functions.

Moreover, the neuropsychologic approach is relevant to several concepts now being discussed by the ILAE Task Force for Classification and Terminology, such as the concept of the epilepsy process, and the potential harm caused by ictal or interictal epileptic discharges.

"Epilepsy process" designates the complex of putative biological mechanisms that gives an epilepsy the intrinsic potential to progress toward a more severe condition in terms of seizures and the associated neurologic and/or psychic defects. Such a progressive course is typically observed in epileptic encephalopathies such as Dravet, West, Lennox-Gastaut, and Doose syndromes: "conditions in which the epileptiform abnormalities themselves are believed to contribute to the progressive disturbance in cerebral function" (2).

When these syndromes are cryptogenic (i.e., not associated with any detectable brain pathology), the results of neuropsychologic examinations are normal at the time of clinical onset and become indicative of progressive impairment during the subsequent course, thus supporting the idea that persistent epileptic activity leads to cognitive impairment, although it is not yet possible to rule out the alternative hypothesis that seizure worsening and cognitive deterioration are both expressions of a still-unidentified underlying progressive disorder. Nevertheless, the possibility that electroencephalographic (EEG) discharges per se can lead to cognitive impairment is strongly supported by the course of Landau-Kleffner syndrome and epilepsy with continuous spike-wave during sleep, in which the extreme activation of epileptiform activity during sleep (Figure 63-1) is associated with cognitive defects that specifically affect language in Landau-Kleffner syndrome.

There is also evidence that, in benign epilepsy with centrotemporal spikes (BECT, the prototype of idiopathic

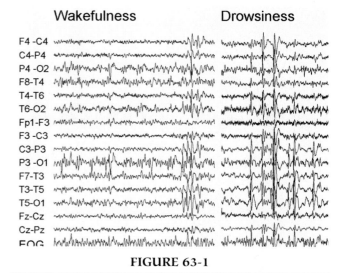

FIGURE 63-1

Epilepsy with continuous spike and waves during sleep (CSWS). (Top) EEG in wakefulness, drowsiness, and sleep stage 2. (Bottom) Results of neuropsychologic verbal (A) and performance (B) tests in twelve subjects during CSWS. The verbal (A1) and performance (A2) tests have been repeated in eight patients after disappearance of CSWS, showing an overall improvement although the impairment of performances was still present in seven patients (from Mira et al. [13]).

benign epilepsies), the particularly pronounced activation of EEG discharges during sleep may be associated with cognitive disturbances. This should lead us to reconsider the idea that BECT is necessarily benign, and introduces the challenging idea of a continuum ranging from idiopathic epilepsies to epileptic encephalopathies. However, when discussing this still open question, it is necessary to consider the possibility that the cognitive impairment is not so much due to the pronounced EEG discharges themselves but to their disruption of normal sleep profiles.

It is certainly true that recently collected data demonstrate that "idiopathic" does not necessarily mean "benign," and to some extent they challenge the very concept of idiopathic. However, it must be borne in mind that, even if it is proved that epileptiform abnormalities can impair cerebral functions, this certainly does not apply to all types of epilepsies: for example, childhood absence epilepsy can present a very large number of EEG discharges (associated with absences or not), but there is no evidence of any cerebral impairment whatsoever.

In addition to epileptic encephalopathies, temporal lobe epilepsy provides another example of epileptogenesis as a process insofar as its natural history is characterized by an initial factor that is thought to set in motion a sequence of biological mechanisms leading to the development of a chronic and often difficult-to-treat condition. Neuropsychologic assessments are sensitive in monitoring the development of the epileptogenic process underlying temporal lobe epilepsy.

EPILEPSY AND MADNESS

The first known written documents on the topic of epilepsy are Babylonian tablets from ca. 1000 BC (Figure 63-2), recently translated by Wilson and Reynolds (3). Since then, the history of epilepsy has been characterized by interpretations based on an interplay of magical concepts and surprisingly lucid intuitions that were applied not only to the seizures themselves but also to the alterations in behavior and character that were more or less legitimately attributed to the person suffering from them.

It would be far beyond the scope of this chapter to try to describe in detail the way in which prejudices about demonic origins were counterbalanced by a scientific view that was remarkably precise even as early as the time of Hippocrates in the fifth century BC, and so I will concentrate on the unexpected evolution that the medicoscientific conception, established by the publication of Tissot's treatise in 1770, underwent during the following 50 years in the hands of some authoritative French psychiatrists. Most of the information contained in this section has been summarized from Avanzini and Assael (4), in which all the quoted references (including Tissot 1770) can be found.

In 1854, Delasiauve published a treatise in which he proposed the hypothesis that epileptic seizures involve

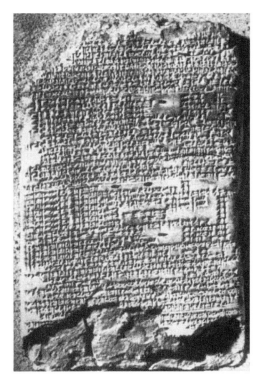

FIGURE 63-2

Tablet describing epilepsy and its therapy in a Babylonian textbook of medicine (from Wilson and Reynolds [3]).

repeated cerebral concussions that, in the long term, lead to severe functional disorders. The mental disturbances considered to be due to epilepsy were various, with mania, a type of mental exaltation ranging from irascibility to uncontrolled fury, more frequently taking the furious form with sudden explosions of delirium, sometimes alternating with ecstatic phases.

According to Delasiauve, "Such observations would explain an ancient opinion recently developed by Bouchet and Cazauvieilh who, on the basis of their symptomatic characteristics and site, believe that mental derangement, hysteria, catalepsy and epilepsy have a number of analogies in their nature: they should be considered alike, interchangeable or as one giving rise to another."

Following the same line of thought, under the heading of epilepsy in his *Nouveau Dictionnaire de Médecine et de Chirurgie Pratique* 1870, André Voisin wrote:

> Epileptics, be they children, adults or elderly, almost always manifest changes in character and intelligence. In general terms, one cannot admit the opinion of some physicians that it is possible to be epileptic and completely healthy in spirit. I do not mean that every epileptic is alienated; but every epileptic is original, full of fancy and difficult to live with and, because of hallucinations, can unpredictably commit irresistible and dangerous acts. The epileptics admitted to hospitals should therefore be put in the charge of a physician responsible for the mad. The main reason for doubting the psychic integrity of certain epileptics who are considered not be deranged is the facility with which almost all of them allow themselves to be dominated by ill-humor, cholera and unseemly instincts.

These incredible statements find their systematic definition in the theory of degeneration, of which epilepsy was considered the most representative example. In support of this thesis, a substantial part of scientific thought had recourse to the major theories of biology beginning to take shape in the second half of the nineteenth century: that is, the theories of evolution and inheritance, from which they derived some subproducts such as the theory of moral degeneration and eugenics.

The fact that these theories found substantial literary legitimacy in such a great novel as *The Brothers Karamazov* is a sign of the strength with which they managed to impose themselves on the intellectual consciousness and imagination of the time. By means of his character with epilepsy, Smerdyakov, Dostoevsky wanted to create the figure of an outcast, someone who personifies the progressive degeneration of humanity and its abjection. And in developing the idea of degeneration through his character, he makes clear use of ideas that, however aberrant, had taken root in the anthropological and psychiatric sciences of the nineteenth century, whose detailed studies of the complex moral and physical structure of persons with epilepsy had led to them becoming archetypes of degenerative and mental disease.

The doctrine of degeneration began to prevail mainly as a result of the work of Bénédict-Augustin Morel, a positivist physician, a friend of Claude Bernard and a reader of Auguste Comte and Jean-Baptiste Lamarck, who was inspired by Prosper Lucas's *Traité philosophique et physiologique de l'hérédité naturelle dans les états de santé et de maladie du système nerveux*. The dominant element of Morel's work reflects a view of the "degenerate" epileptic/madman as the prototype of mankind estranged from the ideal of Eden and from the dominion of the moral over the physical world, somewhat as in the religious concept of original sin

"Degeneration," said Morel,

> constitutes a diseased state and, left to himself, a degenerate being falls into a condition of progressive degradation. He becomes (and I am not afraid of repeating this truth) not only incapable of forming the chain of transmission of progress in humanity but, by his relationships with the healthy part of the population, is the major obstacle to progress. Finally, the duration of his life is limited, like that of every monstrous being.

Morel's Italian disciple Tonnini had this to say:

> One is almost tempted to believe that an epileptic is the scion of a family of lunatics and moral madmen, the first of which are by selection purged prevalently of atavistic phenomena, while preserving those that are degenerative and morbid, and the second are purged of some of the morbid phenomena of the epileptic neurosis.

The identification of moral insanity with epilepsy was authoritatively codified by Burlureaux in the *Dictionnaire encyclopédique des sciences medicales*:

> These are sick people affected by diffuse epilepsy in whom the epilepsy no longer translates into intellectual or convulsive disorders, but into nothing less than moral insanity. They have the instinct of evil driven to its maximum degree; they are perverse from their tenderest infancy, essentially malfactors and dangerous, their moral sense has totally disappeared, nothing touches them and it is much if they are only moved by the fear of castigation. It is from among them that thieves and professional murderers are often recruited.

It is difficult to understand today how such a barbaric theory as that of degeneration could have gained such widespread credit in countries with such great cultural traditions as France, Italy, and Germany, to the point that, in the last decades of the nineteenth century, almost all of the diagnostic certificates of French psychiatric hospitals began with the words "*dégénérescence mentale avec. . . .*"

In addition to the doctrinaire prejudices that sustained the theory of degeneration, the factors that led positivist psychiatry to this gigantic falsification of reality included the particular conditions under which the psychiatrists of the institutes to which the patients with epilepsy were admitted made their observations. Modern psychiatry has in fact demonstrated that many of the psychiatric pictures codified in their treatises only existed inside the lunatic asylums, and that their phenomenological expression was attributable to the condition of institutionalization. This is not the place to discuss the larger question of the role of lunatic asylums in generating rather than remedying mental illness, but in relation to the supposed psychopathology of institutionalized epilepsy patients, it is enough to note Voisin's description: "they [epilepsy patients] would spend their days in the asylums playing cards and sleeping . . ." Did such places offer any kind of alternative?—Yes, of course they did: ". . . unless they were stimulated by the bait of gainful employment"—by which was meant the shameful exploitation to which the inmates of the asylums were subjected. It is significant that in 1870 (22 years after the publication of the *Communist Manifesto* of Marx and Engels), paid work was identified not as a fundamental element of human dignity but an astute means of attracting the attention of an indolent asylum patient.

The psychopathological traits delineated by the exponents of the psychiatry of degeneration (which it may be better to define as degenerated itself) were therefore not attributable to epilepsy, but to the lunatic asylums: "a place in which a person is inexorably crushed by an apparatus intent on reducing him to a pre-postulated stereotype of mental disease." For the rest, the aberrations of positivist psychiatry had relatively little impact on the British epileptological school founded by John Hughlings Jackson at the National Hospital for the Paralysed and Epileptic, an institution whose very name bore the imprint of a different approach to epilepsy in the context of nonrepressive psychiatric culture precipitated by the pioneering work of William and Samuel Tuke, and John Conolly.

What today seems to be the most criticizable aspect of positivist psychiatry is its unjustified generalization of some objective but circumscribed observations aimed at supporting a general theory that was largely based on ideologic assumptions. That the well-documented degeneration induced in some structures of the nervous system by alcohol, syphilis, or other infectious or toxic agents are responsible for alterations in intelligence, character, and behavior does not justify the assumption that every disorder in mental function can be attributed to degeneration, which, unless documented objectively, takes on the value of a metaphysical rather than a scientific category. At our own point in history, when the epistemological pendulum of psychiatry is once again swinging in an organicist direction, the lesson that can be drawn from the psychiatry of degeneration must be borne in mind to avoid the risk that insufficiently controlled, though promising, neurobiological observations are speculatively generalized to support theories that are not yet substantiated by facts.

PSYCHIATRY AND EPILEPSY TODAY

As in the case of any other disease, physicians caring for patients with epilepsy must have the capacity to listen and be sufficiently sensitive to pick up the emotive resonances associated with the disease, and use them when making therapeutic decisions.

It is well known that the chronically ill share many distresses regardless of the particular source of their illness, and that several of the distresses felt by patients with epilepsy are not particular to them. However, what is specific to epilepsy is the dramatic experience of undergoing a seizure (an event that inserts a caesura in the patient's relationship with reality), and the ambivalent reaction of the environment, which is simultaneously hyperprotective and alienating. The seizures that modify the field of consciousness without totally abolishing it arouse greater anxiety than do those that involve a more or less protracted but complete loss of consciousness. It is therefore frequent to encounter greater existential discomfort in patients who are subject to perhaps even the briefest of seizures involving alterations in perceptions, communication, or, more generally, their relationship with reality than in those who suffer from generalized convulsive seizures. The impact of these factors can be such as to generate a structured psychopathological picture that, per se, requires psychotherapy or psychopharmacological treatment.

These considerations do not rule out the possible role of impaired cerebral functions that, as discussed previously, may be due to the pathological process responsible for epilepsy or the consequences of persistent epileptic activity. Our increasingly precise understanding of the cerebral areas involved in emotive or instinctive life and the physiopathology of epilepsy provides a sound scientific foundation for investigating the neurobiological bases of the behavioral alterations associated with epilepsies. I will discuss briefly this important question with specific references to bipolar disorders, personality disorders, psychoses, and psychogenic seizures.

Bipolar Disorders and Epilepsy

In the fourth edition of the *Diagnostic and Statistical Manual of Mental Disorders* (DSM-IV), bipolar disorders (BP) are defined as situations characterized by repeated episodes of mania (BPI) or hypomania (BPII) interspersed with periods of depression (5). They have been assumed to have an endogenous basis on the grounds of the familial and constitutional predisposition recognized since the end of the nineteenth century (6), and a possible pathophysiological relationship with epilepsy has been suggested by the effectiveness of some antiepileptic drugs (AEDs) in treating them. I shall here try to summarize the many findings supporting these assumptions on the basis of the recent update by Schmitz and Trimble published as an *Epilepsia* supplement (7).

Postmortem neuropathological studies of patients with bipolar disorders have revealed structural alterations in the prefrontal and anterior cingulate cortices and the structures of the temporal lobe, consisting of a reduction in the density of (mainly nonpyramidal) neurons and glial cells in the neocortical layers and hippocampus and non-univocally assessed changes in amygdala volume. Some of these data have been confirmed by means of in vivo imaging, which has led to the development of specific projects aimed at systematically characterizing the morphological changes associated with bipolar disorders using advanced magnetic resonance imaging (MRI) techniques, such as diffusion tensor imaging and magnetization transfer imaging with voxel-based morphometry, which seems to be particularly promising as a means of characterizing the neuropathological changes common to both epilepsy and bipolar disorders.

Considerable effort is currently being made to understand the implications of the mood-stabilizing effect of AEDs in bipolar disorders, which is the main reason for assuming that epilepsy and bipolar disorders may share some common pathogenetic mechanisms. It has been claimed that the neurotransmitters, neuromodulators, ion currents, and second messengers thought to be targeted by AEDs are involved in the pathophysiology of both conditions. It is noteworthy that the AEDs most frequently used in bipolar disorders (carbamazepine, valproate, and oxcarbazepine) are all inhibitors of sodium currents, which are also strongly affected by lithium, a very effective mood stabilizer. Lithium replaces sodium, but because it is not effectively removed by the sodium pump, it prevents the cellular reentry of potassium and significantly reduces sodium-activated potassium currents, thus interfering with cell excitability.

However, it should not be forgotten that the sensitivity of a given disorder to a given drug cannot be taken as proof that its pathogenesis depends on the same elementary mechanism on which the drug is known to act, because it is possible that the drug-induced effect on a given cell mechanism simply restores the excitation/inhibition balance perturbed by an independent pathophysiological mechanism.

Despite this reservation, we look forward to learning what else future pharmacological studies may reveal concerning the pathophysiological relationships of epilepsy and bipolar disorders.

Personality Disorders

The nineteenth-century history of epilepsy studies and their use of the concept of degeneration to explain epileptic personality is probably one of the main reasons for the ardent opposition to any attempt to demonstrate a personality disorder characteristic of epilepsy.

The DSM-IV defines a personality disorder as an enduring pattern of inner experience and behavior that deviates markedly from the expectations of the individual's culture. It is certainly possible to identify deviant patterns of inner experience and behavior in patients with epilepsy, but no consistent relationship has been found between a specific pattern and a given type of epilepsy. The most systematic attempt to correlate specific personality features (the "Geschwind syndrome") with a given epilepsy type (temporal lobe epilepsy) was made by Geschwind himself (8).

According to Waxman and Geschwind, the personality profile associated with temporal lobe epilepsy is characterized by alterations in behavior, cognition, and affect that are secondary to an overinvestment of affect in ongoing external stimuli, and are expressed by traits such as religiosity, nascent philosophical interest, an increased sense of personal destiny, circumstantiality, viscosity, hypergraphia, and so forth. The overinvestment of affect would have a neurobiological basis in a process of sensory–limbic hyperconnection due to epilepsy-related plasticity.

However, no consistent relationship between Geschwind syndrome and temporal lobe epilepsy has ever been demonstrated. It is true that some of the eighteen traits that have been described can be identified in some patients with temporal lobe epilepsy, but their frequency is not significantly higher than that observed in the general population. My own personal experience is that "an augmented sense of personal destiny, viscosity, and hypergraphia" are found more often in my colleagues than in my patients.

Epilepsies and Psychoses

A wide-ranging and balanced review of psychoses and epilepsy by Trimble and Schmitz has been published in a comprehensive textbook titled *Epilepsy* (9) and on which this account is largely based. The book describes epidemiological studies whose estimates of the frequency of psychoses in epilepsy vary widely depending on whether they were population-based surveys or based on clinical case series (9). In the first, the prevalence of psychoses does not differ significantly from that found in the general population, whereas it is significantly higher among patients attending specialist centers, probably because of risk factors related to complicated epilepsy or chronic illness (9).

The psychotic symptoms occurring during nonconvulsive status epilepticus are diagnostically important, because it is not exceptional to see patients in whom the epileptic nature of periodic behavioral alterations unassociated with convulsions has never been recognized.

About 25% of the psychoses observed in epilepsy are postictal (9), frequently occurring 1–6 days after repeated seizures or status epilepticus. In most patients, they consist of abnormal mood and paranoid delusions, possibly associated with a typically fluctuating course of confusion. The psychotic symptoms usually remit within days or weeks but may sometimes evolve into chronic psychosis; dopamine is involved in their pathogenesis.

Chronic psychoses that are apparently unrelated to ictal events account for 10–30% of the psychoses observed in epilepsy, and their phenomenology is not different from the psychoses occurring in the absence of epilepsy. The existence of epilepsy-related risk factors and pathogenetic mechanisms, and the identification of specific correlations between epilepsy type(s) and the clinical pictures of the psychoses, are debated matters that have important implications for biological psychiatry and go beyond the scope of my own expertise. Interested readers should refer to the textbook chapters by Trimble and Schmitz (9) and by Engel and Taylor (10).

One particular phenomenon is represented by the psychoses that appear when EEG discharges or seizures are completely suppressed by antiepileptic therapy (forced normalization), or when a patient with previously uncontrolled epilepsy undergoes surgical resection of the epileptogenic area.

Forced Normalization and Alternative Psychosis

According to Landolt's original description (9), forced normalization is characterized by the fact that the recurrence of psychotic states is accompanied by normal EEG findings in comparison with previous and subsequent EEG examinations. Its clinical counterpart of patients who become psychotic when their seizures are controlled and experience the resolution of their psychosis with the return of seizures has been called alternative psychosis by Tellenbach (9). The symptoms of alternative psychoses include hallucinations, delusions, depression, mania, and anxiety.

Postsurgical psychosis following surgery was reported in the Maudsley series (11) and has been observed in anecdotal cases after temporal lobectomy; patients with right-sided lobectomy may be more prone to these psychiatric disturbances (see Trimble and Schmitz [9]). Although no clear relationship between surgical success and psychosis has been demonstrated, this phenomenon suggests a mechanism similar to forced normalization.

The biological mechanisms underlying the apparent antagonism between seizures (or EEG discharges) and psychotic symptoms are not clear; it is likewise unknown why well-documented alternative psychoses occur relatively infrequently even in patients whose EEG discharges have completely disappeared, or what risk factors are associated with occurrence. Furthermore, the findings of similar psychopathological manifestations associated with active epileptic discharges in some cases and the suppression of discharges in others are difficult to reconcile and deserve further controlled studies.

PSYCHOGENIC SEIZURES

One particular aspect of the problem is represented by psychogenically based pseudoepileptic seizures (or pseudoseizures), which can be difficult to identify, especially in patients who are also affected by genuine epileptic seizures. These psychogenic seizures, which are attributable to the Freudian mechanism of the somatic conversion of unconscious conflicts, repropose the much-debated question of the relationship between hysteria and epilepsy, which, once stripped of the academic redundancies of the nineteenth century, can be outlined quite simply. Psychogenic seizures should be considered as a sort of theatrical representation of epileptic seizures in which the director (the unconscious) acts for purposes of protection and defense. Most of the patients whom Charcot and Richet (see Avanzini and Assael [4]) would have considered hysteroepileptic are actually patients with epilepsy who also present somatic conversion seizures, which the unconscious stages *using* the phenomenology characteristic of genuine epileptic seizures as its inspiration. My italics are intended to reflect the metaphorical nature of the terminology, and emphasize that the mechanism of conversion is completely beyond the control of conscious will. Although similar in their external manifestations (and sometimes coexisting in the same subject), epileptic and psychogenic seizures are clearly due to completely different mechanisms, and so terms suggesting equivocal unitary interpretations, such as "hysteroepilepsy," have no sense.

CONCLUSIONS

Cognitive alterations, behavioral disturbances, and psychopathological symptoms can all be associated with different types of epilepsy. Several potentially relevant factors must be taken into account when discussing their origin: the reactive psychological distress caused by the dramatic experience of seizures and the negative attitude of the environment, underlying brain diseases (if any), and seizure- or discharge-dependent brain dysfunctions, all of which may play specific roles individually or in combination. Interest in the relationship between the neurologic and psychiatric dimensions has undergone a rebirth, founded on sound scientific bases that open up new perspectives for interpreting the psychiatric disorders associated with epilepsy.

Nothing survives of the doctrine that made epilepsy patients "prototypes of the degenerative Proteus" other than the memory of a dark period in the cultural history of science, which should however not be forgotten in order to ensure that the resulting aberrations are never repeated. This, indeed, is the role of history. There are many excellent works on the history of epilepsy that readers can profitably consult, starting with Temkin's classic book *The Falling Sickness* (12); what is still missing is a history of persons with epilepsy: a history of the people affected by a disease who have asked (and still ask) science and their fellows to understand their pain and give them the means to overcome it, and a history of the replies that science and their fellows have given them.

References

1. Fisher RS, van Emde Boas W, Blume W, Elger C, et al. Epileptic seizures and epilepsy: definitions proposed by the International League Against Epilepsy (ILAE) and the International Bureau for Epilepsy (IBE). *Epilepsia* 2005; 46:470–472.
2. Engel J Jr. Report of the ILAE Classification Core Group. *Epilepsia* 2006; 47:1558–1568.
3. Wilson JV, Reynolds EH. Texts and documents. Translation and analysis of a cuneiform text forming part of a Babylonian treatise on epilepsy. *Med Hist* 1990; 34:185–198.
4. Avanzini G, Assael BM. Il male dell'anima. L'epilessia tra '800 e '900. Roma: Editori Laterza, 1997.
5. American Psychiatric Association. Diagnostic and statistical manual of mental disorders, fourth edition. Washington, DC: American Psychiatric Publishing, 1994.
6. Kraepelin E. Psychiatrie. Ein lehrbuch für studirende und aerzte. Sechste, vollständing umgearbeitete auflage. I. Band. Allgemeine psychiatrie. II. Band. Klinische psychiatrie. Leipzig: Barth Verlag, 1899.
7. Schmitz B, Trimble MR, eds. Neurobiological links of epilepsy, bipolar disorder, and anticonvulsants. *Epilepsia* 2005; 46(Suppl 4).
8. Waxman SG, Geschwind N. The interictal behavior syndrome of temporal lobe epilepsy. *Arch Gen Psychiatry* 1975; 32:1580–1586.
9. Trimble MR, Schmitz B. The psychoses of epilepsy/schizophrenia. In: Engel J Jr, Pedley TA, eds. Epilepsy. A comprehensive textbook. Vol. 2. Philadelphia: Lippincott-Raven Publishers, 1997:2071–2081.
10. Engel J Jr, Taylor DC. Neurobiology of behavioural disorders. In: Engel J Jr, Pedley TA, eds. Epilepsy. A comprehensive textbook, Vol. 2. Philadelphia: Lippincott-Raven Publishers, 1997:2045–2052.
11. Bruton CJ. The neuropathology of temporal lobe epilepsy. Maudsley Monograph No. 31. Oxford, UK: Oxford University Press, 1988.
12. Temkin O, ed. The falling sickness: a history of epilepsy from the Greeks to the beginnings of modern neurology. Baltimore, MD: The Johns Hopkins Press, 1945:380.
13. Mira L, Oxilia B, Van Lierde A. Cognitive assessment of children with CSWS syndrome: a critical review of data from 155 cases submitted to the Venice colloquium. In: Beaumanoir A, Bureau M, Deonna T, Mira L, et al., eds. *Mariani Foundation Paediatric Neurology Series*. London: John Libbey, 1995:229–242.

Index

Note: An italicized *f* following a page locator indicates a figure.